AF478632

Congestive Heart Failure

Dean T. Mason, MD

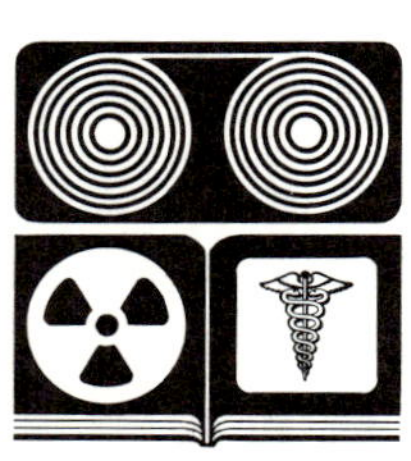

YORKE MEDICAL BOOKS

Dun-Donnelley Publishing Corporation
New York

Congestive Heart Failure

Mechanisms, Evaluation and Treatment

Edited by

Dean T. Mason, MD, FACC

Professor of Medicine
Professor of Physiology
Chief, Cardiovascular Medicine
University of California
School of Medicine
Davis, California

President-Elect, American College of Cardiology

Congestive Heart Failure

First edition

Library of Congress Catalog Card Number: 76-3321

International Standard Book Number: 0-914316-05-2

To my wife, Maureen,
  and my daughters, Kathleen and Alison,
  for their devotion, understanding, patience, equanimity
  and ability to tolerate my schedule

and to my Cardiology Faculty, Fellows and Staff
  whose dedication, tireless efforts, talent, excellence,
  comprehensive teamwork
  and esprit de corps made this book possible.
                              Dean T. Mason, MD, FACC

Contents

Contents

Chapter 1

Introduction to Recent Advances in Pathogenesis and Management of Congestive Heart Failure   **1**
Dean T. Mason

PART I: MECHANISMS

Chapter 2

Structural Conditions in the Hypertrophied and Failing Heart   **13**
Henry M. Spotnitz and Edmund H. Sonnenblick

Chapter 3

Abnormal Biochemistry in Myocardial Failure   **25**
Arnold Schwartz, Louis A. Sordahl, Mark L. Entman, Julius C. Allen, Y. S. Reddy, M. Ann Goldstein, Robert J. Luchi and Leigh E. Wyborny

Chapter 4
Ribonucleic Acid (RNA) Polymerase and Adenyl Cyclase in Cardiac Hypertrophy and Cardiomyopathy   45

Kappiareth G. Nair, Teddy Umali and James Potts

Chapter 5
Myofibrillar Proteins and the Contractile Mechanism in the Normal and Failing Heart   53

Joan Wikman-Coffelt, Claudia Fenner, Antone F. Salel, Teiko Kamiyama and Dean T. Mason

Chapter 6
Effects of Ischemia on the Contractile Processes of Heart Muscle   77

Arnold M. Katz

Chapter 10

Peripheral Circulatory Control Mechanisms in Congestive Heart Failure   **129**

Robert Zelis, John Longhurst, Robert J. Capone, Garrett Lee and Dean T. Mason

Chapter 11

Function of the Hypoxic Myocardium: Experimental and Clinical Aspects   **143**

Ezra A. Amsterdam

Chapter 12

Nature and Significance of Alterations in Myocardial Compliance   **159**

James W. Covell and John Ross, Jr

PART II: EVALUATION

Chapter 16

Cardiac Catheterization in the Clinical Assessment of Heart Disease and Ventricular Performance **225**

Dean T. Mason, Richard R. Miller, Daniel S. Berman, Louis A. Vismara, David O. Williams, Antone F. Salel, Anthony N. DeMaria, Hugo G. Bogren, Gerald L. DeNardo and Ezra A. Amsterdam

Chapter 17

Catheterization Evaluation of Cardiac Function in Acute and Chronic Coronary Artery Disease **273**

Charles E. Rackley, Richard O. Russell, Jr, Roger E. Moraski, John A. Mantle, Bolling J. Feild and McKamy Smith

PART III: TREATMENT

Chapter 21

Ventricular Afterload-Reducing Agents in Congestive Heart Failure Therapy   343

Richard R. Miller, David O. Williams, Anthony N. DeMaria, Ezra A. Amsterdam and Dean T. Mason

Chapter 22

Myocardial Infarction Shock: Mechanisms and Management   365

Ezra A. Amsterdam, Anthony N. DeMaria, James L. Hughes, Edward J. Hurley, Arthur J. Lurie, David O. Williams, Richard R. Miller and Dean T. Mason

The Editor

Dean T. Mason, MD, is Professor of Medicine, Professor Physiology and Chief of Cardiovascular Medicine at the University of California, School of Medicine, Davis, California, and the University of California at Davis-Sacramento Medical Center, Sacramento, California. He came to his present position in 1968 from the National Heart Institute at the National Institutes of Health in Bethesda, Maryland, where he had been Attending Physician and Senior Investigator and Assistant Section Director of Cardiovascular Diagnosis in the Cardiology Branch since 1963. A native of Berkeley, California, Doctor Mason received his MD degree from Duke University School of Medicine in 1958. After completing his Medical Internship and Medical Residency on the Osler Service at the Johns Hopkins University Hospital in Baltimore in 1961, he was Clinical Associate in the Cardiology Branch of the National Heart Institute from 1961 to 1963. Doctor Mason has authored more than 400 original articles on several aspects of cardiovascular science and clinical cardiology; he serves on the Editorial Boards of *The American Journal of Cardiology, Journal of Clinical Investigation, Circulation, Chest, Clinical Pharmacology and Therapeutics, Catheterization and Cardiovascular Diagnosis* and *Heart and Lung.* He is President-Elect of the American College of Cardiology, President of the Western Society for Clinical Research and Member of the American Board of Internal Medicine Cardiovascular Diseases. Doctor Mason is recipient of the American Society for Pharmacology and Experimental Therapeutics' Award in Experimental Therapeutics in 1973, the American Therapeutic Society Research Award in 1965, and the Theodore and Susan B. Cummings Humanitarian Awards in 1972, 1973 and 1975 from the US State Department and the American College of Cardiology.

Contributing Authors

Julius C. Allen, PhD
Associate Professor
Department of Cell Biophysics
Baylor College of Medicine
Texas Medical Center
Houston, Texas

Ezra A. Amsterdam, MD
Associate Professor of Medicine
Director, Coronary Care Unit
Section of Cardiovascular Medicine
University of California
School of Medicine and Sacramento Medical
    Center
Davis and Sacramento, California

Daniel S. Berman, MD
Assistant Professor of Radiology
Director, Nuclear Cardiology
Section of Nuclear Medicine
University of California
School of Medicine and Sacramento Medical
    Center
Davis and Sacramento, California

Hugo G. Bogren, MD
Professor of Radiology
Director, Cardiovascular Radiology
Section of Diagnostic Radiology
University of California
School of Medicine and Sacramento Medical
    Center
Davis and Sacramento, California

Robert Capone, MD
Assistant Professor of Medicine
Brown University
Director, Coronary Care Unit
Rhode Island Hospital
Providence, Rhode Island

H. Neal Coleman, III, MD
Co-Director of Cardiology
Little Company of Mary Hospital
Evergreen Park, Illinois
Associate Professor of Medicine
Rush Medical College
Chicago, Illinois

George Cooper, IV, MD
Fellow, Cardiovascular Medicine
Division of Cardiology
Department of Medicine
Duke University School of Medicine
Durham, North Carolina

James W. Covell, MD
Associate Professor of Medicine and
    Bioengineering
Cardiovascular Division
Department of Medicine
University of California
School of Medicine
San Diego, California

Michael H. Crawford, MD
Assistant Professor of Medicine
Cardiovascular Division
Department of Medicine
University of California
School of Medicine
San Diego, California

Anthony N. DeMaria, MD
Assistant Professor of Medicine
Director, Echocardiography
Section of Cardiovascular Medicine
University of California
School of Medicine and Sacramento Medical
    Center
Davis and Sacramento, California

Gerald L. DeNardo, MD
Professor of Radiology and Medicine
Chief, Section of Nuclear Medicine
University of California
School of Medicine and Sacramento Medical
  Center
Davis and Sacramento, California

Mark L. Entman, MD
Associate Professor of Cell Biophysics and
  Medicine
Baylor College of Medicine
Texas Medical Center
Houston, Texas

Claudia Fenner, BS
Research Biochemist
Section of Cardiovascular Medicine
University of California
School of Medicine
Davis, California

Bolling J. Feild, MD
Fellow in Cardiovascular Medicine
Division of Cardiology
Department of Medicine
University of Alabama Medical Center
Birmingham, Alabama

Margaret Ann Goldstein, PhD
Assistant Professor of Cell Biophysics and
  Medicine
Baylor College of Medicine
Texas Medical Center
Houston, Texas

John F. Gunning, MD
Attending Cardiologist
Royal Victoria Hospital
Sydney, Australia

Carlos E. Harrison, Jr, MD
Associate Professor of Internal Medicine
Mayo Graduate School of Medicine
University of Minnesota
Rochester, Minnesota

James L. Hughes, MD
Fellow in Cardiovascular Medicine
Section of Cardiovascular Medicine
University of California

School of Medicine and Sacramento Medical
  Center
Davis and Sacramento, California

Edward J. Hurley, MD
Professor of Surgery
Chief, Section of Cardiovascular Surgery
University of California
School of Medicine and Sacramento Medical
  Center
Davis and Sacramento, California

Teiko Kamiyama, MD
Research Physiologist
Section of Cardiovascular Medicine
University of California
School of Medicine
Davis, California

Arnold J. Katz, MD
Philip J and Harriet L Goodhart Professor of
  Medicine
Division of Cardiology
Mount Sinai School of Medicine
The City University of New York
New York, New York

Garrett Lee, MD
Assistant Professor of Medicine
Section of Cardiovascular Medicine
University of California
School of Medicine and Sacramento Medical
  Center
Davis and Sacramento, California

John Longhurst, MD, PhD
Fellow, Cardiovascular Medicine
Division of Cardiology
University of Texas Southwestern Medical
  School at Dallas
Dallas, Texas

Robert J. Luchi, MD
Chief, Medical Service
Houston VA Hospital
Professor and Vice Chairman, Department of
  Medicine
Baylor College of Medicine
Texas Medical Center
Houston, Texas

Arthur J. Lurie, MD
Assistant Professor of Surgery
Section of Thoracic Surgery
University of California
School of Medicine and Sacramento Medical
    Center
Davis and Sacramento, California

John A. Mantle, MD
Assistant Professor of Medicine
Division of Cardiology
Department of Medicine
University of Alabama Medical Center
Birmingham, Alabama

Dean T. Mason, MD
Professor of Medicine
Professor of Physiology
Chief, Cardiovascular Medicine
University of California
School of Medicine and Sacramento Medical
    Center
Davis and Sacramento, California

Rashid A. Massumi, MD
Professor of Medicine
Section of Cardiovascular Medicine
University of California
School of Medicine and Sacramento Medical
    Center
Davis and Sacramento, California

Richard R. Miller, MD
Associate Professor of Medicine
Director, Cardiac Catheterization Laboratory
Section of Cardiovascular Medicine
University of California
School of Medicine and Sacramento Medical
    Center
Davis and Sacramento, California

Roger E. Moraski, MD
Assistant Professor of Medicine
Division of Cardiology
Department of Medicine
University of Alabama Medical Center
Birhimgham, Alabama

Kappiareth G. Nair, MD
Director-Professor of Medicine
Head of Cardiology

Seth G.S. Medical College and King Edward VII
    Memorial Hospital
Parel, Bombay, India

Alexander L. Neumann, BS
Research Associate
Section of Cardiovascular Medicine
University of California
School of Medicine and Sacramento Medical
    Center
Davis and Sacramento, California

Robert A. O'Rourke, MD
Associate Professor of Medicine
Director, Clinical Cardiology Section
Cardiovascular Division
Department of Medicine
University of California
School of Medicine
San Diego, California

James Potts, MD
Assistant Professor of Medicine
Department of Medicine
University of Syracuse
School of Medicine
Syracuse, New York

Charles E. Rackley, MD
Professor of Medicine
Director, Myocardial Infarction Research Unit
Division of Cardiology
Department of Medicine
University of Alabama Medical Center
Birmingham, Alabama

Yerradhoddi S. Reddy, PhD
Assistant Professor of Cell Biophysics
Baylor College of Medicine
Texas Medical Center
Houston, Texas

Stanley M. Rosen, MD
Associate Professor of Medicine
Chief, Renal Division
Department of Medicine
University of California
School of Medicine
Irvine, California

John Ross, Jr, MD
Professor of Medicine
Chief, Cardiovascular Division
Department of Medicine
University of California
School of Medicine
San Diego, California

Richard O. Russell, Jr, MD
Professor of Medicine
Division of Cardiology
Department of Medicine
University of Alabama Medical Center
Birmingham, Alabama

Harold L. Rutenberg, MD
Chief, Cardiology
Pennsylvania Hospital
Assistant Professor of Medicine
Temple University Health Science Center
Philadelphia, Pennsylvania

Antone F. Salel, MD
Assistant Professor of Medicine
Director, Lipid Clinic and Cardiovascular
  Engineering
Section of Cardiovascular Medicine
University of California
School of Medicine and Sacramento Medical
  Center
Davis and Sacramento, California

Arnold Schwartz, PhD
Professor and Chairman, Department of Cell
  Biophysics
Head, Division of Myocardial Biology
Baylor College of Medicine
Texas Medical Center
Houston, Texas

Leigh D. Segel, PhD
Research Biochemist
Section of Cardiovascular Medicine
University of California
School of Medicine
Davis, California

McKamy Smith, MD
Fellow in Cardiovascular Medicine
Division of Cardiology
Department of Medicine

University of Alabama Medical Center
Birmingham, Alabama

Edmund H. Sonnenblick, MD
Professor of Medicine
Chief, Division of Cardiology
Albert Einstein College of Medicine at Yeshiva
  University
Bronx, New York

Louis A. Sordahl, PhD
Associate Professor of Biochemistry
Department of Human Biological Chemistry
  and Genetics
University of Texas Medical Branch at
  Galveston
Galveston, Texas

James F. Spann, Jr, MD
Professor of Medicine
Chief, Section of Cardiology
Temple University Health Science Center
Philadelphia, Pennsylvania

Henry M. Spotnitz, MD
Assistant Professor of Surgery
Columbia Presbyterian Hospital
Columbia University College of Physicians and
  Surgeons
New York, New York

Melvin J. Tonkon, MD
Assistant Professor of Medicine
Director, Hypertension Clinic
Section of Cardiovascular Medicine
University of California
School of Medicine and Sacramento Medical
  Center
Davis and Sacramento, California

Teddy Umali, MS
Research Biologist
Department of Medicine
Hospital of the University of Pennsylvania
Philadelphia, Pennsylvania

Zakauddin Vera, MD
Assistant Professor of Medicine
Director, Clinical Electrophysiology
Section of Cardiovascular Medicine
University of California

School of Medicine and Sacramento Medical
  Center
Davis and Sacramento, California

Louis A. Vismara, MD
Assistant Professor of Medicine
Director, Cardiology Clinic
Section of Cardiovascular Medicine
University of California
School of Medicine and Sacramento Medical
  Center
Davis and Sacramento, California

Joan Wikman-Coffelt, PhD
Assistant Professor of Molecular Cardiology
Section of Cardiovascular Medicine
University of California
School of Medicine
Davis, California

David O. Williams, MD
Assistant Professor Medicine
Section of Cardiovascular Medicine
University of California
School of Medicine

Davis, California
Director, Cardiology Service
Martinez VA Hospital
Martinez, California

John F. Williams, Jr, MD
Professor of Medicine
Director, Cardiology Division
University of Texas Medical Branch at
  Galveston
Galveston, Texas

Leigh E. Wyborny, PhD
Instructor, Department of Medicine
Baylor College of Medicine
Texas Medical Center
Houston, Texas

Robert F. Zelis, MD
Professor of Medicine and Physiology
Chief, Division of Cardiology
Milton S. Hershey Medical Center
University of Pennsylvania
Hershey, Pennsylvania

Preface

The purpose of this volume is to present the recent advances and current status of modern knowledge concerning the broad subject of the common denominator of cardiovascular medicine itself: **Congestive Heart Failure.** To most effectively accomplish these objectives, this monograph is organized within the three principal areas of relevant understanding necessary for improved clinical management of this condition: (1) **Mechanisms,** (2) **Evaluation** and (3) **Treatment** of congestive heart failure. While each of the twenty-three chapters comprising this textbook, with hundreds of illustrations and references, provides independent coverage of a specific topic, the chapters are carefully integrated in a synthesized manner to sequentially build upon a purposefully developed body of crucial information to afford a comprehensive overview and appreciation of this multifaceted subject without unnecessary repetition. It should be pointed out that the stimulus for this book was an outgrowth of the eleven articles constituting a recent special issue of *The American Journal of Cardiology.* Where necessary, certain of these original articles have been revised and up-dated. Importantly, the majority of the present volume consists of new material, twelve new chapters in all, with the idea of extending the original symposium on basic research in congestive heart failure to a wide clinically oriented audience of professionals in medicine, including medical students, physicians-in-training, generalists, internists and cardiologists, as well as postgraduate students in the medical sciences and academic basic and clinical investigators.

Emphasis is placed on the elucidation of important concepts and principles of congestive heart failure so that the clinician can approach a particular aspect of the problem logically and, as desired and motivated, may further proceed expeditiously into even greater detail of the matter of interest. In addition, a vigorous effort has been made to select major topics written by investigators well recognized in the field to provide an authorative volume on congestive heart failure. To the fifty-six contributing authors who readily agreed to construct this comprehensive sourcebook, I am deeply grateful for their superb contributions. In effect, this volume represents a textbook of modern cardiology, with congestive heart failure serving as the focal point. In summary, the intent of this volume is to present an overall survey of recent basic and clinical progress in contemporary knowledge of congestive heart failure important in the advancement of patient care.

Dean T. Mason, MD, FACC

Congestive Heart Failure

Introduction to Recent Advances in Pathogenesis and Management of Congestive Heart Failure

Dean T. Mason, MD, FACC

In the past decade, improved understanding of the hemodynamic and mechanical mechanisms of cardiac contraction has provided precise definition of the heart failure state. *Heart failure* is the abnormal condition in which disturbed cardiac performance is primarily responsible for the inability of the heart to pump blood at a rate commensurate with systemic metabolic requirements at rest and during normal activity. Heart failure is considered to be *compensated* when cardiac output is maintained at a normal level by reserve systems inherent in the ventricle, often with congestion and other symptoms attending the operation of these adaptive processes. *Decompensated* heart failure evolves with chronic low cardiac output despite maximal activity of cardiocirculatory protective mechanisms.

Although a complete and detailed elucidation of the fundamental physiologic and molecular derangements causing myocardial failure is not yet available, and despite the substantial controversy concerning certain of its aspects, recent intensive investigation has produced a considerable body of new information that has permitted formulation of improved concepts of the underlying events occurring in heart failure. These advances have been stimulated by contributions from workers in several disciplines, including the anatomist, biochemist, physiologist,

pharmacologist and clinical investigator, through the development of refined techniques and their application to experimental biologic systems and to patients.

The chapters that follow in Part One of this textbook provide a synthesized perspective of the important multidisciplinary findings relating to improved understanding of the heart failure state. Further, the chapters comprising Part Two delineate the important noninvasive techniques and cardiac catheterization approaches available to the clinician for systematic determination of the heart diseases causing congestive heart failure and the degree and nature of cardiac dysfunction. Finally, the chapters of Part Three describe the new principles of management and therapeutic armamentarium in the modern treatment of patients with congestive heart failure.

Part One: Mechanisms of Congestive Heart Failure

Structural Alterations in the Hypertrophied and Failing Heart: Spotnitz and Sonnenblick begin this monograph with an integrated analysis of alterations in myocardial ultrastructure and ventricular macroarchitecture in the hypertrophied and failing heart. The distinctly different morphologic patterns of concentric (pressure overload) and eccentric (volume overload) ventricular hypertrophy in long-term adaptation to excessive hemodynamic burden are correlated with sarcomere and ventricular performance in these two situations. Concerning functional evaluation of the sarcomere—the fundamental contractile unit—these authors direct attention to the significance of concomitant changes in ventricular pressure, volume, mass and thickness, radius of curvature, wall stress and shortening vectors, dispersion of sarcomere lengths, fiber orientation, interfiber slippage and connective tissue skeleton. Although a specific qualitative change in microanatomy is not responsible for heart failure, the quantitative structural alterations accompanying hypertrophy are of functional importance.

Abnormal Biochemistry in Myocardial Failure: One of the most exciting developments in recent years has been the illumination of biochemical processes and subcellular contraction mechanisms in the normal and diseased myocardium. Thus, Schwartz and co-workers provide a comprehensive discussion of modern knowledge and concepts of cardiac muscle metabolism, excitation-contraction coupling and the contractile process itself. The contractile apparatus of the sarcomere consists of four protein aggregates—the primary interacting actin and myosin molecular chains and the modulator proteins troponin and tropomyosin, which inhibit the actin-myosin reaction. Linkage of electrical excitation to mechanical contraction is achieved by delivery of calcium to troponin from the sarcoplasmic reticulum and sarcolemma. The combination of calcium with troponin activates the contractile process by releasing the troponin-tropomyosin inhibition of actin-myosin binding. Contraction occurs by myosin adenosine triphosphatase-regulated cyclic interactions between the actin-myosin linkages, with the development of force and shortening. Adenosine triphosphate energy for operation of the contractile machinery is produced in surrounding mitochondria by the oxidative phosphorylation of circulating free fatty acids and glucose. Present information suggests that disturbance in mitochondrial energy production may contribute to myocardial depression in advanced heart failure secondary to long-standing me-

chanical stress. Current speculation concerning causation relates the impaired contractile state in chronic hemodynamic overload to depressed activities of adenosine triphosphatase-dependent calcium transport in the sarcoplasmic reticulum (relaxing factor) and of myosin adenosine triphosphatase.

Ribonucleic Acid (RNA) Polymerase and Adenyl Cyclase in Cardiac Hypertrophy: Protein synthesis in the myocardium provides a continuously operative system for renewal of fiber structure and enzymatic machinery and a rapidly responsive compensatory mechanism for ventricular hypertrophy induced by excessive cardiac mechanical stress. Three stages comprise the process of protein synthesis: (1) replication in the nucleus—synthesis of deoxyribonucleic acid (DNA); (2) transcription in the nucleus—synthesis of ribonucleic acid (RNA); and (3) translation in the sarcoplasm—specific protein formation on ribosomal aggregates, termed polysomes. Nair and co-workers discuss the pathways of ventricular protein synthesis in hemodynamic overload and in an animal model of cardiomyopathy, the Syrian golden hamster. Large increases in RNA polymerase activity and ribosomes occur during cardiac hypertrophy. Interestingly, myocardial norepinephrine synthesis and adenyl cyclase activity are increased in the hamster with cardiomyoapthy, and a possible connection between cyclic adenosine monophosphate and RNA transcription is considered.

Myofibrillar Proteins and the Contractile Mechanism in the Normal and Failing Heart: Attention most recently has been directed to the function of the contractile proteins themselves in the process of myocardial contraction. In this regard, Wikman-Coffelt and her colleagues delineate the series of studies they have carried out on the properties, structure, enzymatic activity, subunits and regulation of myosin in both normal and abnormal heart muscle. These investigations have led to the concept that the enzymatic function of myosin during contraction is controlled by the subunit composition of whole myosin; light chains within the myosin head appear to suppress adenosine triphosphatase activity contained in the heavy chain portion of the myosin head. Further, the normal left ventricle possesses higher potassium- and calcium-activated levels of myosin adenosine triphosphatase associated with fewer myosin light chains in proportion to heavy chains, compared with the normal right ventricle. In mild experimental hemodynamic overload, myosin enzymatic performance increased in the early hypertrophied, stressed ventricle accompanied by synthesis of relatively more heavy chain than light chain subunits; thus, in the initial stage of mild pulmonic stenosis, the right ventricle developed the properties of the normal left ventricle. Concordant with this view that myosin light chains govern myosin enzymatic function is the finding, in chronic experimental severe aortic stenosis, that myosin adenosine triphosphatase was depressed concomitant with an increase in the proportion of light chains to heavy chains in the myosin heads in the markedly stressed ventricle; therefore, in severe hemodynamic overload, left ventricular myosin developed the characteristics of normal right ventricular myosin.

Effect of Ischemia on Myocardial Contraction: This section of the text examines the problem of ischemic heart failure. The underlying mechanism by which oxygen deprivation causes depression of contractile function is yet to be clarified. However, new insights into this problem have been provided by basic investigations of the effects of hypoxia on the biochemistry and mechanisms of cardiac muscle contraction. Katz considers the possible nature of the primary metabolic aberrations responsible for the rapid mechanical deterioration induced by ischemia. He emphasizes the probable importance of intracellular acidosis with hydrogen ion generation, resulting from enhanced anaerobic glycolysis and accelerated lactate formation. He postulates that hydrogen ions compete for calcium-binding sites on troponin, thereby maintaining the heart in a state of relaxation. Finally, with depletion of adenosine triphosphate, contracture of the myocardium develops.

Alterations in Cardiac Adrenergic Neurotransmitter Activity in Heart Failure: The sympathetic nervous system normally exerts a major regulatory role in the augmentation of cardio-

vascular function in response to increased metabolic needs of the body, and it represents an immediately available compensatory mechanism in support of the failing heart. Although generalized sympathetic activity is increased in heart failure, norepinephrine is reduced paradoxically in the hypertrophied and failing myocardium because of its defective synthesis locally. Rutenberg and Spann review the mechanisms of alterations in cardiac adrenergic neurotransmitter activity in congestive heart failure. The depression of myocardial norepinephrine appears to result from disturbed metabolic function of the neuron rather than from actual loss of sympathetic tissue. Although this defect deprives the dysfunctioning ventricle of rapid inotropic and chronotropic adaptation, it is not causally related to the intrinsic inotropic weakness of the failing myocardium. Adrenergic reserve is partially restored to the failing heart by increased circulating norepinephrine because of its greater synthesis in the peripheral vasculature and adrenal medulla in this condition.

Contractile and Energetic Behavior of Hypertrophied and Failing Myocardium: Myocardial oxygen consumption ($M\dot{V}O_2$) is principally determined by the integration of three related hemodynamic variables: (1) intraventricular systolic tension—primarily governed by systolic pressure and ventricular volume; (2) contractility; (3) heart rate. In this chapter, Cooper and co-workers consider the energetics and mechanical efficiency of the hypertrophied and failing myocardium in experimental ventricular pressure overload. The authors document an increased oxygen cost of developing tension, in conjunction with diminished contractility, in the hypertrophied and failing ventricle. This combination of depressed contractility and paradoxically augmented myocardial oxygen consumption appears to be related to the excessive pressure stress itself, rather than to the hypertrophic response, since these investigators found both contractility and myocardial oxygen consumption to be normal with the same extent and duration of hypertrophy induced by experimental systolic volume overload. It is suggested that the mechanism of the paradoxical increase in myocardial oxygen utilization in ventricular systolic pressure overload is accentuation of nonphosphorylating mitrochondrial respiration as a result of abnormal calcium metabolism in this condition, due to a primary defect of decreased calcium uptake by the sarcoplasmic reticulum with augmented calcium accumulation in the mitochondria as a secondary factor.

Regulation of Cardiac Performance in Heart Disease: Disturbed cardiac performance in clinical heart disease is produced by three possible general types of pathophysiologic mechanisms: (1) disorder of contractility; (2) systolic mechanical ventricular overloading (volume or pressure); and (3) diastolic mechanical inhibition of ventricular loading. In this chapter of the textbook, I describe the regulation of cardiac output in primary inotropic diseases and chronic hemodynamic overloads. The contributions and side effects of preload, hypertrophy and inotropic reserves are discussed. Prolonged hemodynamic stress leads to reduced contractile state, and the concept is formulated that, in cardiomyopathies and systolic mechanical disorders, contractility is the fundamental physiologic variable in heart failure and that the extent of its impairment determines the onset of decompensation. The compensatory mechanisms employed and the critical level of inotropic depression responsible for decompensation are dependent on the specific pathophysiologic condition. The clinical functional classification of congestive heart failure is based largely on symptoms due to operation of compensatory adaptation rather than on those due to derangements of the primary factors of decompensation—cardiac output (crucial hemodynamic variable) and contractility (the fundamental determinant).

Peripheral Circulatory Control Mechanisms in Heart Failure: In addition to the cardiac compensatory mechanisms in heart failure, concomitant adjustments take place in the peripheral vasculature that serve to support regional circulatory function. Thus, with a decrease in cardiac output, systemic vascular resistance increases to maintain normal perfusion pressure, and redistribution of blood flow occurs to sustain the oxygen needs of organs with greater metabolic requirements. In this chapter, Zelis and co-workers deal with the important,

but relatively unappreciated, subject of peripheral circulatory control mechanisms at rest and during exercise in congestive heart failure. In addition to increased sympathetic activity, vascular stiffness due to excess sodium and water in the arteriolar wall and a rise in the level of tissue pressure observed in edema bring about the increased systemic resistance characteristic of the heart failure state. In exercising skeletal muscle in heart failure, the reduced dilator capacity of the resistance vessels leads to increased oxygen extraction, diminished oxygen consumption regionally and probably augmented anaerobic metabolism with lactic acidemia. Concerning the adrenergically influenced partitioning of regional blood flow in heart failure, it is postulated that the afferent reflex limb may originate in active skeletal muscle and baroreceptor responsiveness may be diminished.

Function of the Hypoxic Myocardium: In this chapter, Amsterdam analyzes the determinental effects of inadequate oxygen supply on the mechanical and hemodynamic performance of the heart. An imbalance between myocardial oxygen delivery and demand provokes regional ischemia that, in angina pectoris, leads to reversible ventricular depression; more intense and prolonged discrepancy results in myocardial infarction. A characteristic disorder of cardiac function in ischemic heart disease is abnormal segmental contraction—dyssynergy. The electrocardiogram in clinical coronary disease provides an estimate of the presence, degree and nature of dyssynergy and the status of left ventricular function. The left anterior descending coronary artery is most responsible for maintaining pump integrity. Cardiogenic shock is principally related to the extent of myocardial infarction, with consequent reduction of cardiac output. In addition, a secondary contribution to hypotension may be an inadequate increase in systemic vascular resistance due to competitive reflex vasodilation, initiated by stretch and chemoreceptors within the left ventricular wall.

Alterations in Myocardial Compliance: The diastolic characteristics of cardiac muscle and the whole heart have received relatively less attention than have their contractile properties, and knowledge of the important quality of resting compliance—reciprocal of stiffness—in heart disease has been incomplete. Covell and Ross consider the passive stress-strain relations of the myocardium and ventricle in normal and abnormal conditions. Acute pharmacologically induced changes in contractility do not influence compliance. However, the entire ventricular diastolic pressure-volume curve is displaced to the right in chronic volume overload so that preload compensation can operate with fewer symptoms of congestion. In contrast, acute myocardial infarction results in a leftward shift that tends to increase left ventricular end-diastolic pressure. Clinically, the concentrically hypertrophied ventricle appears to manifest diminished distensibility, but this observation has been difficult to reproduce experimentally. In the assessment of the diastolic pressure-volume relation of the ventricle, the authors introduce the concept of its functional compliance throughout the filling period.

Renal Function and Edema Formation in Congestive Heart Failure: It is now recognized that abnormal renal function in heart disease is the result of cardiac dysfunction rather than the initiating determinant of congestive heart failure. Tonkon and colleagues point out that the fluid and electrolyte derangements in congestive heart failure are multifactorial. Thus, decreased cardiac output is translated into diminished renal perfusion resulting in outer cortical ischemia with an increased percentage of total renal blood flow supplied to the inner cortex and medulla. Glomerular filtration becomes reduced, the filtration fraction is increased, and enhanced reabsorption of sodium and water takes place in the proximal renal tubules. Further, lack of a postulated natriuretic hormone that normally rejects proximal renal tubular sodium reabsorption may play a role in the edematous state. In addition, there is increased activity of the renin-angiotensin-aldosterone humoral system: elevated aldosterone secretion increases sodium reabsorption at the expense of potassium loss in the distal tubules. Inappropriate increased secretion of antidiuretic hormones may also occur and contributes to dilutional hyponatremia. In the early stage of heart failure, increased proximal tubular reabsorption of sodium is the principal factor in fluid

retention, while elevated renin-aldosterone activity critically affects the chronic edematous state.

Part Two: Evaluation of Congestive Heart Failure

Physical Findings in Heart Failure and Their Physiologic Basis: A characteristic constellation of clinical manifestations accompany the congestive heart failure state due to any of the specific types of cardiac disease. O'Rourke and Crawford delineate the physical signs of ventricular dysfunction—pulsus alternans, dicrotic pulse, abnormalities of the jugular venous pulse and abnormal results of chest and abdominal examinations and cardiac auscultation. The methods for the bedside detection of cardiac compensatory mechanisms that are detailed include identification of increased sympathetic activity, ventricular dilation and hypertrophy and increased salt and water retention.

Echocardiographic Evaluation of Cardiac Function: The most important new examining technique in cardiovascular medicine is echocardiography. By providing acoustic images of pulsed ultrasound reflected from the interface of different media, the echogram obtains noninvasively the graphic representation of dynamic cardiac anatomy. In addition to the ability of ultrasound to identify a variety of cardiac diseases, echocardiography also provides a practical and reliable means for the assessment of heart function in terms of both hemodynamic and mechanical properties of cardiac performance. In this chapter, DeMaria and his colleagues describe the echographic methods for obtaining absolute dimensions of cardiac chambers and structures, and for determining the volume, wall thickness, segmental motion and velocity of circumferential fiber shortening of the left ventricle, as well as the size of the left atrium. Evaluation of left ventricular diastolic inflow is also afforded by study of the mitral echogram. The advantages and limitations of echocardiography are emphasized. Further, the new multidimensional echocardiographic techniques that allow the extension of the standard one-dimensional echographic view to three-dimensional analysis of the heart are delineated.

In addition, the authors describe the echographic approach to the definitive examination of cardiomegaly and congestive heart failure of unknown etiology.

Cardiac Catheterization in the Clinical Assessment of Heart Disease and Ventricular Performance: The most important advancement in cardiovascular medicine in the past quarter century has been the development of methods for catheterization of the human heart that can be performed with relative ease and patient safety. Application of cardiac catheterization has provided understanding of the pathophysiologic mechanisms in heart disease, established cardiovascular diagnosis and evaluation of cardiac function on a precise scientific basis, and spearheaded innovations in both medical and surgical therapy of cardiovascular disorders. In this chapter, my colleagues and I at the University of California, Davis, delineate the proper utilization of these techniques in the identification of heart diseases and the assessment of cardiac function in patients with emphasis on the interpretation of the physiologic information obtained from these studies. In regard to the evaluation of ventricular performance, the specific property of cardiac contractility can be determined clinically by variables of pump performance (hemodynamic measures of pressure and flow) and by parameters of the mechanical characteristics of heart muscle (isovolumic indexes utilizing the rate of intraventricular pressure rise or dp/dt and ejection indexes employing fiber shortening rate or V_{CF}). Since there are advantages and limitations with each of the hemodynamic methods and mechanical indexes, it is necessary to select the proper approach according to the conditions of study for assessment of right and left ventricular contractility in intrapatient and interpatient investigations. In addition, the new techniques in nuclear cardiology are described. The recent availability of the Anger gamma scintillation camera, capable of recording wide-field radio-isotopic images over the precordium, provides a means for the assessment of left ventricular ejection fraction and segmental contraction and regional myocardial perfusion and ischemia, as well as a means for detection of acute myocardial infarction.

Catheterization Evaluation of Cardiac Function in Acute and Chronic Coronary Artery Disease: In coronary artery disease, ventricular performance may be impaired acutely due to myocardial infarction or chronically due to long-standing ischemic heart disease. Rackley and co-workers describe the special cardiac catheterization techniques required in the evaluation of patients with coronary disease. In acute myocardial infarction, measurements of hemodynamics and left ventricular filling pressures using the special pervenous Swan-Ganz catheter in the coronary care unit provide vital information in the management of pump dysfunction and in the evaluation of prognosis. Detailed left heart catheterization, including ventriculography and coronary arteriography, allows identification of patients suitable for operative intervention in acute and chronic coronary heart disease with marked congestive heart failure refractory to medical management.

Part Three: Treatment of Congestive Heart Failure

Management of Chronic Refractory Congestive Heart Failure: In some patients with severe, chronic cardiac dysfunction, proper use of the standard therapeutic measures of rest, diet, digitalis and diuretics does not alleviate the congestive heart failure state. In this chapter my colleagues and I delineate that management in such persons is based on firm knowledge of the pathophysiologic mechanisms involved, identification of the specific type of heart disease responsible and correction of extracardiac factors contributing to the unresponsive condition. In general, cardiac catheterization is performed to determine the cause of heart disease and to delineate the extent of abnormal ventricular performance. Cardiac dysfunction should not be allowed to become refractory to medical therapy in congenital heart disease or acquired valvular disorders; surgery is usually carried out electively before symptoms develop in congenital structural disorders and when cardiac symptoms occur with ordinary activity in chronic rheumatic valvular disease. Successful treatment of intractable congestive heart failure due to several depressed ventricular contractility in which operative intervention is not feasible (the specific, idiopathic and ischemic cardiomyopathies) requires the skillful correction of disorders of the four principal determinants of cardiac pump performance: (1) preload; (2) afterload; (3) contractility; and (4) heart rate. In these patients, medical management usually consists of certain therapeutic combinations of digitalis and dopamine to increase depressed inotropic state; diuretics and long-acting nitrates to relieve circulatory congestion; maintenance of ventricular filling pressure at the upper limit of normal with volume expansion if necessary to provide optimal preload; afterload reduction by lowering impedance to left ventricular ejection by peripheral vasodilators such as nitroprusside; and establishment of normal ventricular rate and cardiac rhythm by antiarrhythmic agents, direct current cardioversion and pacemakers. In coronary heart disease, it is necessary to give special consideration to the effects of therapy on myocardial oxygen consumption.

Cardiac Stimulating Agents in Treatment of Heart Failure: In this chapter, Williams discusses advances in the medical treatment of congestive heart failure with positive inotropic agents. The final common pathway for augmenting the inotropic state seems to be enhanced delivery of calcium to troponin, one of the modulator proteins of the contractile apparatus. In general, 2 subcellular mechanisms appear to be potentially available for increasing calcium transport to the contractile proteins, thereby stimulating the process of excitation-contraction coupling. The first is increased transverse tubular influx of calcium by drug action on the sarcolemma (digitalis glycosides). The second mechanism involves pharmacologic alterations of the subcellular beta sympathomimetic system, comprising the beta receptor, adenyl cyclase, cyclic adenosine monophosphate, phosphodiesterase and, apparently, protein kinase-mediated increased intracellular release of calcium from the sarcoplasmic reticulum (catecholamines, glucagon, thyroid hormone, tolbutamide and aminophylline). The possible salutary effects of certain combinations of these agents are considered.

Clinical Pharmacology and Therapeutics of the Digitalis Glycosides: Although the digitalis glycosides have been employed for nearly 2 centuries as the principal drug in the treatment of congestive heart failure, it has become clear only within the past decade that stimulation of ventricular contractile state is the fundamental therapeutic action of these agents. In this chapter my colleagues and I show that the expression of this increase in contractility depends on the type of heart disease and on cardiocirculatory status at the time the glycoside is administered. Therefore, variable and even opposite effects on cardiac output, systemic circulatory dynamics and myocardial oxygen consumption can take place as the result of interplay between direct and indirect cardiac and peripheral vascular effects of digitalis. Radioimmunoassay has established the therapeutic digoxin concentration usually to be between 1 and 2 nanograms per milliliter of serum. Since studies with tritiated digoxin have shown that 80 percent of oral digoxin is absorbed, the total oral digitalizing dose of digoxin has now been lowered to 2 milligrams. Moreover, oral daily maintenance doses of digoxin achieve therapeutic serum concentrations in approximately 7 to 10 days, and therefore, loading doses are no longer recommended except in urgent situations. Renal insufficiency is the most common predisposing factor for digoxin toxicity. The fundamental positive inotropic action of digitalis now appears to be the result of a glycoside-induced increase in transmembrane (sarcolemma-transverse tubular system) influx of calcium. In contrast, transmembrane fluxes of sodium and potassium underlie the electrical properties of the glycosides.

Ventricular Afterload-Reducing Agents in Congestive Heart Failure Therapy: Clinical use of peripheral vasodilator drugs to reduce left ventricular afterload constitutes a new therapeutic approach in the management of congestive heart failure. Miller and his associates describe the two pincipal mechanisms by which such agents can diminish left ventricular wall tension during systole (ventricular afterload). The first mechanism is the reduction of systemic vascular resistance, which decreases aortic impedance to left ventricular ejection and thereby results in greater stroke volume and cardiac output. Since low cardiac output usually increases to the same extent that elevated peripheral vascular resistance decreases, there is little or no decline in systemic arterial blood pressure accompanied by little or no increase in heart rate. The second mechanism is the relaxation of vascular smooth muscle in the systemic venous bed, which causes peripheral pooling of blood volume with diminished venous return to the heart. Consequently, left ventricular filling pressure and end-diastolic volume (ventricular preload) are reduced and pulmonary congestion is relieved. In addition, myocardial oxygen requirements are reduced by the decrease in left ventricular wall tension during contraction resulting from the decreases in both aortic impedance and ventricular end-diastolic volume. The principal vasodilator drugs currently in clinical use for afterload reduction—nitroprusside, phentolamine, nitroglycerin, trimethaphan and long-acting nitrates—exert differential actions on the peripheral arteriolar and venous beds. Nitroprusside and trimethaphan produce balanced relaxing effects on the systemic resistance and capacitance beds, whereas phentolamine has a greater effect on the arterial tree than on the peripheral venous system. In contrast, the action of sublingual nitroglycerin and the long-acting nitrates is exerted almost entirely on the systemic venous bed.

Mechanisms and Therapy of Myocardial Infarction Shock: Cardiogenic shock due to left ventricular pump failure is now the major cause of death in patients hospitalized with acute myocardial infarction. Although implementation of the concept of intensive monitoring in the coronary care unit during the past decade has provided effective managment of potentially lethal ventricular arrhythmias, thereby decreasing mortality in acute myocardial infarction from 30 to 15 percent in many medical centers, efforts to overcome heart failure shock in myocardial infarction have been unsatisfactory, and the remaining hospital deaths are largely the result of this grave complication that is fatal in more than 4 of 5 instances. In this chapter, Amsterdam and his associates show that myocardial infarction shock is chiefly related to extensive loss of left ventricular muscle, although extramyocardial factors may be contributory. Quantitative hemodynamic evaluation by Swan-Ganz catheterization allows accurate assess-

ment of prognosis and provides a physiologic basis for a choice among the available modes of therapy. Treatment consists of rapid blood volume expansion (dextran, saline, dextrose in water), pharmacologic agents (dopamine, norepinephrine), mechanical circulatory assist (intraaortic balloon counterpulsation) and surgical correction of mechanical cardiac defects related to infarction. Evaluation by complete right and left heart catheterization, including left ventriculography and coronary arteriography, for the detection of potentially surgically correctable cardiac abnormalities is carried out in appropriate patients within a few hours when shock remains refractory to medical management and mechanical circulatory assist. Operative procedures that have sometimes been successful include infarctectomy, mitral valve replacement for papillary muscle dysfunction and repair of ventricular septal rupture—usually combined with myocardial revascularization—in certain carefully selected patients after cardiac catheterization.

Clinical Pharmacology and Therapeutics of Antiarrhythmic Agents: The ability to identify and successfully treat cardiac arrhythmias represents one of the principal recent advances in the management of clinical heart disease. Since disorders of cardiac rhythm and conduction commonly accompany and complicate heart failure—particularly pump dysfunction due to coronary disease—my colleagues and I at the University of California, Davis, discuss the pathophysiology of tachyarrhythmias and the clinical application of the antiarrhythmic agents in the final chapter of this textbook on congestive heart failure. Each of the antiarrhythmic drugs depresses disorders of rapid impulse formation (repetitive ectopic pacemaker activity) by reducing diastolic depolarization and automaticity, and they inhibit disorders of impulse conduction (reentry tachyarrhythmias) by altering conduction velocity and refractory period, thus interrupting reciprocal excitation pathways. In unidirectional block, which perpetuates the reentry mechanism, Group I drugs (quinidine, procainamide, propranolol, bretylium and potassium) abate the arrhythmia by producing bidirectional block through slowing of conduction velocity, whereas Group II drugs (lidocaine and diphenylhydantoin) terminate the arrhythmia by abolishing the unindirectional block through enhancement of conduction velocity. In general, supraventricular tachyarrhythmias are treated with digitalis, vagal stimulation, quinidine, procainamide, propranolol and direct current countershock. Ventricular tachyarrhythmias are managed with lidocaine, procainamide, quinidine, propranolol, diphenylhydantoin, bretylium, direct current countershock, and electrical pacemaker ventricular overdrive. Antiarrhythmic agents, particularly in large doses, usually exert a negative inotropic action on the heart apparently by their interference with cardiac cellular transmembrane calcium influx. In contrast, the salutary electrical properties of the antiarrhythmic agents are related to their alterations of cardiac transmembrane fluxes of sodium and potassium. In addition, the antiarrhythmic efficacy of certain drugs such as verapamil may be due to the depression of slow-channel calcium transport into myocardial cells of specialized cardiac tissues.

Acknowledgment: The author wishes to thank Gail Garnas and Leslie Silvernail for their administrative and secretarial assistance.

PART I: MECHANISMS

Structural Conditions in the Hypertrophied and Failing Heart

Henry M. Spotnitz, MD
Edmund H. Sonnenblick, MD, FACC

The purpose of this discussion is not to review the normal structure of heart muscle, which has been noted in detail elsewhere,[1-4] but rather to note those characteristics of the structure of the heart that form the basis for normal function and in their extensions provide the substrate for the development of disease. Our major thesis is that the normal function of the heart can be explained by the rational synthesis of its component parts, especially the sarcomere,[5-7] and that much of dysfunction may reflect limits to the normal physiologic function accompanied by superimposed compensation for abnormal loads. Discussion of myocardial failure involves consideration of not only the structure at the level of the electron microscope but also the macro-construction of fibers in the wall of the heart and their relative disposition to create the ventricular wall. Thus, an integrated analysis at the gross and microscopic level becomes necessary for a more complete structural picture. In addition, it is recognized that many abnormalities in the overstressed heart may be only an accompaniment to the primary process and in and of themselves may not signify a necessary change related to the failing myocardium. Thus, artifacts of secondary changes, postmortem alteration, or fixation require constant consideration, and alterations that may be observed under abnormal conditions need evaluation as to their specific role in the process that is occurring.

Eccentric and Concentric Hypertrophy

When the ventricle is presented with abnormal volume and pressure loads, compensatory responses ensue that involve an increase in ventricular mass. However, this increase in total mass occurs in two distinct patterns, depending on the stress imposed. Thus, when diastolic volume is augmented (for example, by arteriovenous shunting or mitral insufficiency), intraventricular volume increases. Ventricular wall thickness, however, tends to remain the same, whereas the total mass of the ventricle is increased. An increase in synthesis of muscle must ensue to maintain wall thickness when volume is augmented. This condition is termed eccentric hypertrophy[8] (Figure 1). In contrast, when an excess systolic pressure load is applied to the ventricle (as in aortic stenosis or systemic hypertension) the wall becomes thickened, whereas end-diastolic intraventricular volume tends to remain unchanged. This condition is termed concentric hypertrophy.[8]

The effects of eccentric and concentric hypertrophy on ventricular architecture are illus-

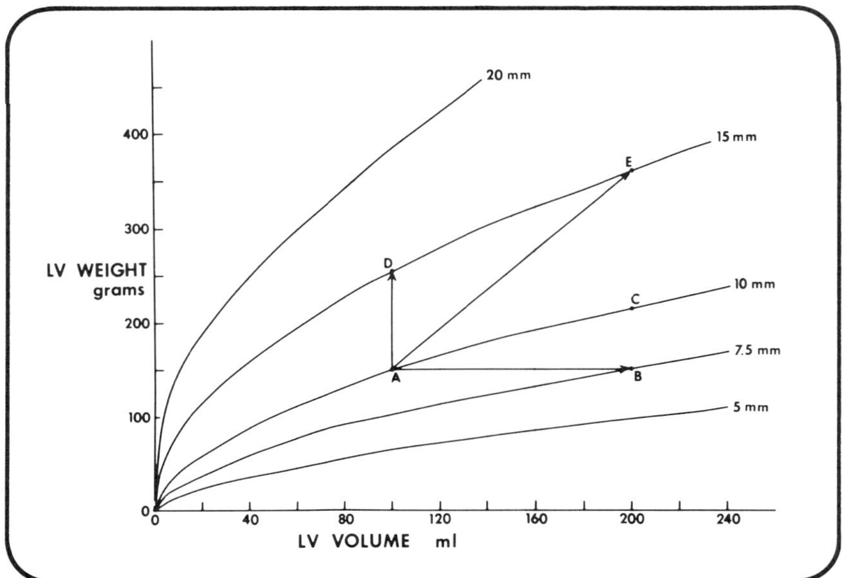

FIGURE 1. The relation of left ventricular weight and volume is illustrated for five different wall thicknesses from 5 to 20 mm. Point A is arbitrarily designated normal. Point B represents the effects of dilatation at constant weight. Point C represents eccentric hypertrophy: dilatation with maintenance of constant wall thickness. Point D represents concentric hypertrophy: increased wall thickness at normal volumes. Point E is decompensated concentric hypertrophy. Small changes in wall thickness are associated with large changes in ventricular weight. Data are derived from a thick-walled spherical model.

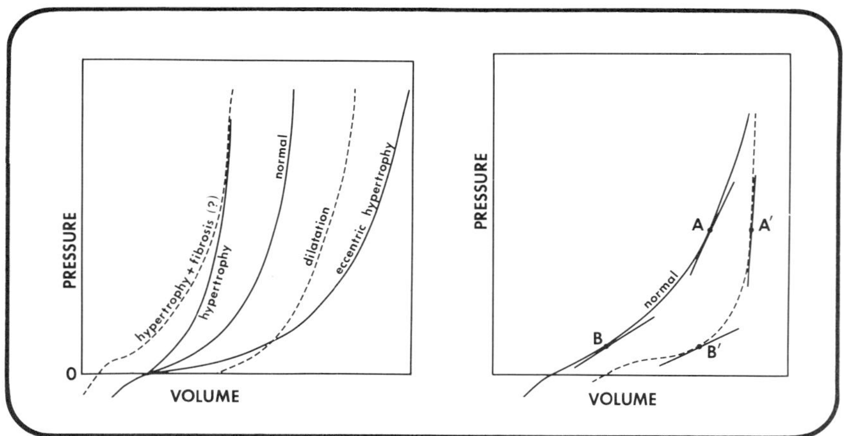

FIGURE 2 (left). Schematic representation of hypothetical effects of pathologic changes on ventricular compliance, dV/dP. An increase in compliance generally shifts the curve to the right, but in the dilated ventricle compliance may be abnormally reduced and yet the curve is still shifted to the right as the result of an abnormally large volume at zero pressure. In concentric hypertrophy the curve is shifted to the left, and compliance appears to be abnormally reduced. However, when the results are normalized for an increase in ventricular mass, intrinsic compliance of the myocardium may be normal in the absence of fibrosis.

FIGURE 3 (right). Hypothetical illustration of abnormal compliance curve in which compliance appears abnormally small (A,A') or abnormally large (B,B') depending on the area of measurement. This indicates the need for full documentation of compliance curves when possible. The figure illustrates as well that the absolute value of ventricular volume may actually be increased while dV/dP decreases.

trated schematically in Figure 1, which is based on a thick-walled spherical model. For the example chosen, normal end-diastolic volume is 100 ml for a normal left ventricle weighing 150 g with a wall thickness of 10 mm (point A). Doubling end-diastolic volume in the absence of hypertrophy produces a 25 percent decrease in wall thickness (point B). To maintain a constant wall thickness during a 100 percent increase in ventricular volume, as occurs in eccentric hypertrophy, a 43 percent increase in ventricular weight is required (point C). In contrast, "concentric" hypertrophy increases wall thickness with little change in end-diastolic volume. For the example shown (point D), a 50 percent increase in wall thickness is associated with a 67 percent increase in ventricular mass. With late decompensation of ventricular performance, concentric hypertrophy is usually followed by dilatation (point E). Figure 1 illustrates the general principle that large changes in ventricular mass are required to produce measurable changes in wall thickness, especially in the presence of ventricular dilatation. Alternatively, rather small changes in ventricular wall thickness are associated with relatively large changes in ventricular mass. Obviously, data on ventricular weight alone will provide an incomplete picture of the pathologic process, but specific knowledge of intraventricular volumes and filling pressures as they existed in life are rarely available along with the myocardial tissue.

Ventricular Compliance

Relative to these changes in structure, alterations in "compliance" of the ventricle are of interest. Physiologically, compliance of the intact ventricle is derived from the passive pressure-volume relation. The "compliance" in itself should express the relation of a change in volume (dV) to a change in pressure (dP). An increase in compliance implies a decreased ventricular diastolic pressure at any given volume. However, since the pressure-volume relation of the ventricle is curvilinear, dV/dP will decrease as the pressure at which it is measured is augmented. Furthermore, doubling wall thickness can double end-diastolic pressure without increasing the linear stresses (in grams per square centimeter of cross-sectional area) in

the myocardium. Compliance of the intact ventricle must therefore be distinguished from the compliance of a square centimeter cross section of the myocardium. If decreased compliance in concentric hypertrophy is normalized for an increase in wall thickness,[9-11] alternative conditions can be distinguished. In the first, dV/dP will be decreased at any given volume due to an increase in muscle mass by itself although the compliance or, conversely, the stiffness of each individual unit of muscle in the wall is normal. Alternatively, fibrosis and scarring in the wall can decrease compliance despite normalization. Precise definition of the term compliance is thus fundamental to analysis of the problem.

In eccentric hypertrophy, the problem of compliance is even more complex (Figure 2). In general, the relation between pressure and volume is shifted to the right so that the volume is augmented for any given filling pressure, and compliance appears to be increased. Large acute increments in filling pressure may induce "stress relaxation" in the ventricular wall, characterized by a decrease in filling pressure although volume is maintained. This apparent increase in compliance is a reversible change. In chronic eccentric hypertrophy, accurate evaluation of compliance may be a complex problem. First, the filling pressure is zero at some finite initial volume, and this point may or may not be shifted to the right (Figure 3). The curve may not be symmetrical or a continuous function; that is, at an increased filling pressure the curve may be very steep (A,A'), whereas at small volumes, the curve may be very flat (B,B'). In this setting, the compliance will be neither decreased nor increased, but merely altered (Figure 3). This dilemma becomes more poignant when viewed in terms of recent studies claiming specific alterations in compliance of the abnormal ventricle. We believe that unless the entire pressure-volume curve can be defined and corrections made for wall thickness, specific definitions of alterations in "compliance" must be considered tentative.

Animal studies have indicated that compliance of the right or left ventricle may appear to be reduced in acute or chronic dilatation of the opposite ventricle. This finding may be a result of displacement of the interventricular septum into the opposite ventricle.[12,13] Similar effects have been postulated to occur in man as well.[14,15]

Systolic and Diastolic Wall Stresses

The physical laws relating ventricular compliance to the linear elastic properties of the myocardial fibers also determine contractile performance of the intact ventricle. Thus, the relation of pressure, volume and wall thickness to forces on the individual fiber in the wall is the same in both systole and diastole. However, the site and mechanism of systolic and diastolic force generation at the level of the myocardial fiber are quite different.[16-18]

In general, an increase in the number of myofilaments bearing a given pressure will decrease the load in any given filament. Conversely, an increase in the number of isotonic filaments will increase ventricular pressure. A second principle of importance in interpreting pathologic changes is the negative effect of dilatation on the mechanical advantage of the myocardial fibers. Thus, increasing volume will decrease ventricular pressure if wall forces remain constant. Similarly, in the dilated ventricle, increased wall forces are required to maintain normal ventricular pressure. As a convenience for simple calculations, the expression $S = PRi/h$, derived from Laplace's law for membranous spheres, has been used.[16] Wall force is expressed as a stress, in grams per square centimeter, and related to ventricular pressure (P), endocardial radius (Ri) and wall thickness (h). Multiplication by a geometric correction factor for thick walls (Ri/Rm) gives $S = PRi^2/(Ro^2 - Ri^2)$ in which Ro = epicardial radius and Rm = midwall radius. This formula has also been widely utilized and embodies the same basic concepts.[18]

It is accordingly clear that concentric hypertrophy can compensate for the pressure-overloaded ventricle by distributing the pressure load over a larger number of contractile elements arranged in parallel. Furthermore, the effect of hypertrophy is to normalize both systolic and diastolic wall stresses, despite an increase in corresponding pressures.[10,11,19] The mechanisms that allow eccentric hypertrophy or dilatation to provide an increase in ventricular reserve are less clear, since dilatation does not by itself improve the mechanical advantage provided by the Laplace law. Nevertheless, since normal stroke volume becomes an ever-diminishing fraction of end-diastolic volume in the dilating ventricle, geometric considerations provide that lesser shortening in the wall is necessary to produce a given stroke volume from a larger end-diastolic volume. Alternatively, the same extent of shortening per segment of ventricular wall will produce a larger stroke volume when end-diastolic volume is augmented. Thus, the increased contractile force requirements in eccentric hypertrophy are partially offset by a decreased requirement for shortening and an increase in the number of contractile elements.

Furthermore, augmentation of end-diastolic volume in valvular regurgitation is generally associated with reduced impedance to ventricular ejection. Ventricular emptying thus tends to be enhanced, and the decrease in ventricular volume reduces ventricular wall forces.[20] Conversely, secondary late failure of contractile function will dissipate this mechanical advantage and may superimpose pressure and volume loads so that concentric hypertrophy may be superimposed on eccentric hypertrophy.

The Laplace relation further indicates that for ventricles of different absolute size, and within different regions of the same ventricle, a given intraventricular pressure will be associated with a constant level of wall stress, so long as the Ri/h value remains constant.[11] Thus, the left ventricular wall is thinnest at the apex, where radius of curvature is smallest. Similarly, dilatation and hypertrophy tend to occur concomitantly.[11] Moreover, the rat and dog have very similar passive pressure-volume curves (left ventricular volume/weight = 0.55 and 0.46 cc/g, respectively, at 12 mm Hg)[1,21] despite a 100-fold difference in ventricular weight (1 vs. 100 g). The fundamental common factor is the maintenance of the same relative proportions of radius and wall thickness. Similarly, systolic wall stresses are the same in both hearts at matched pressures and matched relative volumes. The possible functional significance of a loss of these "normal" proportionality ratios under pathologic conditions remains to be demonstrated.

Sarcomere Lengths

In both skeletal and heart muscle, the sarcomere is the fundamental unit of contraction.[5] Force of contraction for a given degree of activation depends on the relative disposition of two sets of contractile filaments with optimal sarcomere length occurring at 2.2 μ. Previous studies in the dog have shown that normal diastolic sarcomere lengths range from an average of 2.05 to 2.15 μ and that, during systole, the changes in length of the sarcomeres can explain the stroke volume and ejection fraction of the normal heart.[3,7] In addition, alterations in end-diastolic volume induce changes in average sarcomere length, and thus changes in stroke volume, helping to explain the Frank-Starling relation.

It should be recognized that average sarcomere length is a statistical reality. For any given diastolic tension in isolated segments of heart muscle, or for any given distending pressure in the intact heart, there is a dispersion of sarcomere lengths.[1,3,22] Changes in the width and distribution pattern of sarcomere dispersion may occur at average sarcomere lengths greater than 2.3 μ. Heart muscle becomes very stiff beyond this point. Alterations in the pattern of distribution of sarcomere lengths may alter ventricular performance without changing average sarcomere length. Further attention to this point is indicated. It should be remembered that the normal diastolic sarcomere length in the heart encompasses a relatively narrow range. Even at zero filling pressure, sarcomere length averages 1.95 μ.[1] At sarcomere lengths of less than 1.95 μ, a double overlap of thin filaments occurs during contraction and elastic recoil tends to elongate the sarcomere after the end of contraction.

Within any one myocardial cell, sarcomere dispersion tends to be rather narrow, apparently because of an equitable distribution of stresses along myofibrils that span the length of the cell. The optimal sampling for sarcomere dispersion will therefore be obtained by measuring sarcomeres in as many different cells as possible, rather than by measuring multiple sarcomeres within the same cell.

In the thick-walled left ventricle, the distribution of sarcomere lengths across the wall is far more variable than the distribution around the mean at a given depth in the wall. Midwall sarcomere length tends to be the most reproducible, with the narrowest distribution. For a given change in ventricular volume the largest percentage change in radius occurs at the endocardium, and the largest change in sarcomere

length also occurs here.[1,22,23] Conversely, the smallest changes in sarcomere length occur toward the epicardial surface (Figure 4, bottom panel). The thin-walled right ventricle shows relatively little variation from epicardium to endocardium.[4] Complete understanding of the functional limits of the sarcomere requires correlation of force and shortening vectors, sarcomere length, fiber orientation and radius of curvature. This problem has been only partly resolved.[17]

Ventricular Volume Overload

Recent studies have indicated that the upper limits to the ability to increase stroke volume by increasing end-diastolic volume are also set by the sarcomere.[5] What happens then in the acute and chronically dilated ventricle? Whereas the sarcomeres of skeletal muscle can readily be stretched beyond a length of 2.2 μ, leading to dissociation of thick and thin filaments and an enlarging H zone in the center of the sarcomeres,[5] cardiac muscle is relatively stiff.[1] Thus, at that muscle of fiber length in which sarcomeres are 2.2 μ, resting forces to stretch the muscle are rising exponentially. Even in acutely distended heart muscle, it is difficult to elongate sarcomeres further and dissociate the overlap of thick and thin filaments. Rather than much further elongation of individual sarcomeres, major distortions of the myocardium start to occur. This is characterized by loss of register of sarcomeres between fibrils in individual cells and even some necrosis of some of the fibers (Spotnitz WD et al., unpublished observations).

In chronic dilatation, sarcomere dimensions have been studied only under limited controlled conditions. Since human hearts cannot be fixed and studied in such circumstances, one can only speculate as to the crossovers from animal studies. In dogs, aorta to vena caval shunts have been created, leading to left ventricular dilatation.[7] The pressure-volume relations of the left ventricle were shifted to the right with an augmentation of intraventricular volume for any filling pressure, accompanied by little change in ventricular wall thickness. Overall ventricular mass was augmented, attesting to the fact that "eccentric" hypertrophy had occurred. Analysis of sarcomere structure indicated that average midwall sarcomere length was shorter than

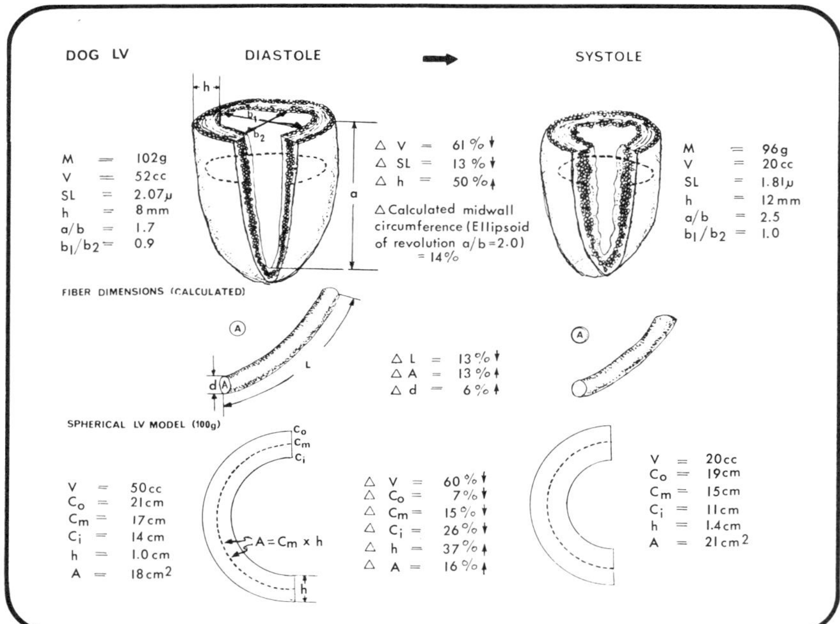

FIGURE 4. Dimensional data derived from experimental study of the dog left ventricle[3,24] are presented for systole and diastole in the **upper panel.** Changes in intraventricular volume (V) measured by Silastic casts, sarcomere length (SL), and wall thickness (h) are indicated. Axial ratios are defined as follows: a/b = ratio of apex/base ventricular axis to the average minor semiaxis at base; b_1/b_2 = the ratio of minor semiaxes at base. The observed increase in the axial ratios from diastole to systole indicates a relative elongation of ventricular shape during systole. b_1/b_2 is close to 1, indicating that approximation of the left ventricle as an ellipsoid of revolution is appropriate. The **center panel** presents derived dimensional changes for midwall fibers based on observed changes in sarcomere length (SL) and circumference. Maintenance of constant fiber volume requires changes in fiber length (L) to be accompanied by equal and opposite changes in cross-sectional area of the fibers (A). The derived change in fiber diameter (d) is based on an assumed cylindrical shape. Data are presented in the **lower panel** for a thick-walled spherical model of the left ventricle of average weight (100 g) with volume changes similar to those observed in the **upper panel.** The theoretical changes in wall thickness (h) and midwall circumference (Cm) closely match observed changes in wall thickness and midwall sarcomere length. Calculated changes in epicardial circumference (Co) are smaller than those calculated for midwall (Cm) and endocardium (Ci). Changes in cross-sectional area of the sectioned hemisphere (A = Cm × h) are similar to the predicted changes in fiber area, indicating little geometric requirement for changes in intercellular space. The changes in ventricular wall thickness (h) are many times larger than the changes in fiber thickness (d), indicating a strong geometric requirement for internal rearrangement in the ventricular wall to permit changes in the wall thickness. **Dashed line** in lower panel represents principal and wall fiber orientation.

would have been expected for the augmentation of volume. Furthermore, sarcomeres were not overstretched but were found to average 2.2 μ in length at normal end-diastolic pressure. Thus, a dissociation of thick and thin filaments did not occur. It appears that dissociation of thick and thin filaments cannot be viewed as a cause of ventricular depression in chronic left ventricular dilatation.[7]

As stated, hypertrophy tends to reduce the force of contraction required of the myocardium, whereas dilation increases it (Laplace relation). Since normal stroke volume represents a smaller fraction of total end-diastolic volume in the dilated heart, a decreased ejection fraction can produce a normal stroke volume. A reduction in the amount of shortening required of the contractile elements thus tends to offset the disadvantages of increased loading.

How can volume be augmented out of proportion to an increase in sarcomere length in chronic distension and eccentric hypertrophy? Many factors may be involved. Ventricular circumference could be increased either by some form of intercellular slippage, with displacement of cells relative to one another and distension of the ventricular collagen "backbone,"[8] or by an increase in the length of the cells.[26] Longitudinal "slippage" of myofibrils relative to one another also appears to occur in some areas of the myocardium. This provides for a somewhat longer cell. New filaments appear to be laid down along the periphery of the fibrils in the cell leading to an increase in fibril cross section with a restoration of fiber diameter. In addition, synthesis of new sarcomeres may be occurring at the intercalated discs that lie at the ends of the cell. In these chronically dilated hearts, the intercalated disc becomes wider and more serpentine and numerous loose filaments are noted in this zone. This may signify growth of new sarcomeres in the area of the intercalated disc.[27] We have found no evidence that new sarcomeres are created from widening Z lines of sarcomeres along the fibrils,[27,28] although some localized thickening of Z lines does occur.

Recently we have found that when isolated segments of heart muscle are stretched acutely in vitro, sarcomeres resist overstretching despite huge increases in resting tension. Some "slippage" is observed in this circumstance. In addition, acute stretching of cardiac muscle produces spotty damage to individual fibers with resultant localized contracture and necrosis. This loss of cells may lead to a vicious cycle when extended to the dilated intact heart and may help to explain the spotty fibrosis commonly observed in chronically dilated hearts (Spotnitz WD et al., unpublished observations).

The right ventricle is normally subjected to reduced resistance to emptying and has a relatively thin wall. When the dog heart is subjected to a long-term combined pressure and volume overload in the form of pulmonic stenosis and tricuspid insufficiency, the structural findings in the right ventricle have been different from those in the left ventricle.[25] Thus, a shift in the pressure-volume relation of the right ventricle ensues, yielding larger diastolic volumes for the same filling pressure. Unlike the sarcomeres in the left ventricle, those in the dilated right ventricle are commonly elongated beyond 2.2 μ, although anticipated H zones are not readily perceived. The animals appear to have rather stable chronic right-sided failure under these circumstances, although the majority of sarcomeres appear to be "overstretched."

Ventricular Pressure Overload

The structural changes that occur in the left ventricle subjected to pressure overloads are limited.[27,29–31] Except early in life, most, if not all, of the increase in ventricular muscle mass results from an increase in the size rather than the number of individual cardiac cells. The increments in deoxyribonucleic acid (DNA) observed in the hypertrophied ventricle can be attributed to hyperplasia of connective tissue rather than of myocardial cells. The manner in which the increase in cell size occurs is still not generally agreed upon. The relative disposition of thick and thin filaments within the sarcomere is not altered.[29] The existence of polysomes and stray filamentous material along the lateral portions of fibrils and at the ends of the cell adjacent to the intercalated disc suggests that synthesis of new sarcomeres may be occurring in these areas.[27,29,31,32] Claims that new sarcomeres evolve from Z line material are yet to be confirmed and have not been uniformly observed, although thickening of Z line substance is commonly observed in hypertrophy and occasionally with normal aging.[28]

In the concentrically hypertrophied heart, intracellular mass is increased without extensive qualitative alterations of the contractile substance, mitochondria, sarcoplasmic reticulum or the T system, even when myocardial failure has supervened.[27,31] Intracellular structures are increased. However, mitochondrial mass is increased somewhat less, in relative proportion, than contractile mass.[31] Although the cross-sectional area of the individual cell is increased, the irregular shape of myofibrils and their tendency to phase into one another makes it difficult to evaluate their size. The membranes of the sarcoplasmic reticulum are spread over the surface of the myofibrils, and the possibility remains that an increase in the diameter of the myofibrils may decrease the relative density of this system which is essential for activation.[33] This event could provide an ultrastructural basis for reduced function that may ensue late in the course of hypertrophy. Studies on this point are required.

Sarcomere length relative to the passive pressure-volume curve has also been analyzed in experimental hypertrophy produced in the left ventricle of the rabbit by aortic banding.[31] The normal relation between sarcomere length and filling pressure was identical to that previously obtained in the left ventricle of the·dog.[1] However, with severe hypertrophy and a thickened left ventricular wall, sarcomere lengths were somewhat shorter for the same filling pressure, although the normal distribution of lengths across the wall was observed.

Coincidental Secondary Changes

A major problem in utilizing structure to characterize pathology is the many possible nonspecific, artifactual or coincidental changes that may not define the underlying etiology. For example, in acute ischemia, swelling of mitochondria is noted quite early with minor dilation of the sarcoplasmic reticulum. These changes may be very marked after 30 minutes of ischemia yet are all readily reversible with restoration of blood flow.[34] Nevertheless, sarcomere structure is often reasonably normal after 2 to 3 hours of ischemia when irreversible damage has already occurred. After a few hours of ischemia, some areas of intracellular contracture may be seen, thereby suggesting that the integrity of surface membranes may be disrupted.

In the experimental hereditary cardiomyopathy seen in the Syrian hamster, most of the alterations in structure that are observed reflect either complete loss of cells with healing or the changes of compensatory hypertrophy. Thus, somewhat enlarged cells, enlarged and scalloped nuclei, a plethora of mitochondria, and widened and more serpentine intercalated discs are commonly seen. The thickness of Z lines of sarcomeres tends to vary from cell to cell. Thus, a qualitative abnormality of structure has yet to be defined to explain the failure of cardiac tissue before the occurrence of extensive ventricular dilatation. Additional difficulty in the analysis of ventricular function at the ultrastructural level is statistical. The normal left ventricle is estimated to contain some 10^{12} or more sarcomeres, and the performance of the intact ventricle reflects a summation of these units. This has already been stressed in previous studies but warrants reiteration.[3]

Ventricular Fiber Orientation

In addition to consideration of ultrastructure, the grosser organization of the wall is of interest. Examination of left ventricular myocardial fiber orientation in serial sections from epicardium to endocardium, beginning tangential to the epicardial surface, has provided useful information regarding the vectors of force distribution in the ventricular wall[17] but has not yet been studied in relation to pathologic lesions.

Indeed, the stability of the fiber matrix when examined from this orientation is remarkable.[22,35] Transitions of fiber angle are gradual throughout the wall, so that abrupt changes in force vectors do not occur. The principal fiber orientation is circumferential at midwall (dashed line, Figure 4) in planes parallel to the ventricular equator. Some 60 percent of the free wall fibers lie within ±22° of this orientation. This midwall band is flanked by fibers that form increasingly oblique spirals toward the epicardium and endocardium. The fibers spiral in opposite directions, so that fibers at the endocardium are inclined at +60° relative to the ventricular equator and 120° oblique to the epicardial fibers, which form an angle at −60° with the midwall fibers. In the transition from diastole to systole, little change of angles within the matrix itself has been observed, although the entire wall shifts some 10° relative to the major ventricular axis. Figure 5 illustrates the vectors that determine force distribution in the free wall of the left ventricle. Fiber orientation strongly favors circumferential forces in the wall, except in the 30 percent closest to the epicardial and endocardial surfaces. The vectors themselves do not represent actual forces. The actual pattern of force distribution also depends on the radius of curvature of the ventricular wall, which has been measured,[17] and the preload and afterload transmitted to sarcomeres at various depths in the ventricular wall. This forms a complex problem, which is as yet only partially resolved.[17] Nevertheless, the ratio of 3.6:1 of force vectors in the circumferential versus the meridional (apex to base) direction is far in excess of the theoretical requirement for ellipsoids of revolution of 2:1 asymmetry. The theoretical ratios are in the range of 1.4 to 2.5.[11,19,35–38] This is believed to indicate a great

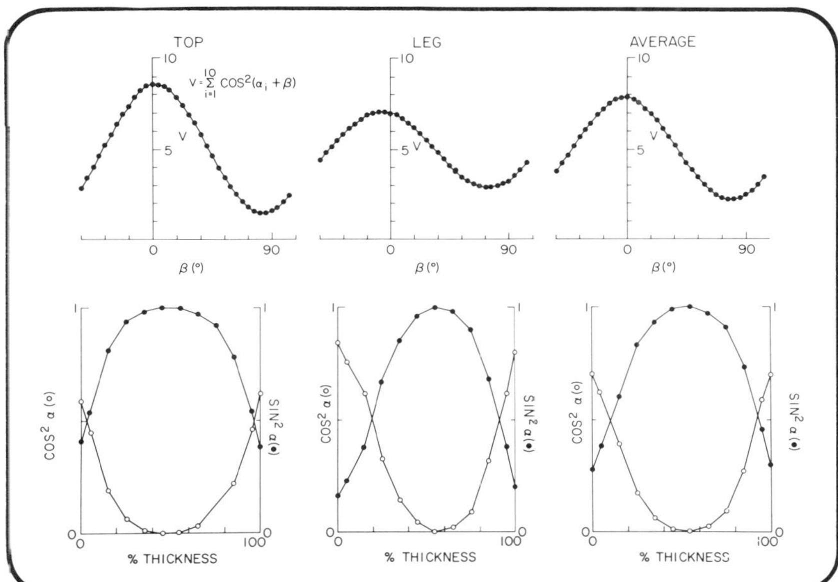

FIGURE 5. Spatial vectors determining force distribution in the ventricular wall. Data are derived for the dog left ventricle. The **lower panels** illustrate squares of the sine and cosine functions for fibers of the free wall as a function of wall thickness. "Top" refers to the basilar half of the free wall, "Leg" to the apical half, "average" to the entire wall. The cosine functions **(dark circles)** when corrected for wall curvature and multiplied by force of fiber contraction will give the magnitude of force in the circumferential direction. The sine function **(open circles)** applies to the apex to base or meridional direction. The great preponderance of fiber orientation for force generation in the circumferential direction is apparent. The vector for apex to base force generation predominates only in the deepest and most superficial regions of the myocardium. The **upper panels** indicate the magnitude of the vector function summated for the entire wall on the ordinate as a function of the angle of inclination from 0° (circumferential direction) to 90° (meridional or apex to base direction) on the abscissa. Averaged for the entire wall, the spatial vector is 3.6 times larger in the circumferential direction than it is in the apex to base direction. Choice of the square of the sine and cosine rather than the first power is controversial.

reserve of myocardium for circumferential contraction, and is thought to be responsible for a recognized elongation of the left ventricle in the transition from diastole to systole, with an increase in the ratio of major to minor semiaxes from 1.7 to 2.5[24] (Figure 4). Major alterations in the fiber matrix have not as yet been reported in abnormal ventricles in which ventricular shape becomes globular[7] despite the excess of circumferential fibers, presumably reflecting a loss of contractility. The pattern of fiber distribution in the right ventricle appears to be similar to that of the left.

Increasing attention to correlation of changes in ventricular dimensions and sarcomere length has also revealed that side-to-side alignment of myocardial fibers across the ventricular wall is an area of paramount importance. Thus, an average change in dog midwall sarcomere length

of 13 percent in the transition from diastole to systole cannot readily explain an associated 30 to 50 percent increase in left ventricular wall thickness[3,21,24] (Figure 4). To reduce the argument to its simplest form, the myocardial fibers are viewed as cylinders of constant volume. A 13 percent decrease in sarcomere length, ventricular circumference and cell length should correspond to a 13 percent increase in cross-sectional area of the myocardial fibers since fiber volume is numerically equal to the product of fiber length and cross section. A 13 percent increase in cross section is geometrically equivalent to a 6 percent increase in the diameter of a cylinder. How then can a 50 percent increase in wall thickness be explained by a 6 percent increase in fiber thickness? Clearly, considerable internal rearrangement must occur in the ventricular wall during systole. Data recently derived

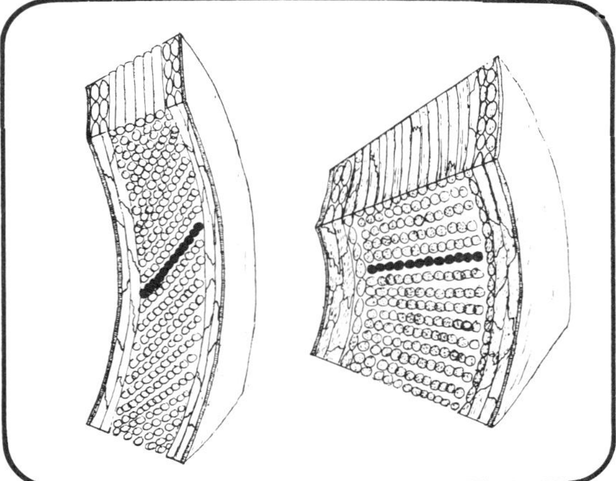

FIGURE 6. Schematic cross sections of left ventricular free wall show the simplest observed form of internal fiber rearrangement, permitting changes in wall thickness many times greater than changes in fiber thickness. Sliding planes within the wall permit fibers in the midwall region (**black dots**) to shift to a more radial alignment in the low volume, thick-walled ventricle (**right**). In the thinner-walled high volume ventricle (**left**), the fibers shift to the apex to base direction permitting the ventricle to increase in height as well as in girth.

from studies of the rat left ventricle suggest that in the range of physiologic volume, increases in wall thickness can be correlated with proportionate increases in the number of fibers aligned side to side from endocardium to epicardium.[21] Changes in intercellular spacing are of lesser significance. Cross-sectional area of the fibers appears to increase linearly with decreases in ventricular radius.[21] This view has similarly been expressed by Hort.[39] A number of possible mechanisms can be invoked for the change in wall thickness, but observations indicate that fiber rearrangements are permitted by sliding planes in the ventricular wall, illustrated in simplest form in Figure 6. The myocardial fibers are actually irregular, rather than circular in cross section, a fact of little importance to the basic argument. These observations are consistent with the apparent stability previously attributed to the matrix of fiber spirals, since the changes take place in perpendicular planes. These geometric constraints apply equally to discussions of transitions from diastole to systole and also to acute ventricular dilatation. In summary, acutely increasing ventricular volume causes the fibers to become smaller in cross section,

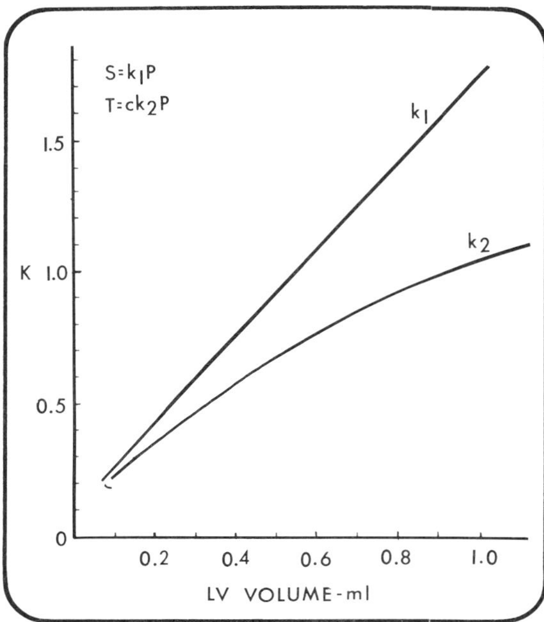

FIGURE 7. The value of K_1 at any ventricular volume multiplied by ventricular pressure (in grams per square centimeter) gives wall stress (in grams per square centimeter) as calculated by the Laplace formula, $S = P(Ri)^2/(Ro^2 - Ri^2)$ (see text). Data show a linear increase of wall stress (line k_1) with volume if pressure remains constant. Calculations are for a 1 g spherical ventricular model in a volume range of 0.1 to 1.0 ml, but are equally valid for a 100 g ventricle in a 10 to 100 ml volume range. Line k_2 is not scaled in absolute units, but indicates the increase in loading *per fiber* (in grams) with increasing ventricular volume, at constant ventricular pressure. An increase in volume from 0.3 to 0.6 ml will increase wall stress (k_1) 82%, while the fiber loading (k_2) increases only 63%. The smaller increase in fiber loading is the result of an increase in the number of fibers per unit cross-sectional area of the wall as ventricular volume increases and fibers get thinner. This is the reverse of systole, when ventricular volume is decreasing and fibers become thicker. Derived data will only apply to that range of ventricular volumes in which changes in fiber and sarcomere length are proportionate to changes in ventricular circumference.

increases the number of fibers per unit of area in the wall itself, and redistributes the fibers to permit degrees of attenuation of the wall considerably greater than corresponding decreases in fiber thickness.

Since internal rearrangement of myocardial fibers appears to be involved in changes in ventricular wall thickness, obliteration of the required cleavage planes in fibrosis and scarring may present an additional impediment to ventricular compliance and cause an increase in myocardial oxygen consumption.

Although ventricular wall forces are generally expressed as stresses, such as those provided by the Laplace relation, the actual force generators of the myocardium are the actin and myosin myofilaments, which essentially can be viewed as a series of linear chords traversing the sarcomere. The force-generating properties of these filaments are not believed to be related to cross-sectional area of the sarcomeres. Furthermore, recent observations suggest that the number of fibers per unit of cross-sectional area of the myocardium increases linearly with ventricular radius.[21] Therefore, although the Laplace formula and its derivatives have certain advantages, they do not accurately express the effects of dilatation on forces at the level of the contractile elements. Appropriate correction of the Laplace formula[21,39] yields the results illustrated in Figure 7. It is apparent that force per fiber increases with ventricular volume, but to a lesser degree than wall stress, so that a 100 percent increase in ventricular volume is associated with an 82 percent increase in wall stress, in grams per square centimeter calculated by the Laplace formula, whereas force, in grams per fiber, increases 63 percent. Thus, a comprehensive understanding of the effects of eccentric or concentric hypertrophy on ventricular performance and myocardial oxygen consumption must include consideration of alterations in the number, size and packing of the myocardial fibers and the elements they contain.[8,38-42] Similar arguments suggest that translation of fiber forces within the ventricular wall are governed by the first power rather than the square of the sine and cosine of the angle of fiber inclination (Figure 5). Under this interpretation, the ratio of circumferential to meridional force vectors discussed is 2.1:1 rather than 3.6:1 for the canine left ventricle.

Summary

Hypertrophy represents a chronic adaptation of the myocardium to diastolic (volume) or systolic (pressure) loads. Resultant "eccentric" and "concentric" hypertrophy is discussed relative to ventricular compliance. The need for defined pressure-volume curves with known ventricular mass and shape in human disease is stressed. Ultrastructural constraints to normal and abnormal function are noted in terms of the sarcomere, and the physiologic features of fiber orientation in the ventricular wall and their implications for normal function are denoted. In the absence of significant qualitative changes in structure in ventricular hypertrophy, the quantitative implications of these changes are noted. As yet, little is known of the fiber orientation and connective tissue skeleton of the heart in either severe hypertrophy or severe myocardial failure with dilatation.

Acknowledgment: This work was supported in part by National Institutes of Health Grants HE11306 and HL05890.

References

1. **Spotnitz HM, Sonnenblick EH, Spiro D:** Relation of ultrastructure to function in the intact heart. Sarcomere structure relative to the pressure-volume curves of the intact ventricles of dog and cat. Circ Res 18:49, 1966

2. **McNutt NS, Fawcett DW:** The ultrastructure of the cat myocardium. J Cell Biol 42:47, 1969

3. **Sonnenblick EH, Ross J Jr, Covell JW, et al:** The ultrastructure of the heart in systole and diastole. Changes in sarcomere length. Circ Res 21:423, 1967

4. **Leyton RA, Spotnitz HM, Sonnenblick EH:** Cardiac ultrastructure and function: sarcomeres in the right ventricle. Amer J Physiol 221:902, 1971

5. **Sonnenblick EH:** Correlation of myocardial ultrastructure and function. Circulation 38:29, 1968

6. **Leyton RA, Sonnenblick EH:** Ultrastructure of the failing heart. Amer J Med Sci 258:304, 1969

7. **Ross J Jr, Sonnenblick EH, Taylor RR, et al:** Diastolic geometry and sarcomere lengths in the chronically dilated canine left ventricle. Circ Res 28:49, 1971

8. **Linzbach AJ:** Heart failure from the point of view of quantitative anatomy. Amer J Cardiol 5:370, 1960

9. **Braunwald E, Ross J Jr:** Ventricular diastolic pressure: an appraisal of its value in the recognition of ventricular failure in man. Amer J Med 34:147, 1963

10. **Rackley CE, Hood WP Jr, Rolett EL, et al:** Left ventricular end-diastolic pressure in chronic heart disease. Amer J Med 48:310, 1970

11. **Sandler H, Dodge HT:** Left ventricular tension and stress in man. Circ Res 13:91, 1963

12. **Kelly DT, Spotnitz HM, Beiser GD, et al:** Effects of chronic right ventricular volume and pressure loading on left ventricular performance. Circulation 44:403, 1971

13. **Taylor RR, Covell JW, Sonnenblick EH, et al:** Dependence of ventricular distensibility on the filling of the opposite ventricle. Amer J Physiol 213:711, 1967

14. **Bernheim PI:** De l'asytolie veineuse dans l'hypertrophie du coeur gauche par stenose concomitante du ventricule droit. Rev Med 30:785, 1910

15. **Dexter L:** Atrial septal defect. Brit Heart J 18:209, 1956

16. **Badeer HS:** Contractile tension in the myocardium. Amer Heart J 66: 432, 1963

17. **Streeter DD, Vaishnav RN, Patel DJ, et al:** Stress distribution in the canine left ventricle during diastole and systole. Biophys J 10:345, 1970

18. **Taylor RR, Ross J Jr, Covell JW, et al:** A quantitative analysis of left ventricular myocardial function in the intact, sedated dog. Circ Res 21:99, 1967

19. **Hood WP, Thomson WJ, Rackley CE, et al:** Comparison of calculations of left ventricular wall stress in man from thin-walled and thick-walled ellipsoidal models. Circ Res 24:575, 1969

20. **Urschel CW, Covell JW, Sonnenblick EH, et al:** Myocardial mechanics in aortic and mitral valvular regurgitation: the concept of instantaneous impedance as a determinant of performance of the intact heart. J Clin Invest 47:867, 1967

21. **Spotnitz HM, Spotnitz WD, Cottrell TS, et al:** Volume related changes in fiber size and position in the normal rat left ventricle (abstr). Circulation 44 suppl II:103, 1971

22. **Hort W:** Makroskopische und mikrometrische Untersuchungen am Myokard verschieden Stark sefullter linker Kammern. Virchow Arch Path Anat 333:523, 1960

23. **Ross J Jr, Yoran C:** Distribution of sarcomere lengths during acute and chronic variations in left ventricular volume (abstr). Circulation 44 suppl II:44, 1972

24. **Ross J Jr, Sonnenblick EH, Covell JW, et al:** The architecture of the heart in systole and diastole. Technique of rapid fixation and analysis of left ventriculary geometry. Circ Res 21:409, 1967

25. **Spotnitz HM, Leyton RA, Kelly DT, et al:** "Overstretched" sarcomeres in subacute volume-pressure loading of dog right ventricles. Circulation 46 suppl II:44, 1972

26. **Laks MM, Morady F, Swan HJC:** Canine right and left ventricular cell and sarcomere lengths after banding the pulmonary artery. Circ Res 24:705, 1969

27. **Bishop SP, Cole CR:** Ultrastructural changes in the canine myocardium with right ventricular hypertrophy and congestive failure. Lab Invest 20:219, 1969

28. **Legato MJ:** Sarcomerogenesis in human myocardium. J Molec Cell Cardiol 1:425, 1970

29. **Richter GW, Kellner A:** Hypertrophy of the human heart at the level of fine structure. J Cell Biol 18:195, 1963

30. **Meesen H:** Ultrastructure of the myocardium. Its significance in myocardial disease. Amer J Cardiol 22:319, 1968

31. **Anversa P, Vitali-mazza L, Visiote D, et al:** Experimental cardiac hypertrophy: a quantitative ultrastructural study in the compensatory stage. J Molec Cardiol 3:213, 1971

32. **Hatt PY, Ledoux Ch, Bonvalet JP:** Lyse et synthese des proteines myocardiques au cours de l'insuffisance cardiaque experimentale. Arch Mal Coeur 58:1703, 1965

33. **Gertz E, Stam AC Jr, Sonnenblick EH:** A quantitative and qualitative defect in the sarcoplasmic reticulum in the hereditary cardiomyopathy of the Syrian hamster. Biochem Biophys Acta Res Comm 40:746, 1970

34. **Buja LM, Levitsky S, Souther SG, et al:** Acute and chronic effects of normothermic anoxia on canine hearts; light and electron microscopic evaluation (abstr). Circulation 42 suppl III: 57, 1970

35. **Streeter DD Jr, Spotnitz HM, Patel DJ, et al:** Fiber orientation in the canine left ventricle during diastole and systole. Circ Res 24:339, 1969

36. **Mirsky I:** Left ventricular stresses in the intact human heart. Biophys J 9:189, 1969

37. **Wong AYK, Rautaharju PM:** Stress distribution within the left ventricular wall approximated as a thick ellipsoidal shell. Amer Heart J 75:649, 1968

38. **Falsetti HL, Mates RE, Grout C, et al:** Left ventricular wall stress calculated from one-plane cineangiography. An approach to force-velocity analysis in man. Circ Res 26:71, 1970

39. **Hort W:** Untersuchengen zur funktionellen Morphologie des Myokards. Klin Wschr 38:785, 1960

40. **Harrison TR, Ashman R, Larson RM:** Congestive heart failure. The relation between the thickness of the cardiac muscle fiber and the optimum rate of the heart. Arch Intern Med (Chicago) 49:151, 1932

41. **Karsner HE, Saphir O, Todd TW:** The state of the cardiac muscle in hypertrophy and atrophy. Amer J Path 1:351, 1925

42. **Shipley RA, Shipley LJ, Wearn JT:** The capillary supply in normal and hypertrophied hearts of rabbits. J Exp Med 65:29, 1937

Chapter 3

Abnormal Biochemistry in Myocardial Failure

Arnold Schwartz, PhD, FACC
Louis A. Sordahl, PhD
Mark L. Entman, MD, FACC
Julius C. Allen, PhD
Y. S. Reddy, PhD
M. Ann Goldstein, PhD
Robert J. Luchi, MD, FACC
Leigh E. Wyborny, PhD

Cardiovascular disease accounts for well over 50 percent of all deaths in the United States. Approximately one of every five persons has some form of cardiovascular ailment, including heart disease, stroke and hypertension. Indeed, cardiovascular disease is truly the "twentieth century epidemic." It is not surprising, therefore, that the U. S. government (under the aegis of the National Heart and Lung Institute) and nongovernmental groups (such as the American Heart Association and the American College of Cardiology) vigorously support attempts to reduce this scourge through basic experimental and clinical research and education and services for physicians and laymen. During the past 20 years, practically every discipline in basic and clinical science has made some contribution to the understanding of the factors that cause cardiovascular disease. Teams of investigators, specializing in pathology, biochemistry, biophysics, virology, pharmacology, physiology and clinical medicine, have combined talents in the battle against this disease.

One of the most serious consequences of all types of cardiovascular ailments involves the function of the heart as a pump. It is well known, for example, that "pump failure" is the probable chief cause of death in cardiovascular disease associated with ischemia and infarction. It is vital then to have a complete understanding of both the molecular architecture of cardiac muscle and all of its functional characteristics. It is the purpose of our chapter to review some of the modern biologic concepts of the normal and abnormal myocardium.

Normal Ultrastructure of the Heart

The ultrastructure of cells from various portions of the heart has been carefully documented by many investigators[1-12] and will be reviewed briefly here. The electron micrograph in Figure 1 and the diagram of the cell in Figure 2 illustrate important microanatomic features. The normal working myocardial cell is surrounded by a membrane called the *sarcolem-*

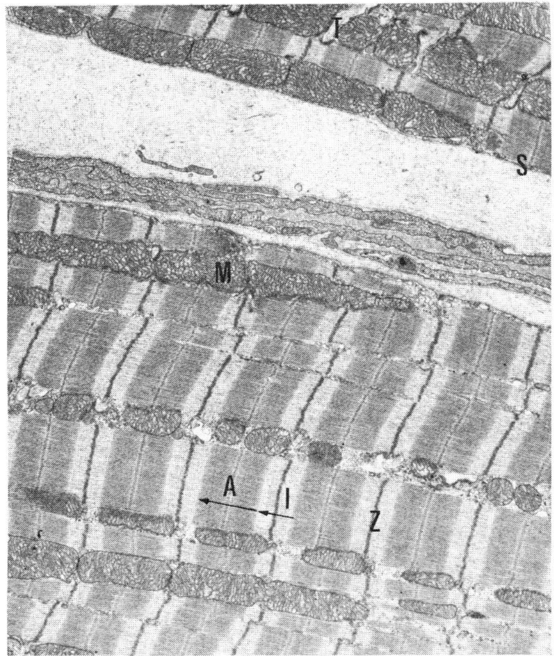

FIGURE 1. Electron micrograph of normal canine myocardium showing functional components in two cells: sarcolemma (S), T system (T), mitochondria (M), A band, I band and Z disc. (Original magnification × 9,000.)

ma. At various junctions, the sarcolemma invaginates deep into the interior of the cell and forms the *T system.* Another thin-walled membranous network, presumably surrounding the myofilament but not extending to the extracellular space, is called the *sarcoplasmic reticulum.* This reticulum is characteristic of mammalian heart and skeletal muscle; there is evidence that reticulum is present in some smooth muscle but absent in amphibian heart muscle, or at least is present to only a small extent. Each myocardial cell is generally separated by junctions that are divided into four types of regions, the *nexuses,* the *desmosomes,* the *fasciae adherentes* and the *undifferentiated regions.*[5] The nexus is now regarded as a gap junction. In the cell junctions, which are called intercalated discs of working myocardium, the transverse segments are occupied for the most part by large fasciae adherentes, and the longitudinal segments have large nexuses; the undifferentiated regions are much less extensive. It has been suggested that the intercalated discs

may become separated (dehiscence) in various pathologic conditions. The so-called bordering lines of each sarcomere are known as the *Z bands.* These bands have not yet been well characterized, although alterations of these areas have been observed in some abnormal states.

Functions of Cardiac Cell Structures: The average mammalian cardiac muscle cell contains an abundance of mitochondria. These organelles are responsible for the conversion of energy-laden foodstuffs into a usable form of energy—adenosine triphosphate (ATP)—that is used for muscle contraction and relaxation, active transport and protein synthesis. Mitochondria also carry out a series of energy-dependent reactions of their own, such as ion transport and synthesis of reduced coenzymes. The sarcolemma and T system are not just structural in nature; the membrane carries out important enzymatic activities, including the maintenance and transport of important monovalent and divalent cations. The sarcoplasmic reticulum has a special function in muscle, namely, sequestra-

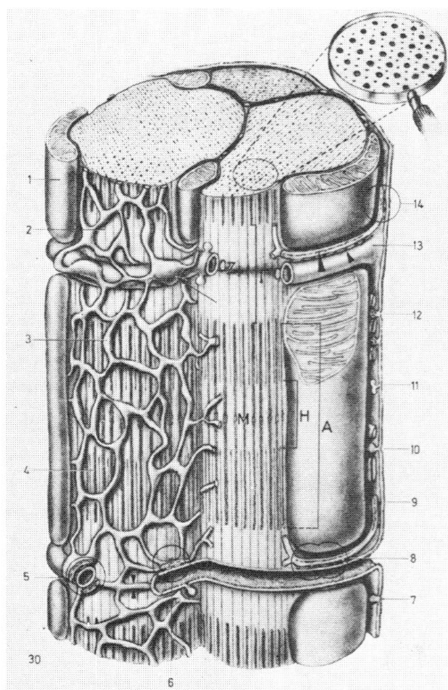

FIGURE 2. Three-dimensional diagram of the ultrastructure of the cardiac cell. (Reprinted by permission from Sommer and Johnson.[13])

tion of intracellular calcium, at a rate and capacity consistent with the process of relaxation. The calcium is generally believed to be released from a specific portion of the sarcoplasmic reticulum called the *cisternae*. In skeletal muscle, which does not require an external source of calcium, it is also believed that portions of the sarcoplasmic reticulum may release enough calcium to effect complete contraction. Heart muscle, however, requires an external source of calcium, as Sydney Ringer pointed out many years ago; hence, some believe that a specific pool of calcium associated with the cell membrane may control the process of contraction, whereas relaxation is carried on chiefly by the sarcoplasmic reticulum binding phenomenon.

The Cardiac Action Potential: Extensive stud-ies employing sophisticated microelectrode techniques have established that the working myocardium shows a specific characteristic action potential that is easily differentiated from electrical activity in skeletal and smooth muscle. It is generally believed that the rising phase (*Phase zero*) of the action potential (pictured in idealized fashion in Figure 3), which coincides with the QRS complex of the electrocardiogram, is probably due to a rapid alteration in sodium permeability. *Phase 2,* the plateau region of the action potential, is believed by some to be associated with a slow inward calcium current. This calcium current may be responsible for the control of cardiac contraction although there is dispute concerning this. *Phase 3* represents repolarization, during which the

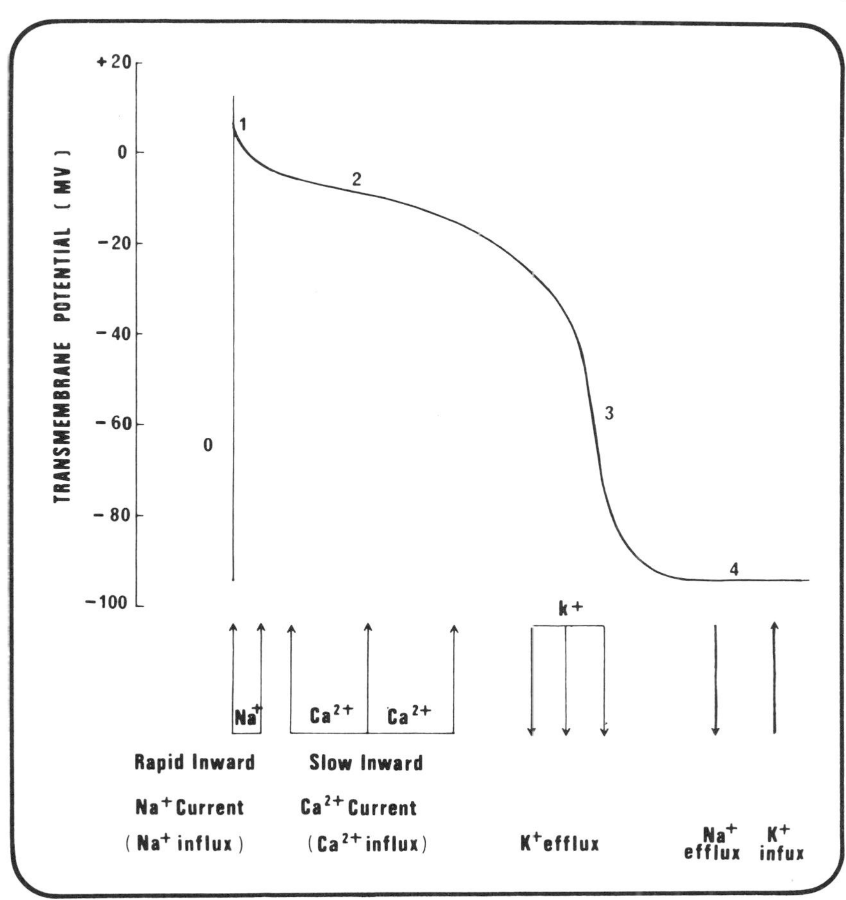

FIGURE 3. Diagram of an idealized ventricular action potential correlating phasic voltage changes with cation flux.

(Reprinted by permission from Naylor and Merrilees.[14])

permeability to potassium is presumably increased so that small but significant amounts of potassium may "leak" out of the cell. *Phase 4* constitutes in part a recovery process during which sodium and potassium are "pumped" back to their original positions by the expenditure of energy derived from cellular metabolism. This classic concept, like all concepts, is constantly being altered. For example, it is quite difficult to determine concentrations and movements of ions in a highly heterogeneous, membrane-filled cardiac cell. Furthermore, the state of intracellular water is not known. Many persons consider that the internal portion of cardiac and skeletal muscle cells consists of highly ordered or structured water molecules. If this is true, then the usual calculations of concentrations become relatively meaningless.

Molecular Nature of Cardiac Contraction: Modern biochemistry has made several important contributions to the understanding of the molecular nature of muscle contraction. The sarcomere (the basic unit of contraction) consists of a number of well defined bands of proteins. The "A" band represents myosin of which there are at least two types: light meromyosin and heavy meromyosin (Figure 4). Heavy meromyosin represents the cross bridge that extends from light meromyosin toward the "I" band. The I band consists of actin, a protein that seems to be attached to the Z line, and two modulator proteins, tropomyosin and troponin. Troponin is now regarded, at least in part, as the calcium receptor at the molecular level. It consists of at least three different proteins or subunits, one of which actively binds calcium with an affinity quite consistent with the contractile process. There are at least two or three additional proteins in the sarcomere with various functions proposed for them. Many more subunits and possibly proteins may have vital functions. It is now believed that the process of muscle contraction really represents a "depression" process.

Figure 5 illustrates a typical model of contraction. Presumably, the cross bridge, with two specific globular subunits at the end, remains unattached to specific sites on actin during diastole, or the relaxed state. This is due to the fact that tropomyosin "covers" the active sites and troponin remains free of calcium binding. During excitation, either enough calcium is released from intracellular sites or enough enters the cell, or both, to bind to troponin and cause a

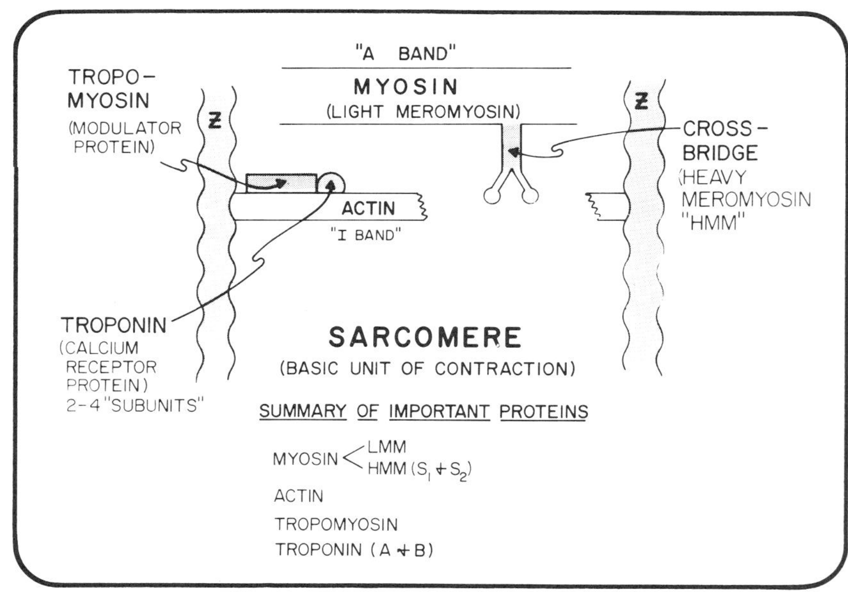

FIGURE 4. Diagram of the contractile element demonstrating the proposed arrangement of the contractile and modulator protein and subunits. LMM = light meromyosin. (Reprinted by permission.[15])

specific change in the molecular conformation. The change results in the exposure of sites on actin to which the globular subunits of the cross bridge can attach. Once attached, the process of isometric tension develops and is followed by the well known sliding process originally described by H. E. Huxley. The energy required for this process is acquired from ATP. It is believed that the splitting of ATP does not occur until after the development of isometric tension.

Excitation-Contraction-Relaxation Coupling Processes: Let us review one possible mechanism for these coupling processes (Figure 6). During each depolarization event, a specific amount of calcium may enter the cell. This calcium, as suggested, might be associated with Phase 2 of the action potential. The calcium interacts with troponin. It is entirely possible that some calcium is also released from specific areas of the sarcoplasmic reticulum. In any event, the calcium-troponin complex changes molecularly, removing tropomyosin from the active site. Thus, calcium acts as a "derepressing agent" that exposes the active sites so that the globular ends of the cross bridge can attach to the sites; this process leads to contraction, as described earlier. Relaxation somehow involves the activation of a complicated enzymatic system that is associated with the sarcoplasmic reticulum and possibly mitochondria,

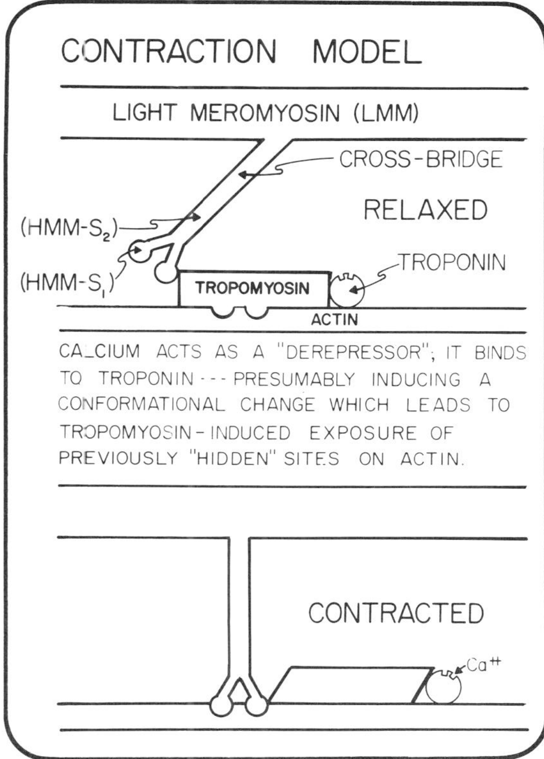

FIGURE 5. Proposed mechanism of interaction of contractile and modulator proteins resulting in calcium-induced contraction.

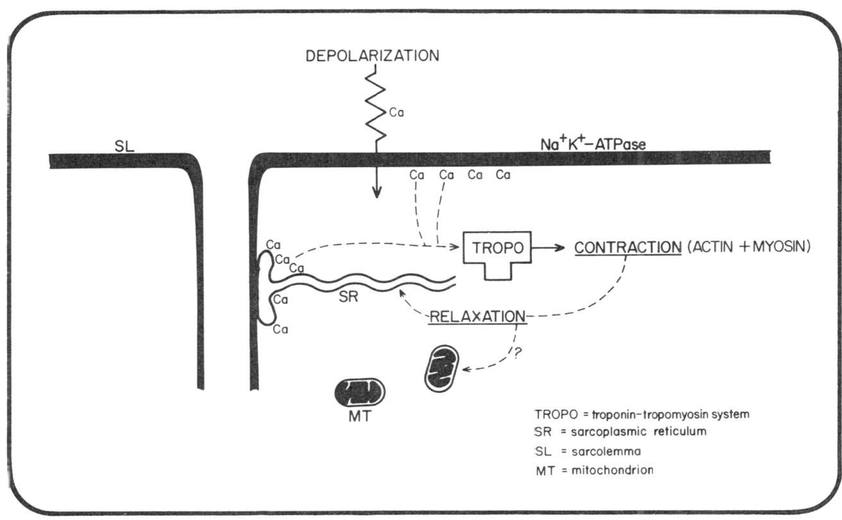

FIGURE 6. Diagram of proposed pathways of calcium flux during contraction and relaxation in the cardiac cell. (Reprinted by permission.[15])

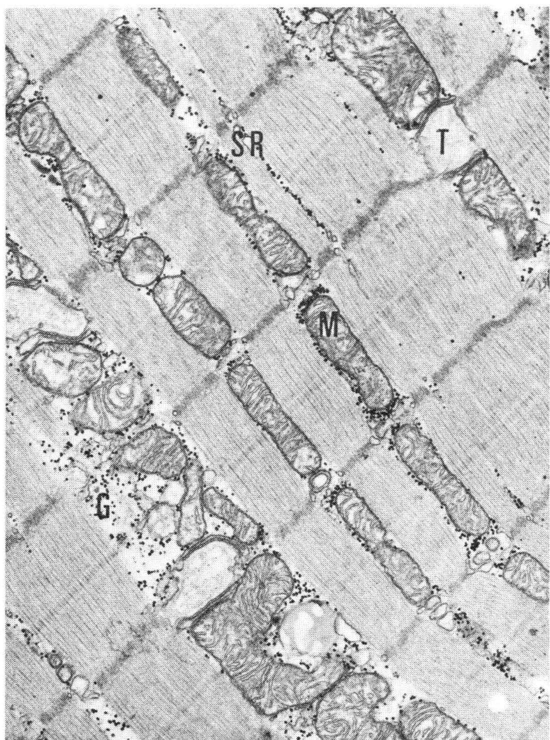

FIGURE 7. Electron micrograph of normal human myocardium showing usual size and distribution of mitochondria (M), glycogen (G), sarcoplasmic reticulum (SR), T system (T) and contractile filaments. (Original magnification × 18,000.) (Reprinted by permission from Sordahl et al.[15])

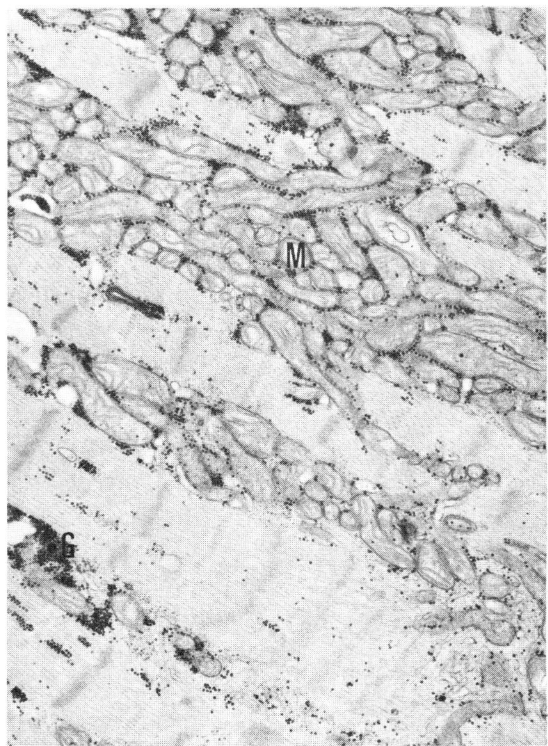

FIGURE 8. Electron micrograph of cardiomyopathic human myocardium showing the numerous small mitochondria grouped together interspersed with deposits of glycogen. (Original magnification × 18,000.)

so that calcium is actively removed from troponin. It has been clearly shown that sarcoplasmic reticulum from mammalian heart muscle can remove enough calcium at a sufficiently rapid rate to cause relaxation in the required time period.[16–18] Thus, the modulator of cardiac tone is probably calcium. The regulation of specific activator intracellular calcium is complex and not entirely understood. However, it is believed that a number of "membranous sinks" compete for the available calcium. These sinks include the cell membrane, sarcoplasmic reticulum, troponin and mitochondria. When calcium is attached to troponin, contraction ensues, and when calcium is unattached to or detached from troponin and attached to some other site, relaxation occurs. It is intriguing to regard a possible aberration in any one of the systems controlling calcium with respect to

pathologic conditions. Each of these systems has been examined, some in greater detail than others, and is discussed in this chapter.

Myocardial Ultrastructure in Hypertrophy and Failure

The ultrastructure of mammalian ventricular myocardium has been observed in normal and experimental animals in various stages of hypertrophy,[19–22] cardiomyopathy[23] and heart failure.[24,25] Extensive structural alterations suggesting a primary lesion have not been seen (Figure 7), even when heart failure was frank. In hypertrophied hearts the morphologic features of individual cells varied but generally reflected an increased functional demand and increased synthetic activity.[25] Glycogen deposits were more numerous (Figure 8). Mitochondria were

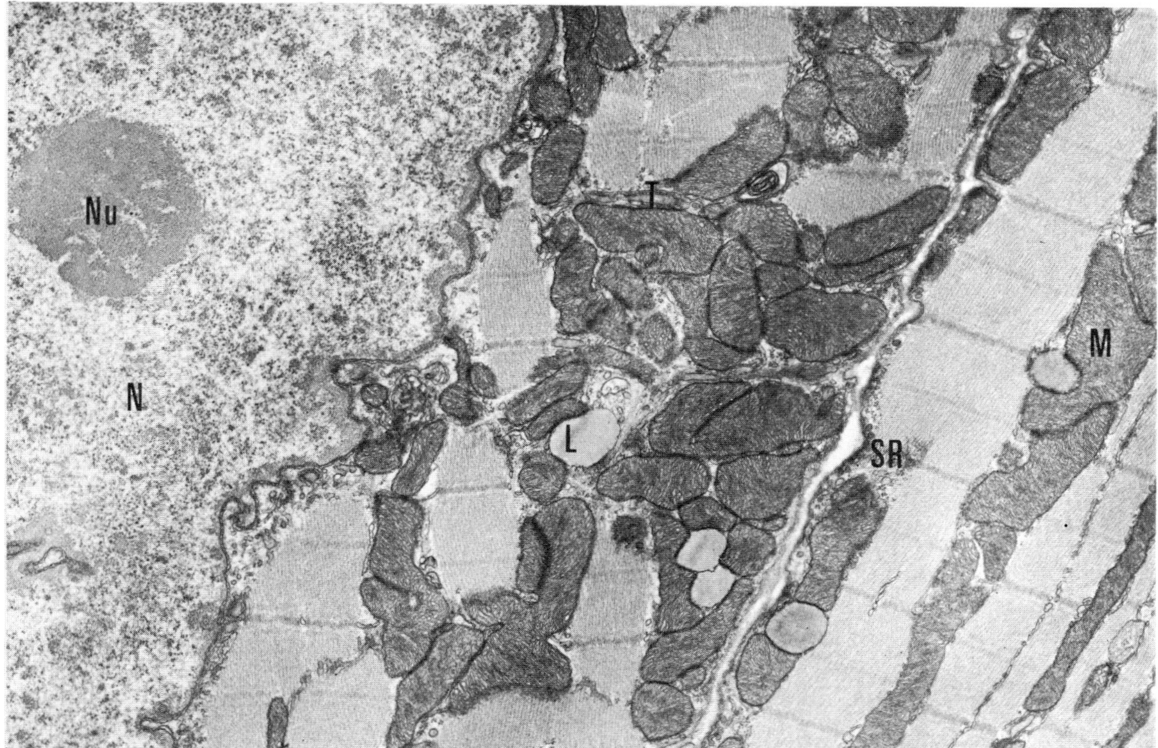

FIGURE 9. Electron micrograph of myocardium of cardio-myopathic Syrian hamster (strain 40.54) showing nucleus (N), nucleolus (Nu), mitochondria (M), lipid (L), T system (T) and sarcoplasmic reticulum (SR). (Original magnification × 14,000.)

normal in appearance but varied considerably in size and number from cell to cell (Figure 9). Mitochondrial profiles were more numerous per unit area of tissue but were smaller in size (Figure 8), and in many instances there was actually a decreased volume of mitochondria per cell.[19,24,25] The nucleus contained numerous ribosomes and a prominent nucleolus (Figure 9). Individual myofibers increased in size by the addition of new sarcomeres. Accumulations of Z substance, believed to be necessary for the formation of new contractile units,[24,26] were observable as widened Z discs in existing sarcomeres and at the sarcolemma with associated thin filaments (Figure 10). The compact wavy appearance of the intercalated disc was lost, and the observed distortion of the longitudinal folds of the disc (Figure 11) was explained by the addition of a new sarcomere nearby.[24,26]

Qualitative changes in ultrastructure have been reported[24,27] but do not appear to be unique to myocardial pathology. Quantitative studies of hypertrophied and failing hearts have revealed additional changes in fine structure that are not readily apparent. Morphometric analysis of the size and distribution of various cellular components has shown significant differences between normal and failing hearts. In the case of mitochondria, for example, changes have been observed in such physiologically important variables as the ratios of surface to volume and of mitochondria to myofibrils.

Mitochondria in Heart Failure

The normal adult heart is an aerobic organ that derives almost all of its useful energy from oxidative reactions catalyzed by mitochondria.

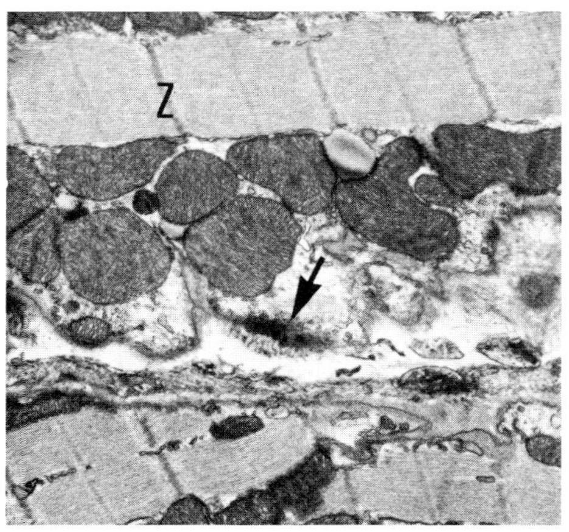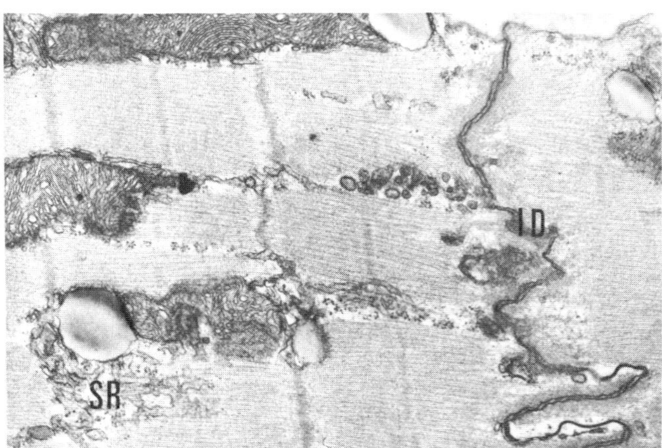

FIGURE 10 (left). Electron micrograph of myocardium of cardiomyopathic Syrian hamster (strain 40.54) showing accumulation of Z substance at the sarcolemma **(arrow)** and Z bands (Z). (Original magnification × 12,000.) **FIGURE 11 (right).** Electron micrograph of myocardium of cardiomyopathic Syrian hamster (strain 40.54) showing folds of intercalated disc (D) and sarcoplasmic reticulum (SR). (Original magnification × 23,000.)

The oxidation of various substrates by the mitochondria generates "energy" in the form of adenosine triphosphate (ATP) from the process of oxidative phosphorylation. Two decades ago techniques[28] for the isolation and assay of mitochondria were developed that allowed discrete in vitro measurements of the primary energy-producing mechanism in both normal and diseased hearts. We have subsequently learned that mitochondria are capable of several energy-utilizing functions,[26] including calcium transport, which is of particular interest to the muscle biochemist.

During the past 12 years, there have been several conflicting reports[30-36] on mitochondrial oxidative phosphorylation (or "energy production") in various animal models of heart failure. For example, findings have differed on whether mitochondrial production of energy is impaired in congestive heart failure. It is probable that the major reasons for these discrepancies involve (1) the severity and type of failure at the time the mitochondria are isolated from the heart, and (2) the quality and method of assay of the mitochondrial preparations.

Heart Failure in Animal Hearts: Our laboratory reinvestigated[37] this problem with the view of obtaining optimal isolation and assay conditions before measuring mitochondrial function in failing hearts. A study[37] utilizing normal heart mitochondria and a variety of techniques re-

vealed that an isolation medium originally formulated by Von Korff[38]—0.18 M potassium chloride, 10 mM ethylenediaminetetraacetic acid (EDTA) and 0.5 percent bovine serum albumin at pH 7.2 and subsequent homogenization with a Polytron shearing device (Brinkmann Instruments)—yielded mitochondria with optimal oxidative phosphorylation capacity measured both manometrically and polarographically. Heart failure in guinea pigs was produced by various degrees of stenosis of the ascending aorta.[32] As shown in Table I, the respiratory control index (RCI = ratio of active phosphorylating respiration to resting respiration) and the rate of oxygen consumption during active phosphorylation (QO_2) were markedly decreased in mitochondria from hearts with severe failure. Our study demonstrated that quantitative differences between normal and experimental respiratory values were greatest when optimal conditions were used. We concluded that *severe* heart failure is characterized by defects in mitochondrial energy production;[37] whether these defects are primary or secondary events in the genesis of congestive failure could not be determined.

Subsequent studies[39] of mitochondria from a genetically linked animal model of heart disease, the cardiomyopathic Syrian hamster, also revealed depression of respiratory activity compared with that of normal control animals (Table II). In addition, mitochondria isolated from the hamsters with severe congestive heart failure had decreased calcium transport capabilities (Table II). These data indicated an impairment both in mitochondrial *energy-producing* mechanism in congestive failure and also in an *energy-utilizing process.* In another study,[40] mitochondria from hamsters with mild-congestive heart failure had only slightly impaired respiratory activity. These mitochondria also accumulated less calcium. The results suggested that changes in mitochondrial oxidative phosphorylation and calcium transport were related to the *severeity* of failure.

Mitochondria from Failing Human Heart: At the time these studies were in progress, fresh tissue from a failing human heart became available through the cardiac transplantation program at this center. In an earlier study of mitochondria from failing human papillary muscles, Chidsey et al.[41] found no impairment of oxidative phosphorylation. However, mitochondria isolated from failing human ventricles[42] exhibited large differences in respiratory activity (Table III). A significant finding was that the rate of oxygen consumption (QO_2) of mitochondria from failing human hearts (Table III) was generally lower than that observed in mitochondria from human hearts with no evidence of cardiovascular disease.[43] Furthermore, studies[42] comparing mitochondria from failing human heart tissue with those isolated from nonfailing hypertrophic human heart tissue (Figure 12) showed a dramatic difference in respiratory activity. Mitochondria from failing human hearts had much lower rates of nicotine

TABLE I

Oxidative Phosphorylation of Normal and "Failed" Cardiac Mitochondria in the Presence of Different Substrates

	Control			Experimental		
	RCI	ADP:O	QO_2	RCI	ADP:O	QO_2
Glutamate	5.0 ± 0.6	2.9 ± 0.1	141 ± 19	2.0 ± 0.3	2.2 ± 0.1	50 ± 5
Succinate	2.2 ± 0.1	1.9 ± 0.1	148 ± 20	1.4 ± 0.1	1.5 ± 0.2	96 ± 19
Glutamate-malate	4.8	3.3	220	3.3	3.2	174
Beta-hydroxy-butyrate	2.5	2.8	115	1.0		104

Control and experimental refer, respectively, to mitochondria from normal and failing guinea pig hearts. Mitochondria were isolated in 0.25 M sucrose, 10 mM Tris, 1 mM EDTA and assayed in the sucrose-Tris medium at 30° C. Values are means of five experiments (glutamate and succinate) or averages of two experiments (glutamate-malate and beta-hydroxybutyrate). The guinea pigs had chronic congestive heart failure. QO_2 = oxygen consumption in nanoatoms O_2/min/mg mitochondrial protein; RCI = respiratory control index. ADP:O = relation of adenosine diphosphate to oxygen efficiency (phosphorylation). (Reprinted from Lindenmayer et al.[37] by permission of the American Heart Association, Inc.)

TABLE II

Oxidative Phosphorylation and Ca++ Uptake of Hamster Heart Mitochondria

Substrate	RCI		ADP:O		QO_2		Ca++ Uptake	
	C	E	C	E	C	E	C	E
Glutamate	8.5 ± 0.8	4.3 ± 0.4	2.92 ± 0.07	3.04 ± 0.25	0.125 ± 0.012	0.092 ± 0.018	...	...
Succinate	2.5 ± 0.5	2.4 ± 0.2	2.06 ± 0.16	1.91 ± 0.19	0.118 ± 0.017	0.093 ± 0.010	419 ± 17	348 ± 17

Each value is the mean of six experiments (glutamate), five experiments (succinate), and four experiments (Ca++ uptake) with the standard error of the mean. C = control hamster heart mitochondria; E = mitochondria from Syrian hamster hearts with congestive failure. Ca++ uptake (nanomoles/mg protein per 30 min, temperature 37° C). QO_2 = oxygen consumption (μatoms/mg protein per min). (Reprinted by permission from Schwartz et al.[39])

TABLE III
Oxidative Phosphorylation Values for Mitochondria Isolated from Recipient Human Cardiac Tissues

	Isolation Medium	Tissue	NADH-Linked Substrates			Succinate		
			ADP:O	RCI	QO$_2$	ADP:O	RCI	QO$_2$
1	KEA	RV + LV	3.0*	10.0	143	2.0	3.3	122*
2	KE	IVS	3.1*	15.3	110	2.0	3.3	75*
		LV	3.1*	15.5	119	2.1	3.3	68*
		RV	3.1*	17.8	140	2.0	3.1	82*
3	KE	RV	3.2	10.0	105	1.9	2.8	86
		FV	0.0	0.0	0	0.0	0.0	0
4	KEA	LV	3.3*	10.0	...	2.5	2.5	...
5	KE	LV	3.3	15.0	125	1.9	5.4	108
6	KE	LV	2.8	8.0	148	2.3	2.0	61
		RV	3.1	9.5	113	2.6	3.6	84
		AW	3.0	8.0	75	2.5	3.7	66
7	KE	LV	3.1	11.0	186	2.0	5.5	270
8	KE	RV + LV	3.1	10.7	148	2.0	5.4	156
9	KE	LV	3.4	13.0	108	...	...	...
		RV	3.5	11.0	73	2.3	3.8	92
10	SE	RV + LV	3.1	6.6	114	2.4	3.5	77
11	KE	Pap	3.4	13.7	79	1.1	5.0	83
		IV	3.5	20.0	130	1.6	5.4	102
		IVS	3.2	13.7	91	1.6	4.1	88
		RV	3.4	20.0	86	1.6	3.4	67
12	KE	LV	2.9*	11.5	117	1.9	3.1	69
		RV	2.8*	5.7	85	2.4	3.2	54

*NADH-linked oxidation carried out in the presence of glutamate-malate; all other values in this category obtained with glutamate as the substrate. Abbreviations for isolation media: KE = 0.18 M KCl, 10 mM EDTA; KEA = 0.18 M KCl, 10 mM EDTA and 0.5 percent bovine serum albumin; SE = 0.25 M sucrose, 10 mM EDTA. Abbreviations for tissues: AW = atrial wall; FV = fibrotic area of left ventricle; IVS = interventricular septum; Pap = papillary muscle; LV = left ventricle; RV = right ventricle; RV + LV = mixture of right and left ventricular sections. QO$_2$ = rate of oxygen consumption in the presence of ADP and expressed as μ atoms/min per mg protein. (Reprinted from Lindenmayer et al.[42])

adenine dinucleotide (NADH)-linked respiratory activity (QO$_2$, Figure 12A) when compared with mitochondria isolated from nonfailing hypertrophic tissues (Figure 12B). These data suggest that values for mitochondrial respiratory activity in normal human cardiac tissue fall somewhere between those obtained for failing and hypertrophied tissues. The markedly increased respiratory activity of mitochondria from hypertrophic tissue (QO$_2$ Figure 12B) may also reflect a quantitative increase in capacity for synthesizing ATP. Increased mitochondrial

performance during compensatory hypertrophy of heart[20,40] and skeletal muscle[44] has been observed. These observations are consistent with the hypothesis of Meerson et al.[45] that increased mitochondrial activity during a stage of "stable hyperfunction" is associated with cardiac compensatory hypertrophy. Although clear-cut similarities are not immediately apparent between mitochondrial activity from failing human hearts and those obtained from various animal models of heart failure, it should be emphasized that the patients were receiving continuous supportive therapy during the course of their disease and most had coronary artery disease. In animal models, failure secondary to left ventricular overload seems most frequently to result in mitochondrial aberrations.[37]

Mitochondrial Function in Compensatory Hypertrophy and Heart Failure: Our laboratory recently developed a new method[46] of producing left ventricular overload by stenosis of the ascending aorta. This procedure involves placing a clip made of Ameroid (a hygroscopic material synthesized from formalin-treated casein) on the aorta of rabbits. Unlike the static constriction that has been produced with clips or ligatures, the hygroscopic Ameroid material slowly swells and produces increasing aortic constriction that results in marked cardiac hypertrophy and eventually congestive failure. The more gradual onset of this overload has permitted temporal studies of mitochondrial function during compensatory hypertrophy and the eventual onset of congestive heart failure.

Mitochondria isolated from hypertrophied nonfailing rabbit hearts had significantly increased respiratory activity (QO$_2$) compared with that of normal control preparations. No changes in phosphorylation—ratio of adenosine disphosphate to oxygen efficiency (ADP:O)—or the "tightness" of respiratory control were observed. However, mitochondria isolated from hearts with congestive failure exhibited respiratory rates near or below normal values, decreased respiratory control and some lowering of phosphorylative efficiency (ADP:O).[18,47] Measurements of calcium uptake in mitochondria isolated from hypertrophied hearts revealed values similar to those of normal control preparations.[18] However, in failing heart preparations, the rate and total uptake of calcium were

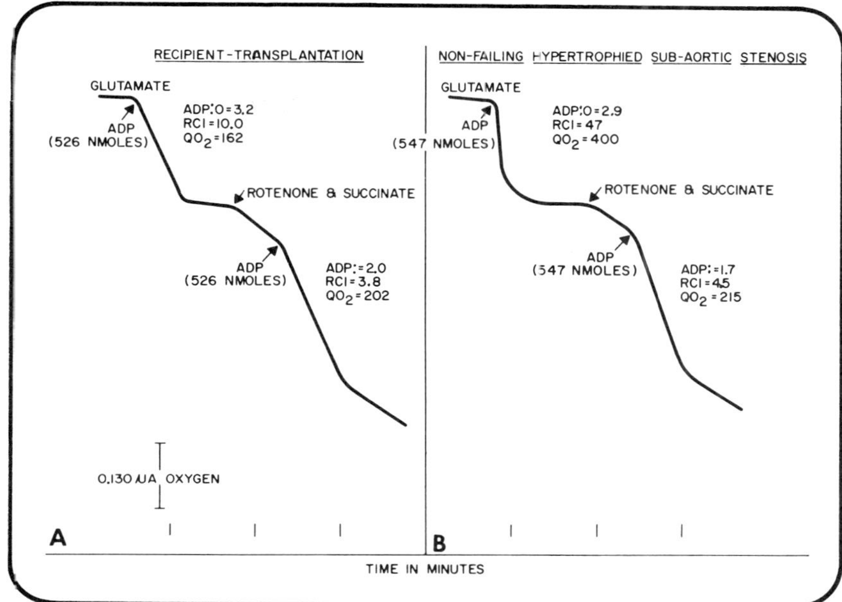

FIGURE 12. Oxygen electrode tracings of human heart mitochondria isolated in 0.18 M KCl, 10 mM EDTA and 0.5 percent bovine serum albumin at pH 7.2. **A,** tracing of mitochondria isolated from a mixture of right and left ventricular sections obtained from a recipient patient in congestive heart failure. **B,** tracing of mitochondria isolated from nonfailing, hypertrophied tissue obtained during surgical correction of subaortic stenosis. The latter is a typical result of four experiments.

markedly decreased. In fact, mitochondria from failing rabbit hearts "released" the calcium taken up, whereas simultaneous measurements of mitochondrial respiration revealed no change in the rate of oxygen consumption during this respiration-supported uptake of calcium.

The increases in mitochondrial respiratory activity during nonfailing compensatory hypertrophy can be interpreted as a compensatory response of the energy-producing mechanism to quantitatively increased production of ATP. Mitochondria from animals with frank congestive failure had respiratory rates at or below normal values. These data are consistent with the hypothesis of Meerson et al.[45] that a stage of "stable hyperfunction" is followed by a final stage of progressive deterioration and failure. The marked depression of mitochondrial respiratory activity in failing heart preparations compared with findings in hypertrophied heart preparations suggests that the mitochondrial activity decreased to a point that was insufficient to meet the energy demands of the hyperfunc-

tioning heart and therefore, contributed to the onset of failure.

Recently, several reports[40,48,49] have proposed a role for mitochondria in the intracellular calcium fluxes involved with excitation-contraction cycles of the heart. The results obtained with mitochondria from the Ameroid rabbit model of failure indicate changes in either the calcium-binding sites or the energy-linked calcium transporting system, especially from hearts with congestive failure. These data suggest that oxidative phosphorylation—the primary function of mitochondria—is sustained until very late in failure, whereas other energy-linked functions—calcium transport—are changing. At present, it cannot be determined whether mitochondria play a primary or secondary role in contributing to congestive heart failure. However, further studies of the energy-linked functions of mitochondria—ion transport, fatty acid oxidations, protein synthesis and so on—may reveal heretofore unsuspected control mechanisms involving cardiac contractility.

Sarcoplasmic Reticulum Relaxing System

Because of the role of calcium in mediating contractile protein interaction, considerable investigation has been devoted to evaluating preparations of myocardial membranes that accumulate calcium. These membrane preparations are presumably fragments of sarcoplasmic reticulum and, as such, have been thought to represent an in vitro index of activator calcium for excitation-contraction coupling. In interpreting the results of these studies, the following should be considered: (1) These membrane preparations isolated by homogenization and differential centrifugation are crude and undoubtedly contain fragments from several subcellular organelles. (2) In all likelihood, there are three major intracellular membrane structures that sequester calcium in vivo—the sarcolemma,[50] mitochondria,[51] and the sarcotubular system (longitudinal sarcoplasmic reticulum).[52] (3) Unlike skeletal muscle, cardiac muscle may derive very little activator calcium from the intracellular sarcoplasmic reticulum and much more from superficial binding sites in the sarcolemma and T system.[50]

Calcium Uptake and Binding in Heart Failure: The accumulation of calcium in myocardial membrane fractions has been studied in a variety of models of congestive heart failure. Initially, accumulation was studied by use of an anionic precipitating agent such as oxalate or phosphate that trapped accumulated calcium yielding an estimate of "calcium uptake." With this technique, defective calcium uptake was demonstrated in failure associated with ischemia,[53] spontaneous, failing heart-lung preparations,[54] pulmonary arterial stenosis,[55] hereditary cardiomyopathy,[56] negative inotropic agents such as barbiturates,[57] quinidine,[58] propranolol,[59] general and local anesthetic agents[60] and bacterial endotoxin.[61]

The use of techniques that require nonphysiologic concentrations of precipitating anions—oxalate, phosphate—has fostered controversy over the applicability of the results to in vivo function. Use of similar techniques in the absence of these anions ("calcium binding") has generally been considered "more physiologic" but likewise has had difficulties. As with studies of calcium uptake, initial studies of calcium binding were performed with the use of $^{45}Ca^{++}$ and by stopping the reaction at various intervals with millipore filtration. Since calcium binding is very rapid, initial binding rates were not obtained and most published data reported the steady state of calcium binding at a later rate (15 seconds, 30 seconds and so on). From these indexes, it was calculated that the "capacity" of the calcium-binding system was adequate to obtain relaxation in vivo and assumed that calcium binding was the actual physiologic process occurring in vivo.

With use of millipore-filtration methods, steady-state "calcium binding" has likewise been shown to be impaired in failure associated with hereditary cardiomyopathy[62] and spontaneous failure in substrate-depleted isolated hearts.[63] The authors of these latter studies stressed the greater sensitivity of "binding" methods in detecting defects in contractility. In fact, Sulakhe and Dhalla[62] did not find a defect in calcium *uptake* in dystrophic hamsters. However, Gertz et al.[56] observed a defect in calcium uptake in a similar species. These discrepancies in the findings of "binding" and "uptake" methods are compounded by the work of Suko et al.[55] in which right ventricular failure in calves (surgically constricted pulmonary artery) was associated with impaired calcium uptake but *not* binding. Further elucidation of these processes is required in order to clarify the discrepancies. However, there is qualitative agreement in the field of calcium transport that strongly suggests the presence of a defect in sarcoplasmic reticulum and that this lesion may contribute to myocardial failure.

A relatively new spectrophotometric method[64] for measuring calcium binding has aided in the characterization of the normal and pathologic physiology of these calcium-binding membranes (Figure 13). Use of the technique has shown that ATP-dependent calcium binding: (1) is sufficiently rapid to effect cardiac relaxation;[66] (2) consists of independent phasic changes with distinct thermodynamic properties and biochemical requirements[67]—that is, the first phase is initiated by ATP and induces calcium binding; the second phase requires calcium binding and allows or "induces" calcium release; and (3) is a saturable system of sites

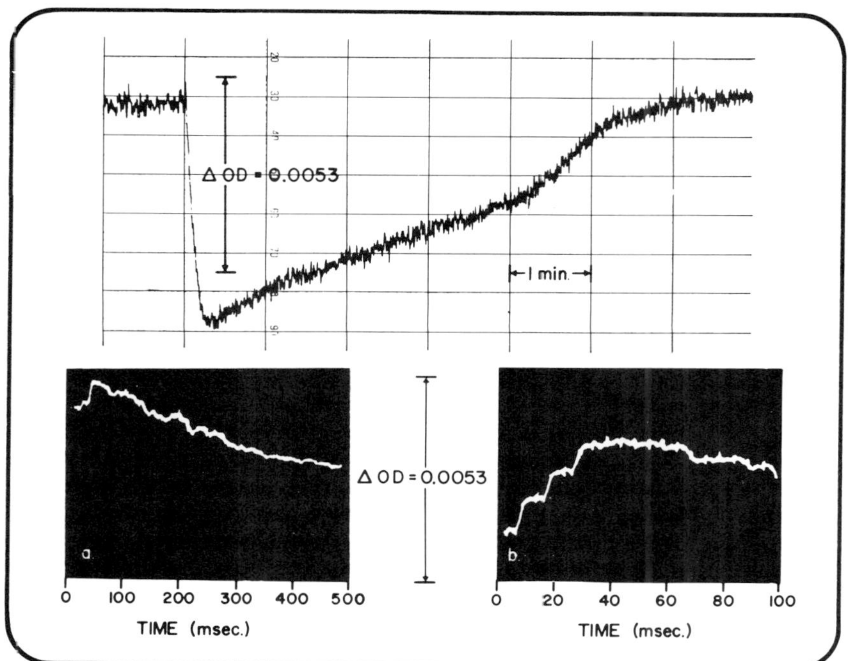

FIGURE 13. Dual-beam spectrophotometric trace of calcium binding and release in cardiac relaxing system. **Upper tracing** shows entire cycle; two **lower tracings,** performed by stopped-flow, show the rapid initial rate of calcium binding. Reaction medium: 0.1 M KCl, 10 mM MgCl$_2$, 20 mM Tris maleate (pH 6.8), 0.2 mM Murexide, 30 mM CaCl$_2$, 0.2 mM ATP at 30° C. (Reprinted by permission from Schwartz.[65])

with each able to function independent of the others in the binding and release process.[66,67]

Once the properties of the normal calcium-binding membranes were defined, it was possible to delineate and characterize further the abnormalities found in such membranes in models of heart failure. The earliest change is a decrease in the rate of calcium release, as studied in cardiac relaxing system isolated from failing human,[16] rabbit,[46] cardiomyopathic hamster[68] (Figures 14-16) and ischemic dog (unpublished observations) hearts. The rate of binding is next attenuated and, later still, the total calcium binding is reduced. Recent evidence from our laboratory suggests, therefore, that calcium release, which is controlled by that phase in the binding-release cycle with the greatest energy of activation, is the most sensitive index of in vivo contractile failure. Alterations in intracellular pH may contribute to the genesis of the defects (Figure 17).

Functional Defect in Sarcotubular System: It would seem logical from the unanimity of these studies that there is a functional impairment in the sarcotubular system (and, perhaps, in the sarcolemmal binding sites). The resulting functional defect is characterized physiologically but the explanation for it in terms of these studies is speculative. At least two possible explanations exist: (1) The sarcotubular calcium pool may actually help control the amount of activator calcium and, therefore, its size, and impairment of release directly decreases calcium supplied to the contractile proteins. (2) The effect is indirect, that is, relaxation and calcium egress—known functions of the sarcoplasmic reticulum in heart tissue—are impaired, primarily causing a secondary change in contractility. A combination of these factors may also be present. However, until further characterization of subcellular fractions is forthcoming such questions remain unanswered.

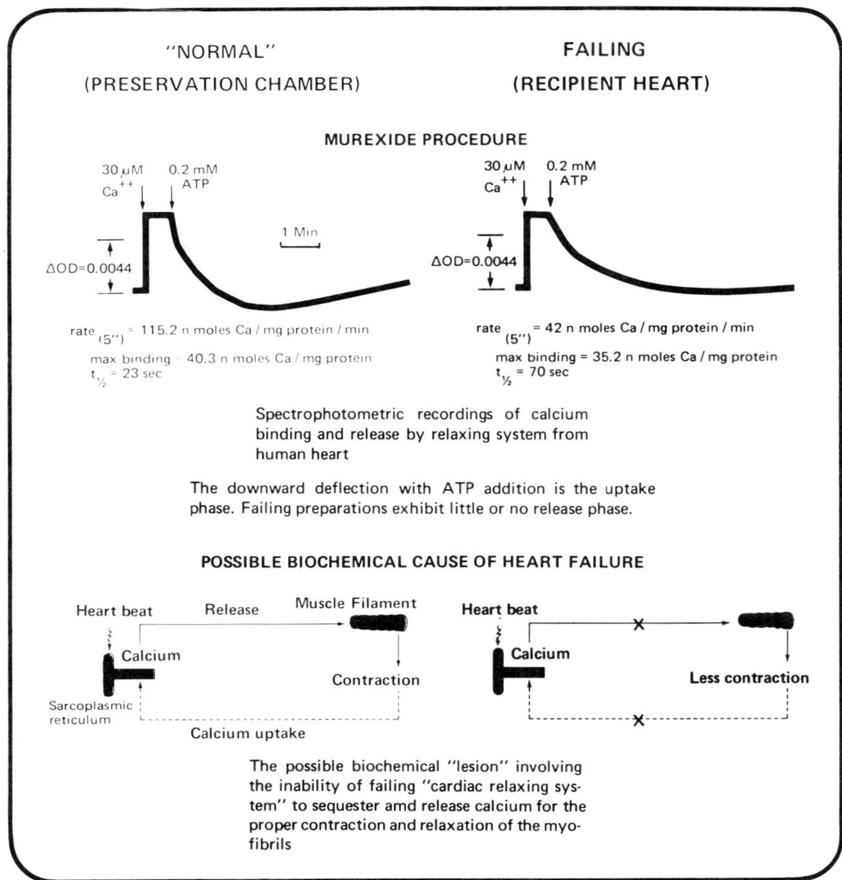

FIGURE 14. Proposed mechanism for heart failure resulting from observed defects in cardiac relaxing system. (Reprinted by permission from Schwartz.[65])

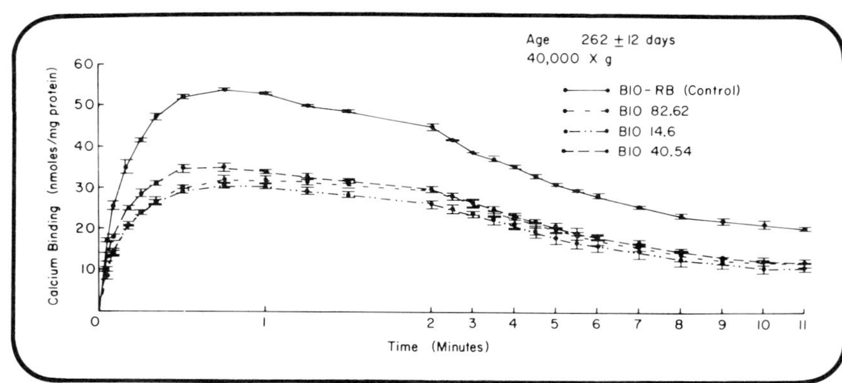

FIGURE 15. Calcium binding by 40,000 g (cardiac relaxing system) of myopathic Syrian hamsters of various strains (Bio-RB = control; Bio 82.62, 14.6 and 40.54 = diseased). All were about 262 days old. Note defective calcium binding by cardiac relaxing system of myopathic strains. Reaction medium as in Figure 13. (Reprinted by permission from Schwartz.[65])

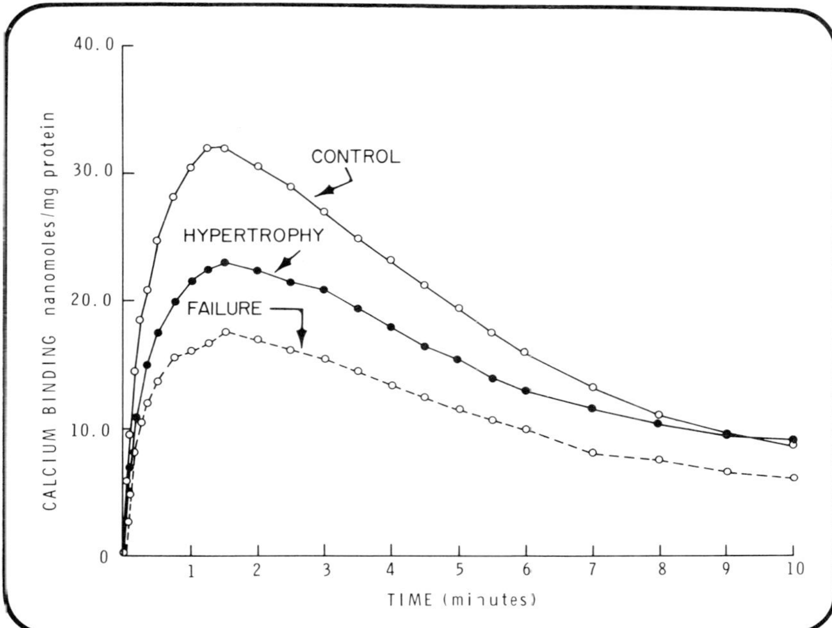

FIGURE 16. Isolated sarcoplasmic reticulum fragments from control, hypertrophied and failing rabbit hearts. Reaction medium as in Figure 13. (Reprinted by permission from McCollum.[69])

Na⁺, K⁺-ATPase

The membrane transport enzyme sodium, potassium adenosine triphosphatase (Na⁺,K⁺–ATPase) is presumed to be directly involved in the active transport of both Na⁺ and K⁺ across the cell membrane.[70] Furthermore, studies from this laboratory[71,72] and others[73,74] have suggested that the enzyme system may be the pharmacologic receptor for cardiac glycosides. Although there is much indirect evidence for this interaction, the mechanism is still controversial.[75]

Despite the acknowledged role of the membrane transport enzyme in active cation transport and its presumed role in the action of cardiac glycosides, very little work has been done on its role, if any, in congestive heart failure. In the single report on this subject, Mead et al.[76] observed that "sarcolemmal" ATPase isolated from either the right or left ventricle of dogs with congestive heart failure induced by progressive pulmonary arterial stenosis[77] was less inhibited by a high concentration of ouabain (10⁻⁴M) than a comparable preparation isolated from control dogs (61 vs. 91 percent). This finding suggests that less of the sarcolem-

mal ATPase activity per gram of tissue is Na⁺, K⁺–ATPase, since the authors defined the preparation as that ATPase activity which, in the presence of Na⁺ and K⁺, is inhibited by ouabain. However, such conclusions are vague. The preparation used[78] is not justifiably a "sarcolemmal" preparation. A complex reorganization of cellular membrane densities in the diseased condition could account for such results, and recovery studies should be performed. Furthermore, the control Na⁺,K⁺–ATPase activity levels were very low for the normal dog heart. Hence we conclude that involvement of Na⁺,K⁺–ATPase in congestive heart failure has not yet been demonstrated.

In a recent report from this laboratory[42] on published biochemical information from recipient hearts obtained during transplantation, Na⁺,K⁺–ATPase was found to be severely depressed. The explanation offered was that, since all these patients had some type of heart failure and were heavily digitalized, the enzyme was depressed because of in vivo binding of the drug, for which experimental precedent has been established.[71,72,74] However, since proper control studies have not been made, it is possi-

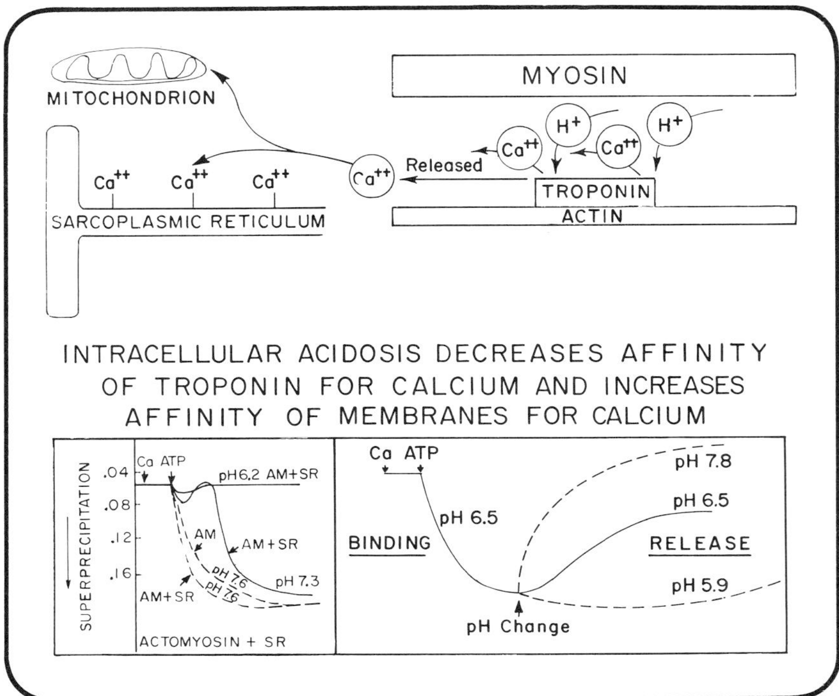

FIGURE 17. Diagram of proposed mechanism of contractile failure resulting from intracellular acidosis. **Upper panel,** diagram of hypothesis. **Lower panel (left),** superprecipitation of myosin B under conditions shown. Note delay in superprecipitation in the presence of sarcoplasmic reticulum when pH is 6.2 (calcium affinity of sarcoplasmic reticulum > calcium affinity of troponin component of myosin B); addition of base to increase pH to 7.3 causes immediate superprecipitation (calcium release by sarcoplasmic reticulum). **Lower panel (right),** calcium binding by sarcoplasmic reticulum showing effect of rapid pH change. Reaction as in Figure 12 with pH as shown; pH is changed at **arrow.** (Reprinted by permission from Schwartz.[65])

ble that depressed Na^+,K^+−ATPase is characteristic of the failing process itself. It must be concluded at present that no definitive work has been performed on Na^+,K^+−ATPase in the failing process and the role of this enzyme system in such disease states remains to be elucidated.

Contractile Proteins in Heart Failure

Contractile ATPase: Correlations have been sought between the reduced contractile performance that occurs during heart failure and the function of the contractile proteins[79–90] (Table IV). Although some of the early studies yielded conflicting results, reports published after 1965 indicate that a functional lesion exists in the contractile proteins.

Several investigators[79–81] have observed a reduction of cardiac myofibrillar ATPase activity in patients with spontaneously occurring heart failure. A similar depression of cardiac myosin ATPase activity was reported by Luchi et al.[90] in dogs with spontaneously occurring heart failure. Since Nebel and Bing[88] found that human beings with heart failure had a myosin with increased ATPase activity, it appears that this problem deserves further investigation.

The presence of a lesion in the contractile proteins during heart failure is also supported in a recent study by Draper et al.[83] who induced congestive heart failure in guinea pigs by constricting the ascending aorta. Hearts from these animals showed a decrease in myofibrillar ATPase activity and in ATPase activity of the actomyosin. It is not clear whether these decreases are a result of a change in myosin or some other contractile proteins.

Troponin-Tropomyosin System: Katz and

TABLE IV
Contractile ATPase from Failing Hearts

Contractile Preparation	Species	Activity Change
Myofibrils	Human	Decrease[79–81]
	Cat	Decrease[82]
	Guinea pig	Decrease[83]
	Dog	No change[84]
Actomyosin	Dog	Decrease[85,86]
	Dog	Increase[87]
	Dog	No change[86]
	Guinea pig	Decrease[83]
Myosin	Human	Increase[88]
	Dog	No change[89]
	Dog	Decrease[90]

Hecht[91] recently pointed out that the increased acidity generally believed to accompany an acute heart attack or an ischemic event could conceivably alter the affinity of troponin for calcium. It is well known that the interaction between calcium and the calcium-binding site on troponin is pH-dependent. This affinity decreases as pH is reduced. During a number of pathologic events it is possible that the metabolism of the heart is shifted to a predominantly glycolytic character. If this were so, the increase in lactic acid would be responsible for the decreased pH.* The troponin-tropomyosin complex may be quite labile and therefore may be one of the first "molecular lesions" accompanying a pathologic process associated with heart disease.

In preliminary studies we examined the tropomyosin-troponin system isolated from acute and chronic "ischemic" dog hearts. Native actomyosin was isolated and both ATPase activity and superprecipitation were studied. Native actomyosin contains the proteins actin, myosin, troponin and tropomyosin. The latter two proteins confer calcium sensitivity to actomyosin. If stored for several weeks, the troponin-tropomyosin system deteriorates and leaves what is known as desensitized actomyosin. The latter substance lacks calcium sensitivity and superprecipitation, therefore, is not sensitive to EGTA. Desensitized actomyosin from our pathologic models behaved in a manner that was statistically similar to that from normal control animals. Conversely, native actomyosin derived from the pathologic models showed defective superprecipitation characterized by a diminution in calcium sensitivity. To determine whether a defect might reside in the troponin-tropomyosin system, we carried out a series of "cross-experiments," combining the normal troponin-tropomyosin complex with "diseased" desensitized actomyosin and "diseased" troponin-tropomyosin complex with normal desensitized actomyosin. These experiments clearly showed that the aberration cited was observed only when the troponin-tropomyosin complex isolated from abnormal hearts was combined with normal or diseased desensitized actomyosin. Consequently, an important defect in contractility failure may involve calcium-binding sites on the troponin-tropomyosin complex.

Summary

The important subcellular systems involved in the regulation of intracellular calcium were studied in normal and in diseased heart muscle. These include mitochondria, fragments of sarcoplasmic reticulum, sodium, potassium adenosine triphosphatase and the tropomyosin-troponin system. Normal and pathologic tissues were obtained from human and animal models. In all specimens taken from areas in which a significant diminution of contractility was measured, one of the earliest defects was found in isolated fragments of sarcoplasmic reticulum. The rate of calcium released from the sarcoplasmic reticulum was decreased, compared with that in control preparations. When the severity of failing process increased, the rate of calcium binding by isolated fragments of sarcoplasmic reticulum was also attenuated. Alterations of intracellular pH may play a role in these early aberrations.

Mitochondria isolated from severely failing hearts were defective with respect to respiration control and calcium accumulation. During "nonfailing" compensatory cardiac hypertrophy, mitochondria exhibited increased rates of respiration and no defect in oxidative phosphorylation. Another significant, albeit preliminary observation of an early defect in "pump failure"

---

*The competitive characteristic of H^+ and Ca^{++} on troponin has now been questioned (Symposium on Calcium-Binding Protiens. Warsaw Poland, 1973).

involved the tropomyosin-troponin system. Isolated, purified actomyosin from cardiac muscle exhibited a significant diminution in calcium sensitivity due to a defect in the tropomyosin-troponin system.

Acknowledgment: This study was supported by U.S. Public Health Service Grants HL 05435, HL 07906, HL 05925, HL 13870, NIH-71-2493, and the American Heart Association, Texas Affiliate, Houston Chapter. Doctor Schwartz is the recipient of Research Career Development Award K3 HL 11875.

References

1. **Leyton RA, Sonnenblick EH:** The ultrastructure of the failing heart. Amer J Med Sci 258:304, 1969
2. **Poche R:** Ultrastructure of heart muscle under pathological conditions. Ann NY Acad Sci 156:334, 1969
3. **Fawcett DW, McNutt NS:** The ultrastructure of the cat myocardium. I. Ventricular capillary muscle. II. Atrial muscle. J Cell Biol 42:1, 1969
4. **Forssmann WG, Girardier L:** A study of the T-system in rat heart. J Cell Biol 44:1, 1970
5. **Kawamura K, James TN:** Comparative ultrastructure of cellular junctions in working myocardium and a conduction system under normal and pathologic conditions. J Molec Cell Cardiol 3:31, 1971
6. **Melax H, Leeson TS:** Fine structure of the endocardium in adult rats. J Cardiovasc Res 1:349, 1967
7. **Legato MJ:** Correlation of ultrastructure and function in the mammalian myocardial cell. Progr Cardiovasc Dis 11:391, 1969
8. **Legato MJ, Langer GA:** The subcellular localization of calcium ion in mammalian myocardium. J Cell Biol 41:401, 1969
9. **Sommer JR, Johnson EA:** Comparative ultrastructure of cardiac cell membrane specializations. A review. Amer J Cardiol 25:184, 1970
10. **Staley NA, Benson ZS:** The ultrastructure of frog ventricular cardiac muscle and its relationship to mechanisms of excitation-contraction coupling. J Cell Biol 38:99, 1968
11. **Hibbs RG, Ferrans VJ:** An ultrastructural and histochemical study of rat atrial myocardium. Amer J Anat 124:251, 1969
12. **Bishop SP:** Ultrastructural alterations in canine myocardial hypertrophy. In, Cardiac Hypertrophy (Alpert N, ed). New York, Academic Press, 1971, p 107
13. **Sommer JR, Johnson EA:** Cardiac muscle: a comparative ultrastructural study with special reference to frog and chicken hearts. Z Zellforsch 98:437, 1969
14. **Nayler WG, Merrilees NCR:** Cellular exchange of calcium. In, Calcium and the Heart (Harris P, Opie LH, ed). London and New York, Academic Press, 1971, p 36
15. **Sordahl LA, et al:** In, Paul D. White Honorary Symposium, The normal and failing heart: action of digitalis on cardiac cell membrane. American College of Cardiology, New York, 1971
16. **Harigaya S, Schwartz A:** Rate of calcium binding and uptake in normal animal and failing human cardiac muscle. Circ Res 25:781, 1969
17. **Besch HR, Schwartz A:** Initial calcium binding rates of canine cardiac relaxing system (sarcoplasmic reticulum fragments) determined by stopped-flow spectrophotometry. Biochem Biophys Res Comm 45:286, 1971
18. **Sordahl LA, McCollum WB, Wood WG, et al:** Mitochondria and sarcoplasmic reticulum function in cardiac hypertrophy and failure. Amer J Physiol 224:497, 1973
19. **Anversa P, Vitali-Mazza L, Visioli O, et al:** Experimental cardiac hypertrophy: a quantitative ultrastructural study in the compensatory stage. J Molec Cell Cardiol 3:213, 1971
20. **Arcos JC, Sohol RS, Sun SC, et al:** Changes in ultrastructure and respiratory control in mitochondria of rat heart hypertrophied by exercise. Exp Molec Path 8:49, 1968
21. **Poche R:** Submikroscopische Beiträge zur Pathologie der Herzmuskelzelle bei Phosphorvergiftung, Hypertrophie, Atrophie, und Kaliummengel. Virchows Arch Path Anat Physiol Klin Med 331:165, 1958
22. **Richter GW, Kellner A:** Hypertrophy of the human heart at the level of fine structure. J Cell Biol 18:195, 1963
23. **Sordahl LA, Crow CA, Kraft GH, et al:** Some ultrastructural and biochemical aspects of heart mitochondria associated with development: fetal and cardiomyopathic tissue. J Molec Cell Cardiol 4:1, 1972
24. **Bishop SP, Cole CR:** Ultrastructural changes in the canine myocardium with right ventricular hypertrophy and congestive heart failure. Lab Invest 20:219, 1969
25. **Meerson FZ:** The myocardium in hyperfunction, hypertrophy and heart failure. Circ Res 25 suppl II:1, 1969
26. **Legato MJ:** Sarcomerogenesis in human myocardium. J Molec Cell Cardiol 1:425, 1970
27. **Meessen H:** Ultrastructure of the myocardium: its significance in myocardial disease. Amer J Cardiol 22:319, 1968
28. **Lehninger AL:** The Mitochondrion, second edition. Baltimore, WJ Benjamin, 1965
29. **Chance B:** Energy-linked Functions of Mitochondria. New York, Academic Press, 1963
30. **Plaut GWE, Gertler MM:** Oxidative phosphorylation studies in normal and experimentally produced congestive heart failure in the guinea pig: a comparison. Ann NY Acad Sci 72:515, 1959
31. **Szekeres L, Schein M:** Cell metabolism of the overloaded mammalian heart in situ. Cardiologia (Basel) 34:18, 1959
32. **Schwartz A, Lee KS:** Study of heart mitochondria and glycolytic metabolism in experimentally induced cardiac failure. Circ Res 10:321, 1962
33. **Wollenberger A, Kleitke B, Raabe G:** Some metabolic

characteristics of mitochondria from chronically overloaded hypertrophied hearts. Exp Molec Path 2:251,1963

34. **Argus MF, Arcos JC, Sardesai VM, et al:** Oxidative rates and phosphorylation in sarcosomes from experimentally-induced failing rat heart. Proc Soc Exp Biol Med 117:380, 1964

35. **Olson RE:** Abnormalities of myocardial metabolism (abstr). Circ Res 14 suppl II:109, 1964

36. **Sobel BE, Spann JF Jr, Pool PE, et al:** Normal oxidative phosphorylation in mitochondria from failing heart. Circ Res 21:355, 1967

37. **Lindenmayer GE, Sordahl LA, Schwartz A:** Reevaluation of oxidative phosphorylation in cardiac muscle from normal animals and animals in heart failure. Circ Res 23:439, 1968

38. **Von Korff RW:** Metabolic characteristics of isolated rabbit heart mitochondria. J Biol Chem 240:1351, 1965

39. **Schwartz A, Lindenmayer GE, Harigaya S:** Respiratory control and calcium transport in heart mitochondria from the cardiomyopathic Syrian hamster. Trans NY Acad Sci 30 suppl II:951, 1968

40. **Lindenmayer GE, Harigaya S, Bajusz E, et al:** Oxidative phosphorylation and calcium transport of mitochondria isolated from cardiomyopathic hamster hearts. J Molec Cell Cardiol 1:249, 1970

41. **Chidsey CA, Weinbach EC, Pool PE, et al:** Biochemical studies of energy production in the failing human heart. J Clin Invest 45:40, 1966

42. **Lindenmayer GE, Sordahl LA, Harigaya S, et al:** Some biochemical studies on subcellular systems isolated from fresh recipient human cardiac tissue obtained during transplantation. Amer J Cardiol 27:277, 1971

43. **Sordahl LA, Liddicoat JE Jr, Diethrich EB, et al:** Respiratory activity of mitochondria from isolated human and dog hearts maintained in a portable preservation chamber. J Molec Cell Cardiol 1:379, 1970

44. **Holloszy JO:** Biochemical adaptations in muscle. Effects of exercise on mitochondrial oxygen uptake and respiratory enzyme activity in skeletal muscle. J Biol Chem 242:2278, 1967

45. **Meerson FZ, Zaletayeva TA, Lagutchev SS, et al:** Structure and mass of mitochondria in the process of compensatory hyperfunction and hypertrophy of the heart. Exp Cell Res 36:568, 1964

46. **Sordahl LA, Wood WG, Schwartz A:** Production of cardiac hypertrophy and failure in rabbits with Ameroid clips. J Molec Cell Cardiol 1:341, 1970

47. **Sordahl LA, Wood WG, Lazarus M, et al:** Alterations in heart mitochondria during hypertrophy and progressive failure: increases and decreases in function and structure. Circ Res 42 suppl II:51, 1970

48. **Haugaard N, Haugaard ES, Lee NH, et al:** Possible role of mitochondria in regulation of cardiac contractility. Fed Proc 28:1657, 1969

49. **Ueba Y, Ito Y, Chidsey CA:** Intracellular calcium and myocardial contractility. Amer J Physiol 220:1553, 1971

50. **Langer GA, Serena SD:** Effects of strophanthidin upon contraction and ionic exchange in rabbit ventricular myocardium: relation to control active state. J Molec Cell Cardiol 1:65, 1970

51. **Patriarca P, Carafoli E:** A study of the intracellular transport of calcium in rat heart. J Cell Physiol 72:29, 1968

52. **Inesi G, Ebashi S, Watanabe S:** Preparation of vesicular relaxing factor from bovine heart tissue. Amer J Physiol 207:1339, 1964

53. **Lee KS, Ladinsky H, Stuckey JH:** Decreased Ca^{++} uptake by sarcoplasmic reticulum after coronary artery occlusion for 60 and 90 minutes. Circ Res 21:439, 1967

54. **Gertz EW, Hess ML, Lain RF, et al:** Activity of the vesicular calcium pump in the spontaneously failing heart lung preparation. Circ Res 20:477, 1967

55. **Suko J, Vogel JHK, Chidsey CA:** Intracellular calcium and myocardial contractility. 3. Reduced calcium uptake and ATPase in the sarcoplasmic reticular fraction prepared from chemically failing calf hearts. Circ Res 27:235, 1970

56. **Gertz EW, Stam AC Jr, Sonnenblick EH:** A quantitative and qualitative defect in the sarcoplasmic reticulum in the hereditary cardiomyopathy of the Syrian hamster. Biochem Biophys Res Commun 40:746, 1970

57. **Briggs FN, Gertz EW, Hess ML:** Calcium uptake by cardiac vesicles: inhibition by amytol and reversal by ouabain. Biochem 345:122, 1966

58. **Fuchs F, Gertz EW, Briggs FN:** The effect of quinidine on calcium accumulation by isolated sarcoplasmic reticulum of skeletal and cardiac muscle. J Gen Physiol 52:955, 1968

59. **Hess ML, Briggs FN, Shinebourne E, et al:** The effect of adrenergic blocking agents on the calcium pump of cardiac sarcoplasmic reticulum. Nature 220:79, 1968

60. **Lain RF, Hess ML, Gertz EW, et al:** Calcium uptake activity of canine myocardial sarcoplasmic reticulum in the presence of anesthetic agents. Circ Res 23:597, 1968

61. **Hess ML, Briggs FN:** The effect of gram negative endotoxin on the calcium uptake activity of sarcoplasmic reticulum isolated from canine myocardium. Biochem Biophys Res Comm 45:917, 1971

62. **Sulakhe PV, Dhalla NS:** Excitation-contraction coupling in the heart. VII. Calcium accumulation in subcellular particles in congestive heart failure. J Clin Invest 50:1019, 1971

63. **Muir JR, Dhalla NS, Ortega JF, et al:** Energy linked calcium transport in subcellular fractions of the failing rat heart. Circ Res 26:429, 1970

64. **Ohnishi T, Ebashi S:** Spectrophotometric measurement of instantaneous calcium binding to the relaxing factor of muscle. J Biochem 54:506, 1963

65. **Schwartz A:** Calcium and the sarcoplasmic reticulum. In Ref 14, p 82

66. **McCollum WB, Besch HR Jr, Entman ML, et al:** Apparent initial binding rate of calcium by canine cardiac relaxing system. Amer J Physiol 223:608, 1972

67. **Entman ML, Bornet EP, Schwartz A:** Phasic components of calcium binding and release by canine cardiac relaxing system (sarcoplasmic reticulum). J Molec Cell Cardiol 4:155, 1972

68. **McCollum WB, Crow C, Harigaya S, et al:** Calcium binding by cardiac relaxing system isolated from myopathic Syrian hamsters (strains 14.6, 82.62 and 40.54). J Molec Cell Cardiol 1:445, 1970

69. **McCollum WB:** Sarcoplasmic Reticulum: A Biochemi-

cal Study of Calcium Binding in Normal and Failing Myocardium. PhD thesis, Baylor College of Medicine, 1971

70. **Skou JC:** Enzymatic basis for active transport of Na^+ across cell membrane. Physiol Rev 45:596, 1965

71. **Besch HR, Allen JC, Glick G, et al:** Correlation between the inotropic action of ouabain and its effects on subcellular enzyme systems from canine myocardium. J Pharmacol Exp Ther 171:1, 1970

72. **Allen JC, Besch HR, Glick G, et al:** H^3-ouabain binding to $Na^+,K^+-ATPase$ and cardiac relaxing system of perfused dog heart. Molec Pharmacol 6:441, 1970

73. **Repke K:** Effect of digitalis on membrane ATPase of cardiac muscle. In, Drugs and Enzymes. Proceedings of 2nd International Pharmacology Meeting. New York, Pergamon Press, 1965, p 65

74. **Akera T, Larsen FS, Brody TM:** Correlation of cardiac $Na^+,K^+-ATPase$ activity with ouabain-induced inotropic stimulation. J Pharmacol Exp Ther 173:145, 1970

75. **Lee KS, Klaus W:** The subcellular basis for the mechanism of inotropic action of cardiac glycosides. Pharmacol Rev 23:193, 1971

76. **Mead RJ, Peterson MB, Welty JD:** Sarcolemmal and sarcoplasmic reticular ATPase activities in the failing canine heart. Circ Res 29:14, 1971

77. **Bishop SP, Cole CR:** Production of externally controlled progressive pulmonic stenosis in the dog. J Appl Physiol 26:659, 1969

78. **Matsui H, Schwartz A:** Purification and properties of a highly active ouabain-sensitive $Na^+,K^+-ATPase$ from cardiac tissue. Biochim Biophys Acta 128:380, 1966

79. **Alpert NR, Gordon MS:** Myofibrillar adenosine triphosphate activity in congestive failure. Amer J Physiol 202:940, 1962

80. **Aras A, Haas G:** ATPase and myokinase activity of myofibrils from normal, hypertrophied and failing human hearts (abstr). Fed Proc Fed Amer Soc Exp Biol 21:132, 1962

81. **Gordon M, Brown AL:** Myofibrillar adenosine triphosphate activity of human heart tissue and congestive failure: effects of ouabain and calcium. Circ Res 18:534, 1966

82. **Chandler BM, Sonnenblick EH, Spann JF, et al:** Association of depressed myofibrillar adenosine triphosphates and reduced contractility in experimental heart failure. Circ Res 21:717, 1967

83. **Draper M, Taylor N, Alpert NR:** Alteration in contractile protein in hypertrophied guinea pig hearts. In Ref 12, p 315

84. **Sommer JR, Spach MS:** Electron microscopic demonstration of adenosine triphosphates in myofibrils and sarcoplasmic membranes of cardiac muscle of normal and abnormal dogs. Amer J Path 44:491, 1964

85. **Miyaharo K:** Studies on actomyosin of heart muscle. Jap Circ J 26:8, 1962

86. **Davis JO, Trapasso M, Yankopoulos N:** Studies of actomyosin from cardiac muscle of dogs with experimental congestive heart failure. Circ Res 7:957, 1959

87. **Benson ES:** Composition and state of protein and heart muscle of normal dogs and dogs with experimental myocardial failure. Circ Res 3:221, 1955

88. **Nebel MI, Bing RJ:** Contractile proteins of normal and failing human heart. Arch Intern Med (Chicago) 111:190, 1963

89. **Olson RE, Ellenbogen E, Iyengar R:** Cardiac myosin and congestive heart failure in the dog. Circulation 24:471, 1961

90. **Luchi RJ, Kritcher EM, Thyrum PT:** Reduced cardiac myosin adenosine triphosphate activity in dogs with spontaneously occurring heart failure. Circ Res 24:513, 1969

91. **Katz AM, Hecht HE:** The early "pump" failure of the ischemic heart. Amer J Med 47:497, 1969

Ribonucleic Acid (RNA) Polymerase and Adenyl Cyclase in Cardiac Hypertrophy and Cardiomyopathy

Kappiareth G. Nair, MD, PhD, FACC
Teddy Umali, MS
James Potts, MD

"The process of protein synthesis which is controlled by the nuclear genetic apparatus constitutes the basis of the building and later also of the renewal of membranes, myofibrils, and the mitochondria as well as the sarcoplasmic reticulum. Thus, the process of protein synthesis is the basis of the plastic endurance of all activity of the myocardial cell."

FZ Meerson[1]

The biochemical mechanisms by which physiologic stimuli such as chronic pressure or volume overload of the heart produce cardiac hypertrophy have been subjected to intensive investigation in recent years.[1-10] By analogy with genetic regulatory mechanisms in bacterial and mammalian systems, Nair et al.[4] suggested that deoxyribonucleic acid (DNA)-dependent ribonucleic acid (RNA) polymerase, a key regulatory enzyme in the control of protein synthesis, played a major role in the early events that occur after an increased work load on the heart. Two models of cardiac hypertrophy were studied. In the first model, left ventricular hypertrophy is produced in rats by creation of supravalvular aortic stenosis using a specially designed silver clip. In the second model, cardiac hypertrophy and myocardial failure occur spontaneously in the Syrian golden hamster (Bio line 14.6), presumably because of a hereditary myopathy. In the former model, changes in heart weight occur within 2 days after aortic banding; in the latter model, increase of heart weight appears only after the third month of life although evidence of myocardial damage may be present during the first month.[11]

This chapter discusses the genetic regulatory mechanisms in cardiac hypertrophy and cardiomyopathy with specific reference to nuclear and nucleolar RNA polymerase. It also suggests a probable cause of cardiomyopathy in the Syrian golden hamster. The interrelation among catecholamines, adenyl cyclase and RNA polymerase is briefly evaluated.

Animal Models of Aortic Stenosis and Cardiomyopathy

Mature female rats of the Sprague-Dawley strain weighing 220 to 240 g were used to produce left ventricular hypertrophy. Syrian hamsters (Bio line 14.6) with dystrophy were obtained from Telaco (Maine). Hamsters from the newborn stage to 180 days of age were used for the study of serial changes in the heart.

Sham-operated littermates served as control animals for the rats, whereas normal healthy hamsters of the same age as the study hamsters served as control animals in this group. The healthy hamsters were obtained from Zucca's hamstery (New Jersey).

The method for banding the aorta above the semilunar valve and the methods for determining heart weight, RNA and DNA content have previously been described in detail.[4]

Biochemical Analyses

RNA Polymerase Assays: Nuclei were isolated from heart muscle homogenates by differential centrifugation using 2.2 M sucrose. The fractionation procedure was based on the method reported by Nair et al.[12] which was modified from the techniques of Widnell and Tata[13] and Chauveau et al.[14] Details of the methods used in heart muscle preparations have been published previously.[12] DNA-dependent RNA polymerase activity was assayed according to the methods of Weiss[15] and Widnell and Tata.[13] The enzyme assay was routinely carried out in duplicate under conditions of reduced ionic strength (polymerase I) and increased ionic strength (polymerase II).[12]

Inhibitory Studies: Alpha amanitine was dissolved in 0.01 M Tris-HCl buffer, pH 7.6, and was used in concentrations ranging from 0.005 to 1 μg/ml of assay mixture.

Adenyl Cyclase Assays: The method of Krishna et al.[16] was followed. Heart muscle was minced finely and passed through a Latapic grinder. It was then homogenized in 15 volumes of ice-cold 0.27 M sucrose in 0.04 M Tris-HCl buffer, pH 7.6. The homogenate was spun at 2,600 revolutions/min for 15 minutes in a Sorvall RC-2B refrigerated centrifuge. The pellet was resuspended in the homogenizing medium and centrifuged at 8,000 revolutions/min for 15 minutes at 0° C. The crude pellet so obtained was used for assay of adenyl cyclase activity. Theophylline, a known inhibitor of cyclic adenosine monophosphate (AMP) phosphodiesterase, was routinely added to all assay mixtures. The incubations were carried out for 10 minutes at 35° C, the reaction being terminated by the prompt addition of excess nonradioactive cyclic 3'5' AMP and subsequent immersion of the incubation tubes in boiling water for 5 minutes. The tubes were centrifuged at 2,500 revolutions/min for 10 minutes, and the supernatant was loaded on to Dowex 50 H$^+$ ion exchange column (0.4 × 3.3 cm). Elution was carried out with distilled water. The first 4 ml of the eluate was discarded, and 0.2 ml each of 0.25 M ZnSO$_4$ and 0.25 M Ba(OH)$_2$ was added to the second 4 ml of the eluate. Cyclic AMP remained in the supernatant after centrifugation. A suitable aliquot was counted in Bray's fluid using liquid scintillation.

RNA and DNA Content: Details of the method for estimating myocardial nucleic acids have been published earlier.[4] Calf thymus DNA (Sigma) and yeast RNA (Sigma) served as standards.

Alterations of RNA Polymerase and Adenyl Cyclase

RNA Polymerase: We have earlier shown that after aortic banding RNA polymerase I activity of the left ventricular myocardium increases sharply, the earliest detectable change occurring after 12 hours in the in vitro system. The peak level is reached on the second day. In nuclei obtained from heart muscle of the Syrian golden hamster (Bio 14.6 strain) there is a sharp increase in RNA polymerase I activity between the fifth and the sixth week of life. By the eighteenth week of life the levels of RNA polymerase activity reach a stable plateau value (Figure 1). In both the rat heart preparations and the nuclear preparations from the myopathic hamster our values for RNA polymerase II activity were random and not quantifiable.

Changes in RNA polymerase I activity were accompanied by an increase in myocardial RNA content (Figure 2). The illustration also shows parallel increases in myocardial DNA content. These changes are qualitatively similar to our findings in ventricular hypertrophy caused by aortic banding.

Alpha amanitine, in concentrations of 0.01 μg/ml of assay mixture, regularly produced far greater inhibition of RNA polymerase II activity than of RNA polymerase I activity (Table I). This differential inhibition caused by alpha amanitine was of the same degree in the myopathic hamsters as in the normal control hamsters.

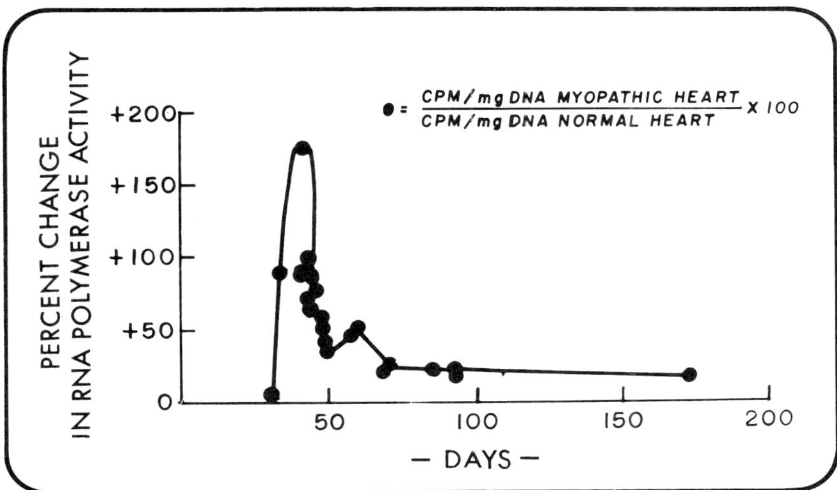

FIGURE 1. RNA polymerase I activity in heart muscle of the Syrian golden hamster with cardiomyopathy. Each **closed circle** represents the mean value of four separate incubation studies. For each assay the hearts of three or four hamsters were pooled. Note the sharp increase in enzyme activity between the fifth and sixth weeks of life.

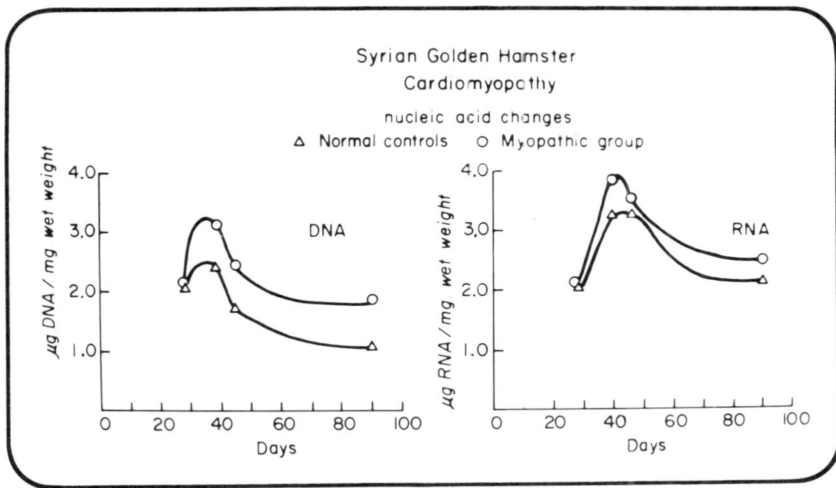

FIGURE 2. Nucleic acid changes in cardiomyopathy. The increases in RNA and DNA (μg/mg wet weight) are maximal around the fifth and the sixth weeks, paralleling the changes in RNA polymerase activity.

Adenyl Cyclase: An increase in myocardial adenyl cyclase activity was noted around the eighth week of life in the myopathic hamsters (Figure 3). This increase seemed to remain sustained until the very late stage (240 days). These results are of a preliminary nature because the number of animals in each group was small (no. = 4 at each day of estimation).

Protein Synthesis in Myocardial Hypertrophy

The myocardium is composed of different types of cells. In addition to the muscle cells there are specialized Purkinje cells, connective tissue cells and endothelial cells. In the process of cardiac hypertrophy all of these cellular ele-

TABLE I
Alpha Amanitine Inhibition of RNA Polymerases

Age (days)	RNA Polymerase I (percent inhibition)		RNA Polymerase II (percent inhibition)	
	Control	Myopathic	Control	Myopathic
32	28.9	21.5	72.5	70.4
45	21.3	22.8	74.4	80.6
50	22.6	20.4	95.0	95.1
71	27.8	26.7	90.0	90.5

ments increase in size or number depending upon their biological abilities at adaptation. Increased protein synthesis is an essential factor in cell growth, and it is not surprising that in experimental cardiac hypertrophy there is an augmented synthesis of RNA and protein in the heart. Once the provocative stimulus to cardiac hypertrophy is removed, some of these changes revert to normal.[18] In general, the changes in RNA and protein content parallel the changes in heart weight.

Various investigations have shown that the increment in RNA and protein content of the myocardium is chiefly due to an accelerated rate of protein synthesis.[1–4,6–8,10] Goldberg has shown in work-induced hypertrophy of skeletal muscle that changes in the rate of RNA and protein turnover may be an operative factor in their accumulation. A similar process probably occurs in heart muscle.

Protein synthesis in the cell takes place on aggregates of ribonucleoprotein particles called polysomes. Each aggregate is made up of units called ribosomes, which are made up of RNA and protein in roughly equal proportions. A special variety of RNA, messenger RNA, holds these ribosomes together in a polysomal cluster. Basically three types of RNA are involved in the process of protein synthesis: (1) ribosomal RNA; (2) messenger RNA; and (3) transfer or soluble RNA. During cardiac hypertrophy it is the ribosomal fraction that increases to a large extent. A proportional increase in messenger RNA and transfer RNA is also very likely.

RNA Polymerase in Ventricular Systolic Pressure Overload

The enzyme RNA polymerase that synthesizes all cellular RNA is located in the cell nucleus. Chromosomal DNA is used as a template to di-

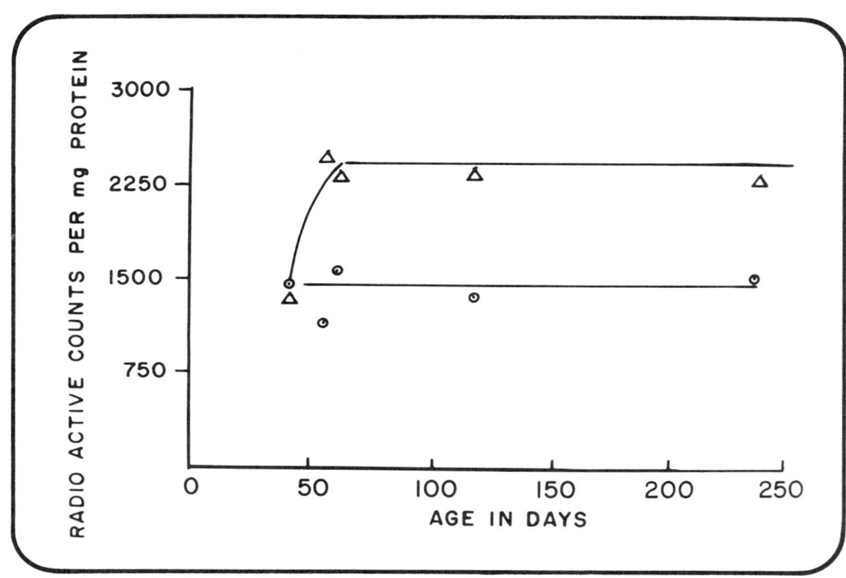

FIGURE 3. Adenyl cyclase activity in the low speed fraction from myocardial homogenates from myopathic (**triangles**) and control (**circles**) hamsters. Note the early increase in enzyme activity around the eighth week of life. Each **trian-** gle or **open circle** represents the mean values from two separate incubations performed in duplicate with the use of pooled hearts from four animals.

rect the synthesis of a specific RNA. With the use of isolated nuclear preparations from heart muscle, Nair et al.[4] showed that within 24 hours after the induction of hypertrophy RNA polymerase activity was increased. These results were later confirmed by Schreiber et al.[20] in perfused guinea pig hearts subjected to a work overload.

Multiple forms of RNA polymerase have been described by several workers.[21–25] Polymerase I is active under conditions of reduced ionic strength, whereas polymerase II is optimally active at a higher level of ionic strength of the incubation medium. Purified nucleoli generally contain polymerase I, whereas polymerase II is found mainly in the nucleoplasmic fraction of the cell nucleus.[22] There may be a third RNA polymerase in the nucleoplasm, but little is known about it at present.[22]

RNA Polymerase in Primary Cardiomyopathy

In an earlier report,[12] we stated that the product of the reaction of polymerase I is ribosomal RNA and that of polymerase II is messenger or DNA-like RNA.[12] Our experiments indicate that the synthesis of ribosomal RNA is greatly accelerated in cardiac hypertrophy. This paper is the first report of increased RNA polymerase activity in the heart muscle of the Syrian golden hamster with myopathy. In this highly inbred line (Bio 14.6 strain), the first signs of muscular weakness appear around the sixtieth day of life. Cardiac lesions such as swelling of muscle fibers, patchy necrosis and pyknotic changes in nuclei may occur as early as the thirtieth day. It is at this time that the first increase in RNA polymerase activity occurs, presumably because of the increased work load imposed on the normal surviving myocardial fibers. It is not clear whether this increased RNA polymerase activity arises entirely from hypertrophying muscle fibers or partly from connective tissue cells.

The differential inhibition of the two polymerases by alpha amanitine is of interest. Nucleoplasmic polymerase, which synthesizes predominantly messenger RNA, is markedly inhibited by this toxic cyclopeptide obtained from the poisonous mushroom Amanita phalloides.[17,26,27] The polymerases from both normal and myopathic animals are inhibited to the same extent, thus indicating no major difference in their behavior. Alpha amanitine should prove to be a powerful tool in further studying the genetic transcriptive mechanisms that are the prelude to protein synthesis.

Adenyl Cyclase in Cardiomyopathy

The increase in myocardial adenyl cyclase activity is of considerable interest. Angelakos et al.[28] have studied the rate of synthesis of norepinephrine in the Bio 14.6 strain of hamsters, and their results indicate that cardiac norepinephrine synthesis is increased two to three times over that of the normal level in the myopathic animals. It is likely that the higher levels of norepinephrine result in increased adenyl cyclase activity of the myocardium.

In conclusion, we suggest the following hypothesis: During the early stages of cardiac hypertrophy in the model of cardiomyopathy under study, there is an increase of RNA polymerase activity with a consequent increase in RNA content of the myocardium. There appears to be a concomitant increase in adenyl cyclase activity of the heart. This is probably due to an initial elevation of the catecholamine content of the myocardium. Although we have not yet measured the levels of cyclic AMP in the heart, the higher levels of adenyl cyclase activity suggest that cyclic AMP may have a crucial role to play in the transcriptive process involving RNA polymerase. Such a role involving the sigma factor has already been demonstrated in bacterial systems.[29] The function of the sigma factor appears to be that of promoting the initiation of transcription at specific sites on the DNA template.[30] Further experimental work along these lines should provide greater insight into the early biochemical events that regulate protein synthesis in cardiac hypertrophy.

Summary

The key enzyme in the genetic process of protein synthesis, ribonucleic acid (RNA) polymerase, is increased in activity during the early stages of cardiac hypertrophy induced by aortic banding. A similar increase in the activity of this enzyme is seen in the cardiomyopathy of the

Syrian golden hamster. There are at least two RNA polymerases in the cell. RNA polymerase I is nucleolar in origin and synthesizes ribosomal RNA under conditions of reduced ionic strength. RNA polymerase II is nucleoplasmic in location and chiefly synthesizes deoxyribonucleic acid (DNA)-like RNA or messenger RNA. The latter enzyme is strongly inhibited by alpha amanitine, a toxic cyclopeptide obtained from the common poisonous mushroom. Increased adenyl cyclase activity in the myocardium of the hamster with cardiomyopathy suggests that catecholamines and cyclic adenosine monophosphate may play an important role in the pathogenesis of the condition.

Acknowledgment: This study was supported by U.S. Public Health Service Grant (Career Development Award) K4-HE-38898, U. S. Public Health Service Program Project Grant HE-08805-07 and the South Eastern Heart Association, Pennsylvania.

The authors wish to thank Doctor J. J. Furth, Department of Biochemistry, University of Pennsylvania, for his generous gift of alpha amanitine.

References

1. **Meerson FZ:** The Myocardium in Hyperfunction, Hypertrophy and Heart Failure (English trans). New York, American Heart Association Monograph No. 26, 1969
2. **Gluck L, Talner NS, Stern H, et al:** Experimental cardiac hypertrophy: concentrations of RNA in the ventricles. Science 144:1244, 1964
3. **Grimm AF, Kubota R, Whitehorn WV:** Ventricular nucleic acid and protein levels with myocardial growth and hypertrophy. Circ Res 19:552, 1966
4. **Nair KG, Cutilletta AF, Zak R, et al:** Biochemical correlates of cardiac hypertrophy. I. Experimental model: changes in heart weight, RNA content, and nuclear RNA polymerase activity. Circ Res 23:451, 1968
5. **Meerson FZ, Kopteva LA, Melechov VV, et al:** Nucleotide content of ribonucleic acid in compensatory hyperfunction and hypertrophy of the heart. Nature (London) 212:927, 1966
6. **Posner BI, Fanburg BL:** Ribonucleic acid synthesis in experimental cardiac hypertrophy in rats. II. Aspects of regulation. Circ Res 23:137, 1968
7. **Schreiber SS, Oratz M, Rothschild MA:** Protein synthesis in the overloaded mammalian heart. Amer J Physiol 211:314, 1966
8. **Gudbjarnason S, Telerman M, Bing RJ:** Protein metabolism in cardiac hypertrophy and heart failure. Amer J Physiol 206:294, 1964
9. **Morkin E, Garrett SC, Fishman AP:** Effects of actinomycin D and hypophysectomy on development of myocardial hypertrophy in the rat. Amer J Physiol 214:6, 1968
10. **Wannemacher RW Jr, McCoy JR:** Regulation of protein synthesis in the ventricular myocardium of hypertrophic hearts. Amer J Physiol 216:781, 1969
11. **Bajusz E, Homburger F, Baker JR, et al:** The heart muscle in muscular dystrophy with special reference to involvement of the cardiovascular system in the hereditary myopathy of the hamster. Ann NY Acad Sci 138:213, 1966
12. **Nair KG, Rabinowitz M, Tu MC:** Characterization of ribonucleic acid synthesized in an isolated nuclear system from rat heart muscle. Biochemistry (Wash) 6:1898, 1967
13. **Widnell CC, Tata JR:** Procedure for the isolation of enzymically active rat-liver nuclei. Biochem J 92:313, 1964
14. **Chauveau J, Moule Y, Rouiller CL:** Isolation of pure and unaltered liver nuclei in morphology and biochemical composition. Exp Cell Res 11:317, 1956
15. **Weiss SB:** Enzymatic incorporation of ribonucleotide triphosphates into the interpolynucleotide linkages of ribonucleic acid. Proc Nat Acad Sci USA 46:1020, 1960
16. **Krishna G, Weiss B, Brodie BB:** A simple sensitive method for the assay of adenyl cyclase. J Pharmacol Exp Ther 163:379, 1968
17. **Nair KG, Umali T:** Increased RNA polymerase activity in the cardiomyopathy of the Syrian hamster (abstr). Circulation 42 suppl III:III-61, 1970
18. **Beznak M, Korecky B, Thomas G:** Regression of cardiac hypertrophies of various origin. Canad J Physiol Pharmacol 47:579, 1969
19. **Goldberg AL:** Protein synthesis during work-induced growth of skeletal muscle. J Cell Biol 36:653, 1968
20. **Schreiber SS, Oratz M, Rothschild MA:** Nuclear RNA polymerase activity in acute hemodynamic overload in the perfused heart. Amer J Physiol 217:1305, 1969
21. **Jacob ST, Sajdel EM, Munro HN:** Presence of two RNA polymerase activities in liver nucleoli. Biochim Biophys Acta 157:421, 1968
22. **Roeder RG, Rutter WJ:** Specific nucleolar and nucleoplasmic RNA polymerases. Proc Nat Acad Sci USA 65:675, 1970
23. **Widnell CC, Tata JR:** Studies on the stimulation by ammonium sulphate of the DNA dependent RNA polymerase of isolated rat liver nuclei. Biochim Biophys Acta 123:478, 1966
24. **Pogo AO:** Modification of ribonucleic acid synthesis in isolated rat liver nuclei by low salt concentrations and specific divalent cations. Biochim Biophys Acta 182:57, 1969

25. **Chambon P, Ramuz M, Mandel P, et al:** The influence of ionic strength and a polyanion on transcription in vitro. Biochim Biophys Acta 157:504, 1968
26. **Novello F, Stirpe F:** Experimental conditions affecting ribonucleic acid polymerase in isolated rat liver nuclei. Biochem J 112:721, 1969
27. **Lindell TJ, Weinberg F, Morris P, et al:** Specific inhibition of nuclear RNA polymerase II by alpha-amanitin. Science 170:447, 1970
28. **Angelakos ET, Carballo L, Daniels J, et al:** Turnover of catecholamines in the heart of dystrophic hamsters (abstr). Circulation 42 suppl III:III-61, 1970
29. **Martelo OJ, Woo SLC, Reimann EM, et al:** Effect of protein kinase on ribonucleic acid polymerase. Biochemistry, (Wash) 9:4807, 1970
30. **Bautz EKF, Dunn JJ, Bautz FA, et al:** Initiation and regulation of transcription by RNA polymerase. In, Lepet t Colloquia on Biology and Medicine No. 1. RNA-polymerase and Transcription. New York, American Elsevier, 1970, p 90

Myofibrillar Proteins and the Contractile Mechanism in the Normal and Failing Heart

Joan Wikman-Coffelt, PhD
Claudia Fenner, BS
Antone F. Salel, MD, FACC
Teiko Kamiyama, MD
Dean T. Mason, MD, FACC

It is now recognized that there is a definite relationship between the fine architecture of heart muscle and the contractile mechanism of the functioning ventricle. Thus, a subcellular structural basis has been established for myocardial mechanical activity and cardiac pump performance in which the fundamental individual contractile unit is the sarcomere. Sarcomeres linked in series constitute the longitudinally arranged myofibrils inside the muscle cell.

The spatial relationships of the various components within the myocardial cell or fiber are shown in Figure 1. The sarcolemma, or external cell membrane, makes deep invaginations into the muscle cell, thereby forming the complex transverse tubular network or T tubules. The T tubules, located adjacent to the ends of the sarcomeres (Z lines), are continuous with the intracellular membrane system, the sarcoplasmic reticulum. The sarcoplasmic reticulum is positioned along the area (A band) of overlapping thick and thin myofilaments of the sarcomeres. The biochemical and biophysical interactions between the thick filaments of myosin molecules and the thin filaments containing actin ag-gregates produce force and contraction of heart muscle. The terminal lateral portions of the sarcomeres (I bands) possess only thin filaments and the center of the sarcomere (H band) consists only of myosin. The energy substrate adenosine triphosphate (ATP), necessary for myosin adenosine triphosphatase (ATPase) during the active state, is manufactured by mitochondria situated near the A bands containing the actin-myosin cross-bridges involved in the chemical and mechanical processes of the contractile reaction.

In the resting state, the myocardial cell is electrically polarized, with the outside of the fiber being positive relative to its interior (Figure 2A). On excitation, the T tubules transmit the electrical impulse internally to the sarcoplasmic reticulum, which results in reversal of polarization across the cellular membranes (Figure 2B). Excitation-contraction coupling takes place with delivery of calcium ion (Ca^{++}) to the contractile proteins by influx of this cation through the T tubules and its release from the lateral sacs of the sarcoplasmic reticulum.[1] During relaxation (Figure 2C), the original polarization of the

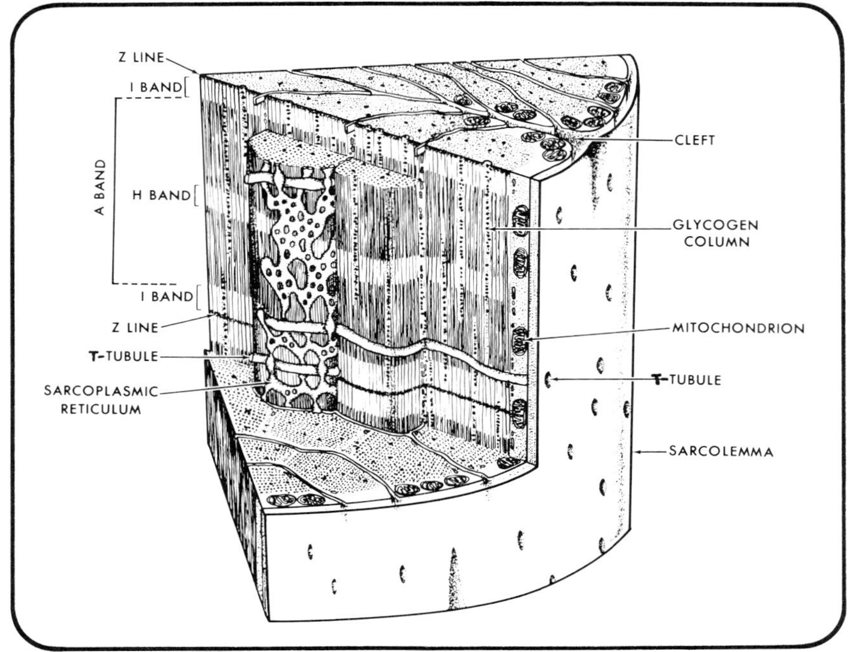

FIGURE 1. Three-dimensional cross-sectional view of a single myocardial cell or fiber.

muscle fiber is restored.[2] Although understanding is incomplete concerning the process responsible for initiating relaxation, passage of Ca^{++} through the sarcoplasmic reticulum involves phosphorylated proteins and is mediated by a transport ATPase associated with this intracellular membrane[3] (Figure 3).

Thin Filaments

The thin filaments consist of an assembly of the proteins actin, tropomyosin and troponin (Figure 4). Figure 4A depicts depolymerized globular actin. During polymerization, globular actin is converted to the fibrous form, re-

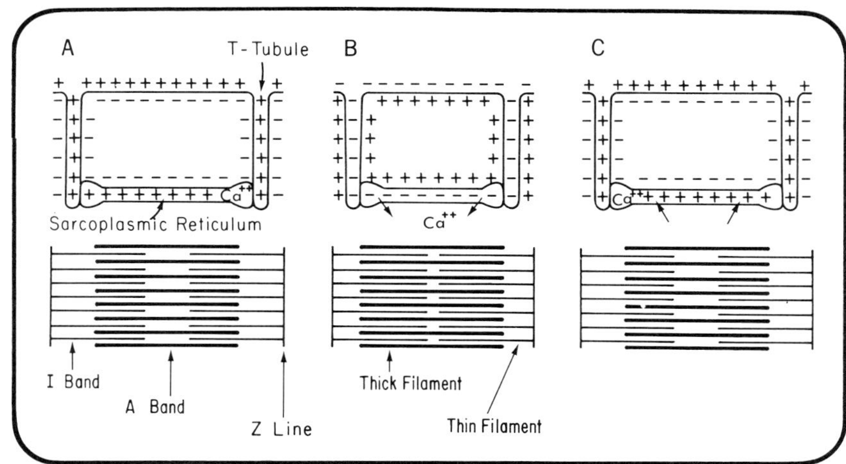

FIGURE 2. Sequence of myocardial intracellular Ca^{++} flux during the cardiac cycle. **A,** the resting state; **B,** the active state of contraction; and **C,** the relaxation process.

sulting in a double helix conformation with seven actin molecules to a turn (Figure 4B). This reaction can be reversed by the addition of calcium and ATP. Tropomyosin is a long, linear molecule composed of two subunits (Figure 4B) spanning seven actin molecules, located alongside the two longitudinal grooves of the double helix of actin (Figure 4C). Troponin is a globular molecule made up of three subunits (Figure 4B) affixed near the end of each tropomyosin molecule[4] (Figure 4C).

The reaction between actin and myosin in vitro continues until all the ATP in the system is exhausted.[2] Control over this process in vivo is exerted by means of troponin and tropomyosin. When actin is "turned on," it reacts with myosin; when "turned off," actin repulses myosin and no reaction takes place.[5,6] The three subunits of troponin are represented by C, I and T in Figure 5. Troponin I alone is capable of inhibiting actin-myosin interaction. Troponin C binds available Ca^{+-} for initiation of contraction. The troponin C-Ca^{++} complex abolishes the inhibitory action of troponin I, thus allowing actin to be turned on. Troponin T binds the troponin subunits to tropomyosin in a defined conformation. Tropomyosin confers calcium sensitivity to troponin, so that in the presence of Ca^{++}, troponin C-Ca^{++} activates actin-myosin linkage by overcoming troponin I inhibition of the contractile process. In the absence of tropomyosin in vitro, troponin C turns on actin whether or not

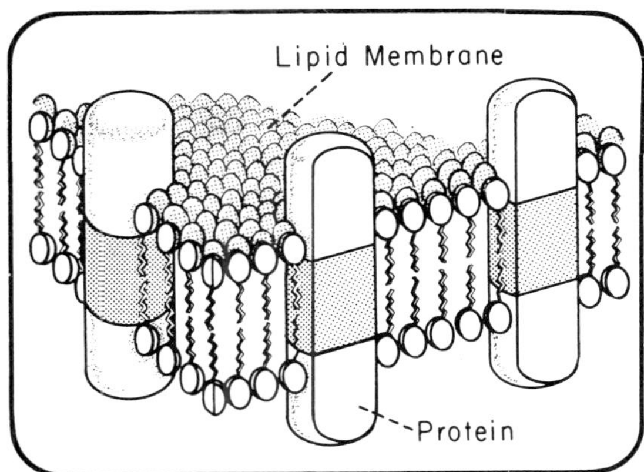

FIGURE 3. Diagramatic representation of the lipid membrane and calcium-binding proteins of sarcoplasmic reticulum.

calcium is present.[4] Since one tropomyosin molecule is complexed throughout the length of seven actin molecules, it appears that the inhibitory action of troponin I is passed down seven actin molecules via tropomyosin, thereby turning off actin, which causes repulsion between actin and myosin.

Thick Filaments

The ultrastructure of the interdigitating thick and thin filaments is illustrated in Figure 6 as they appear in longitudinal section. Three thick and four thin filaments are shown, tropomyosin

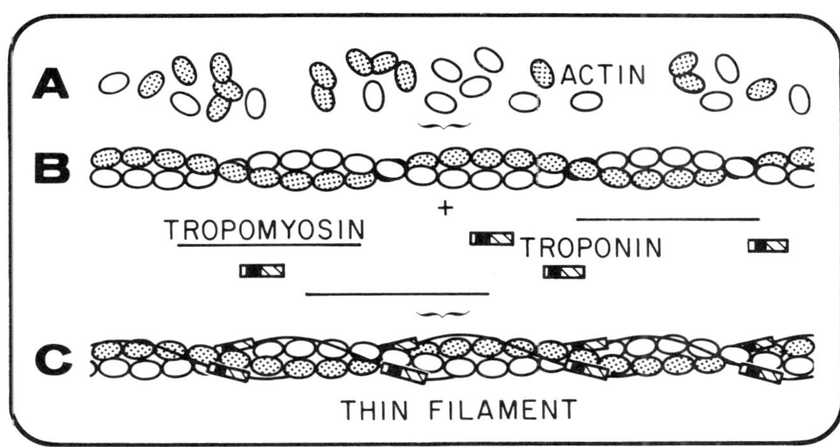

FIGURE 4. Representation of the components of a thin filament. **A,** depolymerized globular actin; **B,** polymerized fibrous actin, tropomyosin and troponin; **C,** the reconstituted thin filament comprised of fibrous actin with tropomyosin alongside the actin grooves and troponin at each turn of the double helix of actin.

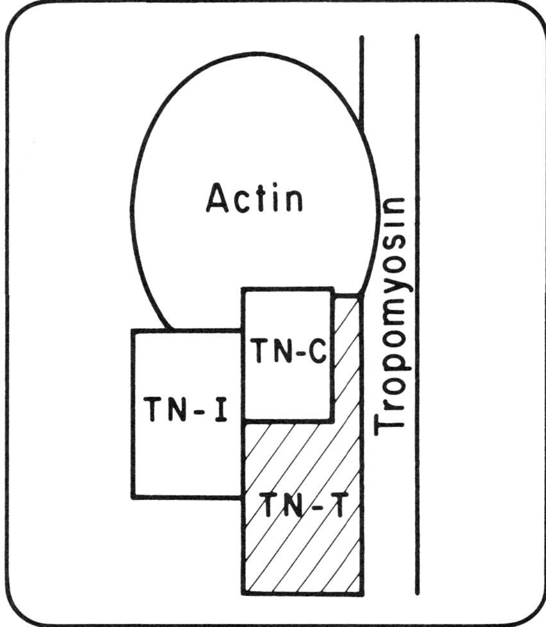

FIGURE 5. Representation of the three subunits of troponin (TN) showing their relation to the other proteins of the thin filament.

is in the groove of the double helix of actin molecules, and troponin is located at every seventh actin molecule. The thick filaments are composed of bundles of myosin molecules, each consisting of a central strand with laterally terminating heads that spiral outward from the core of the cylinder. The myosin molecules comprising the thick filament are grouped sequentially so that the myosin heads spiral along both A band sections of the filament. Only the small midzone (H band) of the filament is without myosin heads. When actin is turned on, the myosin heads establish cross-bridge contact with actin, and enzymatic activity in the myosin heads take place. Figure 7 provides a three-dimensional view of a single thick filament with several pairs of myosin aggregates.

A diagrammatic representation of the manner by which the nomenclature of the myosin fragments has been established is shown in Figure 8. Proteolytic enzymes, such as trypsin, are capable of hydrolyzing covalent bonds between specific amino acids. Thus, trypsin hydrolyzes myosin at its hinge region—referred to as the M bridge—to produce two fragments, light mero-

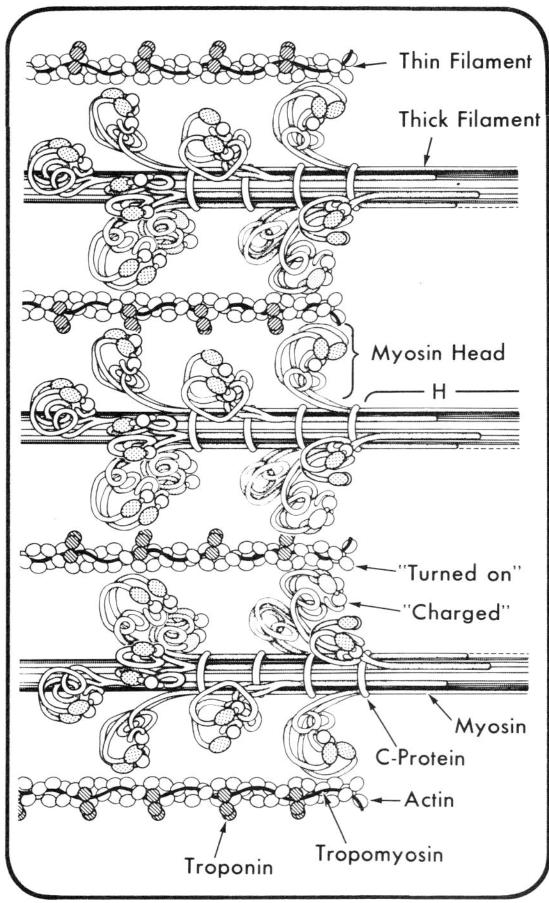

FIGURE 6. Diagrammatic representation of alternating myofilaments in longitudinal view in a portion of a lateral section of thick filaments. H = midzone H band of the thick filaments.

myosin (LMM) and heavy meromyosin (HMM). The ATPase activity of myosin is contained within heavy meromyosin and it is this portion of myosin that forms the cross-bridges with actin. Light meromyosin constitutes the backbone of the thick filaments. Angulation of the head of heavy meromyosin, by changing its degree, results in movement of the thin filaments during contraction; the head angle is located between heavy meromyosin S_1 and heavy meromyosin S_2 as defined by papain digestion of heavy meromyosin (Figure 8). It is specifically in the S_1 component of heavy meromyosin that the ATPase activity of myosin is contained. Further, heavy meromyosin S_1 is referred to as the head of myosin. This myosin head contains the site that reacts with actin. In addition, the S_1 component includes the myosin light chains, which appear to be wrapped inside the myosin head.[7] The light meromyosin region of myosin is approximately 840 Å in length. The remainder of the molecule—heavy meromyosin—is currently thought to be about 460 Å.

Figure 9 shows one of the two heavy chains of myosin; two such chains constitute whole myosin. In this example, the single myosin heavy chain contains two light chains (subunits) in the head region. The heavy chains form a tight helix both in the light meromyosin region and in the heavy meromyosin S_2 region. Heavy meromyosin S_1 is elliptically shaped and not helical in configuration. Each of the two heavy chains of whole cardiac myosin can bind one or more light chains (Figure 9). Importantly, these light chains appear to modulate the activity of myosin ATPase. Figure 10 shows the change from a loose coil to a tight coil that occurs in heavy meromyosin S_2 with the hydrolysis of ATP. As the result of this process, the angulation of the head of myosin increases, thereby moving the heavy meromyosin S_1 head of myosin approximately 100 Å parallel to the light meromyosin backbone (Figure 10B).

Figure 11A is a three-dimensional model of a

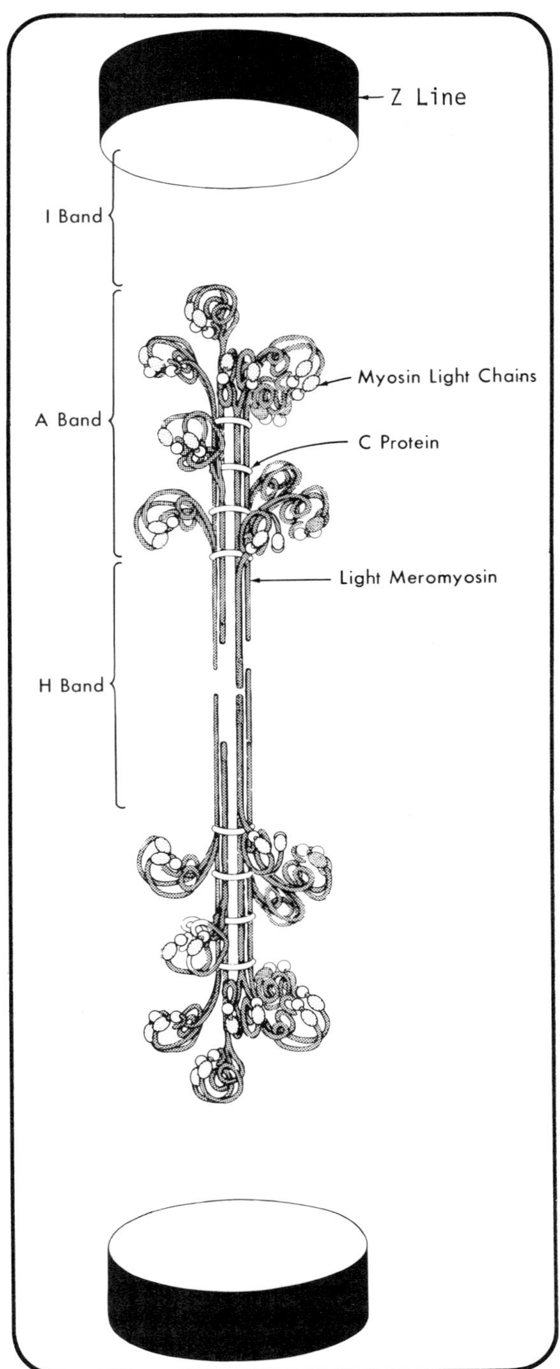

FIGURE 7. Three-dimensional view of a single thick filament containing several pairs of myosin molecules.

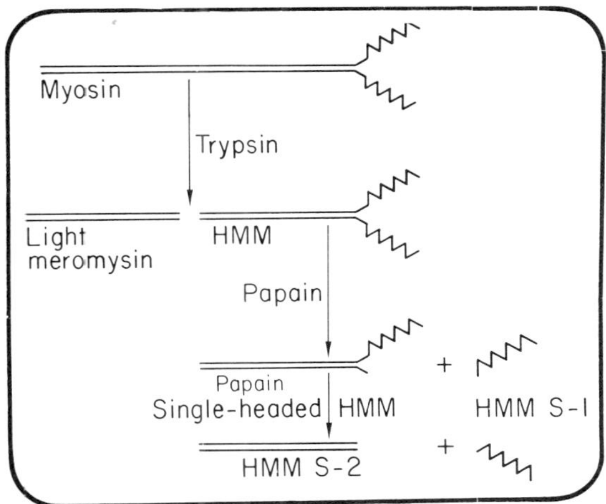

FIGURE 8. Separation of the components of whole myosin by cleavage with proteolytic enzymes. Trypsin produces the two major fragments: light meromyosin and heavy meromyosin (HMM). Papain digestion results in division of heavy meromyosin into its S_2 and S_1 fragments.

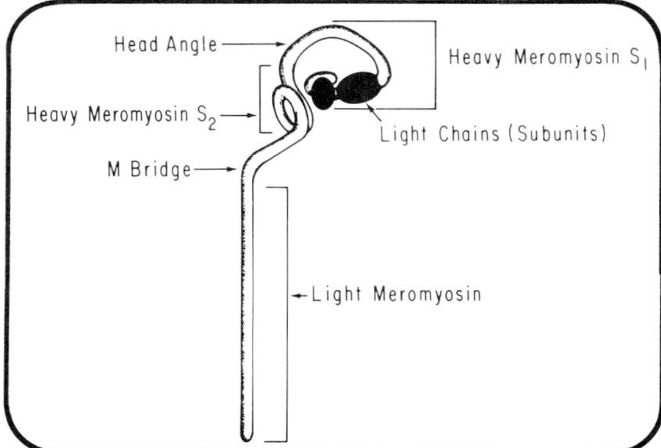

FIGURE 9. Representation of the configuration of one of the two heavy chains of whole myosin. The myosin heavy chain is comprised of light meromyosin and heavy meromyosin. The M bridge is between light and heavy meromyosin, and the head angle between heavy meromyosin S_1 and S_2. In addition, two light chains are bound within the heavy chain myosin head (HMM S_1).

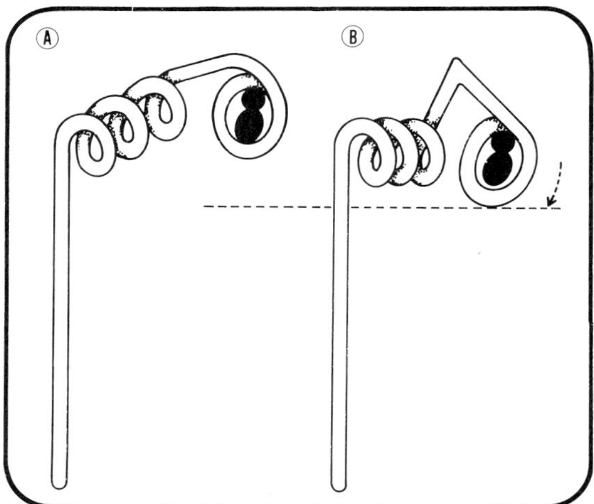

FIGURE 10. Representation of a heavy chain of whole myosin showing the change in the heavy meromyosin S_2 region from a loose coil (**A**) to a tight coil (**B**) during the hydrolysis of ATP by myosin ATPase in the myosin head with heart muscle contraction. With the binding of ATP and cation (**A**) to the myosin head, the M bridge angle increases so that the myosin head makes contact with turned-on actin. Then with hydrolysis of ATP and binding of ADP in the myosin head (**B**), the head angle between heavy meromyosin S_2 and S_1 increases, which results in the inward swivel (**arrow**) of the myosin head (up to the distance indicated by the **broken line**), thereby causing the actin filament to be propelled towards the center of the sarcomere (in the direction of the **arrow**).

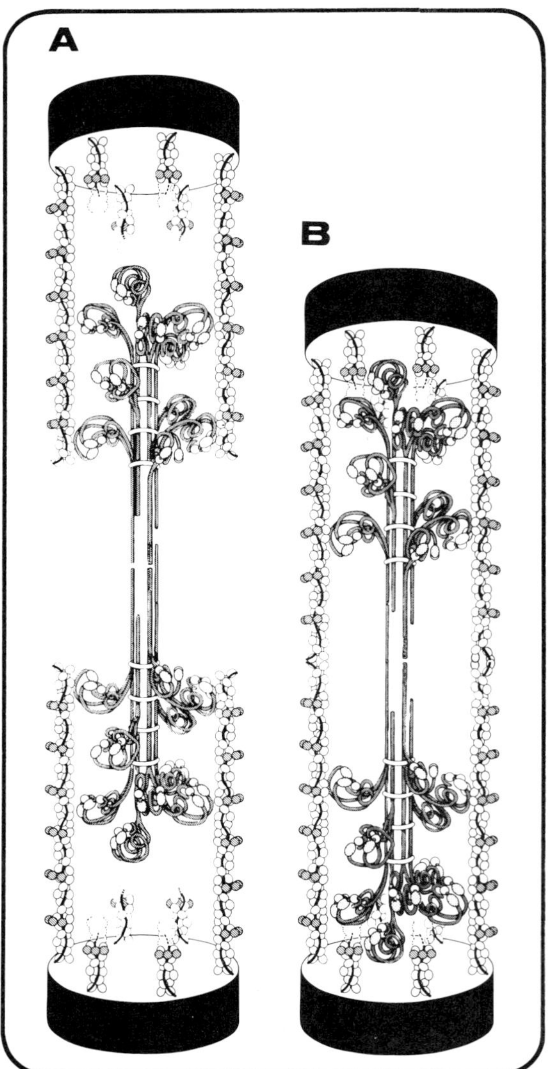

FIGURE 11. Three-dimensional view of a complete thick filament surrounded at each of its ends by six thin filaments, two of which are shown in full length. The lateral limits of the sarcomere are shown by the Z lines (disc-like in appearance in this diagram) to which the lateral ends of the thin filaments are attached. **A,** the sarcomere is in the relaxed state with the central ends of the thin filaments extending only up to the beginning of the central H zone. **B,** with the active state of complete contraction, the central ends of the actin filaments from both sides of the sarcomere are in contract, thereby entirely closing the H zone. In addition, the movement of the thin filaments towards the middle of the sarcomere during systole decreases the distance between the two Z lines; this process underlies cardiac muscle shortening during contraction.

sarcomere in the relaxed state in which the thick filament is shown with two of the six thin filaments that surround it. On contraction, the thin filament moves centrally, thereby closing the area of the H band (Figure 11B). Thus the sequence in Figure 11, A and B, demonstrates the systolic movement of the thin filaments, bringing the Z lines attached to the thin filaments closer together after a series of ATP hydrolysis cycles takes place in the myosin heads during the active state. The Z lines are the terminal ends of the sarcomere and thus demark the zone of contact between the sarcomeres in series. The series of sarcomeres, constituting the myofibrils, are attached to the intercalating discs, which are derivatives of the external cell membrane. From these observations, it is apparent that when the sarcomeres shorten during contraction, the whole cardiac fiber in turn shortens. The proteins that comprise the Z lines are presently being purified and identified; as stated, they are bound tightly to the outer ends of the actin filaments.

The decrease in distance between the Z lines of a single sarcomere upon contraction results in the partial or total disappearance of the I bands, depending on the degree of shortening. Shortening may terminate when myosin is in contact with the Z lines (Figure 11B). However, systolic shortening may terminate before myosin reaches the Z lines, or conversely, contraction may continue to the extreme extent of compressing the thick filaments into a wavy pattern and causing the thin filaments to slip past one another in the H band region.

Myosin ATPase Activity

Two conditions are necessary for myocardial contraction—"charged" myosin and "turned-on" actin. The mechanism by which the thin filaments slide centrally during contraction is under intense investigation. The current postulation is that the driving force is derived from hydrolysis of ATP by myosin ATPase with transfer of the hydrolyzed products, adenosine diphosphatase (ADP) plus inorganic phosphate (P_i), to another region in myosin. It is known that myosin binds ATP and a cation. Then ATP is transferred to another position in myosin and a change in myosin conformation occurs, thus forming a "charged" myosin that can react with a "turned-on" actin.[8]

The sequence of this process of activation of myosin is depicted in Figure 12. With binding of ATP (Figure 12B–1) and cation (Figure 12B–2) to the myosin head, there is an increase in the M bridge angle so that the head of myosin comes in contact with actin[9] (Figure 12B–2). It is further speculated that ATP is hydrolyzed (Figure 12B–3), with the energy from hydrolysis and the transfer of ADP to myosin being utilized to swivel the head from an angle of approximately 90° to one of 45° (Figure 12B–3). This swivel of the myosin heads results in the movement of the thin filaments toward the center of the sarcomere.[10] The products, ADP and P_i, are next shifted to another position in myosin, with P_i being first released and then ADP released from the myosin molecule. Detachment of myosin from actin is achieved only after another ATP is bound to myosin (Figure 12B–4). Finally, the resting state is reached in which ATP is no longer bound to the myosin head (Figure 12B–5). Myosin can then again proceed to the "charged" state by rebinding of ATP and cation to the myosin head, thereby undergoing another hydrolysis cycle.

For each single cycle of contraction, actin is moved approximately 100 Å. To bring the Z line adjacent to the end of the A band, myosin must undergo approximately 35 ATP hydrolysis cycles.[11,12] Thus, as shown in Figure 12A, the total distance the thin filament is moved is 3,500 Å in this example. The precise mechanism by which muscle contraction is terminated remains to be delineated.[13]

In heart muscle, Sonnenblick and Skelton[14] have shown that the extent of diastolic overlap of actin and myosin filaments between sarcomer lengths of 1.5 to 2.2 μ is directly related to the force of contraction, the strongest contraction occurring at the maximal overlap of 2.2μ initial sarcomere length and the weakest at 1.5μ with the minimal overlap (Figure 13). Normally, heart muscle operates at an intermediate point, usually in the upper portion, on the steep ascending limb of its active length-tension curve. Thereby, the muscle can improve its systolic performance by augmenting end-diastolic length.[15] This increase in contractile perfor-

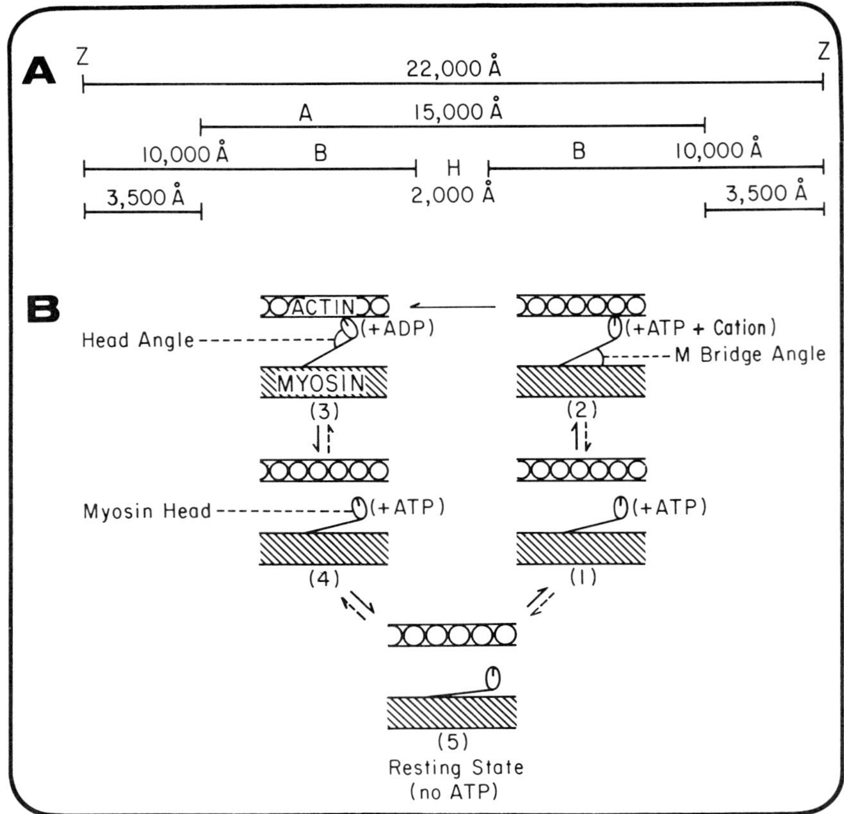

FIGURE 12. A, the spacing of the myofibrillar proteins within the sarcomere (a = thick filament; B = two thin filaments; H = central H zone; Z = two Z lines). **B,** the sequence of the process of activation of myosin. Diagrammed are the configurational changes that occur in heavy meromyosin due to the binding of ATP and cation to the myosin head with hydrolysis of ATP by myosin ATPase, resulting in subsequent movement of the actin filament. **Frames 1** through **4** represent progressive phases of the active state and the resting state is in **frame 5.**

mance is the result of an increase in "turned-on" actin molecules or elevation of myosin ATPase activity, or both.

When myosin ATPase activity is elevated, the number of active actin-myosin cross-bridges formed is increased, depending on the number of "turned-on" actin molecules, the latter being related to the availability of Ca^{++}. An increase in the number of such cross-bridges established during the active state by increased myosin ATPase activity may augment the intensity of the interaction between the thick and thin filaments within the sarcomere, thereby increasing the strength of contraction and the degree of muscle shortening. In addition, these two properties of systole are dependent on end-diastolic muscle length and factors that initiate the process of relaxation.

Rigor Complexes: An exception to the normal events constituting actin-myosin binding just described is the formation of rigor complexes[12] (Figure 14). A rigor complex is formed by an uncharged myosin molecule containing no substrate (ATP) reacting with a turned-off (Figure 14) actin molecule. In this manner, an actin-myosin cross-bridge is established with actin being turned on (Figure 14B) but no mechanical contraction performed. Under these conditions myosin cannot move the thin filament, and the actin is released only with the availability of ATP. Thus, the rigidity of muscle that occurs after death (rigor mortis) results directly from

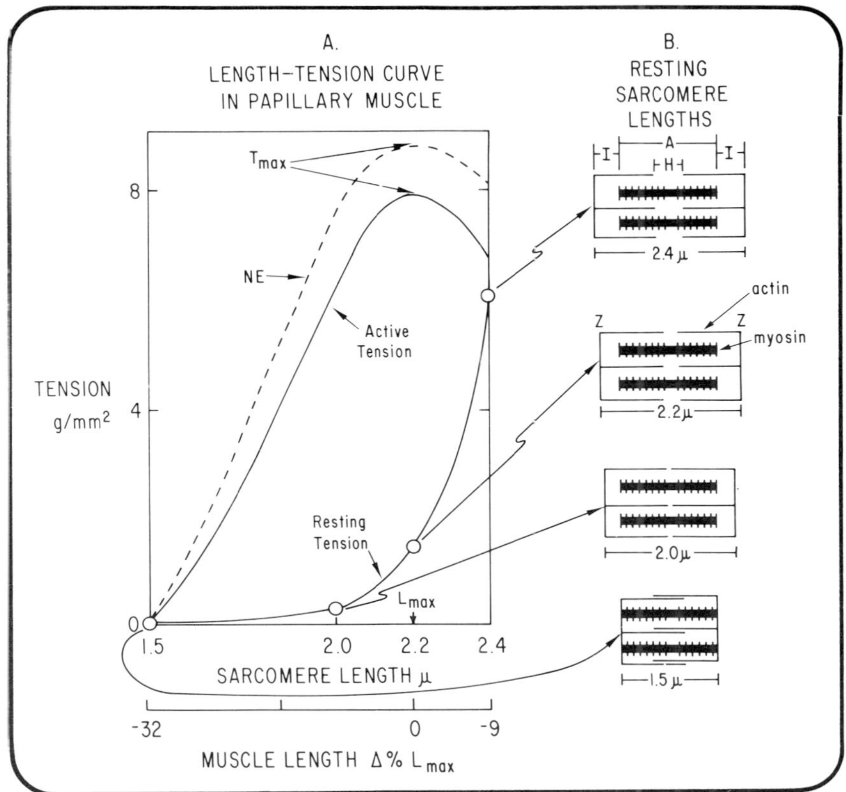

FIGURE 13. **A,** the typical length-tension relationship of normal heart muscle. Given are the relations between active and resting tension development and sarcomere and cardiac muscle length. The active tension curve is elevated by increased contractile state induced by norepinephrine (NE). Tmax = maximal active tension; Lmax = resting muscle length at which Tmax occurs. **B,** resting sarcomere lengths showing relations between actin and myosin filaments at different end-diastolic preloads. (Reprinted by permission from Mason et al.[15])

lack of ATP. When rigor complexes are produced in the presence of low ATP concentrations, it is possible that a few charged myosin molecules form active actin-myosin complexes with turned-on actin molecules, which may result in some movement of the actin filament by myosin-mediated hydrolysis (Figure 14C). The mechanism by which the rigor complex can turn on actin in the absence of calcium has not been clarified (Figure 14B).

Normal Right and Left Ventricles: In studies carried out in our laboratories,[16–18] myosin was purified[16] from normal canine right and left ventricles as well as from skeletal muscle, and the maximal rate of myosin ATPase activity (enzymatic Vmax values) was determined in each tissue. As shown in Figure 15, there were pronounced differences in the enzymatic Vmax values of myosin from the three muscles.[17,18] Myosin ATPase activities dependent on potassium (K^+) and calcium (C^{++}) ions were greater in the normal left ventricle compared with those in the normal right ventricle with various concentrations of ATP (Figure 15, A and B) and with various concentrations of K^+ and Ca^{++} activator cations (Figure 15, D and E). Interestingly, with ammonium ion (NH_4^+) as the activator cation, myosin ATPase activities were similar in the three muscles (Figure 15, C and F). Since myosin ATPase activity varies with temperature, it is important that the enzymatic assay be carried out with this factor constant; myosin ATPase activity rises considerably with increasing temperature (Figure 16).

Right Ventricular Systolic Pressure Overloading: The effects of chronic right ventricular systolic pressure overloading on myosin ATPase activity in the hemodynamically stressed ventricle have been evaluated in a series of canine studies in our laboratories.[19,20] Mild pulmonic stenosis was produced by partial banding of the main pulmonary artery, causing elevation of right ventricular peak systolic pressure to 60 percent above normal. This mild right ventricular pressure overload was found to be accompanied by a progressive increase in enzymatic activity of right ventricular K^+- and Ca^{++}-activated myosin ATPase, which increased to a peak 35 percent above normal values at 5 weeks after induction of mild pulmonic stenosis[19] (Figure 17). Thereafter, the myosin ATPase values became less elevated and were

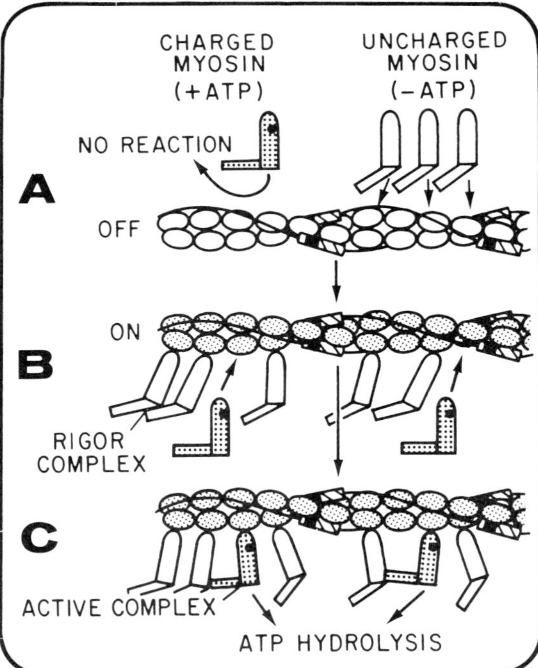

FIGURE 14. Representation of the formation of actin-myosin rigor complexes. **A (right)**, an uncharged myosin (without ATP) is capable of reacting with a turned-off actin filament. **B**, a rigor complex is thereby established with actin being turned on but no mechanical work accomplished. **C**, charged myosin (with ATP) can now react with the turned-on actin to form active actin-myosin complexes, with the result that there is some movement of the actin filament with ATP hydrolysis occurring in the charged myosin heads.

significantly below control values by 16 weeks after banding[19] (Figure 17).

In contrast to mild pulmonic stenosis, chronic severe systolic pressure overload of the right ventricle effected by Jacobson cuff inflation of the main pulmonary artery, elevating right ventricular peak systolic pressure to 300 percent above control, did not result in increased myosin ATPase activity in the stressed ventricle. Instead, K^+- and Ca^{++}-activated right ventricular myosin ATPase decreased to 12 percent below normal values after 6 weeks of severe pressure overloading.[20] Therefore, the effects of chronic systolic pressure overloading on the enzymatic performance of right ventricular myosin are dependent on both the degree and duration of obstruction to pulmonic outflow.

Left Ventricular Systolic Pressure Overloading: The influences of chronic systolic pressure overloading on the canine left ventricle also have been evaluated by investigations in our laboratories.[21,22] Mild aortic stenosis, produced by partial banding of the ascending aorta, caused a peak systolic pressure gradient of 30 mm Hg, which was associated with a mild rise in myosin ATPase activity in the left ventricle after 5 weeks of obstruction.[21] In contrast, chronic experimentally produced marked systolic pressure overloading of the left ventricle, resulting in a peak systolic transaortic outflow pressure gradient of 50 mm Hg, led to a decline in K^+- and Ca^{++}-activated enzymatic Vmax values of left ventricular myosin ATPase after 5 weeks of severe aortic stenosis.[22] In addition, there was further progressive decline in myosin ATPase activity in the stressed left ventricle during the remainder of the period of 16 weeks of severe aortic stenosis.

These observations are consistent with those just described for the right ventricle exposed to pulmonic stenosis and indicate that mild outflow obstruction causes transient increases in myosin enzymatic values in the mildly stressed ventricle whereas severe obstruction to ejection produces sustained declines in myosin ATPase function in the markedly pressure-overloaded ventricle. Thus a differential response to canine myosin ATPase activity takes place in the stressed ventricle in chronic right and left ventricular systolic pressure overloading that is dependent upon the severity and duration of obstruction.

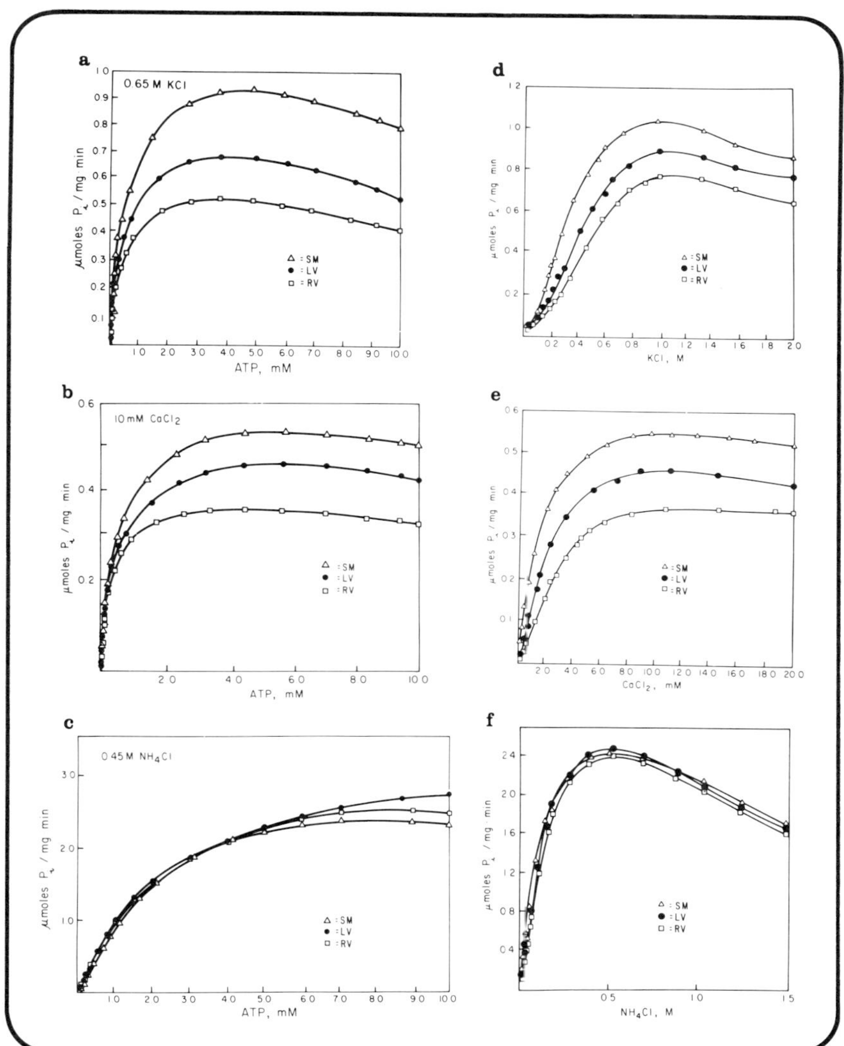

FIGURE 15. Comparative activity of canine myosin ATPase activities from normal left ventricle (LV), normal right ventricle (RV) and skeletal muscle (SM). **A, B** and **C,** myosin ATPase activity is related to increasing concentrations of ATP with the concentration of activator cation constant. **D, E** and **F,** myosin ATPase activity is related to increasing concentrations of activator cation with the concentration of ATP constant. The activator cation is K^+ in **A** and **D,** Ca^{++} in **B** and **E,** and NH_4^+ in **C** and **F.** (Reprinted by permission from Wikman-Coffelt et al.[18])

Subunits of Myosin

In view of these differences in myosin ATPase values—myosin activity in the normal left ventricle being greater than that in the normal right ventricle, and enzymatic performance becoming augmented in hypertrophied muscle in mild ventricular hemodynamic overloading in contrast with marked ventricular pressure overloading—we have undertaken the examination of alterations in the substructure of canine myosin in normal and abnormal conditions to evaluate the possibility that changes in the molecular structure of this contractile protein might provide an explanation for the mechanisms regulating myosin enzymatic function.

When myosin is incubated with the reducing agent sodium dodecylsulfate the enzyme disso-

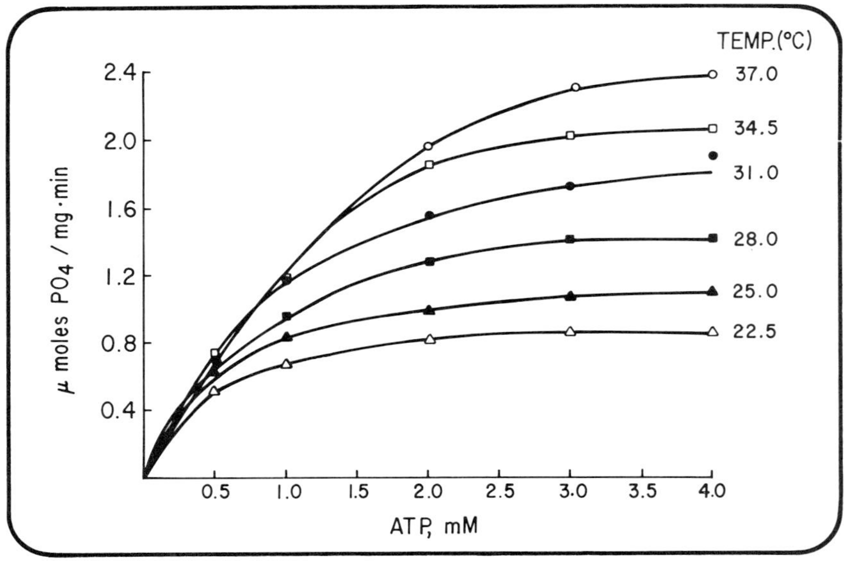

FIGURE 16. Comparative kinetics of normal canine left ventricular myosin ATPase activity at different incubation temperatures. K[+] served as the activator cation.

ciates into its component chains or subunits. In synthesis of these myosin chains, each individual chain is governed by its separate set of messengers during the process of protein translation described subsequently.[23] The various polypeptide chains of myosin are held together by ionic, hydrophobic and disulfide bonds. These chains can then be identified by gel electrophoresis. Further, the light chains of myosin also can be dissociated from whole myosin by treatment with urea. The heavy chains of myosin can then be precipitated by water dilutions, leaving the light chains in solution.

Immunologic Properties: The heavy chains of canine myosin from normal right ventricles, pressure-overloaded hypertrophied right ventricles, and normal left ventricles were observed to be immunologically identical.[18,24,25] Mobility on polyacrylamide electrophoresis was also the same for the three classes of myosin chains found: heavy chains, light chain C_1 and light chain C_2.[18,24,25] Figure 18 demonstrates the electrophoretic mobility of these myosin chains from normal right ventricle and hypertrophied right ventricle.

Proportion of Heavy and Light Chains: Quantification of myosin subunits was accomplished by a new technique using dye-staining of proteins in polyacrylamide gels.[26] Based on the quantified absorbance of Coomassie[®] blue to proteins, the myosin subunits were stained with the dye and fixed in polyacrylamide gels, and the protein concentration was then determined from analysis of the eluted dye. Using this dye elution technique, quantification of myosin subunits in polyacrylamide gels was achieved. The proportion of light chains present in hypertrophied right ventricular myosin and normal left ventricular myosin was the same, light chains constituting 10 percent of total myosin; in contrast, normal right ventricular myosin contained twice the amount of light chains, 20 percent.[25,26] The proportion of light chain C_1 to light chain C_2 was the same for each of these three ventricular tissues.[25,26]

Molecular Weight of Myosin and Myosin Subunits: The molecular weights of canine right and left ventricular myosins were determined by sedimentation equilibrium studies.[27] The molecular weight of normal right ventricular myosin was found to be 574,000; that of normal left ventricular myosin, in which there are fewer light chains, was 524,000. It is postulated that myosin with fewer light chains, such as that from the normal left ventricle compared with that from the normal right ventricle has an al-

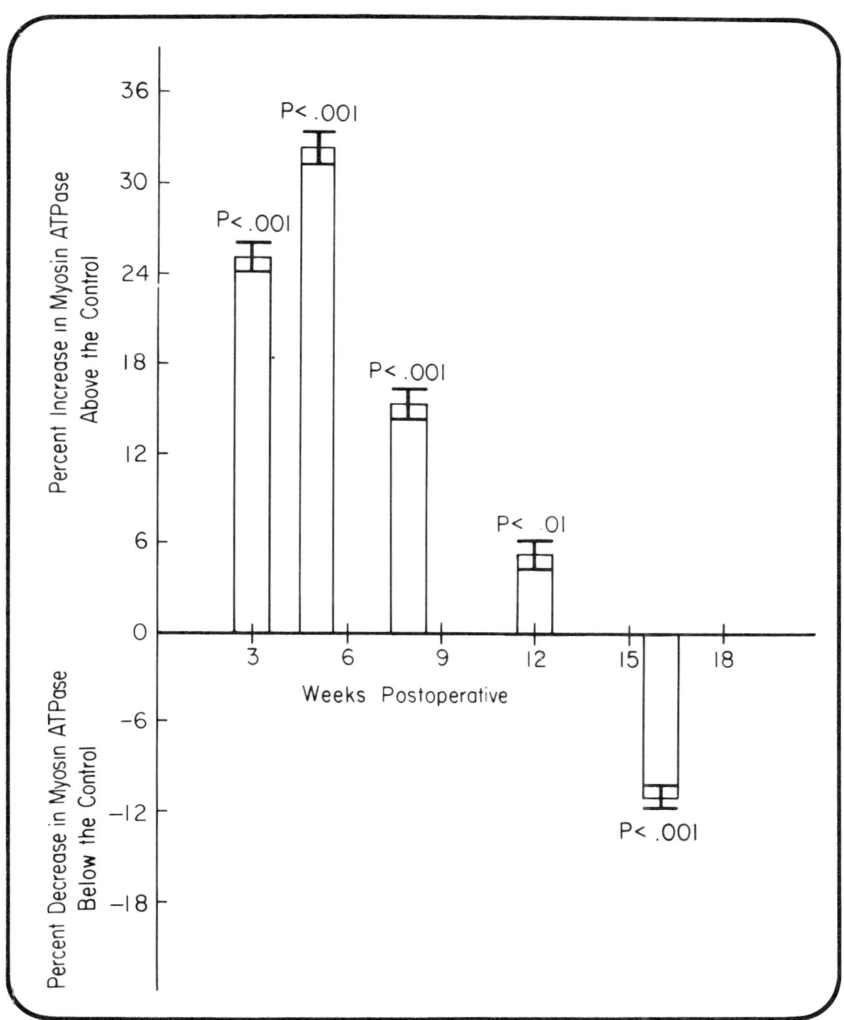

FIGURE 17. Average enzymatic Vmax values for K$^+$-activated right ventricular myosin ATPase in mild pulmonic stenosis experimentally produced in dogs. Weeks postoperative = time after partial pulmonary artery banding. (Reprinted by permission from Wikman-Coffelt et al.[19])

tered molecular conformation, which thereby increases myosin ATPase activity.

The molecular weights of the subunits of canine ventricular myosin were then determined.[18] By converting the protein concentrations of these subunits to moles, it was demonstrated that there was approximately one mole of light chain per mole of heavy chain in both early hypertrophied (from mild pulmonic stenosis) right ventricular myosin and normal left ventricular myosin; however, there were approxi-

mately two moles of light chains per mole of heavy chain in normal right ventricular myosin.[25] From these data, a decrease in myosin light chains was found to be related to an increase in myosin enzymatic activity.

Calcium Binding: It has been shown in skeletal muscle that only one of the myosin light chains binds calcium; the remaining light chains do not.[28] In calcium-binding studies of canine ventricular myosins, we have shown that normal left ventricular myosin binds 1.4 moles

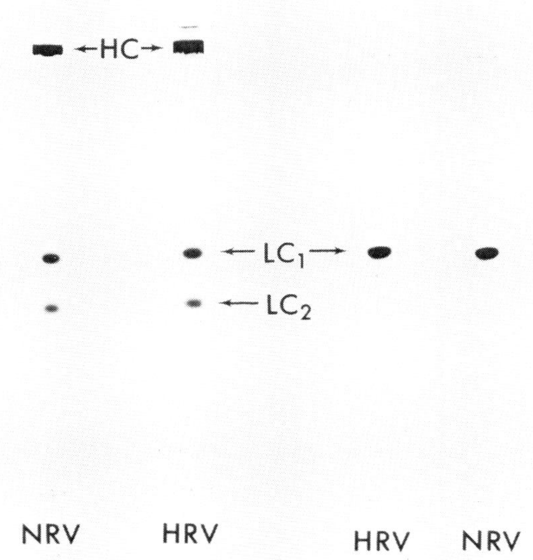

FIGURE 18. Comparative electrophoretic gel (6 percent polyacrylamide) mobility (in 0.1 percent dodecylsulfate) of myosin from normal canine right ventricle (NRV) and from early hypertrophied canine right ventricle (HRV) due to mild pulmonic stenosis. HC = myosin heavy chains; LC$_1$ and LC$_2$ = different myosin light chains. The HC and LC$_1$ and LC$_2$ of NRV and HRV in the two left-hand columns demonstrate that the mobility characteristics of these purified chains are the same in both normal and hypertrophied ventricles. Likewise, isolated LC$_1$ of HRV and NRV in the two right-hand columns shows that this purified light chain retains the same mobility properties in both normal and hypertrophied myocardium.

of calcium per mole of myosin (Figure 19A), whereas normal right ventricular myosin binds twice the amount of calcium, 2.8 moles of calcium per mole of myosin[29] (Figure 19B). The results of these calcium-binding studies are in agreement with our findings of approximately two light chains per heavy chain in normal canine right ventricular myosin and approximately one light chain per heavy chain in normal canine left ventricular myosin (Figure 20). It appears that each of the heavy chains of canine myosin can bind a monomer, dimer or possibly a trimer of their respective light chains; it is probable that specific ventricular myosins under certain conditions comprise a varying combination of these binding characteristics. The top panel of Figure 20 indicates the possibility that two different genes control the production

of myosin subunits—one for heavy chains and one for light chains. There are separate messenger RNA molecules for the light and heavy chains of myosin.[23,30] In addition, we have shown the turnover rate of heavy chains is twice that of light chains in the canine ventricle.[31]

Light Chain Components: With one-dimensional gel electrophoresis, myosin light chains can be separated into two types—C$_1$ and C$_2$. Utilizing a special modification[32] of the technique of two-dimensional polyacrylamide gel electrophoresis,[33] it has been possible to further resolve the canine myosin light chains C$_1$ and C$_2$ into additional components[32] (Figure 21). In each of the panels in Figure 21, the stained one-dimensional gel is shown above the two-dimensional slab gel. Figure 21C illustrates the two-dimensional gel for light chains C$_1$ and C$_2$ of myosin from the normal right ventricle. Figure 21A shows that the myosin light chain C$_1$ from the normal right ventricle is composed of four components on two-dimensional gel electrophoresis.[32] Comparison of Figure 21, A and C indicates that the myosin light chain C$_2$ from the normal right ventricle consists of a single component on two-dimensional gel electrophoresis.[32]

Compared with the four C$_1$ light chain components of myosin from the normal right ventricle myosin (Figure 21C), two-dimensional gel electrophoresis revealed significantly less myosin C$_{1d}$ component from the hypertrophied right ventricle in the early period after mild pulmonic stenosis when right ventricular myosin ATPase activity was elevated[25] (Figure 21, B and D). The concentration of C$_{1d}$ was also found to be low in normal canine left ventricular myosin and in normal canine skeletal muscle myosin; both of these myosins have higher ATPase activities than has normal right ventricular myosin.[18] These series of observations correlating high myosin ATPase activity with reduced levels of myosin light chains strongly suggest that myosin enzymatic activity is modulated by myosin light chains. Moreover, increased myosin enzymatic function appears to be due to reduction of light chain inhibition of myosin ATPase activity.

Phorphorylation of Myosin: In additional canine studies, in vivo phosphorylated ventricular myosin subunits were identified after the injection of radioactive sodium phosphate (^{32}P)

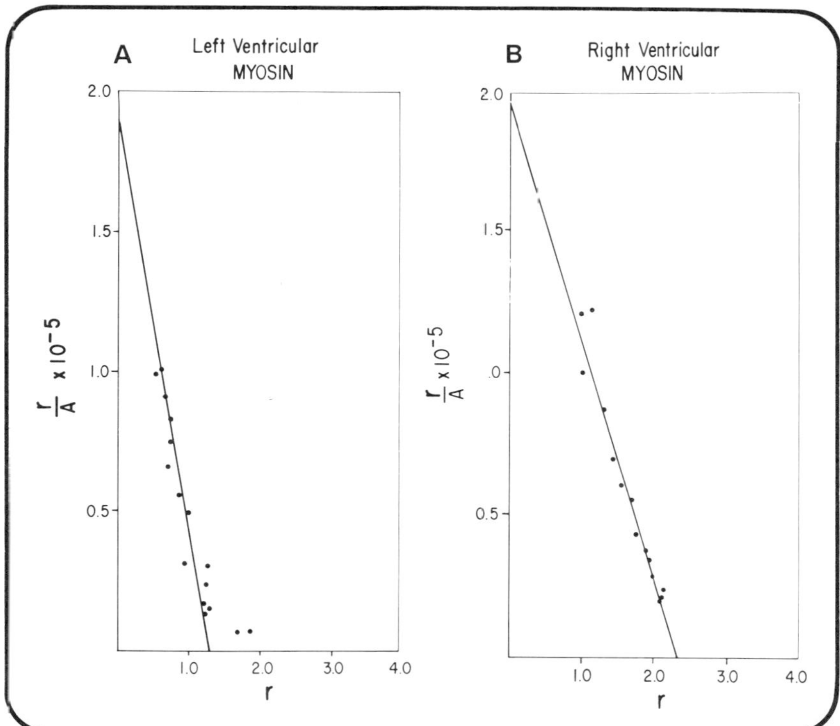

FIGURE 19. Calcium binding (^{45}Ca) in normal canine left ventricular (**A**) and right ventricular (**B**) myosins. The regression line was calculated from the number of calcium-binding sites according to the method of Scatchard with the calcium-binding affinity constant (r) determined by the intercept of the plot with the abscissa.

into normal animals.[34] Two days after injection, at the time of peak protein labeling, the light and heavy chains of cardiac myosin were analyzed for incorporation of radioactivity into these myosin subunits separated by dodecylsulfate gels. The specific activity of purified myosin heavy chains was 20 times greater than that of the light chains in counts per minute/millimole of the myosin subunit.[34] Since bound phosphate in the heavy chains was only 10 times greater than that in the light chains,[34] these findings are consistent with our previous observation that canine cardiac myosin heavy chains have twice the turnover rate of light chains.[31]

Concerning phosphorylation of the isotope in the light chains, 84 percent was incorporated into light chain C_2 and 16 percent into C_1. Two-dimensional gel electrophoresis and isoelectrofocusing were employed to determine isotope incorporation into the various myosin light chain C_1 components; the greatest specific radioactivity was in component C_{1d}.[34] These studies indicate that phosphorylation of myosin subunits occurs during protein synthesis.

In regard to the greater rate of phosphorylation of myosin heavy chains compared with that of light chains, the same results were obtained with canine cardiac fetal tissue cultured in the presence of ^{32}P.[35] In another study of the phosphorylation of cardiac myosin, the moles of bound phosphate were compared with the activity of myosin ATPase in the non-stressed left ventricle of dogs subjected to chronic mild pulmonic stenosis;[19] myosin-bound phosphate was inversely related to the enzymatic activity of myosin.

Mechanism of Myosin ATPase Alterations in Hemodynamic Overload: To conclude this section, a mechanism is postulated by which left ventricular myosin ATPase activity is depressed during chronic severe left ventricular systolic pressure overloading.[22] In dogs with severe ex-

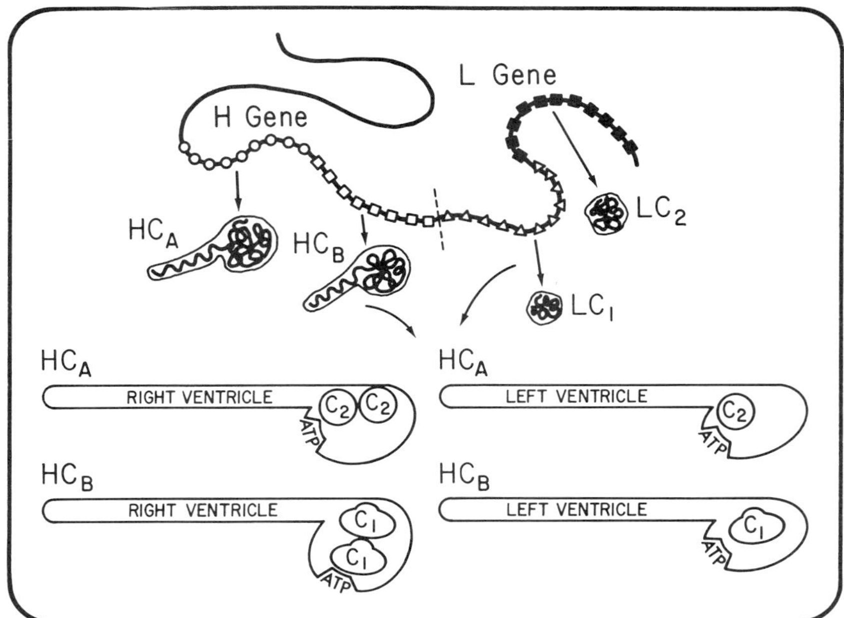

FIGURE 20. Diagrams of normal canine right ventricular myosin (**bottom left**) and of normal canine left ventricular myosin (**bottom right**). The possibility of two different configurations of heavy chains (HC$_A$ and HC$_B$) is illustrated. The **upper panel** suggests two separate genomes for myosin, one for heavy chains (H) and the other for light chains (L). C$_1$ and C$_2$ = the two types of light chains.

perimental aortic stenosis, K$^+$- and Ca^{++}-activated myosin ATPase values progressively decline in the stressed ventricle. The function of myosin in the impaired left ventricle of such hearts becomes similar to that of myosin in the right ventricle of normal hearts. After prolonged severe outflow obstruction, left ventricular myosin simulates normal right ventricular myosin in ATPase activity, proportion of light to heavy chains and degree of calcium binding. Therefore, myosin in the markedly pressure-overloaded left ventricle develops elevations of myosin light chains that appear to suppress myosin enzymatic activity and allow for greater binding of calcium per mole of myosin. Thus in the presence of severe aortic stenosis, abnormal left ventricular myosin undergoes changes in its properties to those of normal right ventricular myosin.

Our findings in dogs with mild pulmonic stenosis[19] are in agreement with the concept that hemodynamic overload induces alterations in myosin ATPase activity through changes in the number of light chains in myosin. Thus, as-

sociated with the elevation of myosin enzymatic activity in the early hypertrophied right ventricle, there was a decrease in the percentage of myosin light chains present in the mildly stressed ventricle. In the case of mild systolic pressure overload, it is suggested that the alterations in myosin chain proportions in the mildly stressed ventricle are the result of the elevation of protein synthesis with disparate turnover rates for light and heavy chains of myosin. Since the turnover rate of heavy chains is greater than that of light chains, the mildly hypertrophied right ventricle develops the myosin chain proportions and greater myosin enzymatic activity of myosin from the left ventricle of normal hearts.

Cardiac Protein Synthesis

The mechanisms of protein synthesis in the heart are generally the same as those in other organs. Protein synthesis in the myocardium provides a continuously operative system for renewal of fiber structure and enzymatic ma-

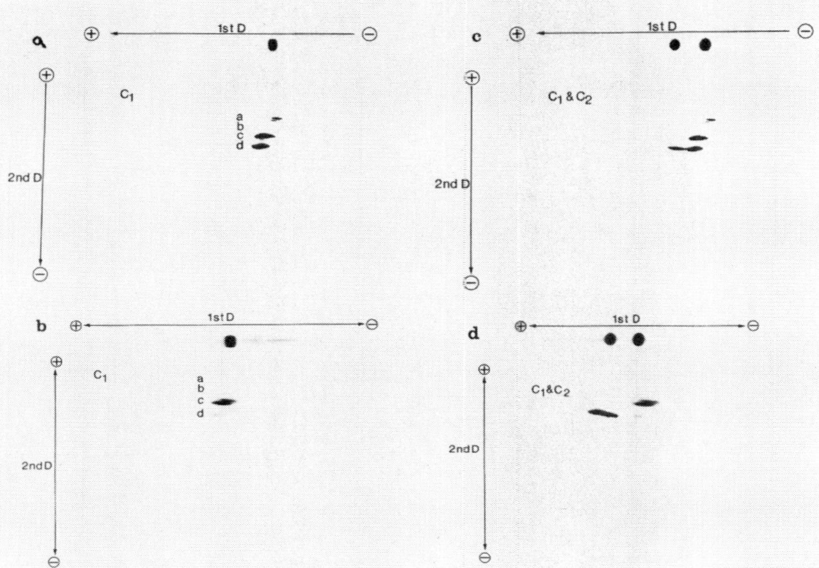

FIGURE 21. Two-dimensional gel electrophoresis patterns (2nd D) of purified canine myocardial myosin light chains. One-dimensional gel electrophoretic patterns (1st D) are shown above each two-dimensional pattern. The patterns of light chain C_1 (**A**) and those of light chains C_1 and C_2 (**C**) from normal right ventricle are shown. For comparison, the patterns of light chain C_1 (**B**) and light chains C_1 and C_2 (**D**) from early hypertrophied right ventricle due to mild pulmonic stenosis at the time right ventricular myosin ATPase activity was elevated are shown. (Reprinted by permission from Wikman-Coffelt et al.[25])

chinery, as well as a rapidly responsive compensatory mechanism for ventricular hypertrophy induced by cardiac mechanical stress. ATP is consumed in the process of protein systhesis, which consists of the stages of: (1) replication in the nucleus (DNA-controlled synthesis of DNA by DNA polymerase); (2) transcription in the nucleus in which nucleoli are centers of RNA activity (RNA synthesis by RNA polymerase on the chromosomal template); and (3) translation involving three types of RNA in the sarcoplasm (formation of specific proteins on ribosomal RNA, directed by messenger RNA containing the genetic code, from amino acids carried by transfer RNA).

Excessive intramyocardial tension appears to be the transducer that couples mechanical systolic overload with increased protein synthesis. Increased muscle mass resulting from chronic elevation of hemodynamic burden is due to hypertrophy rather than hyperplasia of myocardial fibers, although there is some proliferation of connective tissue cells. Activation of all stages of protein synthesis occurs rapidly after hemo-dynamic stress, with increases in DNA in connective tissue cells and elevations of RNA synthesis and incorporation of amino acids into proteins in myocardial cells. For example, even the creation of acute mild pulmonic stenosis in dogs was a potent stimulus for RNA and protein synthesis within 24 hours after pulmonary banding [36] (see Figure 9 in chapter 9), resulting in substantially increased weight of the hypertrophied right ventricle with correspondingly increased myosin content.

Transcription: Transcription is the process by which genetic information, stored in nuclear DNA, is transferred to RNA. The result is the formation of nucleotide polymers containing triplet codons corresponding to those found in DNA. As an example of the regulation of transcription, the process as delineated in a bacterial system involving a repressor[37,38] is depicted in Figure 22. The transcription process of gene control operates in the following manner. A regulatory gene directs the synthesis of a specific protein; the repressor binds to a metabolite or hormone and serves as the regulatory signal.

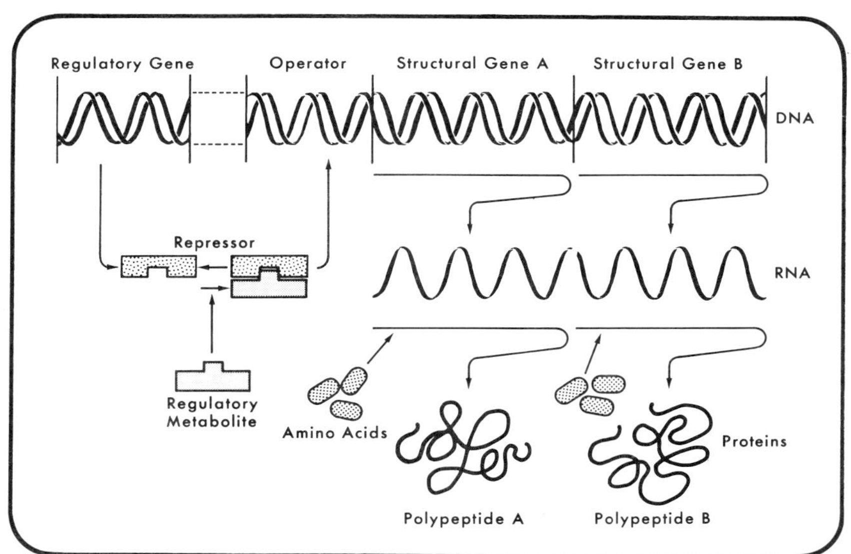

FIGURE 22. Diagram of two genes under one operator constituting a genome and the regulatory gene codes for the repressor, which in turn has the ability to repress or induce transcription of the genome, depending on the presence of certain metabolites in the system.

This binding can either activate or inactivate the repressor, depending on whether the system is repressive or inductive. The repressor in its active state binds the genetic operator and prevents production of messenger RNA from the associated structural gene. In contrast, in an inductive system, the operator remains repressed until the regulatory metabolite complexes with and prevents function of the repressor.[38] It is attractive to apply this model of gene control to the myosin system. Thus, in this transcription system, the cell possesses the ability to respond rapidly to new environmental stress, such as an excessive ventricular hemodynamic burden leading to myocardial hypertrophy. Further, the rapid elevation in RNA synthesis that occurs—for example, in the right ventricle with pulmonic stenosis—may be aided by the availability of an additional factor that acts as an inducer at the transcriptional level.

Translation: Translation is the cellular process through which information that has been transcribed to RNA is utilized to produce proteins (Figure 23). Protein synthesis takes place on cellular particles called ribosomes that travel along the instruction tape of messenger RNA reading the genetic message.[39] The process of translation is divided into three stages: (1) initiation; (2) elongation; and (3) termination. Before the sequence of translation is discussed, it is beneficial to examine the three different types of RNA involved in the process and the respective role of each type of RNA.

Ribosomal RNA (rRNA) is one of the three major types of RNA manufactured during the process of transcription. This type of RNA is transcribed from genes located on chromosomes found in the nucleolus. Initially, a precursor RNA molecule is formed and later cleaved to form an 18S and a 28S RNA subunit. The 28S subunit combines with several types of proteins, moves out of the nucleus and eventually forms the 60S component of the ribosomes. Likewise, the 18S subunit combines with protein, as well as with a smaller 5S RNA molecule, and thus forms the 40S component of the ribosome. The many different proteins that compose the ribosome are in equilibrium with a pool of free ribosomal proteins in the cytoplasm of the cell. Present evidence indicates that the turnover rate varies for each of these proteins.[40]

Messenger RNA (mRNA) is the second of the three types of RNA made in the nucleus and transported to the cytoplasm for production of a protein such as myosin. The mRNA molecules for myosin heavy chains have been purified.[30] It appears that both mRNA and its carrier protein are complexed to the smaller ribosomal subunits when they reach the cytoplasm (Figure 23). When mRNA was purified from the cytoplasm of various cells, it was found to be characterized by its long stretches of polyadenylic acid, one of the four nucleotides comprising RNA. Unlike rRNA and tRNA, mRNA has little tertiary structure and is thus very susceptible to ribonuclease cleavage.

Transfer RNA (tRNA) is the third type of RNA molecule. It is the smallest of the three. Several tRNA varieties have been sequenced, and it was found that the molecule has an overall cloverleaf configuration with about 80 percent of its nucleotides paired. Each amino acid has specific tRNA varieties to which it binds. Further, each amino acid also has a specific aminoacyl-tRNA synthetase enzyme that is responsible for mediating this binding reaction. Certain regions of these individual tRNA molecules contain the anticodon that can match up with the corresponding mRNA codon. This system provides the capacity for accurate recognition between amino acid and code of the mRNA to insure the proper placement of each amino acid in precise sequences in the formation of a specific polypeptide chain.

Specific Protein Synthesis: Protein synthesis is initiated by the complexing of mRNA to the 40S particle of the ribosome. This event is followed by the combination of the 40S particle with the associated mRNA to the larger 60S subunit of the ribosome. To begin translation of the mRNA tape, various soluble initiation factors are required. Certain of these factors, along with guanosine 5'-triphosphate (GTP) and the correct concentration of magnesium (Mg++) and ammonium (NH₄⁺) ions, provide the conditions for the binding of the first tRNA-associated amino acid to the initiating codon of the mRNA.

The complete ribosome contains two binding sites for tRNA. One site, located on the 40S ribosomal subunit, is designated the aminoacyl-tRNA binding site, and the other site on the subunit is referred to as the peptidyl-tRNA binding site. Present evidence indicates that the specific tRNA associated with amino acid formyl-methionine is required for the initiation of translation. It appears that the structure of this molecule enables it to move directly from the aminoacyl site to the peptidyl site on the ribosome, despite the fact it has only one amino acid bound to it. This translocation reaction allows the binding of a new tRNA and associated amino acid to the recently vacated 30S site of the ribosome. It is believed that the hydrolysis of GTP provides the energy needed in this translocation reaction. Two soluble factors, aminoacyl transferase I and II, along with sulfhydryl compounds and Mg++ and NH₄⁺, also play a role in this translocation.

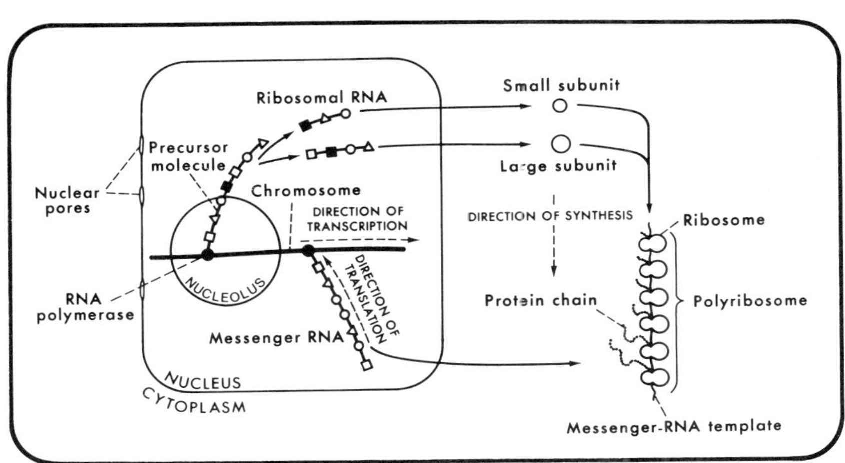

FIGURE 23. Diagram of transcription in the nucleus and translation in the cytoplasm. The transcription of ribosomal RNA is restricted to the nucleolus. The two ribosomal RNA molecules (28S and 18S RNA) are derived from the larger parent precursor molecule, which separates into the two.

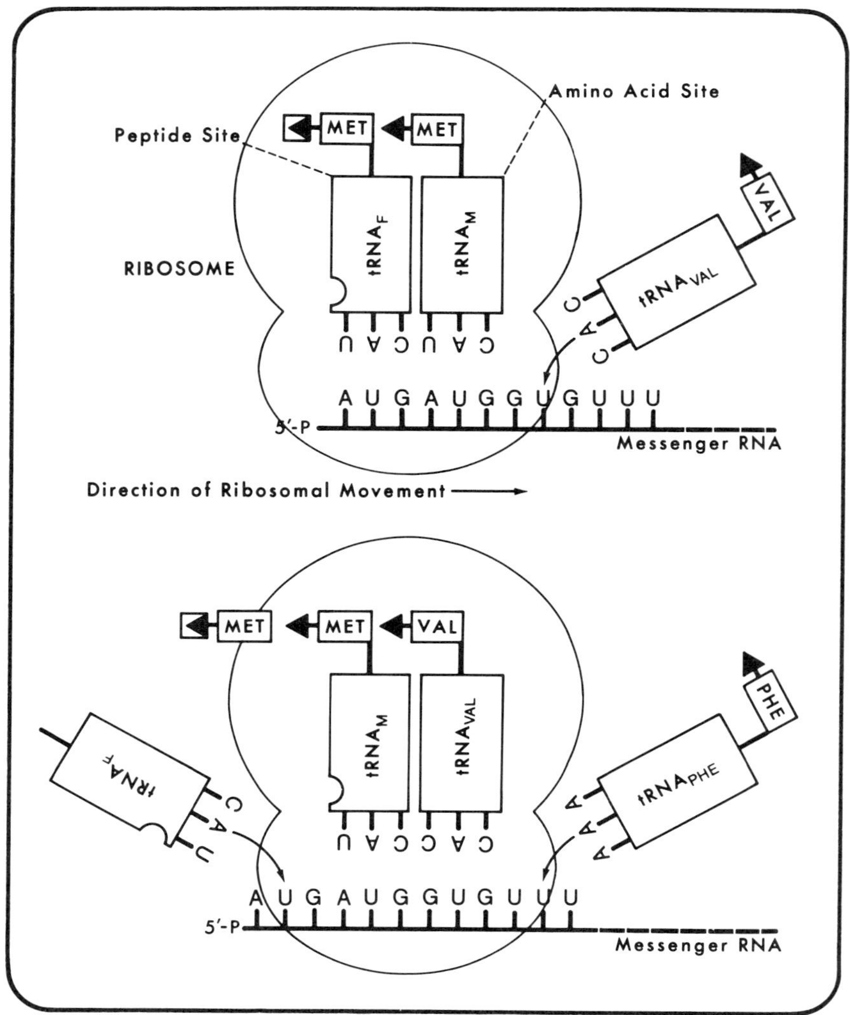

FIGURE 24. Diagram of translation occurring on the messenger RNA complexed to the ribosome. The process of translation begins at the 5' end of the messenger RNA. The transfer RNA molecules are shuttling amino acids to the peptide site to form the growing peptide chain.

The peptide bond formation necessary to bind the two separate amino acids is catalyzed by peptidyl synthetase, located in the 60S ribosomal subunit, and does not require soluble initiation factors or GTP. By continuing the cycle of tRNA binding, peptide bond formation and translocation, it is possible to form peptides containing specific amino acid sequences governed by the code provided by the mRNA (Figure 24).

Protein synthesis is concluded when the ribosome reads a terminator codon located on the mRNA. The terminator codon, in conjunction with certain releasing factors, dissociates the ribosome into its original 40S and 60S subunits and provides for the release of the protein and mRNA. Interestingly, it is possible for several ribosomes to read a single mRNA molecule simultaneously. In this situation, the group of ribosomes is referred to as a polyribosome.

Myosin Synthesis: As described previously, elevation in myosin synthesis is accompanied by augmentation of myosin ATPase activity in certain situations, such as in the stressed ventricle in the presence of mild pulmonic or mild aortic stenosis. At the same time, in these specific hemodynamic situations, the proportion of myosin heavy chains to myosin light chains is increased. In other studies it has been shown that myosin heavy chains have a turnover rate that is twice that of myosin light chains.[31] A phenomenon such as the disparate turnover rates of light and heavy chains of myosin might be the result of regulation at the level of translation or transcription.

A type of regulation at the translational level described for hemoglobin could occur in myosin synthesis. In the case of hemoglobin, there appears to be a selective translation of α or β chains depending on the presence of messenger-specific translational factors.[41] The greater turnover rate of myosin heavy chains might be due to greater affinity or availability of translational factors for the messenger for myosin heavy chains.

Conversely, the greater synthesis of myosin heavy chains in comparison with that of light chains may be due to control at the transcriptional level. As shown in Figure 22, each of the myosin chains might be under different genetic control, so that an activator of one gene would not necessarily be a potent activator of other genes. Gene amplification, which constitutes multiple copies of certain genome sequences, occurs in mammalian tissues. The possibility exists that there is redundancy of genes for myosin chains. Gene duplication facilitates speedy transcription when certain molecules are in great demand, such as occurs with ribosomes. This allows for several simultaneous transcriptions of the same type of molecule at one time. Thus it is speculated that there may be various degrees of gene duplication of the myosin chains (Figure 22), with each of the light and heavy chains having its code in a separate genome controlled by its own operator.

Summary

The hemodynamic function of the heart is dependent on the mechanical properties of its myocardium in which the sarcomere is the basic subcellular contractile unit. The contractile apparatus of the sarcomere consists of four protein molecular aggregates: the primary interacting (1) actin thin filaments and (2) myosin thick filaments and the modulator proteins (3) troponin and (4) tropomyosin, which inhibit actin-myosin reaction. Resting sarcomere length controls the extent of myofilament overlap, which determines the number of actin-myosin binding sites —the subcellular basis for the active length-tension curve. The intensity of interaction between thick and thin filaments regulates contractility. Excitation-contraction coupling is achieved when calcium from the sarcoplasmic reticulum and from outside the cell is delivered to troponin. The combination of calcium with troponin activates the contractile process by releasing troponin-tropomyosin inhibition of actin-myosin binding. Contraction occurs as a result of myosin ATPase-regulated cyclic interactions between the actin-myosin linkages, with the development of myocardial force and shortening.

The enzymatic function of myosin in the contractile process is governed by the subunit composition of whole myosin. Thus, myosin light chains within the heads of myosin appear to suppress the ATPase activity contained in the portion of the heavy chains comprising the myosin heads. Thus, compared with the normal right ventricle, the normal left ventricle possesses higher levels of K^+- and Ca^{++}-activated myosin ATPase associated with fewer myosin light chains in proportion to heavy chains. In mild hemodynamic overload, increased myosin enzymatic function occurred early in the hypertrophied stressed ventricle consequent to the production of relatively more heavy than light myosin subunits. Therefore, in the early period after mild experimental pulmonic stenosis, myosin from the hypertrophied right ventricle develops the properties of normal left ventricular myosin. Consistent with the concept that myosin light chains modulate the enzymatic performance of myosin are the findings in chronic severe canine aortic stenosis; myosin ATPase was depressed and the proportion of light to heavy chains of myosin increased in the markedly stressed left ventricle. Thus, in severe hemodynamic overload, myosin in the heavily stressed left ventricle develops the characteristics of normal right ventricular myosin.

Acknowledgment: This work was supported in part by Research Program Project Grants HL 14780 and AM 16716 from the National Institutes of Health and Research Grants from California chapters of the American Heart Association.

The authors wish to thank Barbara Giles and Leslie Silvernail for their administrative and secretarial assistance and Kathryn Marr and Hal Pullum for their medical artistry.

References

1. **Nakajima Y, Endo M:** Release of calcium induced by depolarization of the sarcoplasmic reticulum. Nature New Biol 246:216, 1973
2. **Hoyle G:** How is muscle turned on and off? Sci Amer 222:84, 1970
3. **Ostwald TJ, MacLennan DH:** Isolation of a high affinity calcium-binding protein from sarcoplasmic reticulum. J Biol Chem 249:973, 1973
4. **Cohen C, Caspar DLD, Johnson JP, et al:** Tropomyosin-troponin assembly. Cold Spring Harbor Sympos Quant Biol 37:287, 1972
5. **Perry SV, Cole HA, Head JF, et al:** Localization and mode of action of the inhibitor protein component of the troponin complex. Cold Spring Harbor Sympos Quant Biol 37:251, 1972
6. **Julian FJ, Sollins MR:** Regulation of force and speed of shortening in muscle contraction. Cold Spring Habor Sympos Quant Biol 37:635, 1972
7. **Lowey S, Slayter HS, Weeds AG, et al:** Substructure of the myosin molecule. J Molec Biol 42:1, 1969
8. **Pepe FA:** The myosin filament: immunochemical and ultrastructural approaches to molecular organization. Cold Spring Harbor Sympos Quant Biol 37:97, 1972
9. **Young M, King MV, O'Hara DS, et al:** Studies on the structure and assembly pattern of the light meromyosin section of the myosin rod. Cold Spring Harbor Sympos Quant Biol 37:65, 1972
10. **Leigh JB, Holmes KC, Mannherz HC, et al:** Effects of ATP analogs on the low-angle x-ray diffraction pattern of insect flight muscle. Cold Spring Harbor Sympos Quant Biol 37:443, 1972
11. **Lymn RW, Huxley HE:** X-ray diagrams from skeletal muscle in the presence of ATP analogs. Cold Spring Harbor Sympos Quant Biol 37:449, 1972
12. **Murray JM, Weber A:** The cooperative action of muscle proteins. Sci Amer 230:59, 1974
13. **Huxley HE:** Muscle 1972: progress and problems. Cold Spring Harbor Sympos Quant Biol 37:689, 1972
14. **Sonnenblick EH, Skelton CL:** Reconsideration of the ultrastructural basis of cardiac length-tension relations. Circ Res 35:517, 1974
15. **Mason DT, Zelis R, Amsterdam EA, et al:** Mechanisms of cardiac contraction: structural, biochemical and functional relations in the normal and diseased heart. In, Pathologic Physiology, fifth edition. (Soderman WA Jr, Soderman WA Sr, ed). Philadelphia, WB Saunders, 1974, p 206
16. **Wikman-Coffelt J, Zelis R, Fenner C, et al:** Comparative purification of myocardial myosin and antigenic specificity of the two light chains. Prep Biochem 3:439, 1973
17. **Fenner C, Mason DT, Zelis R, et al:** Regulatory properties of myocardial myosin. Proc Nat Acad Sci USA 70:3205, 1973
18. **Wikman-Coffelt J, Fenner C, Smith A, et al:** Comparative analyses of the kinetics and subunits of myosin from canine skeletal muscle and cardiac tissue. J Biol Chem 250:1257, 1975
19. **Wikman-Coffelt J, Fenner C, Coffelt R, et al:** Chronological effects of mild pressure overload on myosin ATPase activity in the canine right ventricle. J Molec Cell Cardiol 7:219, 1975
20. **Wikman-Coffelt J, Fenner C, Salel A, et al:** Comparison of mild versus severe pressure overload on the enzymatic activity of myosin in the canine right ventricle. Biochem Med (in press)
21. **Fenner C, Kamiyama T, Salel A, et al:** Differential responses of canine myosin ATPase activity and ventricular gases in the pressure overloaded ventricle dependent upon the degree of obstruction: mild versus severe pulmonic and aortic stenosis. Amer J Cardiol (in press)
22. **Wikman-Coffelt J, Smith A, Walsh R, et al:** Effects of severe pressure overload on the properties of canine left ventricular myosin: mechanism by which myosin ATPase activity is lowered during chronic increased hemodynamic stress. J Molec Cell Cardiol (in press)
23. **Heywood SM, Rich A:** In vitro synthesis of native myosin, actin, and tropomyosin from embryonic chick polyribosomes. In, Papers in Regulation of Gene Activity During Development (Loomis WF, ed). New York, Harper & Row, 1970, p. 163
24. **Wikman-Coffelt J, Zelis R, Fenner C, et al:** Myosin chains of myocardial tissue. I. Purification and immunological properties of myosin heavy chains. Biochem Biophys Res Commun 51:1097, 1973
25. **Wikman-Coffelt J, Fenner C, McPherson J, et al:** Alterations of subunit composition and ATPase activity of myosin in early hypertrophied right ventricles of dogs with mild experimental pulmonic stenosis. J Molec Cell Cardiol 7:513, 1975
26. **Fenner C, Traut R, Mason DT, et al:** Quantification of Coomassie blue stained proteins in polyacrylamide gels based on analyses of eluted dye. Anal Biochem 63:595, 1975
27. **Smith A, Mason DT, Wikman-Coffelt J:** Molecular weight studies of canine cardiac myosins. FEBS Lett 43:104, 1974
28. **Morimoto K, Harrington WF:** Evidence for structural changes in vertebrate thick filaments induced by calcium. J Molec Biol 88:693, 1974
29. **Andreasen T, Fenner C, Mason DT, et al:** Variances in calcium binding of canine right and left ventricular myosins. J Biol Chem (in press)
30. **Orzbykam A, Strohman RC:** Myosin heavy chain mes-

senger RNA from myogenic cell cultures. Proc Nat Acad Sci USA 71: 662, 1974

31. **Wikman-Coffelt J, Zelis R, Fenner C, et al:** Studies on the synthesis and degradation of light and heavy chains of cardiac myosin. J Biol Chem 248:5206, 1973

32. **McPherson J, Traut R, Mason DT, et al:** Resolution of myocardial myosin light chains by two-dimensional gel electrophoresis. J Biol Chem 249:994, 1974

33. **Howard GA, Traut R:** Separation and radioautography of microgram quantities of ribosomal protein by two-dimensional polyacrylamide gel electrophoresis. FEBS Lett 29:177, 1973

34. **McPherson J, Fenner C, Smith A, et al:** Identification of in vivo phosphorylated myosin subunits. FEBS Lett 47:149, 1974

35. **Andreasen T, Castles J, Saito W, et al:** The behavior of fetal canine cardiac cells in culture: synthesis and phosphorylation of myosin. Dev Biol (in press)

36. **Zelis R, Wikman-Coffelt J, Kamiyama T, et al:** Acute right ventricular stress as a stimulus for left ventricular RNA and protein synthesis. In, Recent Advances in Studies on Cardiac Structure and Metabolism, vol 3: Myocardial Metabolism (Dhalla NS, ed). Baltimore, University Park Press, 1973, p 625

37. **Jacob J, Monod J:** Genetic regulatory mechanisms in the synthesis of proteins. J Molec Biol 3:318, 1961

38. **Jacob J, Monod J:** On the regulation of gene activity. Cold Spring Harbor Sympos Quant Biol 26:193, 1963

39. **Wolfe S:** Biology of the Cell. Belmont, California, Wadsworth, 1972, p 264

40. **Dice JF, Schimke RT:** Turnover and exchange of ribosomal proteins from rat liver. J Biol Chem 247:98, 1972

41. **Fuhr J, Natta C:** Hemoglobin synthesis. Nature New Biol 240:274, 1972

Chapter 6

Effects of Ischemia on the Contractile Processes of Heart Muscle

Arnold M. Katz, MD, FACC

. . . and of the sciences, we consider that science which exists for the sake of itself, and for knowledge, to be the more desirable wisdom than the science which exists for the sake of results; and that the former is the more sovereign wisdom . . . for the wise man ought not to be commanded, but to command . . .

Aristotle: Metaphysics, Book I, Chapter I
(PB Katz, translator)

An intensive research program, designed to provide discoveries that will improve the care of patients with acute myocardial infarction, has been developed over the past few years. Based on clinical studies of acute myocardial infarction, and on animal models of this condition, much effort has been directed to the prevention and therapy of the "pump" failure that frequently follows interruption of the coronary arterial circulation. Yet the mechanism by which myocardial ischemia leads to impaired cardiac function remains unknown. It is apparent that the new insights into the mechanism of the rapid deterioration of the ischemic heart primarily represent the by-products of basic biochemical and biophysical studies of cardiac contraction rather than the fruits of "goal-oriented" research. In this chapter, several of these basic areas of investigation will be reviewed briefly to provide an insight into the nature of the defect that impairs the mechanical response of the ischemic heart.

When considering the effects of ischemia on the subcellular processes of heart muscle, it is important to recognize the rapidity of the mechanical deterioration that occurs after coronary occlusion. Complete interruption of coronary flow to a segment of the canine heart is followed within a few seconds by abbreviation of systole and then by failure to contract, so that after less than a minute the ischemic portion of the ventricle bulges outward during systole.[1] These phenomena do not mean that the ischemic myocardium has completely lost the ability to develop tension. Instead, they represent a marked diminution in contractility because the tension generated by the ischemic portion of the ventricle is unable to overcome the intraventricular pressure generated by the normally perfused myocardium. Therefore, to understand the paradoxical motion of the ischemic myocardium, one must define the mechanisms that can cause a rapid decline in myocardial contractility after interruption in coronary blood flow. In this analysis of the myocardial response to ischemia it is useful to refer to four causes defined by Aristotle. The *efficient cause,* that is, the producing agency or the factor that sets into motion the processes that ultimately lead to the loss of contractility in the ischemic myocardium, will be discussed first. The *formal* and *material causes*—the form and matter of the mechanical deterioration—will then be considered together. Finally, and in keeping with this Aristotelian approach, some speculation will be presented as to the nature of the *final cause* of the rapid decline in contractile function, that is, the end that these phenomena may serve in the ischemic myocardium.

Efficient Cause of Impaired Contractility in the Ischemic Myocardium

The rapid decline in myocardial contractility that occurs after coronary arterial occlusion could be due to one or both of two efficent causes: (1) the absence of a substrate or substrates normally supplied by the coronary circulation, or (2) accumulation of one or more metabolites. In terms of substrate delivery, it is almost certain that lack of oxygen is the major consequence of an interruption of coronary blood flow because the mechanical deterioration of the acutely anoxic myocardium is essentially the same as that following ischemia. However, the similarity between the effects of anoxia in the perfused myocardium and those of ischemia do not provide conclusive evidence that the accumulation of metabolites has no role in the mechanical deterioration after coronary occlusion. For example, hydrogen ion, a metabolite implicated in the pathogenesis of ischemic heart failure, may accumulate within the anoxic myocardial cell more rapidly than it can be eliminated from the cell and carried away by an intact circulation. Similarly, extracellular potassium ions, which may also be responsible for the decline in myocardial contractility, can be present in high concentrations in the environment immediately surrounding an anoxic cardiac fiber even though capillary circulation remains unimpared. For these reasons, and because studies of the hypoxic myocardium tend to be more numerous and more complete, the remainder of this chapter will primarily consider the role of myocardial hypoxia as the efficient cause of the early and rapid mechanical deterioration after coronary occlusion.

Myocardial Anoxia: The immediate effect of oxygen deprivaton on the myocardium is a rapid reduction of myocardial oxygen tension.[2] As a result, and because the myocardium lacks significant stores of alternative electron acceptors to permit oxidation of the coenzymes that are reduced during oxidative phosphorylation, lack of oxygen quickly brings the oxidative production of adenosine triphosphate (ATP) to a halt. Although it is tempting to attribute the subsequent decline in myocardial contractility directly to a reduced ATP concentration, this explanation is difficult to reconcile with a number of studies that show little or no decrease of ATP levels in the acutely failing ischemic or anoxic myocardium.[3] Furthermore, the direct effect of depletion of ATP on the cardiac contractile proteins should be the development of rigor (contracture) rather than the systolic bulging of a weakened area of myocardium.[4,5]

Cellular Acidosis: A direct consequence of failure of oxidative regeneration of ATP in the ischemic myocardium is accumulation of the products of continued ATP utilization, notably inorganic phosphate and adenosine monophosphate (AMP). Both of these products accelerate the conversion of glycogen to glucose and the anaerobic glycolytic production of ATP.[3] Enhanced glycolysis is accompanied by marked acceleration of lactate production,[6] with a consequent increase in the production of hydrogen ion. Although it is not now possible to attribute all of the detrimental effects of myocardial anoxia and ischemia to a decrease in cellular pH,[7,8] increased concentration of hydrogen ion is well known to have a marked negative inotropic action on the heart.[4] Therefore, the remainder of this chapter will focus on the role of cellular acidosis in the formal and material causes of the negative inotropic response to ischemia. This emphasis on the actions of hydrogen ion should not be construed to mean that all of the detrimental effects of ischemia can be explained as the result of acidosis, or that the potential negative inotropic action of accumulation of sodium ion or loss of potassium ion is not important.[8] Indeed, our understanding of this important question remains quite incomplete, so that the following discussion represents more of a "model" analysis than a full and valid description of the causes of mechanical failure in the ischemic heart.

Excitation and Entry of Activator Ca⁺⁺ from Extracellular Fluid

Calcium ion is established as the final mediator in the processes of excitation-contraction coupling that link excitation at the cell surface to the initiation of mechanical activity by the contractile machinery of the heart. In the heart, these processes probably involve two sources that make calcium ion available to the contractile proteins—one source is extracellular, the other is intracellular. The first of these sources, the net influx of calcium ion from the extracellular fluid to the intracellular space, appears to be related both to the cardiac action potential and to the "sodium pump." There is evidence that an increase in NA+ in the ischemic heart displaces activator Ca++ from a superficial membrane site;[8] nevertheless, a direct negative inotropic effect of such an increase in cellular Na+ is difficult to reconcile with the view that inhibition of the sodium pump, which normally effects the exchanges of intracellular Na+ for K+ in diastole, causes an increase in intracellular Ca++ (for example, during the positive inotropic action of cardiac glycosides).[9] Thus, inhibition of this ion pump by depletion of ATP cannot now be shown to be directly responsible for the negative inotropic effect of ischemia. Conversely, there is some evidence that the action of the cardiac action potential to modulate this calcium entry may be altered in the ischemic heart.

Cardiac Action Potential Configuration: Although prolonged myocardial ischemia eventually leads to failure of the action potential to propagate, the early and rapid deterioration of contractility in the anoxic[10-14] or ischemic[15] heart is associated with only minor changes in action potential configuration. These abnormalities are primarily an abbreviation of the action potential caused by shortening of the plateau (phase 2).[10-13,15] Preservation of normal resting potential indicates that the K+ -dependent properties (K+ permeability, K+ gradient) of the membrane are not grossly altered, and the lack of major changes in the upstroke of the action potential provides evidence that the Na+ -dependent properties of the membrane, which are responsible for the early and rapid inward current effected by Na+ entry, also remain essentially normal. However, the shortening of the plateau of the action potential indicates that ischemia significantly modifies the ionic processes responsible for the slow inward ionic current that can be measured during this phase of the action potential. In the heart, at least part of this slow inward current appears to be carried by Ca++.[16-19] Evidence that slight modifications of the plateau of the cardiac action potential can have profound effects on contractility[20] supports the possibility that the early detrimental effects

of ischemia are due to a reduction in an inward movement of Ca++ when the plateau of the action potential is shortened. It must be emphasized, however, additional evidence is needed to confirm these speculations that ischemia-induced abbreviation of the action potential and a reduction in net calcium ion influx represent formal and material causes for the early failure of the ischemic myocardium.

Excitation-Contraction Coupling

Release of Activator Ca++ from Intracellular Stores

Release of calcium ion from intracellular stores is a second mechanism by which Ca++ is made available to activate the contractile proteins of the heart during excitation-contraction coupling. These intracellular stores of Ca++ appear to be located in the sarcoplasmic reticulum, a system of internal membranes that envelops the myofibrils. It remains to be defined what role, if any, Ca++ associated with mitochondria has in excitation-contraction coupling. In the hearts of some animals, such as the frog, and in certain fetal or neonatal mammalian hearts in which the sarcoplasmic reticulum is apparently absent, the Ca++ utilized in excitation-contraction coupling is probably derived entirely from the extracellular fluid or subsarcolemmal structures. However, in skeletal muscle, the onset of contraction is too rapid for Ca++ diffusing from the extracellular fluid to provide for excitation-contraction coupling. In the adult human heart, as in most mammalian hearts, a sarcoplasmic reticulum is present, although it is less extensive than that in skeletal muscle. Whereas the role of intracellular, as opposed to extracellular, sources of Ca++ in cardiac excitation-contraction coupling remains uncertain, there is reason to believe that Ca++ derived from extracellular sources during cardiac contraction serves to increase the amount of Ca++ available for release by the sarcoplasmic reticulum in subsequent contractions. Thus, alterations in Ca++ entry may act to modulate stores for Ca++ release, whereas the Ca++ released by the sarcoplasmic reticulum would be directly responsible for development of tension.

Sarcoplasmic Reticulum: The in vitro properties of the sarcoplasmic reticulum of the heart remain normal after brief periods of ischemia,[8,21] but acidosis increases the Ca++ affinities of the sarcoplasmic reticulum of both cardiac[22] and skeletal muscle,[23] indicating that the release of Ca++ from intracellular stores is reduced when the ischemic heart becomes acidotic. This decrease in the ability of the sarcoplasmic reticulum to accept and release Ca++ represents another formal and material cause for impaired contractility after coronary occlusion.

Influence of Activator Ca++ on the Cardiac Contractile Proteins

Following the premise that cellular acidosis is the efficient cause of the precipitous decline in myocardial contractility after coronary arterial occlusion, the effects of hydrogen ion on the contractile proteins of the heart will be reviewed briefly. In this discussion, two aspects of the interactions of certain myofibrillar proteins will be discussed: (1) the primary interaction between actin and myosin that gives rise to contraction; and (2) the response to Ca++ of troponin and tropomyosin, the modulatory proteins, that serves to control the primary interaction.

Actin and Myosin: The essential contractile properties of muscle can be reproduced in vitro by two of the proteins of the myofibril—actin and myosin. These properties—hydrolysis of ATP (which liberates chemical energy) and syneresis (a process of shrinkage analogous to shortening)—can be demonstrated in actomyosins reconstituted from highly purified actin and myosin. Cardiac myosin, like skeletal-muscle myosin, exhibits an "anomaly" in the curve defining the relation between adenosine triphosphatase (ATPase) activity and pH.[4,24] The "anomaly" is manifest by a reduction in ATPase activity as pH increases from 6.0 into the neutral range, followed by an increase in activity as pH becomes more alkaline than approximately 7.5 (Figure 1). Actomyosin and myofibrillar ATPase activity, like that of myosin, exhibits a similar "trough" at neutral pH. If these observations are applicable to the situation in the intact

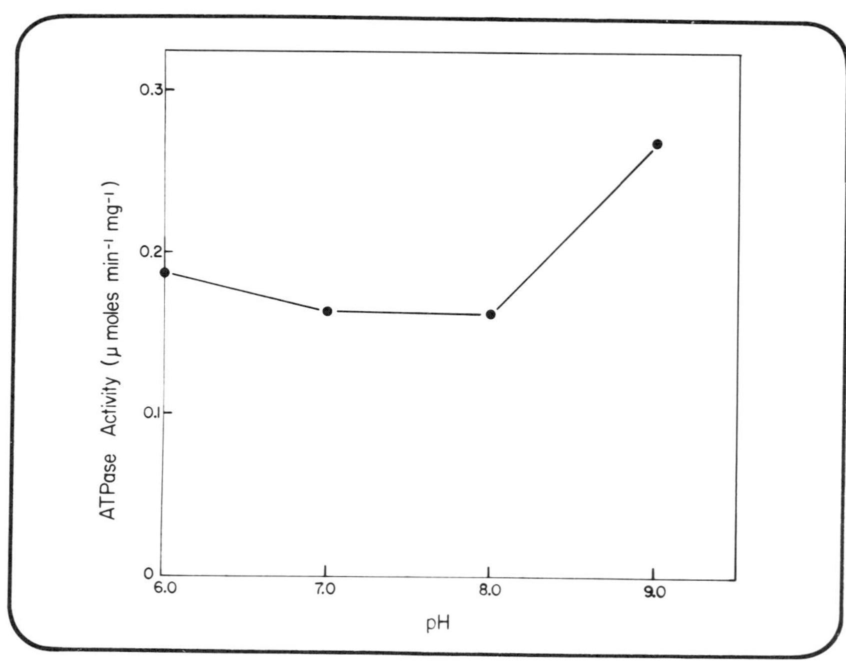

FIGURE 1. Dependence of cardiac myosin ATPase activity on pH. Reactions were carried out in 10 μM calcium chloride, 2 mM ATP, 0.25 M potassium chloride and 20 mM Tris-hydrochloride. (Based on data of Tada et al.[24])

heart, they fail to define an inhibitory effect of acidosis on the rate of energy turnover by the contractile proteins of the ischemic heart.

Troponin and Tropomyosin: A third salient property of muscle, the initiation of contractile activity by micromolar amounts of Ca^{++}, is not seen in actomyosins reconstituted from only actin and myosin. Ca^{++} sensitivity is, instead, a property that is conferred on actomyosin when two modulatory proteins, troponin (a complex of three distinct proteins) and tropomyosin, are bound to actin.[4] In the Ca^{++}-sensitive actomyosins reconstituted from actin, myosin, troponin and tropomyosin, the action of Ca^{++} is mediated by its binding to a high affinity calcium-binding site on troponin C, one of the constituents of troponin. When Ca^{++} is not available for binding to troponin C, the troponin and tropomyosin bound to the actin filament inhibit (repress) the primary interaction between actin and myosin thereby maintaining the heart in a state of relaxation. The function of Ca^{++}, effected by its binding to troponin C, is to abolish (derepress) this inhibitory action of the modulatory proteins, thereby effecting the final step in excitation-contraction coupling. An action of hydrogen ion to displace the Ca^{++} bound to troponin, previously deduced from studies of the Ca^{++} sensitivity of ATPase activity and tension development in cardiac fibers extracted from glycerol,[25,26] has now been demonstrated directly (Table I).[27] These findings indicate that even when the normal amount of Ca^{++} is made available for excitation-contraction coupling, the development of acidosis can impair contractility by displacing Ca^{++} from its binding site on troponin, thus providing another formal and material cause for loss of contractility.

Final Cause of Rapid Loss of Contractility in the Ischemic Myocardium

The precipitous reduction in mechanical function after coronary occlusion, although clearly detrimental to the organism as a whole, has certain advantages for the ischemic area of the myocardium. By attenuating mechanical activity, the most costly of the ATP-utilizing functions, this decline in myocardial contractility conserves chemical energy for other energy-

TABLE I
Effects of pH on the Calcium Affinity of Skeletal Troponin

pH	Calcium-Troponin Binding Constant
8.5	8.0×10^6
8.0	4.0×10^6
7.5	2.2×10^6
7.0	1.0×10^6
6.5	0.4×10^6

Decreasing values for the calcium-troponin binding constant under acid conditions indicate that an increased H^+ concentration causes less Ca^{++} to be bound to this critical regulatory site. (Based on data from Fuchs et al.[27])

consuming reactions that are important in the preservation of myocardial integrity, thereby delaying the development of necrosis. Furthermore, if excitation-contraction coupling were not quickly attenuated, it is likely that the ischemic myocardium would soon deplete its high energy phosphate stores, thereby producing a state of rigor. This state of rigor is not fully reversible,[5] nor is it possible to reestablish perfusion once contracture develops.[28] By contrast, the loss of contractility due to failure of excitation-contraction coupling is probably fully reversible, at least in its early stages, on reperfusion with oxygenated blood.

Recently, Bing et al.[29] have provided evidence that pretreatment of rat myocardium at the alkaline pH of 7.8, followed by 60 minutes of hypoxia, preserves tension during the hypoxic period. Recovery after reoxygenation, however, is impaired in that rigor develops and less tension is regained. Conversely, pretreatment at pH 6.8 reduces tension during hypoxia but increases tension recovered after reoxygenation and prevents the appearance of rigor. These data lend credence to the concluding paragraph of this chapter.

Summary

Myocardial contractility declines precipitously after coronary arterial occlusion. The *efficient cause* of this phenomenon is probably the hypoxia-induced decrease in aerobic adenosine triphosphate (ATP) production by the ischemic myocardium. The *formal* and *material causes* of this negative inotropic effect are less clearly understood. A decrease in influx of calcium ion, due to sodium pump inhibition in the ischemic heart, is difficult to reconcile with evidence that Ca^{++} influx is enhanced under other conditions (for example, administration of cardiac glycosides) that also impair this ion pump. Shortening of the plateau of the action potential after coronary arterial occlusion may be associated with decreased systolic Ca^{++} influx from the extracellular fluid, but additional evidence is needed to corroborate this view. A state of acidosis, resulting from the lactate production that occurs when the ischemic myocardium shifts to anaerobic pathways of energy production, may impair contractility by increasing the tightness of Ca^{++} binding to the sarcoplasmic reticulum of the heart. The increased intracellular hydrogen ion concentration could also exert a negative inotropic effect by displacing Ca^{++} from its binding site on troponin, which is the Ca^{++}-sensitizing protein of the contractile apparatus. The *final* cause of the early depression in mechanical energy production by the ischemic myocardium may be the conservation of chemical energy for the more important task of delaying irreversible rigor and necrosis, thereby preserving myocardial integrity.

Acknowledgment: This study was supported by the New York Heart Association and the National Institutes of Health Research Contract 72-2973-M.

Doctor Katz wishes to dedicate this chapter, especially his wife's translation of Aristotle and his introductory paragraph, to his father, Doctor Louis N. Katz, whose life was devoted to the pursuit of basic knowledge of the diseases of the heart and blood vessels.

References

1. **Tennant R, Wiggers CJ:** The effect of coronary occlusion on myocardial contraction. Amer J Physiol 112:351, 1935
2. **Sayen JJ, Sheldon WF, Pierce G, et al:** Polarographic oxygen, the epicardial electrocardiogram and muscle contraction in experimental acute regional ischemia of the left ventricle. Circ Res 6:779, 1958
3. **Katz AM:** Effects of interrupted coronary flow upon myocardial metabolism. Progr Cardiovasc Dis 10:450, 1968
4. **Katz AM:** The contractile proteins of the heart. Physiol Rev 50:63, 1970
5. **Katz AM, Tada M:** The "stone heart": a challenge to the biochemist. Amer J Cardiol 29:578, 1972
6. **Williamson JR:** Glycolytic control mechanisms. II. Kinetics of intermediate changes during the aerobic-anoxic transition in perfused rat heart. J Biol Chem 241:5026, 1966
7. **Case RB, Nasser MG, Crampton RS:** Biochemical aspects of early myocardial ischemia. Amer J Cardiol 24:766, 1969
8. **Nayler WG, Stone J, Carson V, et al:** Effect of ischemia on cardiac contractility and calcium exchangeability. J Molec Cell Cardiol 2:125, 1971
9. **Besch HR Jr, Schwartz A:** On a mechanism of action of digitalis. J Molec Cell Cardiol 1:195, 1970
10. **Trautwein W, Dudel J:** Aktionspotenial und Kontraktion des Herzmuskels in Sauerstoffmangel. Pflueger Arch 263:23, 1956
11. **Webb JL, Hollander PB:** Metabolic aspects of the relationship between the contractility and membrane potential of the rat atrium. Circ Res 4:618, 1956
12. **Coraboeuf E, Gargouil Y-M, Lapland J, et al:** Action de l'anoxie sur les potentiels electriques des cellules cardiaques de mammiferes actives et inertes (tissu ventriculaire isole de Cobaye). Compt Rend Acad Sci Paris 246:3100, 1958
13. **Trautwein W, Gottstein W, Dudel J:** Der Actionsstrom der Myokardfaser in Sauerstoffmangel. Pflueger Arch 260:40, 1954
14. **MacLeod DP, Daniel EE:** Influence of glucose on the transmembrane action potential of anoxic papillary muscle. J Gen Physiol 48:887, 1965
15. **Kardesch M, Hogancamp CE, Bing RJ:** The effect of complete ischemia on the intracellular electrical activity of the whole mammalian heart. Circ Res 6:715, 1958
16. **Hagiwara S, Nakajima S:** Difference in Na and Ca spikes as examined by application of tetrodotoxin, procaine and manganese ions. J Gen Physiol 49:793, 1966
17. **Reuter H:** The dependence of slow inward current in Purkinje fibers on extracellular calcium concentration. J Physiol (London) 192:479, 1967
18. **Reuter H, Beeler GW Jr:** Calcium current and activation of contraction in ventricular myocardial fibers. Science 163:399, 1969
19. **Beeler GW Jr, Reuter H:** Membrane calcium current in ventricular myocardial fibres. J Physiol (London) 207:191, 1970
20. **Wood EH, Heppner RL, Weidmann S:** Inotropic effects of electric currents. I. Positive and negative effects of constant electric currents or current pulses applied during cardiac action potentials. II. Hypotheses: calcium movements, excitation-contraction coupling and inotropic effects. Circ Res 24:409, 1969
21. **Lee KS, Ladinsky H, Stuckey JH:** Decreased Ca^{2+} uptake by sarcoplasmic reticulum after coronary occlusion for 60 and 90 minutes. Circ Res 21:439, 1967
22. **Nakamaru Y, Schwartz A:** Possible control of intracel-

lular calcium metabolism by [H+]: sarcoplasmic reticulum of skeletal and cardiac muscle. Biochem Biophys Res Commun 41:830, 1970

23. **Nakamaru Y, Schwartz A:** The influence of hydrogen ion concentration on calcium binding and release by skeletal muscle sarcoplasmic reticulum. J Gen Physiol 59:22, 1972

24. **Tada M, Bailin G, Bárány K, et al:** Proteolytic fragmentation of bovine heart heavy meromyosin. Biochem 8:4842, 1969

25. **Schadler MH:** Proportionale Aktivierung von ATPase-Aktivitat und Kontraktinonsspannung durch Calcium-ionen in isolierten contraktilen Strukturen verschiedener Muskelarten. Arch Ges Physiol 296:70, 1967

26. **Katz AM, Hecht HH:** The early "pump" failure of the ischemic heart. Amer J Med 47:497, 1969

27. **Fuchs F, Reddy Y, Briggs FN:** The interaction of cations with the calcium-binding site of troponin. Biochim Biophys Acta 221:407, 1970

28. **Cooley DA:** Ischemic contracture of the heart: "Stone heart." Amer J Cardiol 24:575, 1972

29. **Bing OHL, Brooks WW, Nesser JV:** Heart muscle viability following hypoxia: protective effect of acidosis. Science 180:1297, 1973

Alterations of Cardiac Sympathetic Neurotransmitter Activity in Congestive Heart Failure

Harold L. Rutenberg, MD, FACC
James F. Spann, Jr, MD, FACC

The sympathetic nervous system represents a major control mechanism in the moment to moment regulation of the normal circulatory response to the changing metabolic requirements of the tissues. This system provides a sensitive mechanism for rapid alteration of myocardial contractility, heart rate and peripheral venous and arterial tone. The sympathetic nervous system occupies a crucial role in the responses of man to physical exercise; the increases in heart rate, stroke volume, cardiac output, left ventricular work and velocity of muscle fiber shortening that occur with exercise are due in part to augmented sympathetic activity.[1-3] Further, many of the normal cardiovascular responses to exercise can be drastically altered by sympathetic blockade.[2,3] Tachycardia, diaphoresis, peripheral vascular constriction and suppression of formation of urine are well known clinical expressions of increased sympathetic nervous system activity in congestive heart failure. Since the sympathetic nervous system is of obvious importance in understanding the concept of cardiac reserve, many investigators in recent years have studied this system in congestive heart failure, in which cardiac reserve is limited and alterations in circulatory responses are evident. It is well appreciated that the sympathetic nervous system is of considerable importance in the regulation of peripheral arterial and venous tone as well as cardiac function. However, this chapter will concentrate on the direct influences of the sympathetic nervous system on the normal and failing heart.

Normal Pathways of Sympathetic Stimulation

Nerve terminals from the network of sympathetic nerves that supply the cardiovascular system can be found in arteries, veins and all chambers of the heart, including the conduction system as well as the myocardium. Stored in the nerve terminals are large concentrations of the neurotransmitter norepinephrine; stimulation of these nerves results in the discharge of this norepinephrine, which acts upon the cardiac cellular beta receptor mechanism, to exert effects dependent upon the site of stimulation. Increases in heart rate occur with stimulation of the sinoatrial node, increased velocity of conduction occurs through the atrioventricular junctional tissues, and augmentation of myocardial contractility occurs when the beta receptors are stimulated in the myocardium. It is thought that these effects are mediated indirectly through the activation of adenyl cyclase with resultant formation of adenosine 3',5' phosphate (cyclic AMP) within the cells.[4,5] However, some have postulated that the increased contractility is due to a direct effect of norepinephrine in increasing the rate of uptake of calcium by the sarcoplasmic reticulum.

The synthesis of norepinephrine, as well as uptake and binding of circulating norepinephrine, is also accomplished within these neurons. Synthesis of norepinephrine by these nerve endings probably accounts for 80 to 90 percent of that catecholamine in the heart.[7,8] The major pathway in this synthesis involves the uptake from the blood of the amino acid precursor tyrosine by the nerve endings. Tyrosine hydroxylase, present in the mitochondria, catalyzes the first transformation to dihydroxyphenylalanine (dopa), which is in turn transformed by a cytoplasmic decarboxylase enzyme to dopamine. The final step in biosynthesis occurs in a specialized subcellular particle, the granulated vesicle, where the enzyme dopamine beta oxidase converts dopamine to norepinephrine.[9] Tyrosine hydroxylase is believed to be the major enzyme regulating the rate of synthesis in this sequence.[10] Circulating norepinephrine is taken up by these nerve endings and accounts for the remaining 10 to 20 percent of cardiac norepinephrine in the nerves. The catecholamine from both synthesis and uptake is retained in a physiologically inactive form in the storage granules.[11] Wurtman[12] has characterized these granules as a tissue buffer system not unlike serum protein buffers that bind circulating hormones. Thus, these granules bind and store norepinephrine and retard its diffusion into the neuronal cytoplasm protecting it from enzymatic destruction by monoamine oxidase, which is present within the neuron. The granules release the stored catecholamine from the neuronal cell when stimulated by action potentials along the sympathetic nerve terminals. The granules have the further important function of uptake of free norepinephrine either previously released from the granule[13] or circulating locally. Thus, by retaining the norepineph-

rine in a chemically unchanged but physiologically inert form, these granules may provide one mechanism for the termination of the action of norepinephrine. Two enzymes are responsible for the destruction of norepinephrine. Part of this retained norepinephrine may be subsequently discharged slowly from the nerve to be catabolyzed by the extraneuronal tissue enzyme catechol O-methyltransferase.[14] Some of the norepinephrine is inactivated within the nerve by monoamine oxidase, the major intraneuronal catabolizing enzyme.[15]

Sympathetic Activity in Heart Failure

Effect of Exercise: During physical exercise in normal man, augmented sympathetic activity can be estimated by measuring the changes in arterial plasma norepinephrine concentration, since a portion of norepinephrine released at the nerve terminals enters the circulating blood. In normal subjects, moderate muscular exercise is associated with an elevation of arterial norepinephrine from an average control level of 0.28 μg/liter to an exercise level of 0.46 μg/liter, a change of borderline significance.[16] In patients with congestive heart failure, there is good evidence for increased resting values of arterial plasma norepinephrine concentration, and in these subjects moderate exercise elevated the arterial norepinephrine from an average control value of 0.63 μg/liter to the exercise value of 1.73 μg/liter.[16] Values in patients with heart disease but without evidence of heart failure did not differ from normal. From these studies it was concluded that the excessive augmentation of plasma norepinephrine concentration during exercise in patients with heart failure reflected an increased response of the sympathetic nervous system to exercise and that this increased response may have had an important supportive role in such patients.

Urinary Excretion of Norepinephrine: The daily urinary excretion of norepinephrine has been examined and compared in normal persons, patients with heart disease without congestive failure and patients with congestive heart failure as an estimation of the overall level of sympathetic activity.[17] Excretion of norepinephrine averaged 22 μg/day in both of the first two groups and was significantly increased in the patients with heart failure, averaging 46 μg/day in patients with functional class III status (New York Heart Association classification) and 58 μg/day in patients with class IV status. Thus, further evidence for augmented activity of the sympathetic nervous system, reflected in increased urinary excretion of norepinephrine at rest, has been provided.

Myocardial Concentrations of Norepinephrine: Given this apparent increased level of sympathetic autonomic activity in patients with heart failure, the subsequent finding of depletion of norepinephrine in human myocardial tissue removed at the time of corrective cardiac surgery was of interest.[17,18] The concentration of norepinephrine in the atrial appendages averaged 1.77 μg/g in 34 patients who had not had heart failure before operation. In 49 patients with heart failure, the norepinephrine concentration in the atrial tissue was significantly less, averaging only 0.49 μg/g ($P < 0.01$). In the 26 patients who had or had experienced heart failure and then underwent mitral valve replacement, the norepinephrine concentration in left ventricular papillary muscle averaged 0.52 μg/g. Comparison of the norepinephrine concentrations in the ventricular and atrial tissues in the individual patients revealed a significant positive correlation ($P < 0.05$). In the 12 patients whose atrial concentrations were less than 0.40 μg/g, the ventricular concentrations averaged only 0.27 μg/g. In the 15 patients whose atrial concentration exceeded 0.40 μg/g, the ventricular concentrations were higher, averaging 0.73 μg/g.

There is now abundant evidence for the depletion of cardiac norepinephrine stores in experimentally induced heart failure. Thus, in left heart failure produced by constriction of the ascending aorta of the guinea pig[19,20] or in right heart failure induced in the dog by production of pulmonary stenosis and tricuspid insufficiency[21] or in right ventricular hypertrophy with or without heart failure produced by different degrees of pulmonary arterial constriction in the cat,[22,23] there is a profound reduction in cardiac norepinephrine concentration (Figure 1). This depletion of norepinephrine is present in both the right and left ventricles regardless of which ventricle is subjected to the primary hemodynamic burden. The total content of cardiac nor-

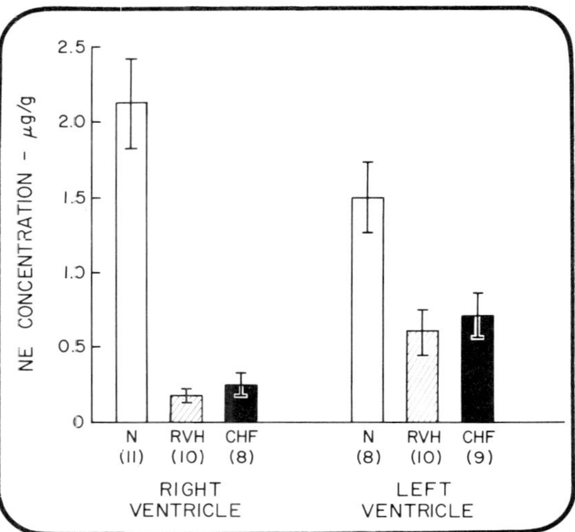

FIGURE 1. The average norepinephrine concentration of the right and left ventricles of normal cats and cats with right ventricular hypertrophy (RVH) and congestive heart failure (CHF). **Vertical lines with cross bars** equal ± 1 standard error of the mean. Numbers in parentheses equal number of animals in each group. (Reprinted by permission of the American Heart Association, Inc. from Spann et al.[23])

epinephrine is also profoundly depressed (Figure 2, C and D), reflecting a true depletion of norepinephrine in heart failure rather than dilution of a normal complement of norepinephrine by hypertrophy of the heart. The ventricular myocardium of cats in which hypertrophy is produced without the occurrence of congestive heart failure also shows this depletion (Figure 1).

In cardiac hypertrophy induced in rats by prolonged intense physical exercise on treadmills, cardiac norepinephrine concentration remains unchanged,[24] thus suggesting that the hemodynamic burden of markedly increased afterload might be an important consideration in the depletion of cardiac norepinephrine stores. Recently, LaFarge et al.[25] demonstrated in the innervated dog heart an increased rate of norepinephrine efflux from the coronary sinus when left ventricular peak pressure was acutely increased by 100 mm Hg by clamping of the ascending aorta. They postulated that such increased peak left ventricular pressures may be one mechanism explaining depletion of cardiac norepinephrine. Increases in left ventricular

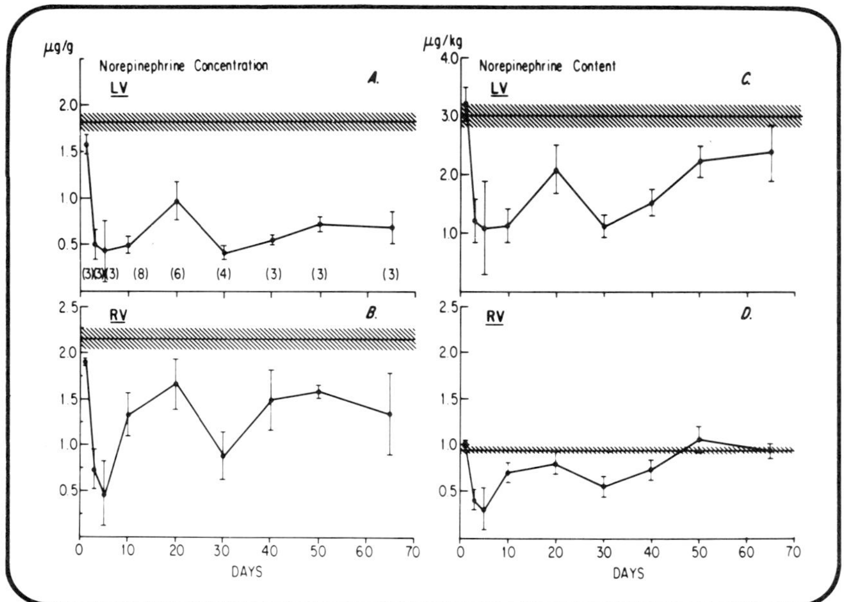

FIGURE 2. Time course of changes in norepinephrine concentration in μg/g (**A** and **B**) and time course of changes in total norepinephrine content in each ventricle expressed as μg/kg body weight (**C** and **D**). **Solid circles** and **vertical bars** represent the mean values ± 1 standard error of the mean obtained from animals with congestive heart failure. **Horizontal lines** and **hatched areas** represent the mean ± 1 standard error of the mean obtained from 15 normal animals. Numbers in parentheses at bottom of panel A refer to the number of animals sacrificed at each point in time that provided the data shown in all four panels. (Reprinted by permission of the American Heart Association, Inc. from Spann et al.[20])

end-diastolic pressure up to 49 mm Hg did not affect efflux of norepinephrine, and induced increases in heart rate produced changes in efflux of only borderline significance.

The time required after onset of heart failure for depletion of cardiac norepinephrine has been determined in the guinea pig[20] (Figure 2). Although the left ventricular norepinephrine concentration was not depressed 1 day after operation, it had fallen to values that averaged 22 percent of control at 5 days after aortic constriction and remained depressed for the 65 day observation period. In contrast to the depletion observed in the heart, there was no significant change in renal norepinephrine stores when the group with congestive failure was considered as a whole, thereby suggesting that adrenergic nerves in other tissues need not be affected by the heart failure state. However, in a few animals, depression of renal norepinephrine accompanied profound depression of cardiac norepinephrine stores.[20]

Mechanisms of Cardiac Norepinephrine Depletion

Defect in Neuronal Binding of Norepinephrine: As has been described, the nerve terminals are complex structures involved in synthesis, uptake, binding, storage and release of norepinephrine. Most of these functions have been studied in an effort to determine the mechanisms by which cardiac norepinephrine is depleted. The defect in neuronal binding of norepinephrine was determined by measurement of the norepinephrine retained in the hearts and kidneys after infusion of *l*-norepinephrine in a group of normal guinea pigs and a group with congestive failure.[20] Figure 3 shows the elevations of norepinephrine concentrations in the heart and kidneys produced by the infusion of norepinephrine in 14 control animals and in 13 guinea pigs in which the aorta had been constricted 10 days previously. In the normal animals, the renal and left and right ventricular concentrations of norepinephrine rose to peak values at the completion of the infusion; the concentrations declined over the ensuing 3 hours to values that approached the control levels. In contrast, the increase in the ventricular concentrations in the animals with heart failure was minimal, whereas the renal norepinephrine in this group increased in a manner similar to that observed in the normal group. Thirty minutes after completion of the infusion in the normal animals, the left ventricular norepinephrine concentration had increased by 1.16 μg/g, an increment above control that was significantly greater than that noted in animals with aortic constriction (0.32 μg/g) (P <0.01). Similarly, in the right ventricle the augmentation of norepinephrine concentration observed 30 minutes after completion of the infusion was greater in the normal animals than in those with heart failure. Thirty minutes after the infusion, the plasma norepinephrine concentrations were comparable in the two groups, averaging 0.029 ± 0.011 μg/ml in the control animals and 0.033 ± 0.014 μg/ml in the constricted animals. Also, when tracer quantities of tritium-labeled *dl*-norepinephrine were injected into these animals, similar results were observed. One hour after injection of tritium-labeled *dl*-norepinephrine, the left ventricles of the normal guinea pigs contained an average of 0.76 ± 0.01 μc/g, whereas this value was only 0.37 ± 0.05 μc/g in the animals with aortic constriction. Thus, if the depletion of norepinephrine in the human heart is also associated with such a defect of uptake and binding, it is unlikely that repletion of these stores could be accomplished by administration of catecholamines.

Turnover Rate of Intraneuronal Norepinephrine (Abnormality of Uptake or Binding): To investigate the net turnover rate of intraneuronal norepinephrine, a small dose of radioactive norepinephrine was administered to normal guinea pigs and those with heart failure, and its turnover was determined by monitoring the specific activity in the left ventricle for 72 hours.[20] In both groups of animals, the decline of specific activity was complex and exhibited two exponential components. This finding is similar to the observations of other investigators[26,27] and is compatible with the presence of a multicompartmental distribution of norepinephrine.

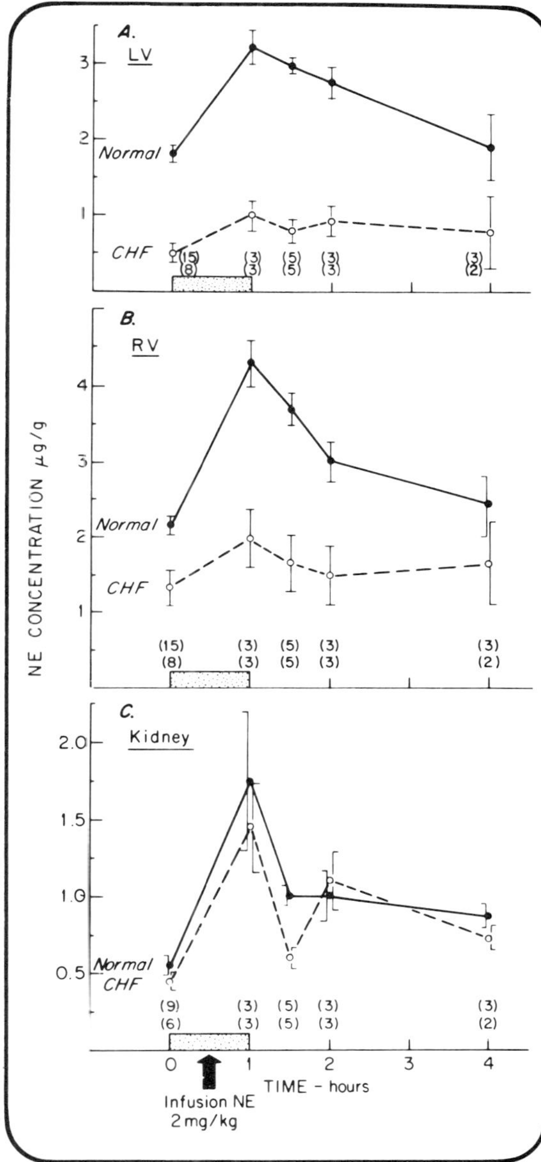

FIGURE 3. Effects of infusion of norepinephrine (NE) on the concentrations of norepinephrine in the left ventricles (LV) (**A**), right ventricles (RV) (**B**) and kidneys (**C**) of normal guinea pigs (**solid lines and circles**) and guinea pigs with congestive heart failure (CHF, **open circles and broken lines**). **Vertical bars** represent ± 1 standard error of the mean. **Stippled areas** represent duration of infusion, and the numbers in parentheses refer to the number of animals in each group sacrificed at the various times. (Reprinted by permission of the American Heart Association, Inc. from Spann et al.[20])

The absolute levels of specific activity and the rates of disappearance were essentially identical in the normal animals and those with heart failure, indicating that the relative net turnover rates were the same, although the absolute net turnover rates were reduced in the animals with heart failure. Thus, in the animals with failure, the smaller increment of norepinephrine in the heart after infusion cannot be explained by a more rapid net turnover of norepinephrine, but must be interpreted as an abnormality of uptake or binding, or both; it is likely that this defect is, in part, responsible for the observed depletion of norepinephrine stores. In view of the smaller norepinephrine stores, the presence of a normal net turnover rate also indicates that the rate of formation in the ventricle must actually be reduced in the group with heart failure.

Defect in Norepinephrine Synthesis: A defect in synthesis of norepinephrine in the failing heart has been reported by Pool et al.,[28] who demonstrated a severe defect in the rate-limiting enzyme system necessary for the synthesis of norepinephrine. Tyrosine hydroxylase activity in the right ventricles of dogs with right-sided congestive heart failure and severe cardiac norepinephrine depletion was reduced from 3.3 $\pm$ 0.7 mμmole/g per hour in the controls to 0.4 $\pm$ 0.1 mμmole/g per hour in the animals with heart failure. In the right atria this enzyme activity was reduced from 4.9 $\pm$ 1.0 mμmole/g per hour in normal animals to 0.5 $\pm$ 0.2 in the dogs with heart failure. Furthermore, a significant positive correlation was evident when the norepinephrine concentration and tyrosine hydroxylase activity were related to each other in the individual chambers of both normal and failing hearts.

Krakoff et al.[29] investigated the role of the enzymes that inactivate norepinephrine, catechol O-methyltransferase and monoamine oxidase, in experimental cardiac hypertrophy and congestive heart failure in cats. Although some differences existed in enzyme activity in the control and failure groups, the investigators concluded that such differences could not account for the striking reduction in cardiac norepinephrine content that occurs in heart failure.

Mechanisms of Defects in Synthesis, Uptake and Binding of Norepinephrine: The demonstration of defects in synthesis, uptake and binding of norepinephrine by the sympathetic neurons of the failing heart raises the question of possible mechanisms responsible for these abnormalities, whether they be simple alterations in the nerve terminals or actual reduction in the total number of nerve endings.

Falck et al.[30] described a fluorescence technique whereby the localization of adrenergic nerves can be studied histochemically, and Jacobowitz et al.,[31] using this technique, demonstrated parallel decreases in norepinephrine content of the myocardium and fluorescence of catecholamine-containing fibers after denervation by mediastinal neural ablation. Vogel et al.[32] recently demonstrated a similar correlation in calves with experimental heart failure in which reduced norepinephrine content paralleled the absence of fluorescence in terminal adrenergic fibers. The heart failure preparation used by these investigators was that of left pulmonary arterial ligation in a high altitude environment; this combination evokes progressive pulmonary hypertension and heart failure. Ligation of the left pulmonary artery does not result in pulmonary hypertension at sea level, and therefore animals in these studies can recover from heart failure by returning to sea level environments. Of considerable interest, recovery from heart failure in two animals was associated with both the restoration of cardiac norepinephrine concentration and normal histochemical appearance of adrenergic nerve distribution within 28 days of returning to sea level, and substantial changes toward the normal were noted within 10 days. This has been the first finding to suggest that the abnormalities in heart failure, whether of storage, uptake, binding or synthesis, may be reversible and perhaps are more likely due to a metabolic dysfunction of the neuron rather than to actual anatomic loss of neural elements. Further investigation of this important question of recovery of cardiac norepinephrine stores when heart failure is relieved is needed.

Mathes et al.[33] and Mathes and Gudbjarnason[34] studied storage and metabolism of norepinephrine after experimental myocardial infarction. In brief, they found a marked decline in cardiac norepinephrine, in both the infarcted and noninfarcted regions. Cardiac norepinephrine was completely absent from the infarcted area at 4 days after infarction in dogs. In the noninfarcted tissue, there was a marked reduction of cardiac norepinephrine during the first 10 days after infarction, and this depletion occurred in both ventricles and, to a lesser extent, in both atria. Cardiac norepinephrine content began to increase in these areas 2 weeks after infarction until normal levels were reached at 6 weeks. These workers could find no correlation between tissue levels of norepinephrine and left ventricular function as reflected by the rate of rise of the first derivative of left ventricular pressure (dP/dt) and concluded that the decline and recovery of left ventricular function were followed rather than preceded by similar alterations in norepinephrine content. They also studied the myocardial retention and subcellular distribution of endogenous and exogenous norepinephrine and showed that this remained unaltered; approximately 60 percent was in the particulate fraction and 14 percent was in the soluble fraction both when cardiac norepinephrine content was normal and when it was at its lowest point 10 days after infarction.[33] This return to normal may testify to the possible reversibility of depleted norepinephrine stores.

Doyle[35] advanced an interesting hypothesis concerning the mechanism of depletion of norepinephrine from the myocardium. He found that both sodium depletion and sodium loading lower cardiac catecholamine levels in rats and suggested that the disturbance of uptake and storage of catecholamines in hypertension and in heart failure may be related to distrubances in sodium distribution.

Cardiac Norepinephrine and Contractile Function

The effect of cardiac norepinephrine depletion on the contractile function of the heart has been studied;[23] a profound depression of the intrinsic contractile state of cardiac muscle isolated from the hearts of cats with pulmonary arterial constriction and overt congestive heart failure was demonstrated. This depression was characterized by a downward shift of the force-velocity curve with substantial reduction of the intrinsic speec of contraction (Vmax) from the normal value of 0.90 ± 0.08 muscle lengths/sec to 0.34 ± 0.06 in the animals with failure (Figure 4A), reduction of maximal active tension

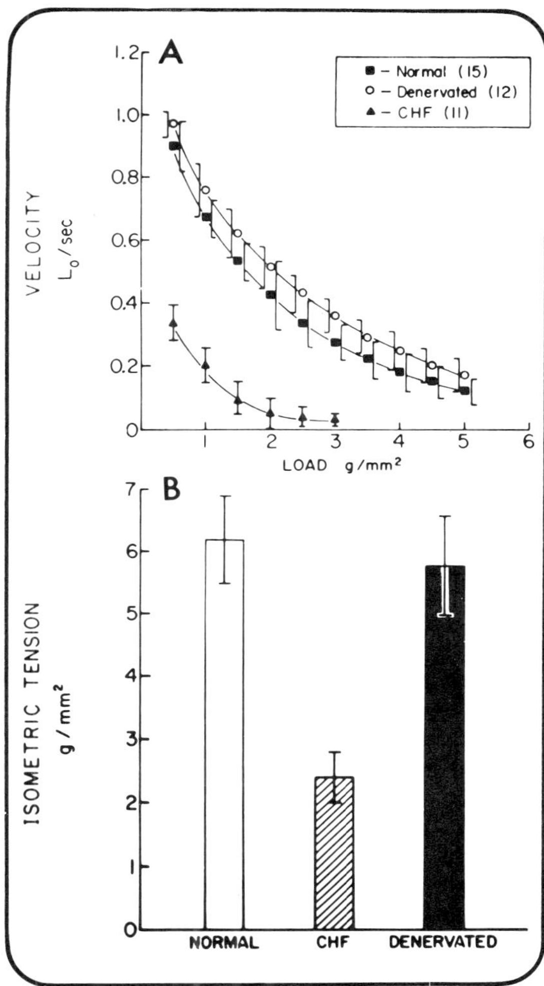

FIGURE 4. Ventricular contractile state. **A,** Average force-velocity relation in right ventricular papillary muscles isolated from normal cats (N) and cats with congestive heart failure (CHF) and denervation. Velocity is expressed on the ordinate as muscle lengths (L₀)/sec and total load is expressed on the abscissa as g/mm². **B,** average maximal active tension developed at the apex of the length-tension curve in isolated right ventricular papillary muscles from the three groups of cats, expressed as g/mm . All **vertical bars** equal ± 1 standard error of the mean, and each number in parenthesis represents the number of animals in that group.

from the normal value of 6.2 ± 0.7 g/mm² to 2.4 ± 0.4 (Figure 4B), and depression of the maximal rate of tension development (df/dt) from 30 ± 5 g/mm²/sec to 10 ± 3. The ventricles from which these failing muscles were removed were depleted of cardiac norepinephrine stores, having an average concentration of 0.23 ± 0.004 μg/g compared with the normal value of 2.13 ± 0.30. To assess the possibility that the cardiac norepinephrine depletion itself was responsible for the intrinsic depression of contractile performance in the failing heart muscle, the contractile state of cardiac muscle removed from hearts depleted of norepinephrine by a mechanism other than heart failure was examined.[36] In 12 cats, cardiac norepinephrine depletion was produced by chronic cardiac denervation; the contractile function of papillary muscles isolated from these hearts was studied in the same manner as the muscles from the failing hearts. The cardiac norepinephrine concentrations of the cardiac denervated animals were reduced to levels of 0.006 ± 0.003 μg/g, a value even lower than the values in the heart failure group. However, the contractile function of cardiac muscle from the norepinephrine-depleted, denervated heart was not depressed (Figure 4, A and B). It was concluded that cardiac stores of norepinephrine are not fundamental for maintaining the basic contractile state of the myocardium and that the cardiac norepinephrine depletion that occurs in congestive heart failure is not responsible for the intrinsic depression of cardiac contractility in failing heart muscle. These conclusions have recently been corroborated in a series of experiments utilizing the isolated rat heart.[37]

Effect of Circulating Norepinephrine on Failing Heart: It has been found that the norepinephrine-depleted cardiac muscle from the failing heart is supersensitive to exogenous norepinephrine.[23] The inotropic effect of *l*-norepinephrine was studied in the muscles from eight normal cats and six cats with pulmonary arterial constriction and depletion of right ventricular norepinephrine to a concentration of 0.39 μg/g or less. All muscles responded to norepinephrine with an increase in tension, and the increments were actually greater in muscles from the cats with pulmonary arterial constriction. For example, at a concentration of 10^{-7} M of *l*-norepinephrine, the increment in isometric force averaged 1.47 ± 0.23 g/mm^2 in muscles from cats with pulmonary arterial constriction, a value significantly greater than that observed in the normal muscles, 0.84 ± 0.20 g/mm^2 (P

<0.005). Thus, the dose-response curve was shifted upward, signifying an increased responsiveness to norepinephrine. Since the circulating arterial norepinephrine concentration is increased in heart failure[16] and the failing heart muscle is not only responsive to exogenous norepinephrine but even supersensitive to its positive inotropic effects, the circulating catecholamines may play an important role in supporting the contractile function of the failing heart. If this is true, it would be expected that agents that block the cardiac beta sympathetic receptor sites would intensify heart failure in certain circumstances. Clinical experience with the beta adrenergic receptor blocking agent propranolol has shown that in patients with advanced cardiac disease, congestive heart failure can appear or increase when propranolol is administered.[38] Vogel and Chidsey[39] demonstrated increases in plasma levels of norepinephrine after propranolol was given to calves in heart failure over and above the increases noted in heart failure alone; they suggested that this finding testifies to the generalized adrenergic stimulation from extracardiac sources, primarily the adrenal medulla, which serves to sustain cardiac performance in the failing heart.

Cardiac Norepinephrine Depletion and Transmission of Sympathetic Impulses: The question of whether the cardiac norepinephrine depletion interferes with transmission of sympathetic impulses to the heart has been examined by Covell et al.[40] in dogs with severe cardiac norepinephrine depletion and right heart failure due to tricuspid insufficiency and pulmonary stenosis. The chronotropic and inotropic responses to graded stimulation of the sympathetic nerves in 6 dogs with chronic right ventricular failure were compared with the responses of 13 normal animals. The responses of heart rate and right ventricular contractile force to stimulation of the right cardioaccelerator nerve were sharply reduced in dogs with heart failure when these responses were compared with the responses in control animals. Furthermore, it was shown that the myocardium of the dogs with heart failure responded directly to exogenously administered norepinephrine. From these observations it may be concluded that the quantity of neurotransmitter released per nerve impulse is drastically reduced in experimental heart failure with cardiac norepinephrine depletion. Since the maximal responses to nerve stimulation were very small in the failing heart, it would appear that even an abnormal increase in the impulse traffic along the cardiac sympathetic nerves would not substantially augment the contractile state of the failing myocardium. Thus, an important mechanism that could improve myocardial force development and velocity of contraction in the failing heart and thereby provide compensation for the intrinsic defect of cardiac muscle function is seriously impaired in the failing heart. The myocardium apparently becomes more and more reliant upon circulating catecholamines from extracardiac sources to maintain its performance.

Sympathetic-Parasympathetic Interactions in the Heart

Any discussion of the cardiovascular sympathetic nervous system would be incomplete without some attention to the possible effects and interactions induced upon that system by the parasympathetic nerves. Levy[41] recently reviewed the complex nature of sympathetic-parasympathetic interaction in the heart and discussed the ramifications of this dual innervation wherein complicated interactions, favored by anatomic proximity of nerve endings of both systems, can occur between the systems. Thus, it has been well known that the cardiac acceleration produced by strong sympathetic stimulation can be overpowered by relatively weak vagal activity.[42] Moreover, the usual slight negative inotropic effect of acetylcholine on ventricular muscle may be magnified to a pronounced depression of myocardial contractility during increased activity of cardiac sympathetic nerves or infusion of exogenous norepinephrine.[43] Whether this might be due to a cholinergic-induced reduction in the amount of norepinephrine released or to an attenuation of the magnitude of response to a given adrenergic stimulus is still unsettled, and other mechanisms might indeed be possible. Cholinergic interventions themselves have been shown to be capable of releasing cardiac norepinephrine.[44] Although acetylcholine exerts a negative inotropic effect similar to that of vagal stimulation on ventricular myocardium when

used in small doses, Buccino et al.[45] demonstrated a positive inotropic effect of acetylcholine on isolated papillary muscle of the cat when that drug was used at higher concentrations. This effect was independent of cardiac norepinephrine stores, and they postulated that there may be two distinct cholinergic receptors in the myocardium. LaRaia and Sonnenblick[46] recently demonstrated that the negative inotropic effects of cholinergic agents were associated with negative changes in adenyl cyclase activity and cyclic adenosine monophosphate (AMP) whereas opposite effects were noted for norepinephrine, thus possibly implicating that enzyme system as the final mediator of both autonomic influences. Grodner et al.[47] postulated that acetylcholine may interfere with the ability of norepinephrine to increase intracellular cyclic AMP.

Although it has been reported[48] that myocardial acetylcholine content is normal in hypertrophied, failing left ventricles of experimental animals in which cardiac norepinephrine stores have been depleted by 75 percent and that such hearts show a normal response to vagal stimulation, Eckberg et al.[49] recently demonstrated a reduced degree of parasympathetic influence on sinoatrial node automaticity in patients with heart failure as determined by vagal blockade with atropine. Moreover, these investigators found that baroceptor-induced slowing of the heart rate provoked by phenylephrine was markedly attenuated in patients with heart disease. Both of these findings point to a marked abnormality in parasympathetic cardiovascular regulation in heart disease and may evoke further interest and experimentation in delineating these abnormalities.

Summary

The sympathetic nervous system exerts an important direct effect on cardiac function, which is mediated by the release at the terminal sympathetic nerve endings of the neurotransmitter norepinephrine. These nerve terminals are complex structures involved in synthesis, uptake, binding and storage as well as release of norepinephrine. The evidence for alteration of many of these functions in congestive heart failure, which is characterized by depletion of myocardial norepinephrine stores, is reviewed. Although cardiac norepinephrine depletion alone is not responsible for the intrinsic depression of cardiac contractility in failing heart muscle, this depletion probably removes a potentially important compensatory mechanism for augmenting myocardial force development and velocity of contraction in the failing heart.

Evidence for parasympathetic-sympathetic system interactions as they affect the heart, as well as alterations in the parasympathetic nervous system in heart failure, is also presented briefly.

Acknowledgment: This work was supported in part by U.S. Public Health Service Training Grant 2T01 HE 05712-06A1.

References

1. **Ross J Jr, Linhart JW, Braunwald E:** Effects of changing heart rate in man by electrical stimulation of the right atrium: studies at rest, during exercise, and with isoproterenol. Circulation 32:549, 1965

2. **Epstein SE, Robinson BF, Kahler RL, et al:** Effects of beta-adrenergic blockade on the cardiac response to maximal and submaximal exercise in man. J Clin Invest 44:1745, 1965

3. **Sonnenblick EH, Braunwald E, Williams JF Jr, et al:** Effects of exercise on myocardial force-velocity relations in intact unanesthetized man: relative roles of changes in heart rate, sympathetic activity, and ventricular dimensions. J Clin Invest 44:2051, 1965

4. **Murad F, Chi YM, Rall TW, et al:** Adenyl cyclase. III. Effect of catecholamines and choline esters on the formation of adenosine 3',5'-phosphate by preparation from cardiac muscle and liver. J Biol Chem 237:1233, 1962

5. **Robinson GA, Butcher RW, Øye I, et al:** Effect of epinephrine on adenosine 3',5' phosphate levels in the isolated perfused rat heart. Molec Pharmacol 1:168, 1965

6. **Shinebourne EA, Hess ML, White RJ, et al:** The effect of noradrenaline on the calcium uptake of the sarcoplasmic reticulum. Cardiovasc Res 3:113, 1969

7. **Chidsey CA, Kaiser GA, Braunwald E:** Biosynthesis of norepinephrine in isolated canine heart. Science 139:828, 1963

8. **Spector S, Sjoerdsma A, Zaltzman-Nirenberg P, et al:** Norepinephrine synthesis from tyrosine-C^{14} in isolated perfused guinea-pig heart. Science 139:1299, 1963

9. **Potter LT, Axelrod J:** Properties of norepinephrine storage particles of rat heart. J Pharmacol Exp Ther 142:299, 1963

10. **Levitt M, Spector S, Sjoerdsma A, et al:** Elucidation of the rate-limiting step in norepinephrine biosynthesis in the perfused guinea pig heart. J Pharmacol Exp Ther 148:1, 1965

11. **Potter LT, Axelrod J:** Subcellular localization of catecholamines in tissues of rat. J Pharmacol Exp Ther 142:291, 1963

12. **Wurtman JR:** Catecholamines. New Eng J Med 273:637, 1965

13. **Hertting G, Axelrod J:** Fate of tritiated noradrenaline at sympathetic nerve endings. Nature (London) 192:172, 1961

14. **Axelrod J:** O-methylation of epinephrine and other catechols in vitro and in vivo. Science 126:400, 1957

15. **Kopin IJ:** Storage and metabolism of catecholamines: role of monoamine oxidase. Pharmacol Rev 16:179, 1964

16. **Chidsey CA, Harrison DC, Braunwald E:** Augmentation of the plasma norepinephrine response to exercise in patients with congestive heart failure. New Eng J Med 267:650, 1962

17. **Chidsey CA, Braunwald E, Morrow AG:** Catecholamine excretion and cardiac stores of norepinephrine in congestive heart failure. Amer J Med 39:442, 1965

18. **Chidsey CA, Braunwald E, Morrow AG, et al:** Myocardial norepinephrine concentration in man: effects of reserpine and of congestive heart failure. New Eng J Med 269:653, 1963

19. **Spann JF Jr, Chidsey CA, Braunwald E:** Reduction of cardiac stores of norepinephrine in experimental heart failure. Science 145:1439, 1964

20. **Spann JF Jr, Chidsey CA, Pool PE, et al:** Mechanism of norepinephrine depletion in experimental heart failure produced by aortic constriction in the guinea pig. Circ Res 17:312, 1965

21. **Chidsey CA, Kaiser GA, Sonnenblick EG, et al:** Cardiac norepinephrine stores in experimental heart failure in the dog. J Clin Invest 43:2386, 1964

22. **Spann JF Jr, Buccino RA, Sonnenblick EH:** Production of right ventricular hypertrophy with and without congestive heart failure in the cat. Proc Soc Exp Biol Med 125:522, 1967

23. **Spann JF Jr, Buccino RA, Sonnenblick EH, et al:** Contractile state of cardiac muscle obtained from cats with experimentally produced ventricular hypertrophy and heart failure. Circ Res 21:341, 1967

24. **Östman I, Sjöstrand NO:** Effect of prolonged physical training on the catecholamine levels of the heart and the adrenals of the rat. Acta Physiol Scand 82:202, 1971

25. **LaFarge CG, Monroe RG, Gamble WJ, et al:** Left ventricular pressure and norepinephrine efflux from the innervated heart. Amer J Physiol 219:519, 1970

26. **Kopin IJ, Hertting G, Gordon EK:** Fate of norepinephrine-H^3 in the isolated perfused rat heart. J Pharmacol Exp Ther 138:34, 1962

27. **Montanari R, Costa E, Beaven MA, et al:** Turnover rates of norepinephrine in hearts of intact mice, rats, and guinea pigs using tritiated norepinephrine. Life Sci 2:232, 1963

28. **Pool PE, Covell JW, Levitt M, et al:** Reduction of cardiac tyrosine hydroxylase activity in experimental congestive heart failure. Circ Res 20:349, 1967

29. **Krakoff LR, Buccino RA, Spann JF Jr, et al:** Cardiac catechol O-methyltransferase and monoamine oxidase activity in congestive heart failure. Amer J Physiol 215:549, 1968

30. **Falck B, Hillarp NA, Thieme G, et al:** Fluorescence of catecholamines and related compounds condensed with formaldehyde. J Histochem Cytochem 10:348, 1962

31. **Jacobowitz D, Cooper T, Barner HB:** Histochemical and chemical studies of the localization of adrenergic and cholinergic nerves in normal and denervated cat hearts. Circ Res 20:289, 1967

32. **Vogel JHK, Jacobowitz D, Chidsey CA:** Distribution of norepinephrine in the failing bovine heart. Circ Res 24:71, 1969

33. **Mathes P, Cowan C, Gudbjarnason S:** Storage and metabolism of norepinephrine after experimental myocardial infarction. Amer J Physiol 220:27, 1971

34. **Mathes P, Gudbjarnason S:** Changes in norepinephrine stores in the canine heart following experimental myocardial infarction. Amer Heart J 81:211, 1971

35. **Doyle AE:** Endogenous-catecholamine content of cardiac muscle in sodium-loaded and sodium-depleted rats. Lancet 1:1399, 1968

36. **Spann JF Jr, Sonnenblick EH, Cooper T, et al:** Cardiac norepinephrine stores and the contractile state of heart muscle. Circ Res 19:317, 1966

37. **Dhalla NS, Naidu KJR, Bhagat B, et al:** Biochemical basis of heart function. 1. Relation of catecholamine stores and contractile force in an isolated rat heart. Cardiovasc Res 5:376, 1971

38. **Stephen A:** Unwanted effects of propranolol. Amer J Cardiol 18:463, 1966

39. **Vogel JHK, Chidsey CA:** Cardiac adrenergic activity in experimental heart failure assessed with beta receptor blockade. Amer J Cardiol 24:198, 1969

40. **Covell JW, Chidsey CA, Braunwald E:** Reduction of the cardiac response to postganglionic sympathetic nerve stimulation in experimental heart failure. Circ Res 19:51, 1966

41. **Levy MN:** Sympathetic-parasympathetic interactions in the heart. Circ Res 24:437, 1971

42. **Samaan A:** Antagonistic cardiac nerves and heart rate. J Physiol (London) 83:332, 1935

43. **Hollenberg M, Carriere S, Barger AC:** Biphasic action of acetylcholine on ventricular myocardium. Circ Res 16:527, 1965

44. **Hoffmann F, Hoffman EJ, Middleton S, et al:** Stimulating effect of acetylcholine on the mammalian heart and the liberation of an epinephrine-like substance by the isolated heart. Amer J Physiol 144:189, 1945

45. **Buccino RA, Sonnenblick EH, Copper T, et al:** Direct positive inotropic effect of acetylcholine on myocardium. Evidence for multiple cholinergic receptors in the heart. Circ Res 19:1097, 1966

46. **LaRaia PJ, Sonnenblick EH:** Autonomic control of cardiac C-AMP. Circ Res 28:377, 1971

47. **Grodner AS, Lahrtz HG, Pool PE, et al:** Neurotransmitter control of sinoatrial pacemaker frequency in isolated rat atria and in intact rabbits. Circ Res 28:867, 1970

48. **Meerson FZ:** The myocardium in hyperfunction, hypertrophy, and heart failure. Circ Res 25 suppl II:143, 1969

49. **Eckberg DI, Drabinsky M, Braunwald E:** Defective cardiac parasympathetic control in patients with heart disease. New Eng J Med 285:877, 1971

Chapter 8

Contractile and Energetic Behavior of Hypertrophied and Failing Myocardium

George Cooper, IV, MD
J. F. Gunning, MB, MRACP
C. E. Harrison, MD, FACC
H. N. Coleman, III, MD, FACC

Although the hypertrophy process is a fundamental mechanism whereby the heart compensates for an increased load, the description of its effects on myocardial contractile and energetic behavior has begun only recently. Various aspects of the contractile activity and the energetics of the hypertrophied and failing myocardium have interested many investigators.[1-9] In recent studies of papillary muscles[10] from hypertrophied right ventricles, as well as of intact hypertrophied right ventricles,[11] Spann and his co-workers characterized myocardial contractility in terms of force-velocity relationships and quantitated a depression of myocardial contractility in both myocardial hypertrophy and hypertrophy that had decompensated into the congestive heart failure state. Subsequent studies by Bing et al.[3] have confirmed these findings. In contrast, Cooper et al.[12] recently investigated hypertrophy induced by a volume overload and described entirely normal myocardial contractile behavior. Since the contractile state has been identified as a major determinant of myocardial energy utilization,[13,14] it might be expected that hypertrophied myocardium, with or without superim-

posed heart failure, would have an altered pattern of myocardial energy utilization. Accordingly, we present our recent findings concerning the mechanics of contraction and the oxygen consumption ($M\dot{V}O_2$) of hypertrophied and failing myocardium.

Production of Right Ventricular Hypertrophy and Failure

Right ventricular hypertrophy and right ventricular hypertrophy with congestive heart failure were produced in adult cats weighing 1.5 to 3.0 kg by the method of Spann et al.[10] In brief, anesthetized cats underwent left thoracotomy, and chronic pressure overload was imposed on the right ventricle by constricting the main pulmonary artery with a circular clip. Clips with internal diameters of 3.5 and 2.8 mm were used to reduce the circumference of the pulmonary artery to approximately 20 and 10 percent of normal, respectively.[10] This procedure produces both hypertrophy of the right ventricle and the right ventricular papillary muscles[10] and, with the 2.8 mm clip, a congestive heart failure syndrome characterized by increased right ven-

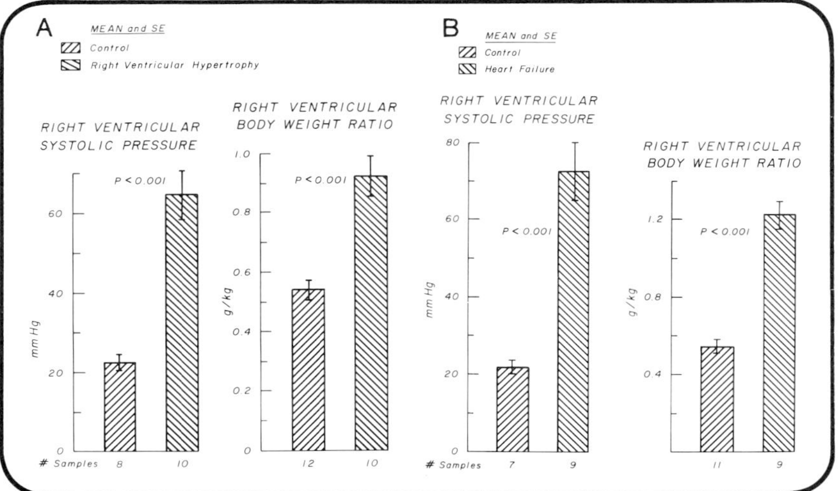

FIGURE 1. A, comparison of average values for ± 1 standard error of the mean (SEM) for right ventricular systolic pressure and ratio of right ventricular weight to body weight from a group of control cats and a group of cats with right ventricular hypertrophy after pulmonary arterial constriction. (Reproduced by permission from Bajusz.[19]) **B,** the same comparisons between the control group and a group of cats with right ventricular hypertrophy and congestive heart failure produced by pulmonary arterial constriction. (Reproduced by permission from Gunning and Coleman.[42])

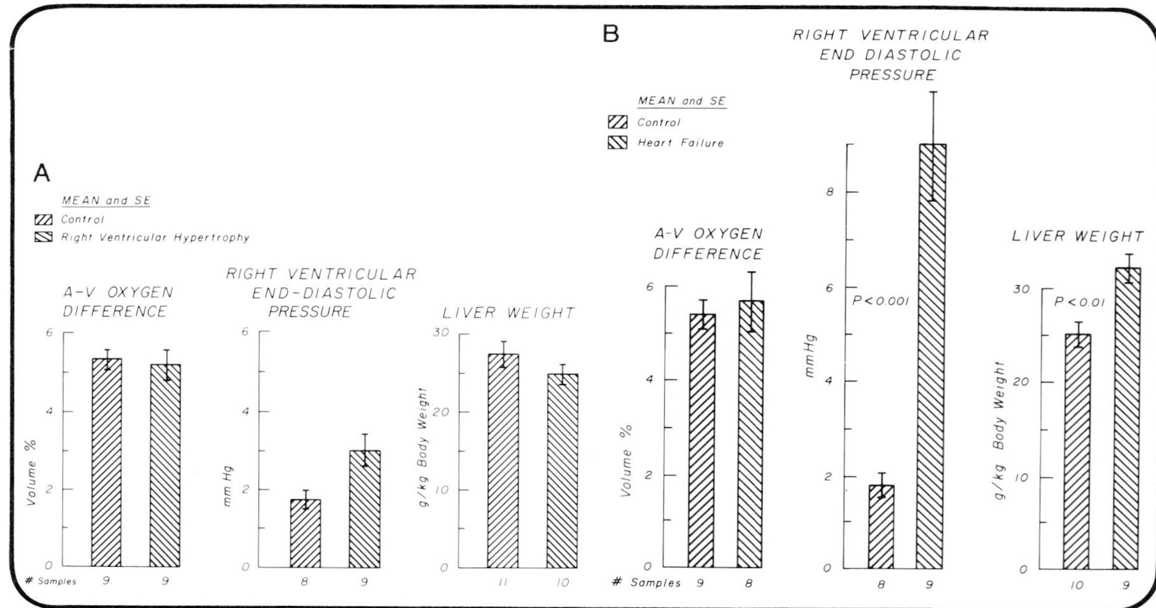

FIGURE 2. A, comparison of average values ± 1 SEM for arteriovenous oxygen difference, right ventricular end-diastolic pressure, and ratio of liver weight to body weight from a group of control cats and a group of cats with right ventricular hypertrophy after pulmonary arterial constriction. (Reproduced by permission from Bajusz.[19]) **B,** the same comparisons between the control group and a group of cats with right ventricular hypertrophy and congestive heart failure produced by pulmonary arterial constriction. (Reproduced by permission from Gunning and Coleman.[42])

tricular end-diastolic pressure, ascites and pleural effusion. After a convalescent period of 25 to 82 days, anesthesia was again induced with intraperitoneal pentobarbital (25 mg/kg), and the hemodynamic status was determined in the 10 cats with right ventricular hypertrophy without congestive failure (RVH), 9 cats with right ventricular hypertrophy with congestive failure (CHF) and 12 cats in the control group.

After these determinations, papillary muscle was rapidly excised from each of the right ventricles and transferred to a Petri dish containing oxygenated Krebs-Ringer's solution. Ties of noncapillary 4–0 silk were placed on the ends of each muscle, which was then mounted from the bottom of the central tubular chamber of a Lucite® muscle bath. Details of this apparatus and procedures for simultaneous measurement of myocardial mechanics and oxygen consumption ($M\dot{V}O_2$) have been presented previously.[15]

Right Ventricular Hypertrophy

Hemodynamics: The findings documenting right ventricular hypertrophy in the cats that underwent operation are shown in Figure 1A. The ratio of right ventricular weight to body weight was increased from 0.54 ± 0.03 standard error of the mean (SEM) g/kg in control cats to 0.93 ± 0.07 in the operated cats ($P < 0.001$). Right ventricular systolic pressure increased from 22 ± 2 mm Hg to 64 ± 6 ($P < 0.001$). The absence of evidence of congestive heart failure is seen in Figure 2A. There was no significant difference between control cats and those that underwent operation in arteriovenous mixed oxygen difference, right ventricular end-diastolic pressure or the ratio of liver weight to body weight. No ascites, pleural effusions or enlarged systemic veins were found in the cats that underwent constriction of the pulmonary artery with 3.5 mm clips.

Mechanics of Contraction and $M\dot{V}O_2$ of Papillary Muscles: The mechanics of contraction of the 10 hypertrophied and 12 control muscles of similar average cross-sectional area (0.90 and 0.92 mm²) were assessed from isotonic force-velocity curves and from isometric contractions at various muscle lengths.

Isotonic force-velocity relations for the two groups of muscles are shown in Figure 3A. The average values for preload, determining initial muscle lengths, were similar (0.44 ± 0.02 g/mm² in the control group and 0.52 ± 0.03 in the group with hypertrophy). In the upper panel the force-velocity curve from the hypertrophied muscles is shown to be depressed downwards and to the left, with a decreased velocity of shortening at all loads. The maximal measured velocity at preload is significantly depressed from 1.35 ± 0.07 muscle lengths/sec in the control group to 0.94 ± 0.08 in the hypertrophy group ($P < 0.01$). In the lower panel, shortening, and thus external work, the product of shortening times load, was not significantly depressed in the hypertrophied muscles.

Figure 4A shows the $M\dot{V}O_2$ values corresponding to the afterloaded contractions of Figure 3A. In hypertrophied muscles, the average oxygen consumption for any given level of load is within normal limits.

Average length-tension curves for control and hypertrophied muscles are shown in Figure 5A. The average resting length-tension curves for the two groups of muscles are similar, with a resting tension at maximal length (Lmax) of 0.87 ± 0.14 g/mm² (control) and 1.00 ± 0.12 (hypertrophy). Average developed tension at Lmax was decreased in the hypertrophied muscles, but the difference was not statistically significant (6.19 ± 0.55 g/mm² and 4.90 ± 0.54, $P > 0.1$). The time course of isometric tension development for the two groups of muscles was analyzed in terms of the maximal rate of tension development and the time from onset of tension development to peak tension at Lmax. The maximal rate of rise of tension at Lmax was significantly depressed from 34.1 ± 3.3 g/mm²/sec in the control muscles to 22.3 ± 2.3 in the hypertrophied muscles ($P < 0.01$). The time to peak tension was significantly greater in the hypertrophied muscles compared with the control (354.5 ± 9.4 msec and 302.4 ± 5.4, respectively, $P < 0.01$), despite the fact that less tension was being developed.

Oxygen consumption was determined for five levels of tension development on each length-tension curve for 12 control and 10 hypertrophied muscles. The relationship between tension development and $M\dot{V}O_2$ in these isometric contractions is presented in Figure 6A. The relationship between $M\dot{V}O_2$ and isometric devel-

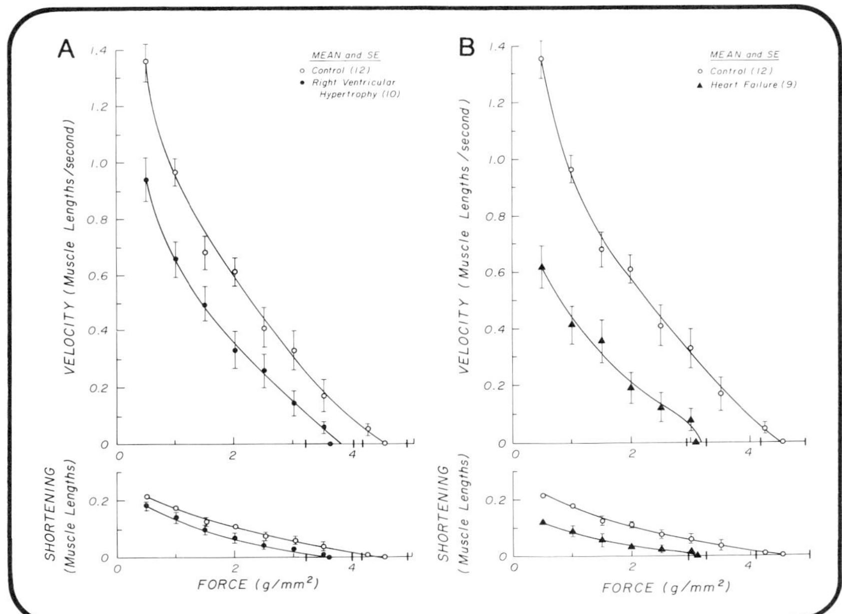

FIGURE 3. A, (upper panel) comparison of average force-velocity relations ± 1 SEM for papillary muscles obtained from 12 control cats and 10 cats with right ventricular hypertrophy; **(lower panel)** extent of shortening normalized in terms of muscle lengths plotted versus force. (Reproduced by permission from Bajusz.[19]) **B,** the same comparisons between the control group and a group of cats with right ventricular hypertrophy and congestive heart failure. (Reproduced by permission from Gunning and Coleman.[42])

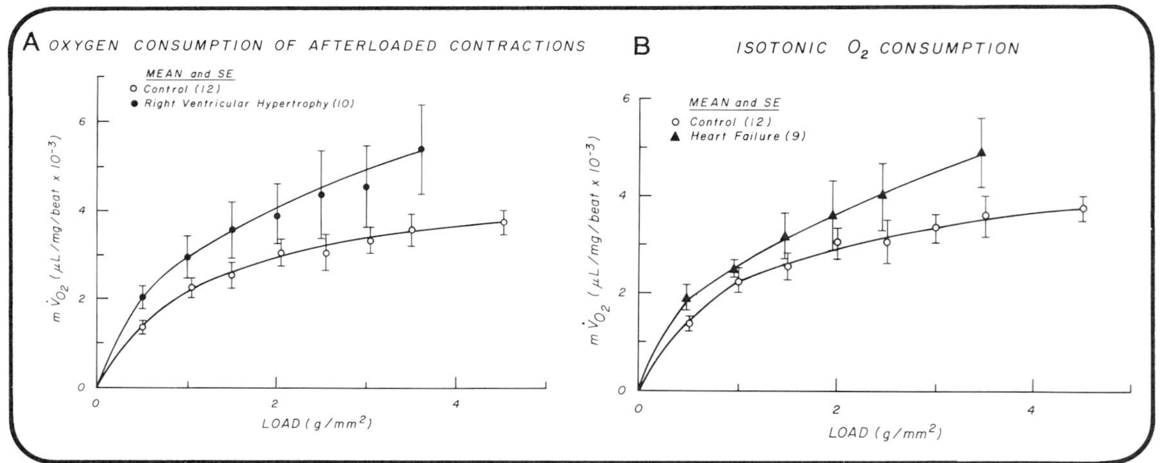

FIGURE 4. A, comparison of average oxygen consumption values ± 1 SEM for the 12 control and 10 papillary muscles with right ventricular hypertrophy depicted in Figure 3A. (Reproduced by permission from Bajusz.[19]) **B,** comparison of average oxygen consumption values ± 1 SEM for the 12 control muscles and 9 muscles with hypertrophy and congestive heart failure depicted in Figure 3B. (Reproduced by permission from Gunning and Coleman.[42])

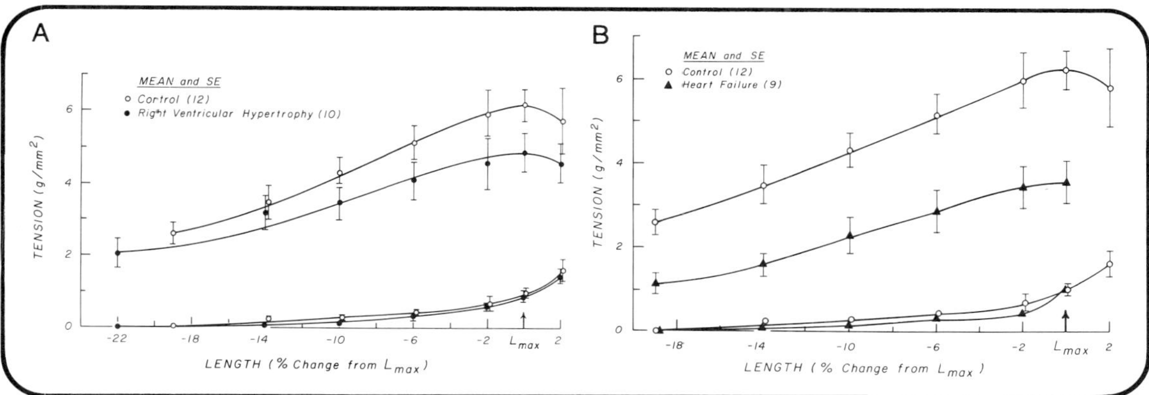

FIGURE 5. A, comparison of average length-tension relations ± 1 SEM for papillary muscles obtained from 12 control cats and 10 cats with right ventricular hypertrophy after pulmonary arterial constriction. **B,** comparison of average length-tension relations ± 1 SEM for papillary muscles from the 12 control right ventricles and 9 with hypertrophy and congestive heart failure. (Reproduced by permission from Gunning and Coleman.[42])

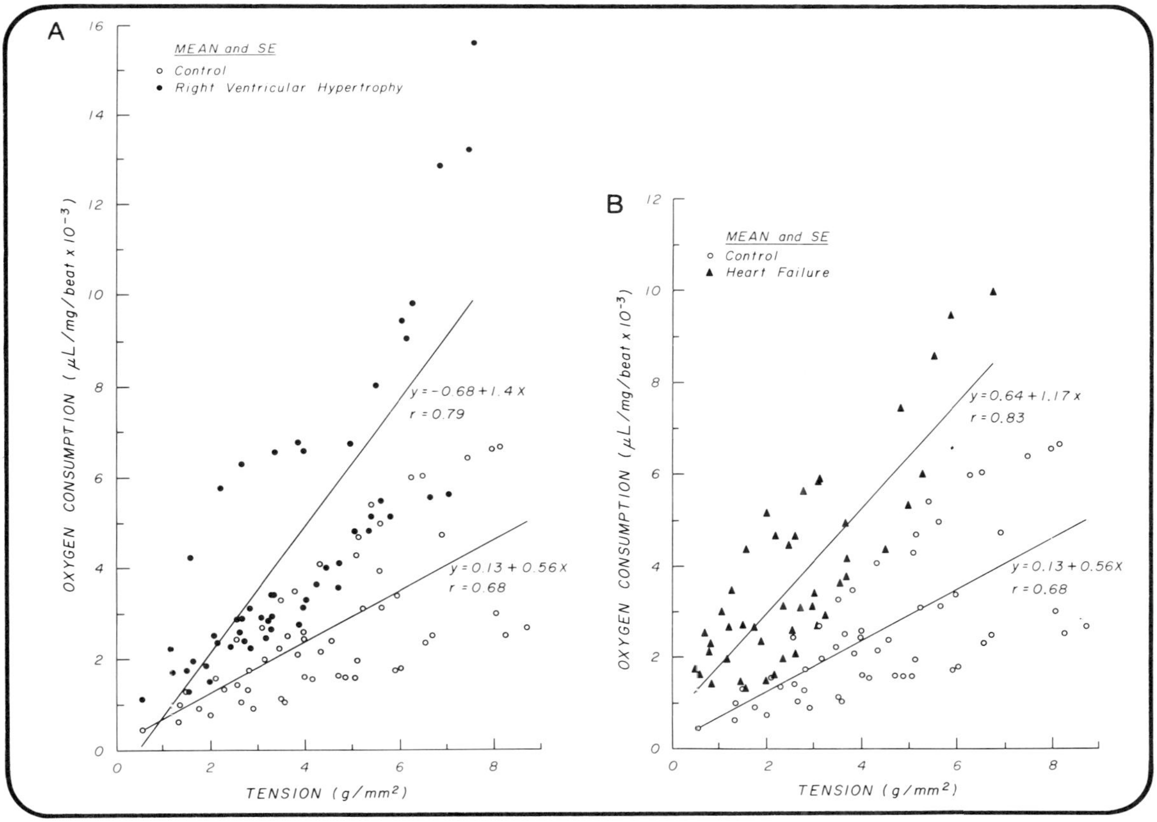

FIGURE 6. A, relation between peak isometric tension development and M$\dot{V}$O$_2$ The relationship between tension and M$\dot{V}$O$_2$ for control muscles is described from the least squares regression equation Y = 0.13 + 0.56 X; for muscles with right ventricular hypertrophy, Y = −0.68 + 1.40 X (see text). (Reproduced by permission from Bajusz.[19]) **B,** the same relationship for the muscles with hypertrophy and congestive heart failure, where Y = 0.64 + 1.17 X. (Reproduced by permission from Gunning and Coleman.[42])

oped tension for normal muscles is described by the least squares linear regression equation Y = 0.13 + 0.56 X (r = 0.68, number of points = 55) and for the hypertrophied muscles by Y = −0.68 + 1.40 X (r = 0.79, number of points = 52) (Figure 6A). The following statistical analysis was applied. The slopes of the regression lines relating $M\dot{V}O_2$ and isometric developed tension for the individual muscles of each group were calculated. The two groups of slopes obtained were then compared, using both the Student t test and the nonparametric rank sum test. The mean slope for the normal muscles was 0.63 ± 0.08 nL O_2/mg/beat/g/mm^2 of tension and for the hypertrophied muscles, 1.28 ± 0.27. This difference is significant (P <0.01). Thus, the oxygen cost per unit of tension development was significantly increased in the hypertrophied muscles. Further evidence that the $M\dot{V}O_2$ of isometric contractions was greater in hypertrophied muscles is seen when the $M\dot{V}O_2$ per gram of tension developed at the peak of the length-tension curves is compared. The $M\dot{V}O_2$/g/mm^2 of tension developed was 1.13 nL/mg/beat for the hypertrophied muscles and 0.61 for the control muscles (P<0.01).

Resting Oxygen Consumption of Papillary Muscles: Resting oxygen consumption was determined in 11 control and 8 hypertrophied muscles. The $M\dot{V}O_2$ was increased from 2.07 ± 0.19 μL/mg/hour in the control muscles to 3.42 ± 0.45 in the hypertrophied muscles (P<0.01).

Right Ventricular Failure

Hemodynamics: In Figure 1B the mean values ± standard error of the mean (SEM) for right ventricular systolic pressure for a group of 9 animals with reduction of the pulmonary arterial lumen to 10 percent of normal (2.8 mm clip) are compared with those of a control group. The average peak systolic pressure was significantly increased from 22 ± 2 mm Hg to 73 ± 7 (P <0.001). The ratio of right ventricular weight to body weight was significantly increased from 0.54 ± 0.08 g/kg to 1.22 ± 0.08 in the cats with pulmonary arterial constriction (P<0.001). The average arteriovenous oxygen difference was unchanged in cats with hypertrophy and heart failure (Figure 2B). However, average right ventricular end-diastolic pressure (1.9 ± 0.2 mm

Hg in the control group and 9.0 ± 1.1 in the group with hypertrophy and heart failure) and the ratio of liver weight to body weight (27.8 ± 1.1 g/kg in the control group and 31.7 ± 1.5 in the group with hypertrophy and heart failure) were significantly increased (P <0.01) in pulmonary arterial constriction. The hemodynamic burden imposed by pulmonary arterial constriction was evidenced in all cats by enlarged systemic veins, central venous congestion of the liver by gross examination and ascites. In addition, 4 cats had bilateral pleural effusions at the time of study. The severity of the heart failure state is indicated by the 60 percent mortality between operation and study in these cats.

Mechanics of Contraction and $M\dot{V}O_2$ of Papillary Muscles: The mechanics of contraction were determined for 9 muscles from the heart failure group and compared with those of 12 normal control muscles of similar average cross-sectional area (0.90 mm^2 in the control muscles and 0.75 in those with heart failure). In Figure 3B, upper panel, the average force-velocity curves for the two groups of muscles are plotted. These relationships were obtained from similar initial muscle lengths, as established by average preload values of 0.44 g/mm^2 in the control group and 0.52 in the group with heart failure. The force-velocity curve from the muscles with failure was depressed, with decreased velocity of shortening at all loads. The maximal measured velocity with only the preload was decreased from 1.35 ± 0.07 muscle lengths/sec in the control group to 0.62 ± 0.06 in the group with failure (P <0.001). In addition, the extent of shortening, and thus external work, the product of shortening times load, was significantly depressed in the muscles with failure. The $M\dot{V}O_2$ values corresponding to the force-velocity mechanics in Figure 3B are shown in Figure 4B. The average $M\dot{V}O_2$ for afterloaded contractions of failing muscles was not significantly different from the $M\dot{V}O_2$ obtained in normal papillary muscles.

The average length-tension relationship for muscles with heart failure is compared with that of control muscles in Figure 5B. The average resting length-tension relations for the two groups are similar, with resting tensions at Lmax of 1.00 ± 0.14 g/mm^2 in the control group and 0.99 ± 0.12 in the group with heart failure. The active developed tension at Lmax in failing muscles was significantly depressed from a control value of 6.19 ± 0.55 g/mm² to 3.55 ± 0.53 (P <0.01). Analysis of the maximal rate of tension development at Lmax revealed a decrease in dF/dt from 34.1 ± 3.3 g/mm²/sec in the control group to 14.7 ± 0.2 in the group with heart failure (P <0.001). The time from onset of tension development to peak tension at Lmax was prolonged in heart failure muscles from a control value of 302 ± 5 msec to 370 ± 15 (P <0.001).

The $M\dot{V}O_2$ of isometric contractions at various resting tensions is plotted in Figure 6B. The relationship between $M\dot{V}O_2$ and isometric developed tension for normal muscles is described by the least squares linear regression equation $Y = 0.64 ± 1.17 X$ ($r = 0.83$, number of points = 45). The slope of each regression line is significantly different from zero (P <0.01). To evaluate the difference in slopes the following statistical analysis was applied. The slopes of the regression lines relating $M\dot{V}O_2$ and isometric developed tension for the individual muscles in each group were calculated. The two groups of slopes obtained were then compared using both the Student t test and the nonparametric rank sum test. The slopes of the two groups were significantly different (P <0.05, rank sum test; P <0.01, Student t test). The mean slope for normal muscles was 0.63 ± 0.08 nL O₂/mg/beat/g/mm² of tension, and for the failing muscles, 1.06 ± 0.12.

Resting Oxygen Consumption of Papillary Muscles: Resting oxygen consumption was satisfactorily determined in 11 control and 8 heart failure muscles. This basal oxygen consumption was elevated from 2.07 ± 0.19 μL/mg/hour in the control muscles to 4.27 ± 0.53 in the heart failure muscles (P <0.001).

Effect of Acetylstrophanthidin on Papillary Muscles: Acetylstrophanthidin, added to the perfusate in a final concentration of $2 × 10^{-7}$ g/ml for 4 muscles with heart failure, augmented contractility, with a shift of the force-velocity relation upward and to the right. Maximal measured velocity of shortening (preload) was augmented by 63, 42, 48 and 103 percent in the 4 muscles after the addition of acetylstrophanthidin. Maximal rate of rise of isometric tension at the apex of the length-tension curve was like-

wise augmented by 36, 55, 64 and 105 percent, respectively. In all muscles, $M\dot{V}O_2$ during isometric contractions was augmented for matched levels of tension development after the addition of acetylstrophanthidin. Tension was matched by decreasing initial muscle length after the addition of acetylstrophanthidin.[15] This relationship in a typical experiment is shown in Figure 7. The oxygen consumption of hypertrophied myocardium is increased at any given level of tension development after the addition of acetylstrophanthidin.

Altered Contractility and Muscle Mechanics in Ventricular Systolic Pressure Overload

The advent of cardiac catheterization and measurement of myocardial oxygen consumption ($M\dot{V}O_2$) instigated the initial investigations[6,16] of the relationships between the heart's metabolism and clinical heart failure states and thus reopened the search initiated by Harrison et al.[17] for a biochemical basis for congestive heart failure. In these initial studies of patients with heart failure, the values of $M\dot{V}O_2$ were not changed from normal. Subsequently, however, it became apparent from a series of investigations[14,18] that (1) $M\dot{V}O_2$ is determined by multiple factors that are principally the mechanical events of contraction, and (2) no precise analysis of mechanical events had been possible in these initial studies of $M\dot{V}O_2$ during heart failure. Of further interest are recent studies defining depression of myocardial contractility in terms of reduced intrinsic velocity of contraction in experimental myocardial hypertrophy in both the presence[10,11] and absence[3] of congestive failure. Since in these studies myocardial contractility was defined in terms of the depressed velocity of contraction—a major determinant of $M\dot{V}O_2$—our investigation focused on determining myocardial metabolism through measurements of $M\dot{V}O_2$ during an experimental hypertrophy-heart failure state induced by pressure overload.

In these studies, Spann's technique[10] of pulmonary arterial constriction was utilized to produce right ventricular pressure overload, resulting in right ventricular hypertrophy with and without congestive heart failure. As shown

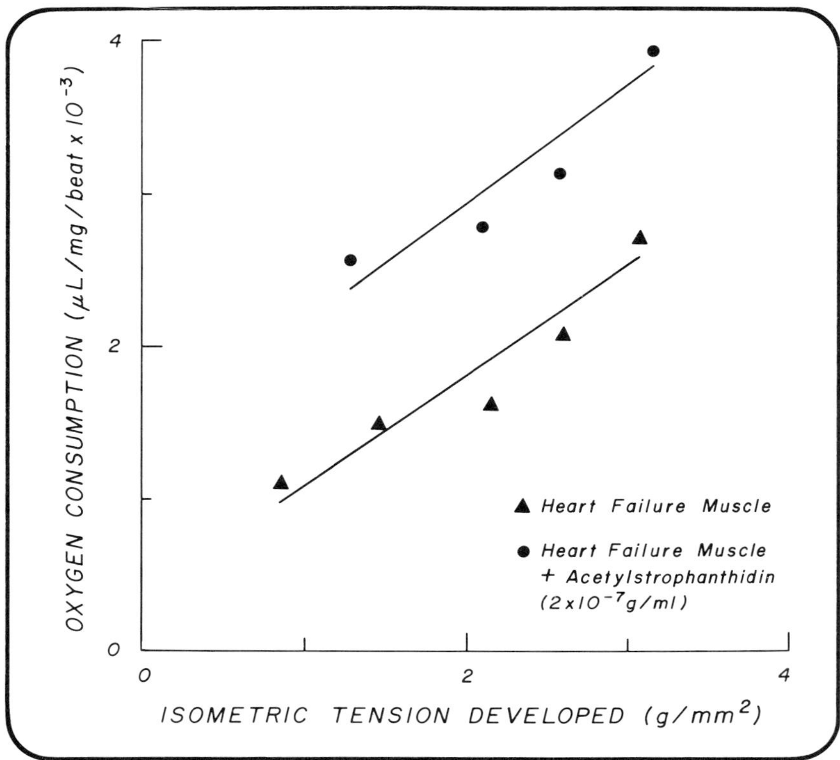

FIGURE 7. Effects of acetylstrophanthidin in increasing $M\dot{V}O_2$ of isometric contractions from a muscle with conges- tive heart failure at a constant level of tension development. (Reproduced by permission from Gunning and Coleman.[42])

in Figures 1B and 2B, this technique resulted in many features common to clinical heart failure states, including a two-fold increase in the ratio of right ventricular weight to body weight, elevated right ventricular end-diastolic pressure, an increase in the ratio of liver weight to body weight, and systemic fluid accumulation. The hypertrophy-failure state was associated with a profound depression of myocardial contractile mechanics, with depression of both the average force-velocity curves (Figure 3B) and the average length-tension curves (Figure 5B). These changes are of the same order of magnitude as those reported for this experimental hypertrophy-failure state by Spann et al.[10] Similar, but less dramatic, depression of the contractile state in experimental hypertrophy without congestive heart failure was noted in our experiments and in those of Spann et al.,[10] and similar results have been reported by Bing et al.[3] and by Gunning and Coleman.[19]

Myocardial Oxygen Consumption in Ventricular Systolic Pressure Overload

The unexpected finding in this investigation was a paradoxical increase in the $M\dot{V}O_2$ of the isometric contractions of hypertrophied and hypertrophied-failing myocardium. This finding was present both at the apex of the length-tension curve when the average $M\dot{V}O_2$ of isometric contractions was expressed per average gram of tension development and when all $M\dot{V}O_2$ values for isometric contractions were evaluated over the range of the length-tension curve. Thus, $M\dot{V}O_2$ per contraction per gram of tension development was effectively doubled in the hypertrophied-failing myocardium from 0.57 to 1.17 nL/mg per contraction per gram of tension development. Similar findings were demonstrated for right ventricular hypertrophy without congestive heart failure with an average $M\dot{V}O_2$ per gram of tension development of 1.40 nL/mg per contraction per gram of tension development. Although the precise values are dependent on both the rate of stimulation and the temperature, these factors were the same for all experiments. Thus, these findings clearly delineate a striking metabolic abnormality associated with experimental hypertrophy and failure induced by a pressure overload.

When isotonic contractions were evaluated, the average velocity of shortening of hypertrophied myocardium was strikingly depressed. In addition, the extent of shortening, and thus the amount of external work performance by hypertrophied muscles, was depressed. Based on depression of these two mechanical factors determining $M\dot{V}O_2$, it would be reasonable to predict that the average $M\dot{V}O_2$ of isotonic contractions of the hypertrophied and hypertrophied-failing myocardium would also be depressed. This expectation was not realized; the $M\dot{V}O_2$ of afterloaded isotonic contractions of hypertrophied and failing muscles was entirely normal. These results undoubtedly reflect interactions among the multiple factors determining the $M\dot{V}O_2$ of isotonic contractions —tension, external work and velocity—but are consistent with the increased oxygen cost of developing tension shown for the isometric contractions of these muscles.

These results are unique in showing a paradoxical relationship between velocity of contraction and $M\dot{V}O_2$, in contrast with previously reported parallel increments in $M\dot{V}O_2$ and contraction velocity in the chronically augmented myocardial contractile state associated with experimental hyperthyroidism.[20] Similarly, Graham et al.[21] reported parallel decrements in $M\dot{V}O_2$ and velocity of contraction in acute myocardial depression and failure, findings that also contrast with those reported here.

Mitochondrial Function in Ventricular Systolic Pressure Overload

The level of $M\dot{V}O_2$ represents the sum of overall myocardial energy utilization, since it is generally accepted that myocardial metabolism is aerobic in character. This premise assumes normal coupling of oxidative phosphorylation to the production of adenosine triphosphate (ATP) in mitochondria. The effects of experimental myocardial hypertrophy and heart failure on this aspect of mitochondrial function have been the subject of conflicting reports. Mitochondrial energy production has been described as normal[22-24] or impaired.[25-27] Sobel et al.[28] utilized a hypertrophy preparation identical to that used in our experiments and reported normal mitochondrial energy production in the presence of depressed contractility. These findings subsequently were critically reviewed by Schwartz,[27] who noted that mitochondria from Sobel's study demonstrated low respiratory control indexes; he suggested that the mitochondria may have been damaged by the proteinase procedure utilized in their isolation. This subject also received critical analysis by Lindenmayer et al.,[23] who stressed that mitochondrial respiration was altered in advanced and severe heart failure, whereas it was generally normal in hypertrophy or mild congestive heart failure. This concept was based on the demonstration by Lindenmayer et al.[25] of normal or even increased mitochondrial respiratory control indexes in the presence of stable experimental hypertrophy and gains support from the findings of Chidsey et al.[22] of normal mitochondrial function in human cardiac hypertrophy and failure states. Another insight into the energy production of mitochondria may be gained from measurements of high energy phosphate stores (ATP and creatine phosphate) in various experimental models of hypertrophy and congestive heart failure. Based on these studies,[29,30] it is generally accepted that the energy stores are either normal or slightly reduced in the presence of hypertrophy and congestive heart failure, thus eliminating depleted energy stores as the biochemical mechanism mediating depressed myocardial contractility.

Increased energy utilization (ATP and creatine phosphate degradation) by myofibrils and a dissociation of the usual relationship between velocity of contraction and $M\dot{V}O_2$ offer an alternative explanation for the observed increase in $M\dot{V}O_2$ in the hypertrophied-failing myocardium. This hypothesis gains credence from the report of Gunning and Coleman[19] of increased $M\dot{V}O_2$ associated with tension development in hypertrophied muscles in the absence of congestive heart failure and also from the reports of Chidsey et al.[22] and Schwartz[27] of

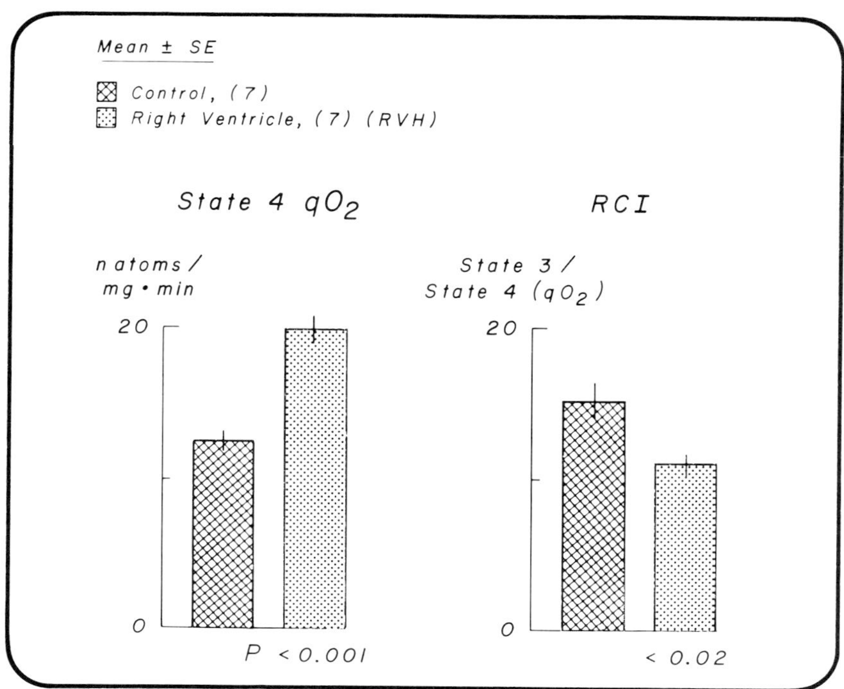

FIGURE 8. Summary of two oxidative indexes of mitochondria obtained simultaneously from control hearts and the right ventricles of experimental hearts. State 4 qO_2 = rate of oxygen consumption after ADP phosphorylation is complete, that is, nonphosphorylating mitochondrial respiration; RCI = respiratory control index, a measure of the degree of coupling of oxidation to phosphorylation. (Reprinted from Cooper et al.[32] by permission of the American Heart Association, Inc.)

normal mitochondrial energy production in stable hypertrophy. Of considerable interest are the results of Pool et al.,[31] who measured the ATP utilization of metabolically blocked papillary muscles from an identical experimental preparation of hypertrophy. These authors concluded that both contractility and ATP utilization were depressed in hypertrophied and failing myocardium. However, the experimental design used in this study made comparisons between the control and hypertrophy-failure groups difficult, and the authors were unable to evaluate the significant differences in ATP utilization between the two groups because of wide variations in data from muscles of each group.

Subsequent studies by Cooper et al.[32] have shown a more severe depression of contractile indexes in this same preparation of myocardial hypertrophy without congestive heart failure and have again demonstrated the paradoxical relationship between depressed contractile state and augmented $M\dot{V}O_2$. Concomitant investiga-

tions of the same right ventricles have shown (Figure 8) that there is a marked increase in nonphosphorylating state 4 respiration of mitochondria isolated from the hypertrophied right ventricles and, because the rate of oxidative phosphorylation (state 3) was only slightly elevated, a reduction of the respiratory control index (the ratio of state 3 to state 4 respiratory rates). A linear correlation ($r = 0.91$) between the increase in papillary muscle respiration and mitochondrial state 4 respiration (Figure 9) suggests a mechanism for the paradoxical energetics of pressure hypertrophied myocardium: in individual experiments the degree of increased papillary muscle respiration relates directly to the degree of nonphosphorylating respiration of mitochondria isolated from the same right ventricle. This reconciles the present findings with those of Pool et al.,[31] since a relationship between ATP utilization rate and nonphosphorylating respiration in the myocardium is unnecessary.

Calcium Metabolism in Ventricular Systolic Pressure Overload

Further consideration of this metabolic abnormality led to an investigation of the calcium metabolism of hypertrophied myocardium, since calcium accumulation by mitochondria has been postulated as one of the primary determinants of nonphosphorylating respiration.[33] After oligomycin had been added to block oxidative phosphorylation of the mitochondria, ruthenium red was used to block mitochondrial calcium uptake. This was found to return the nonphosphorylating respiration of mitochondria from pressure-hypertrophied myocardium to normal (Figure 10). Additional studies by Cooper et al.[34] have demonstrated increased calcium cycling by the mitochondria of intact hypertrophied myocardial cells and have related this to one aspect of abnormal contractile state.

These studies do not suggest a primary abnormality of mitochondrial function in pressure overload hypertrophy. Rather, they may be put in perspective by considering reports of decreased calcium uptake by the sarcoplasmic reticulum of hypertrophied and failing myocardium.[35-38] Coupling this finding with the demonstration of increased calcium content of mitochondria isolated from pressure-hypertrophied myocardium,[39] we suggest that the augmented calcium cycling and resultant increased nonphosphorylating respiration of mitochondria from pressure hypertrophied myocardium may account for the abnormal whole muscle energetics of this preparation. However, it is likely that this is the result of a primary defect in the normal cation biochemistry of the sarcoplasmic

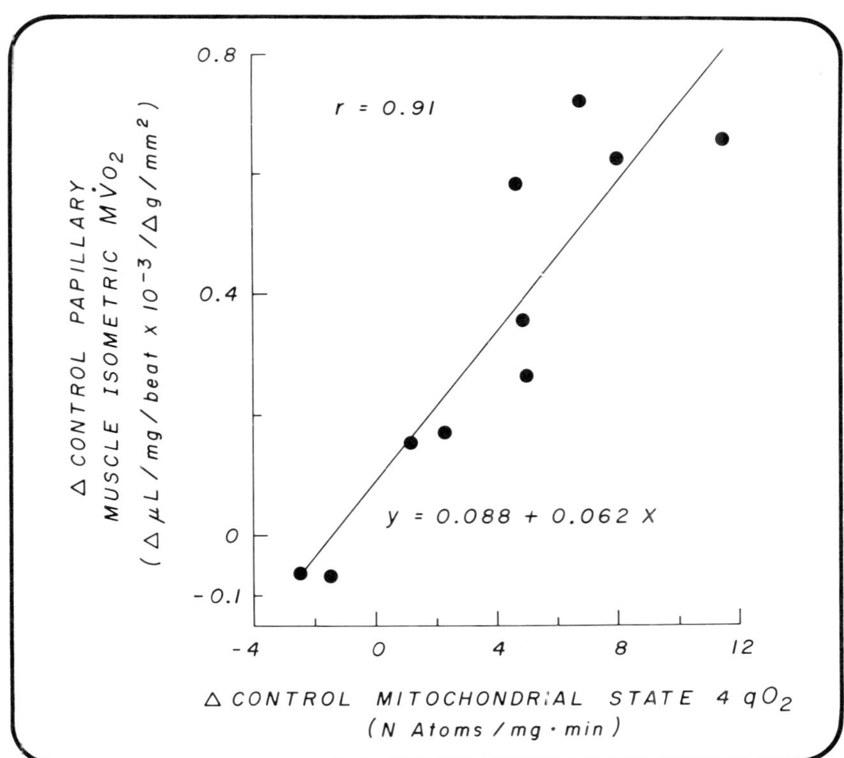

FIGURE 9. Relationship between papillary muscle isometric oxygen consumption (MV̇O₂) and mitochondrial state 4 oxygen consumption (qO₂) in material from the same right ventricles. The linear regression equation and the correlation coefficient for these 10 experiments are shown. (Reprinted from Cooper et al.[32] by permission of the American Heart Association, Inc.)

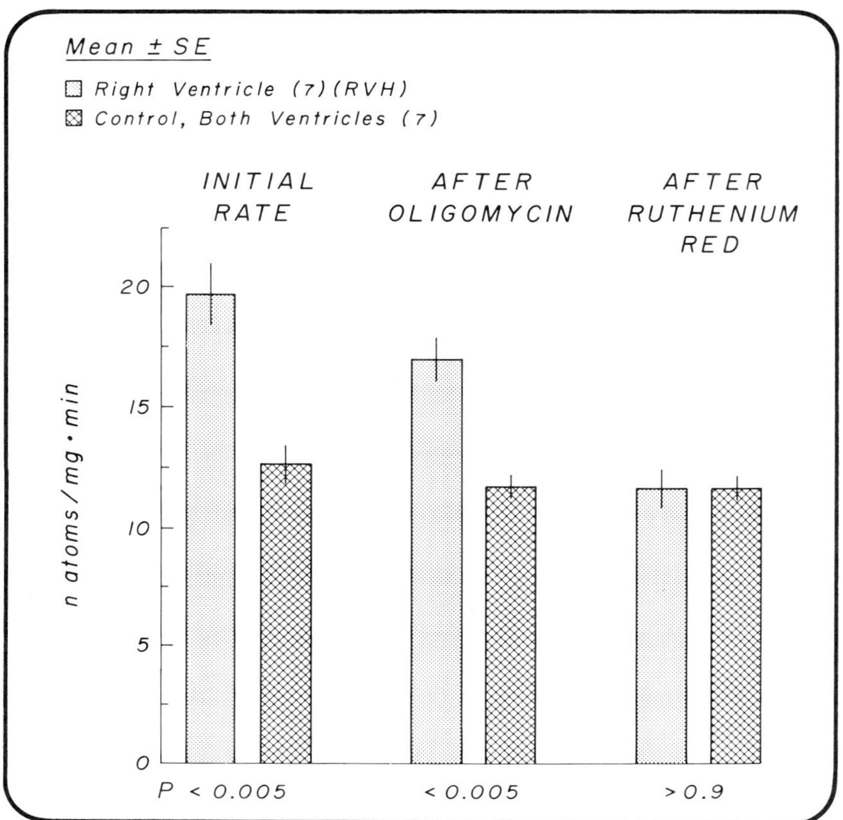

FIGURE 10. Summary of state 4 qO_2 values of mitochondria obtained simultaneously from control hearts and the right ventricles of experimental hearts. This shows that after phosphorylating respiration was blocked by oligomycin, the blockade of mitochondrial calcium uptake by ruthenium red normalized the respiratory rate of mitochondria from the hypertrophied myocardium. (Reprinted from Cooper et al.[32] by permission of the American Heart Association, Inc.)

reticulum of pressure-hypertrophied myocardium rather than the result of some primary disturbance of mitochondrial function.

Ventricular Systolic Volume Overload

It is of critical importance to know whether these findings have any relevance to clinical disease states. Two additional studies, although strictly applicable only to the model employed, bear on this question. First, a study by Cooper et al.[12] demonstrated that ventricular and papillary muscle hypertrophy induced by volume overload does not result in any of the contractile and energetic abnormalities just described above for a comparable degree and duration of hypertrophy induced by pressure overload. Thus, the nature of the inducing stress rather than the hypertrophy process itself must be responsible for the abnormalities described for myocardial hypertrophy induced by pressure overload.

Reversibility of Contractility and Metabolic Alterations in Hemodynamic Overload

Second, Cooper and Satava[40] have recently described a method that allows reversal of pressure overload hypertrophy. Detailed studies of this state[41] demonstrate that all of the morphologic, contractile, and metabolic abnormalities associated with myocardial hypertrophy induced by pressure overload are fully reversible, at least before deterioration into the congestive heart failure state. Taken together, these findings suggest that the contractile and energetic abnormalities of pressure-hypertrophied myocardium are the result of a labile functional derangement produced by the pressure overload itself. A delineation of the detrimental factor(s) inherent in the pressure stress might be of considerable clinical importance in view of the frequent deterioration of stable, compensatory myocardial hypertrophy into the congestive heart failure state.

Summary

Several recent studies have shown that myocardium hypertrophied by a pressure overload exhibits depressed indexes of contractility; further deterioration occurs when congestive heart failure is superimposed. In the cat, measurement of isotonic contractions of isolated right ventricular papillary muscles hypertrophied by pulmonary arterial banding revealed decrements in both the velocity and extent of shortening against any given afterload. Measurement of isometric contractions showed a reduction in the maximal active tension generated, an increase in the time required to reach peak tension and a decrease in the rate of tension development. Because these contractile indexes have been defined as determinants of the oxygen consumption ($M\dot{V}O_2$) of isolated myocardium, the $M\dot{V}O_2$ of isotonic and isometric contractions in this same preparation of pressure-stressed hypertrophied and failing myocardium was examined. It was found that both for hypertrophied myocardium and for hypertrophied and failing myocardium, the expected parallel decrements of contractile indexes and $M\dot{V}O_2$ did not obtain. The $M\dot{V}O_2$ of isotonic contractions was normal, and the $M\dot{V}O_2$ of isometric contractions was increased. This combination of depressed contractility and paradoxically augmented $M\dot{V}O_2$ is apparently related to the pressure stress rather than to the hypertrophic response, as we have found normal contractile indexes and $M\dot{V}O_2$ with the same extent and duration of hypertrophy induced by a volume overload. More recent studies demonstrate that the mechanism for the increased $M\dot{V}O_2$ of pressure-hypertrophied myocardium lies in increased nonphosphorylating respiration by its mitochondria as a result of abnormal calcium metabolism.

Acknowledgment: This work was supported in part by Grants HL 13706 and HL 12997 from the National Heart and Lung Institute, Grant AM 01005 from the National Institute of Arthritis and Metabolic Diseases and a grant from the Minnesota Heart Association.

References

1. **Alexander N, Goldfarb T, Drury DR:** Cardiac performance of hypertensive aorta-constricted rabbits. Circ Res 10:11, 1962
2. **Beznak M:** Cardiac output in rats during the development of cardiac hypertrophy. Circ Res 6:207, 1958
3. **Bing OHL, Matsushita S, Fanburg DL, et al:** Mechanical properties of rat cardiac muscle during experimental hypertrophy. In, Cardiac Hypertrophy (Alpert N, ed). New York, Academic Press, 1971, p 361
4. **Bing RJ:** Metabolism of the heart. Harvey Lect 50:27, 1954
5. **Bishop SP, Altschuld RA:** Evidence for increased glycolytic metabolism in cardiac hypertrophy and congestive heart failure. In Ref 3, p 567
6. **Blain JM, Schafer J, Siegle AL, et al:** Studies in myocardial metabolism in congestive failure. Amer J Med 20:820, 1956
7. **Butzschneider HJ, Bücherl E, Frank A, et al:** Über die Energetik des normalen und hypertrophischen isolierten Saügetierherzens. Arch Ges Physiol 251:458, 1952
8. **Meerson FZ, Pshennikova MG:** Effect of hypertrophy on the contractile function of the heart. Biull Eksp Biol Med 59:34, 1965
9. **Wollenberger A:** Energy metabolism of the failing heart and the metabolic action of cardiac glycosides. Pharmacol Rev 1:311, 1949
10. **Spann JF Jr, Buccino RA, Sonnenblick EH, et al:** Contractile state of cardiac muscle obtained from cats with experimentally produced ventricular hypertrophy and heart failure. Circ Res 21:341, 1967
11. **Spann JF Jr, Covell JR, Eckberg DL, et al:** Myocardial contractile state in hypertrophy and congestive failure. Studies in intact heart and isolated muscle. Circulation 36 suppl II:241, 1967
12. **Cooper G, Puga FJ, Zujko KJ, et al:** Normal myocardial function and energetics in volume-overload hypertrophy in the cat. Circ Res 32:140, 1973
13. **Sonnenblick EH, Ross J Jr, Covell JW, et al:** Velocity of contraction as a determinant of myocardial oxygen consumption. Amer J Physiol 209: 919, 1965
14. **Coleman HN:** Determinants of myocardial energy utilization. In Ref 3, p 485
15. **Coleman HN:** Role of acetylstrophanthidin in augmenting myocardial oxygen consumption. Circ Res 21:487, 1967

16. **Gudbjarnason S, Hayden RC, Wendt VE, et al:** Oxidative reduction in heart muscle: theoretical and clinical considerations. Circulation 26:937, 1962

17. **Harrison TR, Pilcher C, Ewing G:** Studies in congestive heart failure. IV. The potassium content of skeletal and cardiac muscle. J Clin Invest 8:325, 1930

18. **Graham TP, Covell JW, Sonnenblick EH, et al:** Control of myocardial oxygen consumption: relative influence of contractile state and tension development. J Clin Invest 47:375, 1968

19. **Gunning JF, Coleman HN:** The effects of hypertrophy on myocardial energy utilization. In, Myocardiology, vol I (Bajusz E, Rona G, ed). Baltimore, University Park Press, 1972, p 190

20. **Skelton CL, Coleman HN, Wildenthal K, et al:** Augmentation of myocardial oxygen consumption in hyperthyroid cats. Circ Res 27:301, 1971

21. **Graham TP, Ross J Jr, Covell JW, et al:** Myocardial oxygen consumption in acute experimental cardiac depression. Circ Res 21:123, 1967

22. **Chidsey CA, Weinbach EC, Pool PE, et al:** Biochemical studies of energy production in the failing human heart. J Clin Invest 45: 40, 1966

23. **Olson RE:** Abnormalities of myocardial metabolism. Circ Res 14 suppl II:109, 1964

24. **Plaut GWE, Gertler MM:** Oxidative phosphorylation studies in normal and experimentally produced congestive heart failure in guinea pigs: a comparison. Ann NY Acad Sci 72:515, 1959

25. **Lindenmayer GE, Sordahl LA, Schwartz A:** Reevaluation of oxidative phosphorylation in cardiac mitochondria from normal animals and animals in heart failure. Circ Res 23:439, 1968

26. **Schwartz A, Lee KS:** Study of heart mitochondria and glycolytic metabolism in experimentally induced cardiac failure. Circ Res 10:321, 1962

27. **Schwartz A:** Studies on mitochondria from normal, hypertrophied, and failing myocardium. In Ref 3, p 511

28. **Sobel BE, Spann JF Jr, Pool PE, et al:** Normal oxidative phosphorylation in mitochondria from the failing heart. Circ Res 21:355, 1967

29. **Minton PR, Zoll PM, Norman LR:** Levels of phosphate compounds in experimental cardiac hypertrophy. Circ Res 8:924, 1960

30. **Pool PE, Spann JF Jr, Buccino RA, et al:** Myocardial high energy phosphate stores in cardiac hypertrophy and heart failure. Circ Res 21:365, 1967

31. **Pool PE, Chandler BM, Spann JF Jr, et al:** Mechanochemistry of cardiac muscle. IV. Utilization of high energy phosphates in experimental failure in cats. Circ Res 24:313, 1969

32. **Cooper G, Harrison CE, Puga F, et al:** Mechanism for the abnormal energetics of pressure-induced hypertrophy of cat myocardium. Circ Res 33:213, 1973

33. **Rasmussen H:** Mitochondrial ion transport: mechanism and physiological significance. Fed Proc 25:903, 1966

34. **Cooper G, Sack DW, Coleman HN, et al:** Abnormal mitochondrial calcium metabolism in pressure hypertrophied myocardium. Circulation 48 suppl IV:11, 1973

35. **Schwartz A, Sordahl LA, McCollum WB:** Studies on mitochondria and the muscle relaxing system. In Ref 19, p 12

36. **Harigaya S, Schwartz A:** Rate of calcium binding and uptake in normal animal and failing human cardiac muscle. Circ Res 25:781, 1969

37. **Gertz EW, Hess ML, Lain RF, et al:** Activity of the vesicular calcium pump in the spontaneously failing heart-lung preparation. Circ Res 20:477, 1967

38. **Suko J, Vogel JHK, Chidsey CA:** Intracellular calcium and myocardial contractility. Circ Res 27:235, 1970

39. **Ito Y, Chidsey CA:** Intracellular calcium and myocardial contractility. J Molec Cell Cardiol 4:507, 1972

40. **Cooper G, Satava RM:** A method for producing reversible long-term pressure overload of the cat right ventricle. J Appl Physiol (in press)

41. **Cooper G, Satava RM, Harrison CE, et al:** Normal myocardial function and energetics after reversing pressure-overload hypertrophy. Amer J Physiol 226:1158, 1974

42. **Gunning JF, Coleman HN:** Myocardial oxygen consumption during experimental hypertrophy and congestive heart failure. J Molec Cell Cardiol 5:25, 1973

Chapter 9

Regulation of Cardiac Performance in Clinical Heart Disease

Interactions Between Contractile State, Mechanical Abnormalities and Ventricular Compensatory Mechanisms

Dean T. Mason, MD, FACC

Recent findings obtained from experimental and clinical studies on the control of force and velocity of ventricular contraction have made clear that the function of the intact heart is normally governed by intimate integration of four principal determinants that regulate stroke volume and cardiac output:[1-3] (1) preload (ventricular end-diastolic volume); (2) contractility (variable force of ventricular contraction independent of loading); (3) afterload (intraventricular systolic tension during ejection); and (4) heart rate. The first two determinants are fundamental intrinsic mechanisms inherent in the contractile machinery of the myocardium; the latter two are largely under extrinsic autonomic modulation. When considering cardiac function in certain disorders, it is important to add an additional determinant, one that adversely affects ventricular performance:[4] (5) dyssynergy or abnormal temporal sequence of ventricular contraction.

The terms cardiac function and ventricular performance are used in the general sense to refer to combined action of these determinants of cardiac output and not necessarily to the single determinant, contractility itself. The disturbed mechanisms operative in all types of clinical heart disease can be evaluated and accurately characterized within the framework of isolated or composite disorders of these five major determinants of cardiac performance. The recent development of improved techniques and concepts for the assessment of cardiac function in patients by both hemodynamic methods[5-11] and myocardial mechanics[2,3,12-15] has provided the means for differential analyses of the nature and degree of importance of the roles of each of these fundamental determinants and their interrelations with cardiac compensatory mechanisms governing stroke output in heart disease.

Contractile and Mechanical Abnormalities

Clinical heart disease can be broadly classified on a pathophysiologic basis according to three general types of cardiac functional abnormalities: (1) primary contractility disturbance, as in idiopathic or ischemic myocardial disease;

(2) diastolic mechanical inhibition of cardiac performance (ventricular underloading) in which left ventricular hypertrophy does not develop, as in restricted ventricular filling in mitral stenosis or pericardial tamponade; and (3) systolic mechanical ventricular overloading characterized by excessive pressure loading, as in aortic stenosis or essential hypertension, or increased volume loading, as in mitral or aortic regurgitation. Congestive heart failure in systolic ventricular overloading and in primary inotropic disorders occurs when there is substantial depression of contractility; decompensation ensues when the impairment of contractile state becomes particularly severe.[2]

Contractility

In the evaluation of the principal determinants of cardiac performance in heart disease, it has been possible to measure precisely ventricular preload (end-diastolic pressure, volume and tension)[10] and afterload (Laplace relation in which systolic tension and stress are directly equated with the product of ventricular systolic pressure and radius and inversely related to wall thickness)[12] and to characterize the nature and extent of dyssynergy.[4] However, it has been considerably more difficult to assess accurately the contractile state of the intact human heart.

Pump and Muscle Performance Characteristics: There are two general approaches to the evaluation of contractility and function of the heart: its pump (hemodynamics) and muscle (mechanics) performance characteristics. In the traditional approach of pump analysis, qualitative examination of directional differences in inotropism are provided by the standard hemodynamic variables of cardiac output, stroke volume, systolic ejection rate and ventricular end-diastolic pressure and the more complex measurements of ventricular end-diastolic volume, ejection fraction, stroke work, stroke power and ventricular mass in the basal state and also by their evaluation within the background of the Frank-Starling principle of ventricular function curves relating systolic performance to preload.[2,3,10,16]

More recently it has become possible to quantify contractility clinically by the second approach, in terms of muscle mechanics that describe the force, velocity and length properties of the ventricular myocardium. In the numerical assessment of contractile state, the mechanical events occurring during both the isovolumic and ejection phases of systole have been characterized. Thus, measures of inotropic state have been developed along two general lines: (1) isovolumic indexes utilizing dP/dt (rate of rise in ventricular pressure)[13] and (2) ejection indexes employing V_{CF} (circumferential fiber-shortening rate).[12]

Ejection and Isovolumic Indexes of Contractile State: At present, there is considerable discussion concerning the advantages and limitations of derived mechanical variables in the examination of contractile state. Because it has been difficult to evaluate the validity and sensitivity of various indexes of contractility in the intact heart since there is no standard measure of this property of the myocardium with which they can be compared, much of the discussion has consisted of circular reasoning. Nevertheless, certain isovolumic and ejection mechanical indexes appear to provide quantitative data that permit estimation and comparison of basal contractile state among different patients. The ejection measures include V_{CF} at peak tension[12] and mean V_{CF} determined angiographically[17] and by echocardiography.[18]

The isovolumic indexes applicable in interpatient studies include (1) $(dP/dt_{CPIP})/LVEDVI$,[13] in which CPIP is developed isovolumic pressure common to each ventricle (usually 50 mm Hg), and LVEDVI is left ventricular end-diastolic volume index; (2) extrapolated Vmax (maximal V_{CE}) from total pressure-velocity curves[14,19,20] using V_{CE} (contractile element velocity) calculated as $(dP/dt)/(K \cdot IP)$ in which K is the series elastic stiffness constant and IP is total isovolumetric pressure; (3) peak measured V_{CE} (Vpm)[21] also calculated as $(dP/dt)/(K \cdot IP)$; and (4) extrapolated Vmax or V_{CE} at 10 mm Hg of developed pressure from developed pressure-velocity curves[22,23] employing developed pressure for IP in the V_{CE} equation. Although physiologic changes in preload, compliance variations, dyssynergy, nonisovolumic systole (mitral regurgitation) and segmental necrosis may considerably affect loaded V_{CE} before aortic valve opening, the accompanying alterations of the slope of the total and developed pressure-V_{CE} curves are such that extrapolated Vmax is undisturbed or minimally influenced.[3,24–28] Thus it now appears that the problems previously cited largely represent "biological noise" concerning the clinical application of Vmax from isovolumic pressure-velocity curves as an index estimating contractile state. Conversely, the use of peak measured V_{CE} (Vpm) in these situations is limited since loaded V_{CE} is substantially affected. Also, in these particular conditions there may appropriately be marked disparity between ventricular hemodynamic performance and contractility assessed as Vmax.[29]

Depression of Contractility and Congestive Heart Failure: Of the five principal determinants of cardiac function, one of the basic concepts formulated in this report is that the fundamental abnormality in congestive heart failure due to myocardial disease or mechanical systolic overload is depression of ventricular contractility.[2] The final clinical expression of deteriorating cardiac performance due to severely impaired contractile state is the inability of the heart to maintain a normal cardiac output in the basal state despite a marked increase in ventricular filling pressure:[30,31] decompensated congestive heart failure (functional class IV, New York Heart Association classification). Compensated congestive heart failure occurs when ventricular function is depressed with moderately reduced contractile state but the resting cardiac output is preserved with a marked (class III) or moderate (class II) increase in pulmonary and systemic venous pressures. Lesser degrees of cardiac and inotropic dysfunction are observed in primary and secondary ventricular hypertrophy without heart failure when a normal cardiac output is maintained at rest and during physical activity in the absence of circulatory congestion (class I).

Compensatory Mechanisms

When systolic pressure or volume overloading or a primary defect in contractility is imposed upon the heart, there are three principal compensatory mechanisms available that provide a limited amount of ventricular reserve for the direct support of cardiac function and its fundamental goal of maintaining a normal resting level of cardiac output: (1) Frank-Starling

principle; (2) ventricular hypertrophy; and (3) sympathetic nervous system.[2,31] Deleterious symptoms necessarily accompany the operation of these compensatory mechanisms in their primary role of sustaining basal stroke volume, and these symptoms restrict the extent to which the adaptive systems can be employed.

Frank-Starling Principle: The Frank-Starling preload mechanism of ventricular dilation is immediately utilized to aid the ventricle in maintenance of cardiac output in the presence of an excessive systolic hemodynamic (particularly volume) overload or primary inotropic disturbance (Figure 1). The increased end-diastolic volume permits more forceful contraction, and the greater ventricular size allows ejection of a larger stroke volume with less shortening of the circumferential fibers. Conversely, the effectiveness and the reserve capacity of the Frank-Starling system are encroached upon when contractile state is diminished, since its ascending limb becomes less steep and flattened with its apex decreased in amplitude so that the reduced maximal stroke volume possible must be delivered at an abnormally high level of end-diastolic pressure (Figure 1). Thus, the failing ventricle in patients has a lowered and depressed function curve and exhibits decreased systolic response to preload increments.[16] Further, operation of the Frank-Starling preload mechanism by the ventricles for maintaining cardiac output is obligatorily associated with pulmonary and systemic congestion and increased myocardial systolic tension; thus, the price for use of this reserve system is dyspnea and peripheral edema and increased cardiac oxygen needs.

The clinically dysfunctioning left ventricle does not usually perform for long periods of time on the descending limb of the Frank-Starling curve, although the descending portion can be demonstrated in severe failure by interventions that transiently augment preload.[32] Importantly, in chronic left ventricular dilation, excessive muscle fiber stretch does not result in disengagement of the actin-myosin overlap region in the sarcomere but rather causes slippage among myofibrils,[33] thereby aiding the preload mechanism in developing systolic tension without reducing the number of cyclic interactive force-generating sites among the contractile

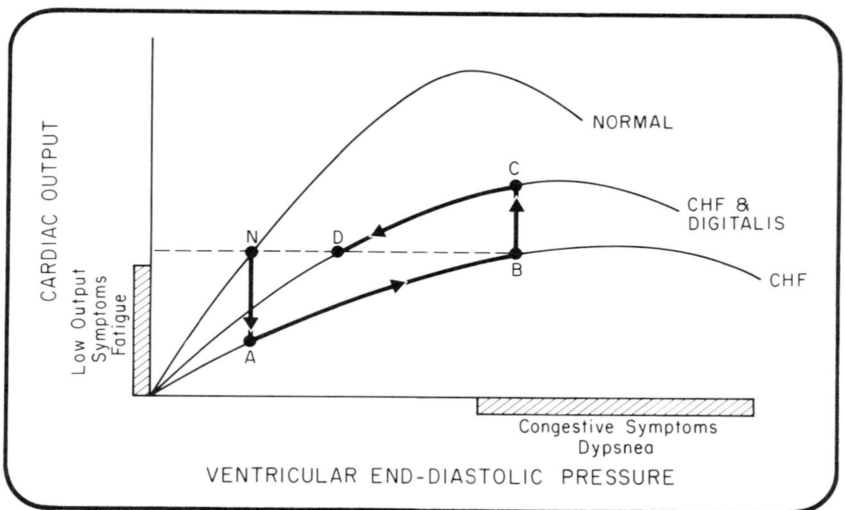

FIGURE 1. Operation of the Frank-Starling mechanism in the preload compensation for heart failure. The three curves represent ventricular function curves in normal, congestive heart failure (CHF) and heart failure after treatment with digitalis. Points N through D indicate in sequence: depression of contractility with decompensated heart failure (A), Frank-Starling compensation (B), increase in contractility with digitalis (C), and reduction in use of Frank-Starling preload compensation that digitalis allows (D). Points N, D and B indicate the same cardiac output on the vertical axis, but each point is at a different end-diastolic pressure on the horizontal axis. The excessive end-diastolic pressures causing congestive symptoms and the lowered levels of cardiac performance resulting in low output symptoms are shown by the **hatched areas.**

proteins. Further, hypertrophy occurring concomitantly in the chronically dilated ventricle results in longer myofibrils with more sarcomeres in series; therefore, at increased end-diastolic volumes there is greater total extent of ventricular thick and thin filament interface as well as retention of some preload reserve within the sarcomeres.[34]

Ventricular Hypertrophy: Increase in the number of contractile units by development of ventricular hypertrophy provides a relatively quickly responsive second compensatory system in support of cardiac output in systolic mechanical (particularly pressure) overloading and in contractile state impairment. Thus, protein synthesis is stimulated by excessive intramyocardial tension, which appears to serve as the mechanical-biochemical transducer or coupling mechanism responsible for accelerated production of ventricular mass.[10,35,36] Since extensive ventricular hypertrophy results in relative myocardial ischemia due to cardiac oxygen demands in excess of delivery capacity of even the normal coronary circulation, angina pectoris may attend marked use of the hypertrophy reserve mechanism. In addition to the increase in oxygen requirements because of greater muscle mass, myocardial oxygen utilization is also enhanced by the Frank-Starling and adrenergic adaptive mechanisms. Thus, at a given ventricular mass, myocardial oxygen consumption is principally determined directly by three hemodynamic variables:[37,38] (1) intramyocardial systolic tension (governed mainly by systolic pressure and cardiac size); (2) heart rate; and (3) contractile state. Ventricular dilation and increased sympathetic activity raise the first two of these factors above normal levels in heart disease.

In adult patients with compensated primary and secondary ventricular hypertrophy, it has recently been shown that even before the onset of circulatory congestion, contractile state is moderately reduced as measured by total isovolumic pressure Vmax, peak measured V_{CE} and $(dP/dt_{CPIP})/LVEDVI$ inotropic indexes[39] (Figure 2). In comparison, contractility is markedly decreased in patients with ventricular hypertrophy and congestive heart failure. Thus clinically, as well as experimentally,[40,41] there is a spectrum of decreasing contractile state between ventricular hypertrophy without failure and hypertrophy with decompensated failure, the latter condition manifest by a low basal level of cardiac output despite a marked increase in end-diastolic pressure. Although the hypertrophy adaptive system is associated with some decline in contractility per muscle unit, cardiac compensation with normal cardiac output at rest is supported by generation of additional myocardial contractile units, so that stroke volume is maintained with moderately increased end-diastolic pressure. The concept is developed that inotropic integrity is the crucial determinant of congestive heart failure; when this fundamental property (contractility) becomes too severely depressed in systolic mechanical overload or primary myocardial disease, cardiac decompensation results (low basal cardiac output with poor organ perfusion and resting fatigue) in spite of maximal use of all three compensatory mechanisms with their consequent effects of marked circulatory congestion and additional associated symptoms.

Sympathetic Nervous System: Besides ventricular dilation and hypertrophy reserves, the dysfunctioning heart has immediately available some inotropic support provided by adrenergic activity. Thus, the ventricles are richly innervated by sympathetic fibers in which increased impulse traffic, through release of its endogenous neurotransmitter, norepinephrine, and consequent myocardial beta receptor stimulation, is capable of improving contractility and increasing frequency of contraction. There is abundant evidence that sympathetic activity is augmented in congestive heart failure.[42] Paradoxically, however, norepinephrine is reduced in the hypertrophied myocardium[43,44] because of its defective synthesis,[45] and the dysfunctioning ventricle is largely deprived of this rapidly responsive compensatory mechanism.[46] Thus, the abnormally performing ventricle clinically shows increased impairment of the contractile state during cardiac sympathetic stimulation accompanying leg exercise[16] and forearm isometric[47,48] exercise. Conversely, adrenergic support is partially restored to the failing heart as the result of increased circulating norepinephrine because of its increased synthesis in the peripheral vasculature[49] and adrenal medulla.[50] The

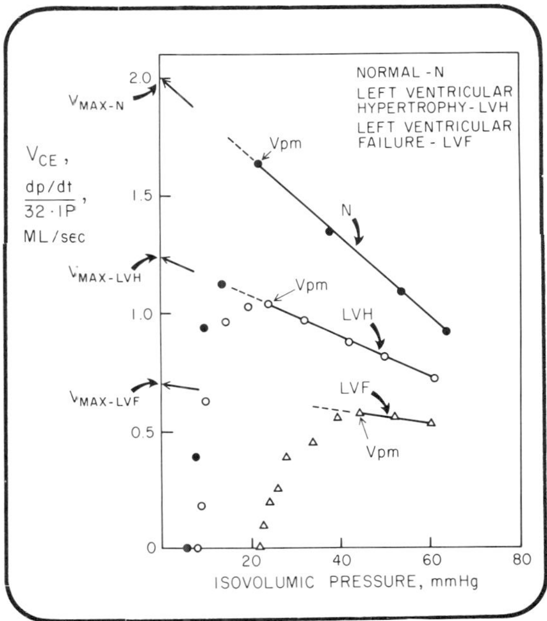

FIGURE 2. Representative clinical comparison of the left ventricular pressure-velocity relation at 5 msec intervals during isovolumic contraction in the normal heart (N) and in aortic stenosis with left ventricular hypertrophy without failure (LVH) and with failure (LVF). Contractile element velocity (V_{CE}) is expressed in muscle lengths (ML)/sec. IP in the V_{CE} equation[14] and pressure on the horizontal axis are total isovolumic pressure. The **diagonal broken lines** indicate linear extrapolation of the isovolumic segments to Vmax (V_{CE} at zero load). Vpm = peak measured V_{CE}.

symptoms accompanying utilization of sympathetic assistance include tachycardia, tachyarrhythmias and those due to redistribution of peripheral blood flow such as excessive sweating, cool skin and oliguria.

Digitalis Inotropic Response and Rationale of Glycoside Use: Concerning the response of contractility mechanisms in the failing heart, the absolute increment response is reduced to positive inotropic stimulation by digitalis, increasing heart rate and paired electroaugmentation in the chronically systolic pressure-overloaded ventricle.[40] However, in this condition, the chronically catecholamine-depleted myocardium demonstrates supersensitivity to blood-borne norepinephrine.[40] After acute depression of the normal ventricle by anesthesia or by beta adrenergic blockade, the positive inotropic response to digitalis is enhanced.[51] In contrast, in

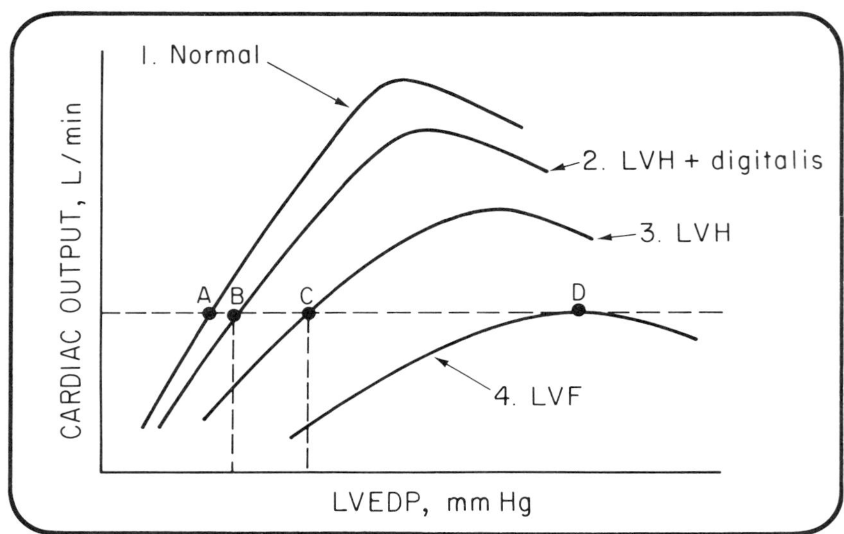

FIGURE 3. Ventricular function curves relating cardiac output to left ventricular end-diastolic pressure (LVEDP) in the normal heart (1), left ventricular hypertrophy (LVH) with (2) and without (3) digitalis, and in left ventricular failure (LVF) (4). Points A, B, C and D on these curves indicate the level of LVEDP **(vertical broken lines)** necessary to achieve normal resting cardiac output **(horizontal broken line).**

the acutely depressed hypoxic myocardium, the ability of digitalis to increase contractile state is impaired.[52,53]

The finding that contractile state is reduced in the hypertrophied and dilated ventricle without overt congestive heart failure[39] establishes the rationale for the application of digitalis in certain patients in this setting.[54] Thus, the glycoside elevates the depressed hypertrophied ventricular function curve toward normal so that cardiac output remains at a normal level with considerably less increase in end-diastolic pressure (Figure 3). Thereby exertional dyspnea is relieved and there is sparing of Frank-Starling reserve, as well as diminished use of the hypertrophy and adrenergic compensatory systems. In addition, the favorable effects of digitalis on the conservation of cardiac reserve

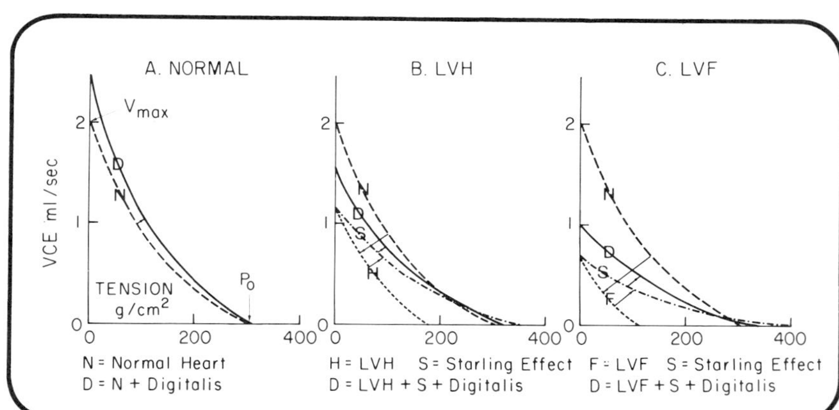

FIGURE 4. Effects of digitalis on force-velocity relations in the isovolumic left ventricle of the normal heart **(A)**, left ventricular hypertrophy (LVH) **(B)** and left ventricular failure (LVF) **(C)**. Vmax quantifies contractile state and P_0 maximal isovolumic tension. S = Frank-Starling compensatory mechanism.

mechanisms in nonfailing hypertrophy and in the failing heart can be appreciated within the ventricular force-velocity perspective[55] (Figure 4). Also, it has been shown experimentally that the positive inotropic support provided by digitalis is capable of reducing the degree of ventricular hypertrophy resulting from chronic pressure overload.[56] In regard to myocardial oxygen requirements of the failing heart and digitalis, it is important to point out that, despite the increased oxygen cost of increasing contractile state per se,[57] the overall glycoside effect is to improve cardiac efficiency and reduce myocardial oxygen consumption since the predominant indirect action of the agent is to diminish heart size, thereby decreasing intramyocardial systolic tension[37] (Figure 5).

Primary vs. Secondary Hypertrophy

The inotropic state and compensatory mechanisms in primary cardiomyopathy have recently been compared with those in ventricular hypertrophy secondary to chronic pressure overloading in aortic stenosis.[58] The possibility was considered that quantitative differences in contractility and utilization of reserve mechanisms might exist between the primarily and secondarily hypertrophied ventricles. The results of this investigation are shown in Figure 6 in which the contractile state and compensatory systems for cardiac output maintenance are compared in patients with these two lesions. In

response to pressure overload in compensated aortic stenosis, the ventricle principally employs the hypertrophy mechanism for supporting cardiac output. Although the inotropic state of this secondarily hypertrophied muscle is somewhat diminished,[58–60] cardiac output is sustained in chronic excessive pressure loading by development of more contractile units without increasing end-diastolic volume.[61,62]

In contrast, in patients with compensated cardiomyopathy who have depressed inotropism as the basic derangement, cardiac output is maintained by operation of both the Frank-Starling and hypertrophy compensatory mechanisms[53,63–65] (Figure 6). In these patients, normal cardiac output and, thereby, compensation are accomplished, although the contractile state is more greatly depressed than in aortic stenosis, since in cardiomyopathy the ventricle does not eject against a severe mechanical abnormality opposing the velocity and extent of fiber shortening. In decompensated congestive heart failure due to primary myocardial disease, cardiac output is reduced when the contractile state becomes further depressed to a very low level despite additional maximal utilization of dilation and hypertrophy compensation. In aortic stenosis, there is decompensation with decline of cardiac output when the adverse effects of chronic left ventricular outflow obstruction on the myocardium reduce contractility more than in the compensated state, in spite of further marked hypertrophy and, with the onset of de-

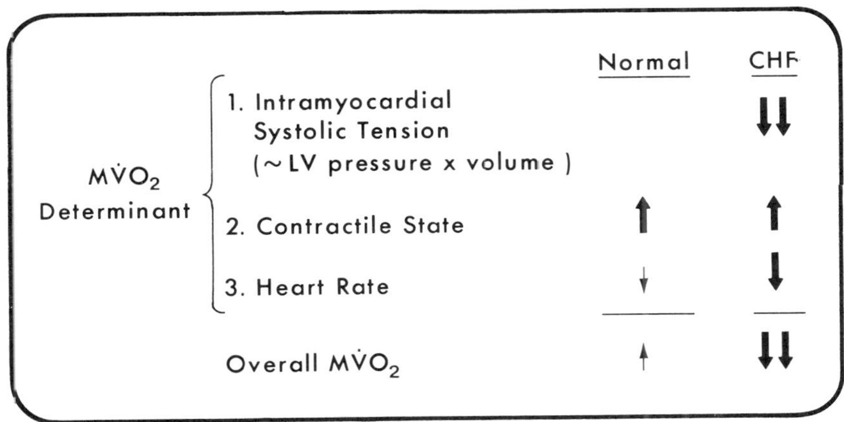

FIGURE 5. Effects of digitalis on the major hemodynamic-related determinants of myocardial oxygen consumption (MVO₂) in the normal and failing heart (CHF).

	V_{max}	LVEDV	LVH
CARDIOMYOPATHY (primary LV inotropic defect)	↓↓↓	↑	↑
MITRAL REGURGITATION (primary LV volume overload)	↓↓	↑↑	↑
AORTIC STENOSIS (primary LV pressure overload)	↓	0	↑↑↑

FIGURE 6. Compensatory mechanisms for maintaining normal cardiac output in chronic primary and secondary left ventricular hypertrophy (LVH). LV = left ventricle; LVEDV = left ventricular end-diastolic volume.

compensated failure, the development of ventricular dilation. Thus, compensation is maintained in cardiomyopathy and aortic stenosis by relatively dissimilar degrees of use of preload and hypertrophy reserve mechanisms. Decompensation occurs when normal basal cardiac output cannot be delivered because the contractile state has fallen below a certain critical level in both primary hypertrophy and hypertrophy secondary to chronic pressure overloading; this critical level is lower in primary cardiomyopathy.

Pressure vs. Volume Overload

In further clinical studies, contractility and compensatory mechanisms were compared in adult patients with chronic ventricular pressure and volume overloading.[9,10,63,65–67] Importantly, in compensated volume overload due to long-standing mitral or aortic regurgitation, contractility is more depressed than in chronic aortic stenosis[67] (Figure 6). In addition, in long-term volume overload, cardiac output is maintained by both the dilation and hypertrophy mechanisms whereas compensation is obtained by marked use of hypertrophy reserve alone in aortic stenosis. However, preload remains highly important for maintenance of cardiac output in the hypertrophied nondilated ventricle, as evidenced in this condition by the function of atrial systole as a booster pump for enhancement of ventricular filling in late diastole.[68] The finding that, in chronic left ventricular dilation, conversion of atrial fibrillation to normal sinus rhythm

usually does not substantially increase cardiac output represents poor atrial contraction and reduced Frank-Starling reserve in this setting.

In both chronic volume overloading and primary cardiomyopathy, Frank-Starling and hypertrophy reserves are used to maintain cardiac output (Figure 6). Decompensated heart failure occurs when there is further reduction in contractility, but to a lesser degree in volume overloading than in cardiomyopathy. Thus, resting cardiac output cannot be maintained at a normal level when contractile state declines to a precarious value. This crucial inotropic level is lowest in primary cardiomyopathy, intermediate in chronic volume overloading and least reduced (but considerably diminished compared with normal) in chronic excessive ventricular pressure loading.[39,58,67]

Acute vs. Chronic Volume and Pressure Overload: It is of interest that in short-term studies of volume overload in experimental animals, there has been marked ventricular dilation with minimal to moderate hypertrophy and little to no adverse effect on contractile state.[69,70] These findings are in contrast to results of experimental studies on ventricular pressure overload for short periods in which hypertrophy is severe and contractility at least moderately depressed.[40,41,71] Thus, in hemodynamic overload of relatively short duration, volume overload does not encroach upon contractile state to the same degree as in excessive acute pressure loading. However, the reverse is the case in long-standing hemodynamic overload. There is substantially greater reduction of inotropic state in

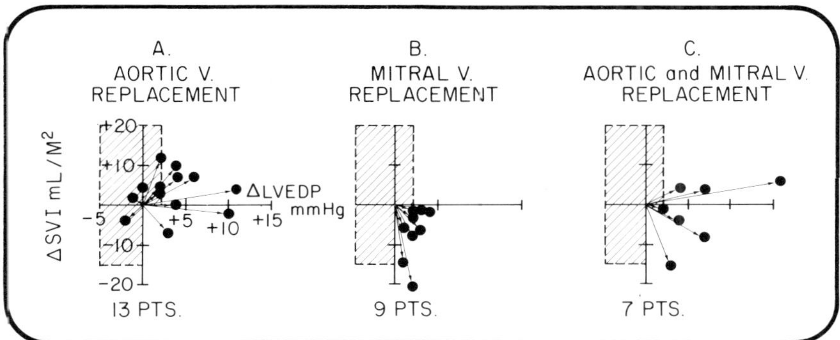

FIGURE 7. Relations between changes in stroke volume index (Δ SVI) and LVEDP that accompanied supine exercise after aortic valve (V.) **(A)**, mitral valve **(B)** and combined aortic and mitral valve **(C)** replacement. Each **arrow** and **closed circle** indicates the changes which occurred in individual patients (pts). **Hatched area** shows range of values observed in normal subjects. (Reproduced by permission of the American Heart Association, Inc. from Mason et al.[72]).

chronic volume overloading than in chronic pressure overloading.[67] Also, the depression of left ventricular contractile state in patients is less reversible after operative correction of the mechanical abnormality in chronic volume overloading than after correction of a long-standing excessive pressure burden[72] (Figure 7). It is likely that with excessive myofibrillar slippage occurring in the chronically dilated and overstretched ventricle, contractile state becomes markedly and largely irreversibly depressed. On the basis of these observations in acute and chronic hemodynamic overload, depression of inotropic state is temporally closely associated with development of hypertrophy secondary to pressure overloading, probably more so in adults than in children;[73] by contrast, in ventricular dilation, a substantial period of time is necessary for depression of contractility, which eventually becomes more severely impaired than in chronic pressure overload.

From these data, it is suggested that the basic abnormal physiologic variable in chronic congestive heart failure is depressed contractility (impaired primarily or by hemodynamic overload secondarily), and that normal resting cardiac output can be achieved by use of reserve mechanisms until contractile state becomes depressed below a critical level. Decompensated congestive heart failure is defined as the inability of the heart to maintain normal cardiac output in the basal state. Within the spectrum of clinical pathophysiology, chronic systolic mechanical abnormalities themselves do not cause decompensation; rather, the consequent degree of inotropic disturbance appears to be the decisive determinant precipitating decompensated heart failure. The compensatory mechanisms and the extent to which they are utilized differ in primary myocardial disease and systolic mechanical overload, and the depressed level of contractile state below which normal cardiac output cannot be maintained depends upon the chronic pathophysiologic process involved. The degree of inotropic reserve prior to the onset of decompensation is progressively greater in, respectively, systolic pressure overloading, systolic volume overloading and primary cardiomyopathy.

Comparison of Volume Overloads

Aortic vs. Mitral Regurgitation: The recent recognition that alterations in instantaneous impedance to ejection and ventricular fiber tension during ejection (afterload) are important determinants of the dynamics of cardiac contraction[74] has provided appreciation of differences in cardiac performance in conditions of systolic mechanical volume overloading. Thus in mitral compared with aortic regurgitation with equivalent total and effective stroke volumes, left ventricular function is more disturbed with greater end-diastolic pressure and volume in aortic regurgitation. In the latter entity, the entire total stroke volume must be delivered into the physiologically high pressure ascending aorta, whereas the regurgitant volume in mitral insufficiency is immediately ejected into the low pressure left atrium.[74] These findings concerning the greater afterload burden operative on the left ventricle in aortic incompetence emphasize the clinical observation of poorer cardiac tolerance in this condition chronically with marked extent of utilization of preload and hypertrophy reserves, contrasted to chronic mitral insufficiency in which similar systolic volume overload is accompanied by considerably less ventricular mass and systolic tension or afterload.

Ventricular Septal Defect vs. Patent Ductus Arteriosus: In additional studies on differences in cardiac performance in systolic volume overloading, it has been shown that left ventricular function is substantially less compromised in ventricular septal defect than in patent ductus arteriosus at the same level of abnormally increased pulmonary blood flow.[75] Thus, in ventricular septal defect the shunted flow is ejected directly into the low pressure right ventricle, whereas in patent ductus arteriosus the entire left ventricular stroke output must be ejected into the high pressure aorta prior to shunting. Therefore, at identically elevated pulmonary to systemic flow ratios, in patent ductus arteriosus

the left ventricular end-diastolic pressure and volume are greater, duration of ejection is prolonged and ventricular ejection rate and fraction are less increased and there is greater ventricular midwall systolic tension, contractile element work and power than in ventricular septal defect[75] (Figure 8). In ventricular septal defect the lesser increase of end-diastolic pressure and volume, greater increase in ejection rate and fraction, lesser increase in tension early in systole and in contractile element work and power throughout systole contrasted to patent ductus arteriosus, and the shorter ejection period with more rapid fall in tension than normal in ventricular septal defect, are the result of greater reduction in instantaneous impedance to left ventricular emptying in ventricular septal defect than in patent ductus.[75–78]

From these observations concerning the dynamics of ventricular contraction, ventricular septal defect is similar to mitral regurgitation and patent ductus arteriosus is similar to aortic regurgitation. Thus, although each of these four conditions of systolic volume overload encroach on ventricular performance, cardiac function is more disturbed in aortic insufficiency and patent ductus arteriosus. Further, since

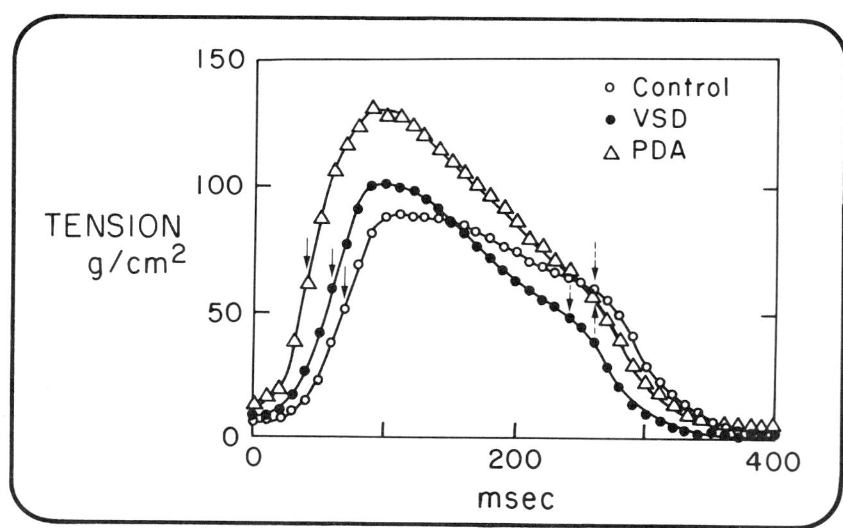

FIGURE 8. Comparison of instantaneous left ventricular wall tension at 5 msec intervals in a normal heart, ventricular septal defect (VSD) and patent ductus arteriosus (PDA) in an open chest canine preparation utilizing external left to right shunts. The ventricular septal defect and patent ductus arteriosus were separately, acutely induced and compared at equal 2:1 pulmonary to systemic flow ratios. Aortic valve opening is indicated by the **solid arrows (left)** and aortic closure by the **broken arrows (right)**.

resistance to ejection is more reduced in mitral regurgitation and ventricular septal defect, their integrated ventricular systolic tension is similar to normal whereas left ventricular afterload is substantially increased above normal in aortic regurgitation and patent ductus.[74,75] In regard to myocardial oxygen consumption, cardiac energy costs are considerably greater in pressure overloading in which ventricular systolic tension and afterload are markedly more increased than in volume overloading.[38,79–82] Further, comparing different types of systolic volume overloads in those conditions in which impedance offered to ejection is considerably reduced, such as mitral regurgitation and ventricular septal defect, there is a smaller increase in cardiac oxygen requirements than in those conditions in which systemic resistance is decreased by a smaller degree, as in patent ductus and aortic regurgitation.

Systolic Pressure Overloading: It is likely that important differences in ventricular dynamics also pertain in comparison of various types of systolic pressure overload. Thus quantitative dissimilarities in ventricular mechanics, loading, contractility, oxygen consumption and utilization of compensatory mechanisms are suggested in different types of aortic stenosis, coarctation of aorta and systolic and diastolic hypertension. Although pure systolic hypertension due to diminished aortic compliance has been generally regarded as unimportant in the development of ventricular dysfunction, recent evidence indicates that this condition increases cardiac outflow impedance and systolic tension during ejection, thereby raising ventricular afterload.[83] Whereas the response to acute pressure overload includes ventricular dilation,[41,84,85] in chronic conditions of increased pressure loading compensation is maintained with delivery of normal stroke output by utilization of hypertrophy reserve alone.[41,61,62]

Left Ventricle in Right Heart Overload

It has been traditionally considered that the left ventricle is uninvolved in conditions of purely right ventricular systolic hemodynamic overloading. Recent experimental and clinical evidence, however, indicates that certain biochemical and functional changes take place in the unstressed left ventricle in primary right heart systolic mechanical overload. Thus, left ventricular norepinephrine is reduced,[40,86] myofibrillar ATPase activity diminished[87] and hydroxyproline increased[88] in conjunction with their greater alterations in the right ventricle in experimental pulmonic stenosis. Further, it has been shown that ribonucleic acid (RNA) and protein synthesis increase in the canine left ventricular free wall, in addition to greater increases in the right ventricle, one day after pulmonary arterial banding[89] (Figure 9). In these studies, right ventricular contractile state was diminished and, interestingly, left ventricular inotropism tended to be reduced as well.[90] The mechanism for stimulation of hypertrophy in the unstressed ventricle appears to be the result of interconnecting muscle bundles between the two ventricles.

In chronic cor pulmonale, a modest decrease in left ventricular contractile state has been suggested in some patients,[91,92] although underloading of the left ventricle largely due to increased pulmonary vascular resistance has been the only disturbance of left heart function in other patients with chronic pulmonary disease.[93–96] In pure mitral stenosis, the left ventricle, in addition to reduced filling, is sometimes associated with moderate decline in performance as a result of posterior-basal dyssynergy caused by extension of mitral valvular chordae tendineae calcification into this area.[97] Left ventricular function may be mildly reduced in clinical pulmonic valvular stenosis[98] and contractile state moderately depressed in tetralogy of Fallot.[99] Also, there is a mild decrease of left ventricular function in large atrial septal defects,[98,100,101] partly as a result of diminished left ventricular filling in some patients.[101] In the study of right and left ventricular function, the contractile state can be evaluated simultaneously in both chambers by isovolumic developed pressure-velocity curves which allow description of a descending limb at relatively small amplitudes of isovolumic pressure[102] (Figure 10).

In addition, ventricular distensibility is normally somewhat dependent on the degree of filling of the opposite ventricle. Large increases in right ventricular diastolic volume lead to reduced compliance of the left ventricle due to the common interventricular septum.[103–105]

From all of these findings, it is clear that abnormalities in left ventricular function often accompany primary right ventricular systolic overload. However, these changes in the unstressed left ventricle are usually mild in degree and unlikely to account for pulmonary congestion and left ventricular decompensation.

Ventricular Unloading Therapy in Severe Heart Failure

Finally, the potential salutary effects of producing alterations in ventricular loading with peripheral vasodilator drugs are becoming rec-

ognized in the treatment of cardiac dysfunction in certain clinical conditions. In heart failure due to chronic essential hypertension, reduction of excessive afterload with nitroprusside has resulted in improved left ventricular function.[106] Recently, the value of this type of therapy using nitroprusside, which results in reduced impedance to left ventricular ejection, has been extended to patients with pump failure due to chronic coronary heart disease with[107] and without[108] mitral regurgitation. More particularly, the principle of ventricular unloading is now undergoing evaluation in experimental[109–110] and clinical[111–117] acute coronary artery

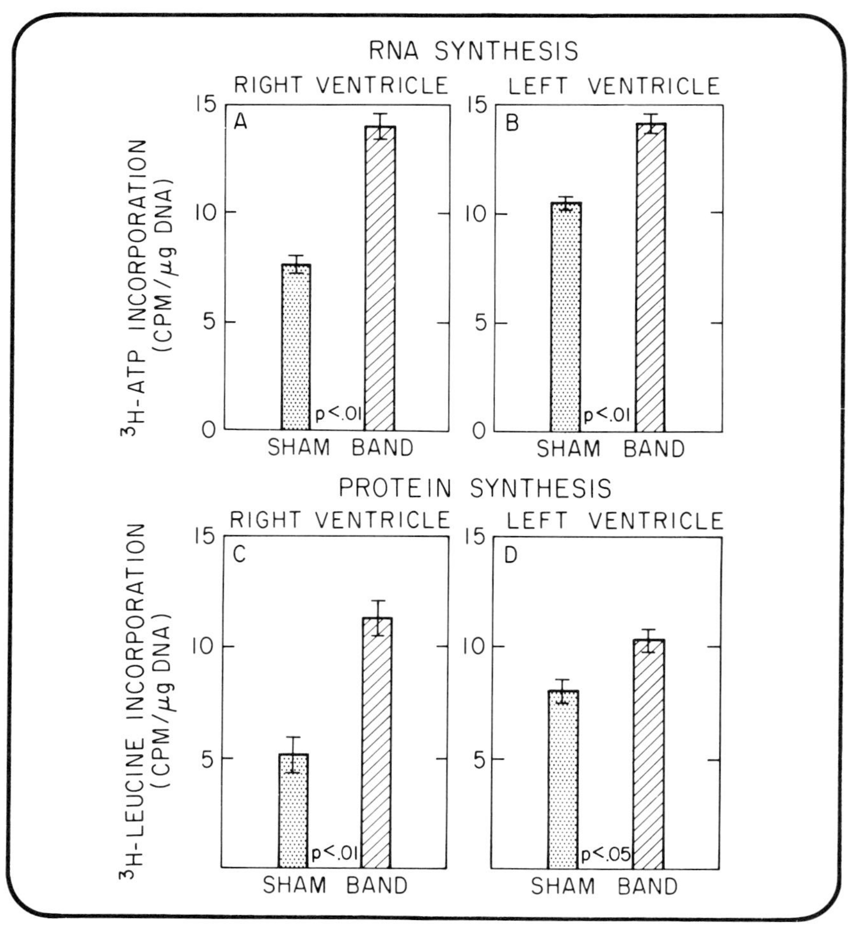

FIGURE 9. Ribonucleic acid (RNA) (**A** and **B**) and protein (**C** and **D**) synthesis in free walls of right (**A** and **C**) and left (**B** and **D**) ventricles of sham-operated dogs and dogs with pulmonary artery banding 24 hours postoperatively. RNA synthesis was determined by ^{3}H-adenosine triphosphate incorporation into acid-insoluble material from nuclear preparation and protein synthesis by ^{3}H-leucine incorporation into acid-insoluble material from postmitochondrial supernatant. Incorporation is expressed as counts/min per μg deoxyribonucleic acid (CPM/μg DNA).

disease by use of nitroprusside, phentolamine or nitroglycerin to diminish myocardial wall tension and oxygen consumption, thereby reducing ventricular ischemia and infarct size with attendant enhancement of cardiac performance and lessened frequency of tachyarrhythmias. Concerning the actions of nitroglycerin, the benefit observed with normotensive myocardial infarction appears to be primarily related to a decrease in preload[114] or possibly improved blood flow to ischemic areas by increased collateral circulation.[110] When associated sympathetic-induced increases in heart rate and contractility are prevented and coronary perfusion pressure is maintained with simultaneous administration of methoxamine or phenylephrine[110] or is augmented by concomitant external counterpulsation,[116] the efficacy of nitroglycerin and nitroprusside appears to be enhanced. The synergistic effects of phenylephrine and balloon counterpulsation in experimental cardiogenic shock[118] suggests that carefully adjusted combinations of phenylephrine,

nitroglycerin and counterpulsation might be beneficial in some patients with acute myocardial infarction. In other patients with acute or chronic ischemic heart disease, the judicious combined use of nitroprusside or phentolamine to reduce afterload, with volume expansion to maintain preload when necessary, and external positive-pressure diastolic counterpulsation applied to the lower extremities appears to provide optimal alterations of ventricular loading and improved myocardial perfusion, which result in augmentation of lowered cardiac output. The clinical application of this new important concept of ventricular unloading management in congestive heart failure is described in detail in chapter 21.

Conclusions

The central theme to which principles formulated in this report are united is that the primary objective of the interaction of cardiac compen-

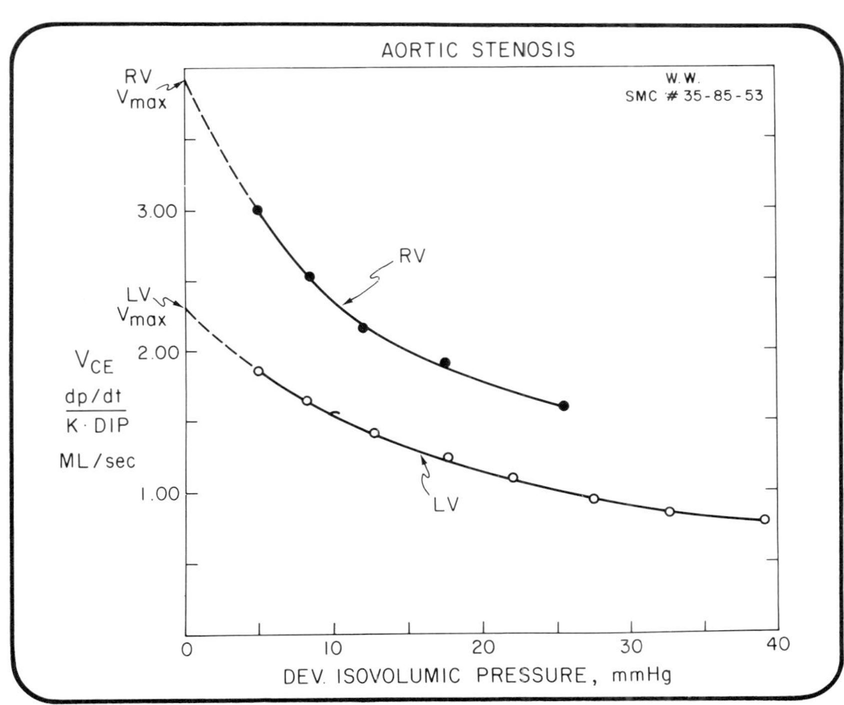

FIGURE 10. Simultaneous right (RV) and left (LV) ventricular isovolumic pressure-velocity relations at 5 msec intervals in a patient with severe aortic stenosis. DIP in the V_{CE} equation[3,102] and pressure on the horizontal axis are developed (dev) isovolumic pressure. K = 32/muscle length.

satory mechanisms with systolic hemodynamic and contractile state abnormalities in clinical heart disease is to maintain resting cardiac output at a normal level. The initial symptoms accompanying cardiac dysfunction are related to the unfavorable side effects resulting from operation of preload, hypertrophy and sympathetic reserves in performace of their compensatory roles, and the late symptoms accompanying congestive heart failure are due to low cardiac output which is the last hemodynamic variable to become abnormal in the basal state when ventricular function is impaired. The amount of reserve these protective mechanisms provide for cardiac output support is inherently limited and, in addition, the deleterious symptoms attending their use restrict the extent to which they can be employed. When cardiac mechanical and contractile disturbances exceed the reserve of the compensatory mechanisms (contractility being the critical variable), the heart is unable to maintain normal basal cardiac output (decompensated congestive heart failure). In compensated heart failure, pulmonary congestion results from increased use of the Frank-Starling mechanism of ventricular dilation prior to the reduction of cardiac output.

Relation between Altered Hemodynamics and Clinical Manifestations: From these observations, the clinical manifestations of advancing heart failure develop initially (functional class II) with dyspnea on more than ordinary activity (early use of Starling preload mechanism), fatigue with moderate or greater activity (reduced response of cardiac output with exercise due to diminished contractility), exertional angina pectoris (ventricular hypertrophy with attendant rise in myocardial oxygen consumption) and excessive tachycardia and sweating with exercise (augmented sympathetic discharge). The clinical picture worsens (class III) with dyspnea, fatigue, angina, tachycardia and sweating with ordinary mild activity (further depression of contractile state with increased use of compensatory mechanisms). Finally, these symptoms become very severe and occur even at rest (class IV) with the addition of weakness, cachexia, mental confusion, oliguria and hypotension (due to reduced resting cardiac output and poor organ perfusion despite maximal use of all compensatory mechanisms). Thus in func-

tional class I (minimal cardiac dysfunction without symptoms), class II (congestion with moderate activity) and in class III (congestion with mild activity), heart failure is compensated (normal basal cardiac output), and in class IV (congestion at rest) decompensation occurs (lowered resting cardiac output).

There may be considerable overlap between the relations of altered hemodynamics and clinical features. Thus, when diuretic therapy reduces congestive symptoms and concurrently reduces utilization of the Starling principle, class III symptoms may be converted to those of class II with reduced cardiac output at rest. Further, it is recognized that these functional classifications of patients comprise a continuum rather than discrete categories. It is evident from these considerations of correlation of clinical signs and symptoms with pathophysiologic mechanisms that the standard clinical functional classification of congestive heart failure is more coupled to symptoms consequent to secondary factors (compensatory mechanisms) in this condition rather than to the crucial hemodynamic variable (cardiac output) and the fundamental cause (depressed contractility) of decompensation.

Summary

Cardiac function in clinical heart disease is governed by ventricular (1) preload, (2) contractility, (3) afterload, (4) heart rate, and (5) dyssynergy. The major types of pathophysiologic abnormalities include inotropic disturbances, systolic mechanical pressure and volume overloads and diastolic mechanical ventricular underloading. In contractility and systolic mechanical disorders, the cardiac compensatory mechanisms of (1) Frank-Starling principle, (2) ventricular hypertrophy, and (3) sympathetic nervous system furnish substantial but limited protective reserve for maintaining cardiac output. Assessment of cardiac performance by pump (hemodynamics) and muscle (isovolumic and ejection mechanics) characteristics, including measurements of inotropic indexes of contractile force and velocity properties, provides quantitative analysis of ventricular function determinants and compensatory system interactions in heart disease.

Congestive heart failure is compensated when resting cardiac output is maintained at normal levels by the adaptive reserves with their deleterious early effects: dyspnea (preload rise), angina pectoris (increased mass) and tachycardia (adrenergic activity). Decompensated congestive heart failure is the inability of the heart to deliver normal basal cardiac output with attendant late symptoms of fatigue at rest and body organ failure despite maximal use of protective reserves. The compensatory responses utilized and the critical level of depressed contractility causing decompensation are dependent on the specific pathophysiologic condition. Thus, the fundamental variable in congestive heart failure is inotropic integrity of which its abnormal degree determines decompensation in chronic heart disease. Compensation can be sustained by reserve mechanisms at a lower inotropic state in cardiomyopathy than in systolic mechanical disorders. Concerning the systolic overloads, volume overload can be compensated for at a more depressed level of contractility than can pressure overload. The standard classification of clinical function in congestive heart failure is based more on early symptoms consequent to secondary adjustments (compensatory mechanisms) than on disturbances of the primary factors of decompensation: cardiac output (crucial hemodynamic variable) and contractility (the fundamental determinant).

Acknowledgment: This work was supported in part by Research Program Project Grant HL 14780 from the National Heart and Lung Institute, National Institutes of Health.

The author wishes to thank Barbara Giles, Karen Sime and Leslie Silvernail for their administrative and secretarial assistance and Kathryn Marr and Hal Pullum for their medical artistry.

References

1. **Braunwald E, Ross J Jr, Sonnenblick EH:** Mechanisms of Contraction of the Normal and Failing Heart. Boston, Little, Brown, 1968, p 77

2. **Mason DT, Spann JF Jr, Zelis R, et al:** Alterations of hemodynamics and myocardial mechanics in patients with congestive heart failure: pathophysiologic mechanisms and assessment of cardiac function and ventricular contractility. Progr Cardiovasc Dis 12:507, 1970

3. **Mason DT, Zelis R, Amsterdam EA, et al:** Clinical determination of left ventricular contractility by hemodynamics and myocardial mechanics. In, Progress in Cardiology (Yu PN, Goodwin JF, ed). Philadelphia, Lea & Febiger, 1972, p 121

4. **Herman MV, Gorlin MV:** Implications of left ventricular asynergy. Amer J Cardiol 23:538, 1969

5. **Dodge HT, Sandler H, Ballew DW, et al:** The use of biplane angiography for the measurement of left ventricular volume in man. Amer Heart J 60:762, 1960

6. **Dodge HT, Hay RE, Sandler H:** An angiographic method for directly determining left ventricular stroke in man. Circ Res 11:739, 1962

7. **Rackley CE, Dodge HT, Coble YD, et al:** A method for determining left ventricular mass in man. Circulation 29:666, 1964

8. **Dodge HT, Sandler H, Baxley WA, et al:** Usefulness and limitations of radiographic methods for determining left ventricular volume. Amer J Cardiol 18:10, 1966

9. **Rackley CE, Behar VS, Whalen RE, et al:** Biplane cineangiographic determinations of left ventricular function: pressure-volume relationships. Amer Heart J 74:766, 1967

10. **Dodge HT, Baxley WA:** Left ventricular volume and mass and their significance in heart disease. Amer J Cardiol 23:528, 1969

11. **Russell RO, Porter CM, Frimmer M, et al:** Left ventricular power in man. Amer Heart J 81:799, 1971

12. **Gault JH, Ross J Jr, Braunwald E:** Contractile state of the left ventricle in man: instantaneous tension-velocity-length relations in patients with and without disease of the left ventricular myocardium. Circ Res 22:451, 1968

13. **Mason DT:** Usefulness and limitations of the rate of rise in intraventricular pressure (dp/dt) in the evaluation of myocardial contractility in man. Amer J Cardiol 23:516, 1969

14. **Mason DT, Spann JF Jr, Zelis R:** Quantification of the contractile state of the intact human heart: maximal velocity of contractile element shortening determined by the instantaneous relation between the rate of pressure rise and pressure in the left ventricle during isovolumic systole. Amer J Cardiol 26:248, 1970

15. **Mason DT, Braunwald E, Covell JW, et al:** Assessment of cardiac contractility: the relation between the rate of pressure rise and ventricular pressure during isovolumic systole. Circulation 44:47, 1971

16. **Ross J Jr, Gault JH, Mason DT, et al:** Left ventricular performance during muscular exercise in patients with and without cardiac dysfunction. Circulation 34:597, 1966

17. **Karliner JS, Gault JH, Eckberg D, et al:** Mean velocity of fiber shortening: a simplified measure of left ventricular myocardial contractility. Circulation 44:323, 1971

18. **Cooper RH, O'Rourke RA, Karliner JS, et al:** Comparison of ultrasound and cineangiographic measurements of the mean rate of circumferential fiber shortening in man. Circulation 46:914, 1972

19. **Mason DT, Spann JF Jr, Zelis R:** The maximum intrin-

sic velocity of the myocardium (Vmax) in man: estimation from the rate of pressure rise and intraventricular contraction. Circulation 38 suppl 6:134, 1968

20. **Wolk MJ, Keefe JF, Bing OHL, et al:** Estimation of Vmax in auxotonic systoles from the rate of relative increase of isovolumic pressure: (dP/dt)KP. J Clin Invest 50:1276, 1971

21. **Mirsky I, Pasternac A, Ellison RC:** General index for the assessment of cardiac function. Amer J Cardiol 30:483, 1972

22. **Urschel CW, Henderson AH, Sonnenblick EH:** Model dependency of ventricular force-velocity relations: importance of developed pressure. Fed Proc 29:719, 1970

23. **Grossman W, Haynes F, Paraskos JA, et al:** Alterations in preload and myocardial mechanics in the dog and in man. Circ Res 31:83, 1972

24. **Capone RJ, Mason DT, Amsterdam EA, et al:** The effect of mitral regurgitation and ventricular aneurysm on Vmax calculated from pressure-velocity data during "isovolumic" systole. Circulation 44 suppl II:96, 1971

25. **Falsetti HL, Mates RE, Greene DG, et al:** Vmax as an index of contractile state in man. Circulation 43:467, 1971

26. **Zelis R, Amsterdam EA, Mason DT:** "Isometric" Vmax as an index of contractility independent of series elastic and fiber shortening: implications concerning pressure-velocity data in myocardial fibrosis, valvular regurgitation, ventricular aneurysm and ventricular septal defect. Circulation 44 suppl II:89, 1971

27. **Zelis R, Salel AF, CApone RJ, et al:** Evaluation of muscle function in the human myocardium by contractility measurements: coronary artery disease. In, Sonderdruck aus Das Chronick Kranke Herz; Grundlagen Funktionellen Diagnostik und Therapie (Roskamm H, Reindell H, ed). Stuttgart, F. K. Schattauer Verlag, 1973, p 379

28. **DeMaria A, Kamiyama T, Peng CL, et al:** Alterations of ventricular function and myocardial contractility indices by ventricular asynchrony. Clin Res 21:414, 1973

29. **Salel A, Mason DT, Amsterdam EA, et al:** Marked depression of myocardial contractility in patients with angina pectoris before left ventricular hemodynamic failure. Clin Res 20:210, 1972

30. **Spann JF Jr, Mason DT, Zelis RF:** Recent advances in the understanding of congestive heart failure. I. Mod Conc Cardiovasc Dis 39:73, 1970

31. **Spann JF Jr, Mason DT, Zelis RF:** Recent advances in the understanding of congestive heart failure II. Mod Conc Cardiovasc Dis 39:79, 1970

32. **Ross J Jr, Braunwald E:** The study of left ventricular function in man by increasing resistance to ventricular ejection with angiotensin. Circulation 29:739, 1964

33. **Ross J Jr, Sonnenblick EH, Taylor RR, et al:** Diastolic geometry and sarcomere lengths in the chronically dilated canine left ventricle. Circ Res 28:49, 1971

34. **Ross J Jr, McCullagh WH:** Nature of enhanced performance of the dilated left ventricle in the dog during chronic volume overloading. Circ Res 30:549, 1972

35. **Hood WP Jr:** Dynamics of hypertrophy in the left ventricular wall of man. In, Cardiac Hypertrophy (Alpert NR, ed). New York, Academic Press, 1971, p 445

36. **Laks MM, Morady F, Garner D, et al:** Relation of ventricular volume, compliance and mass in the normal and pulmonary arterial banded canine heart. Cardiovasc Res 6:187, 1972

37. **Covell JW, Braunwald E, Ross J Jr, et al:** Studies on digitalis. XVI. Effects on myocardial oxygen consumption. J Clin Invest 45:1535, 1966

38. **Braunwald E:** Control of myocardial oxygen consumption: physiologic and clinical considerations. Amer J Cardiol 27:416, 1971

39. **Mason DT, Spann J Jr, Zelis R, et al:** Comparison of the contractile state of the normal, hypertrophied and failing heart in man. In, Ref 35, p 443

40. **Spann JF Jr, Buccino RA, Sonnenblick EH, et al:** Contractile state of cardiac muscle obtained from cats with experimentally produced ventricular hypertrophy and heart failure. Circ Res 21:341, 1967

41. **Kraft-Hunter F, Cothran LN, Hawthorne EW:** Early ventricular adjustments to a chronically increased afterload. In, Ref 35, p 407

42. **Chidsey CA, Braunwald E, Morrow AG:** Catecholamine excretion and cardiac stores of norepinephrine in congestive heart failure. Amer J Med 39:442, 1965

43. **Chidsey CA, Braunwald E, Morrow AG, et al:** Myocardial norepinephrine concentration in man: effects of reserpine and of congestive heart failure. New Eng J Med 269:653, 1963

44. **Spann JF Jr, Chidsey CA, Pool PE, et al:** Mechanism of norepinephrine depletion in experimental heart failure produced by aortic constriction in the guinea pig. Circ Res 17:312, 1965

45. **Pool PE, Covell JW, Levitt M, et al:** Reduction of cardiac tyrosine hydroxylase activity in experimental congestive heart failure. Circ Res 20:349, 1967

46. **Covell JW, Chidsey CA, Braunwald E:** Reduction of the cardiac response to postganglionic sympathetic nerve stimulation in experimental heart failure. Circ Res 19:51, 1966

47. **Kivowitz C, Parmley WW, Donoso R, et al:** Effects of isometric exercise on cardiac performance: the grip test. Circulation 44:994, 1971

48. **Krayenbuehl HP, Rutishauser W, Schoenbeck M, et al:** Evaluation of left ventricular function from isovolumic pressure measurements during isometric exercise. Amer J Cardiol 29:323, 1972

49. **Kramer RS, Mason DT, Braunwald E:** Augmented sympathetic neurotransmitter activity in the peripheral vascular bed of patients with congestive heart failure and cardiac norepinephrine depletion. Circulation 38:629, 1968

50. **Vogel JHK, Chidsey CA:** Cardiac adrenergic activity in experimental heart failure assessed with beta receptor blockade. Amer J Cardiol 24:198, 1969

51. **Vatner SF, Higgins CB, Patrick T, et al:** Effects of cardiac depression and of anesthesia on the myocardial action of a cardiac glycoside. J Clin Invest 50:2585, 1971

52. **Kent KM, Goodfriend TL, McCallum ZT, et al:** Inotropic agents in hypoxic cat myocardium: depression and potentiation. Circ Res 30:196, 1972

53. **Amsterdam EA, Choquet Y, Lenz J, et al:** Attenuation

of positive inotropic action of digitalis by hypoxia and comparison with isoproterenol. Circulation 46 suppl II:124, 1972

54. **Mason DT, Spann JF Jr, Zelis R:** New developments in the understanding of the actions of the digitalis glycosides. Progr Cardiovasc Dis 11:443, 1969

55. **Sonnenblick EH, Williams JF, Glick G, et al:** Studies on digitalis. XV. Effects of cardiac glycosides on myocardial force-velocity relations in the nonfailing heart. Circulation 3:532, 1966

56. **Williams JF Jr, Braunwald E:** Studies on digitalis. XI. Effects of digitoxin on the development of cardiac hypertrophy in the rat subjected to aortic constriction. Amer J Cardiol 16:534, 1965

57. **Coleman HN:** Role of acetylstrophanthidin in augmenting myocardial oxygen consumption: relation of increased O_2 consumption to changes in velocity of contraction. Circ Res 21:487, 1967

58. **Mason DT, Spann JF Jr, Zelis R, et al:** Comparison of inotropic state and compensatory mechanisms between patients with primary and secondary ventricular hypertrophy. Circulation 42 suppl III:85, 1970

59. **Levine HJ, McIntyre KM, Lipana JG, et al:** Force-velocity relations in failing and nonfailing hearts of subjects with aortic stenosis. Amer J Med Sci 259:79, 1970

60. **Simon H, Krayenbuehl HP, Rutishauser W, et al:** The contractile state of the hypertrophied left ventricular myocardium in aortic stenosis. Amer Heart J 79:587, 1970

61. **Grant C, Greene DG, Bunnell IL:** Left ventricular enlargement and hypertrophy. Amer J Med 39:895, 1965

62. **Baxley WA, Dodge HT, Sandler HA:** Quantitative angiocardiographic study of left ventricular hypertrophy and the electrocardiogram. Circulation 37:509, 1968

63. **Bunnell IL, Grant C, Greene DG:** Left ventricular function derived from the pressure-volume diagram. Amer J Med 39:881, 1965

64. **Miller GAH, Kirklin JW, Swan HJC:** Myocardial function and left ventricular volumes in acquired valvular insufficiency. Circulation 31:374, 1965

65. **Dodge HT, Baxley WA:** Hemodynamic aspects of heart failure. Amer J Cardiol 22:24, 1968

66. **Dodge HT, Sandler H, Hay RE:** Left ventricular pressure-volume loops in man with valvular heart disease. Circulation 24:920, 1961

67. **Mason DT, Salel A, Amsterdam EA, et al:** The evaluation of pump and muscle function in patients with left ventricular pressure and volume overloads. Circulation 44 suppl II:126, 1971

68. **Braunwald E:** The hemodynamic significance of atrial systole. Amer J Med 37:665, 1964

69. **Taylor RR, Covell JW, Ross J Jr:** Left ventricular function in experimental aortocaval fistula with circulatory congestion and fluid retention. J Clin Invest 47:1333, 1968

70. **Cooper G, Puga FJ, Zujko KJ, et al:** Normal myocardial function and energetics in volume-overload hypertrophy in the cat. Circ Res 32:140, 1973

71. **Bing OHL, Matsushita S, Fanburg BL, et al:** Mechanical properties of rat cardiac muscle during experimental hypertrophy. In, Ref 35, p 361

72. **Mason DT, Ross J Jr, Gault JH, et al:** Combined prosthetic replacement of the mitral and aortic valves: pre- and postoperative hemodynamic studies including left ventricular responses to muscular exercise. Circulation 35 suppl I:15, 1967

73. **Graham TP, Jarmakani JM, Canent RV Jr, et al:** Evaluation of left ventricular contractile state in childhood: normal values and observations with a pressure overload. Circulation 44:1043, 1971

74. **Urschel CW, Covell JW, Sonnenblick EH, et al:** Myocardial mechanics in aortic and mitral valvular regurgitation: the concept of instantaneous impedance as a determinant of the performance of the intact heart. J Clin Invest 47:867, 1968

75. **Mason DT, Zelis R, Spann JF Jr, et al:** Alterations of left ventricular performance and myocardial mechanics in patent ductus arteriosus and ventricular septal defect. Clin Res 16:240, 1968

76. **Jarmakani MM, Edwards SB, Spach MS, et al:** Left ventricular pressure-volume characteristics in congenital heart disease. Circulation 37:879, 1968

77. **Jarmakani MM, Graham TP, Canent RV, et al:** Effect of site of shunt on left heart-volume characteristics in children with ventricular septal defect and patent ductus arteriosus. Circulation 40:411, 1969

78. **Jarmakani JM, Graham TP, Canent RV Jr:** Left ventricular contractile state in children with successfully corrected ventricular septal defect. Circulation 45 suppl I:102, 1972

79. **Evans CL, Matsuoka Y:** Effect of various mechanical conditions on the gaseous metabolism and efficiency of the mammalian heart. J Physiol (London) 49:378, 1915

80. **Sarnoff SJ, Braunwald E, Welch GH Jr, et al:** Hemodynamic determinants of oxygen consumption of the heart with special reference to the tension-time index. Amer J Physiol 192:148, 1958

81. **Urschel CW, Covell JW, Graham TP, et al:** Effects of acute valvular regurgitation on the oxygen consumption of the canine heart. Circ Res 23:33, 1968

82. **Sonnenblick EH, Skelton CL:** Oxygen consumption of the heart: physiological principles and clinical implications. Mod Conc Cardiovasc Dis 40:9, 1971

83. **Urschel CW, Covell JW, Sonneblick EH, et al:** Effects of decreased aortic compliance on performance of the left ventricle. Amer J Physiol 214:298, 1968

84. **Tsakiris AG, Vandenberg RA, Banchero N, et al:** Variations in left ventricular end-diastolic pressure, volume and ejection fraction with changes in outflow resistance in anesthetized intact dogs. Circ Res 23:213, 1968

85. **Liedtke AJ, Pasternac A, Sonnenblick EH, et al:** Changes in canine ventricular dimensions with acute changes in preload and afterload. Amer J Physiol 223:820, 1972

86. **Chidsey CA, Kaiser GA, Sonnenblick EH, et al:** Cardiac norepinephrine stores in experimental heart failure in the dog. J Clin Invest 43:2386, 1964

87. **Chandler BM, Sonnenblick EH, Spann JF Jr, et al:** Association of depressed myofibrillar adenosine triphosphatase and reduced contractility in experimental heart failure. Circ Res 21:717, 1967

88. **Buccino RA, Harris E, Spann JE Jr, et al:** Response of

myocardial connective tissue to development of experimental hypertrophy. Amer J Physiol 216:425, 1969

89. **Zelis R, Wikman-Coffelt J, Kamiyama T, et al:** Left ventricular RNA and protein synthesis following right ventricular stress. Circulation 46 suppl II:65, 1972

90. **Zelis R, Wikman-Coffelt J, Kamiyama T, et al:** Acute right ventricular stress as a stimulus for left ventricular RNA and protein synthesis. In, Recent Advances in Studies on Cardiac Structure and Metabolism, vol 3: Myocardial Metabolism (Dhalla NS, ed). Baltimore, University Park Press, 1973, p 625

91. **Rao BS, Cohn KE, Eldridge FL, et al:** Left ventricular failure secondary to chronic pulmonary disease. Amer J Med 45:229, 1968

92. **Baum GL, Schwartz A, Llamas R, et al:** Left ventricular function in chronic obstructive lung disease. New Eng J Med 285:361, 1971

93. **Williams JF Jr, Childress RH, Boyd DL, et al:** Left ventricular function in patients with chronic obstructive pulmonary disease. J Clin Invest 47:1143, 1968

94. **Davies H, Overy HR:** Left ventricular function in cor pulmonale. Chest 58:8, 1970

95. **Khaja F, Parker JO:** Right and left ventricular performance in chronic obstructive lung disease. Amer Heart J 82:319, 1970

96. **Frank MJ, Weisse AB, Moschos CB, et al:** Left ventricular function, metabolism, and blood flow in chronic cor pulmonale. Circulation 47:798, 1973

97. **Heller SJ, Carleton RA:** Abnormal left ventricular contraction in patients with mitral stenosis. Circulation 42:1099, 1970

98. **Salel A, Mason DT, Amsterdam E, et al:** Abnormalities of left ventricular contractility in isolated right ventricular pressure overload. Amer J Cardiol 29:288, 1972

99. **Jarmakani JM, Graham TP Jr, Canent RV Jr:** Left ventricular contractile state in children following successful corrective surgery for isolated ventricular septal defect and tetralogy of Fallot. Circulation 44 suppl II:92, 1971

100. **Flamm MD, Cohn KE, Hancock EW:** Ventricular function in atrial septal defect. Amer J Med 48:286, 1970

101. **Graham TP Jr, Jarmakani JM, Canent RV Jr:** Left heart volume characteristics with a right ventricular volume overload: total anomalous pulmonary venous connection and large atrial septal defect. Circulation 45:389, 1972

102. **Salel AF, Kamiyama T, Peng CL, et al:** Pressure-velocity curves in the evaluation of right ventricular contractility. Circulation 46 suppl II:216, 1972

103. **Taylor RR, Covell JW, Sonnenblick EH, et al:** Dependence of ventricular distensibility on filling of the opposite ventricle. Amer J Physiol 213:711, 1967

104. **Kelly DT, Spotnitz HM, Beiser GD, et al:** Effects of chronic right ventricular volume and pressure loading on left ventricular performance. Circulation 44:403, 1971

105. **Urschel CW, Bemis CE, Serur J, et al:** The influence of right ventricular filling pressure on left ventricular pressure and dimension. Circulation 43 suppl II:125, 1971

106. **Rodriguera E, Guiha N, Cohn JN:** Left ventricular function in hypertensive heart failure. Circulation 44 suppl II:129, 1971

107. **Chatterjee K, Parmley WW, Swan HJC, et al:** Beneficial effects of vasodilator agents in severe mitral regurgitation due to dysfunction of subvalvular apparatus. Circulation 48:464, 1973

108. **Miller RR, Vismara LA, Amsterdam EA, et al:** Clinical use of sodium nitroprusside in chronic ischemic heart disease: effects on peripheral vascular resistance and venous tone and on ventricular volume, pump and mechanical function. Circulation 51:328, 1975

109. **Redwood DR, Smith ER, Epstein SE:** Coronary artery occlusion in the conscious dog: effects of alterations in heart rate and arterial pressure on the degree of myocardial ischemia. Circulation 46:323, 1972

110. **Smith ER, Redwood DR, McCarron WE, et al:** Coronary artery occlusion in the conscious dog: effects of alterations in arterial pressure produced by nitroglycerin, hemorrhage, and alpha-adrenergic agonists on the degree of myocardial ischemia. Circulation 47: 51, 1973

111. **Majid PA, Sharma B, Taylor SH:** Phentolamine for vasodilator treatment of severe heart-failure. Lancet 2:719, 1971

112. **Franciosa JA, Guiha NH, Limas CJ, et al:** Improved left ventricular function during nitroprusside infusion in acute myocardial infarction. Lancet 1:650, 1972

113. **Gold HK, Leinback RC, Sanders CA:** Use of sublingual nitroglycerin in congestive failure following acute myocardial infarction. Circulation 46:839, 1972

114. **Williams DO, Otero J, Lies J, et al:** Hemodynamic effects of nitroglycerin in acute myocardial infarction: decrease in preload at the expense of cardiac output. Amer J Cardiol 33:178, 1974

115. **Kelly DT, Delgado DE, Taylor DR, et al:** Use of phentolamine in acute myocardial infarction associated with hypertension and left ventricular failure. Circulation 47:729, 1973

116. **Chatterjee K, Parmley WW, Ganz W, et al:** Hemodynamic and metabolic responses to vasodilator therapy in acute myocardial infarction. Circulation 53:1183, 1973

117. **Shell WE, Sobel BE:** Protection of ischemic myocardium by reduced ventricular afterload. New Eng J Med 291:481, 1974

118. **Feola J, Limet R, Glick G:** Synergistic effects of phenylephrine and counter pulsation in canine cardiogenic shock. Amer J Physiol 224:1044, 1973

Chapter 10

Peripheral Circulatory Control Mechanisms in Congestive Heart Failure

Robert Zelis, MD, FACC
John Longhurst, MD
Robert J. Capone, MD, FACC
Garrett Lee, MD
Dean T. Mason, MD, FACC

With the development of congestive heart failure, there is a progressive reduction in the contractile state of the myocardium. With this reduction in contractility comes a deterioration of the function of the heart as a pump.[1-3] A variety of central compensatory control mechanisms come into play in an attempt to maintain circulatory homeostasis. These include the development of myocardial hypertrophy, that is, an increase in the number of contractile units, an increase in ventricular end-diastolic fiber length to optimize actin-myosin interaction and an increase in circulating catecholamines in an effort to increase myocardial contractility. These compensatory mechanisms are used to various degrees depending upon the etiologic mechanisms responsible for the production of heart failure.[2,4-7] When central compensatory mechanisms ultimately fail, various peripheral circulatory mechanisms act to conserve the limited cardiac output.[8-13] These mechanisms are most noticeable during exercise, which is the most important physiologic stress encountered by the patient with heart disease. During exercise a normal heart can adequately pump the entire venous return at a higher level of pressure to perfuse adequately the various regional circulations and satisfy their metabolic require-

ments. In contrast, the cardiac output response to exercise in patients with congestive heart failure is severely limited and results in an exaggerated increase in left ventricular filling pressure, little change in blood pressure and inadequate perfusion of vital organs. Since the cardiocirculatory response to exercise is complex, it is desirable to examine individually the various local metabolic and neurogenic factors governing the peripheral circulations for a better understanding of how the body attempts to maintain circulatory homeostasis in heart failure (Figure 1).

Local Control of Skeletal Muscle Blood Flow in Congestive Heart Failure

Reactive Hyperemia Response: During exercise two factors are important in determining regional blood flow: (1) a generalized sympathoadrenal discharge; and (2) the production of local vasodilator metabolites in exercising muscle. To evaluate the response of the skeletal muscle circulation to local metabolic factors in a setting that would not be dependent upon the ability of the heart to augment its output, the reactive hyperemia response was studied.[12] Reactive hyperemia is the large increase in regional blood flow that occurs after release of

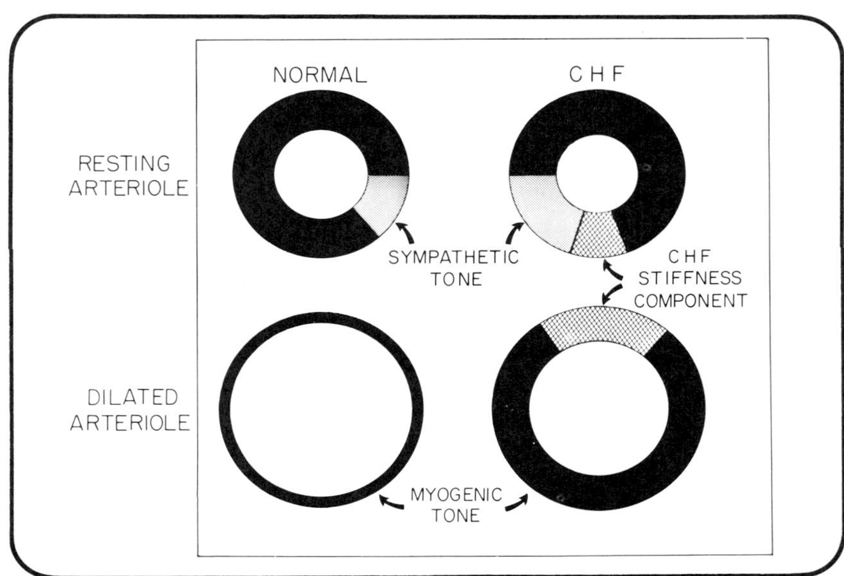

FIGURE 1. Diagrammatic representation of the components determining arteriolar tone at rest and with metabolic vaso-dilation (**horizontal rows**) in normal subjects and in patients with congestive heart failure (CHF) (**vertical columns**). The internal cross-sectional areas have been drawn to scale on the basis of blood flow data. At rest there is increased sym-pathetic arteriolar tone in symptomatic patients with congestive heart failure. With metabolic vasodilatation, sympatholysis occurs and the stiffness component in congestive heart failure becomes important in limiting ex-cessive regional blood flow. (Reprinted by permission from Zelis and Mason.[8])

temporary circulatory arrest (Figure 2A). The reactive hyperemia blood flow in the forearm is principally determined by the accumulation of local vasodilator substances if the subject does not have atherosclerotic arterial disease.[14–17] Blood flow to a limb can easily be measured by the noninvasive technique of venous occlusion plethysmography with a simple mercury-in-rub-ber strain gauge plethysmograph.[18,19] With this device it was demonstrated that forearm blood flow in patients with congestive heart failure was considerably reduced during the resting state when compared with flow in normal sub-jects.[12,20,21] Systemic blood pressure was unal-tered in these subjects, thus indicating that forearm arteriolar constriction was present in patients with heart failure under basal metabol-ic conditions. More important, it was noted that the increase in blood flow that was seen after restoration of the circulation to the ischemic forearm (reactive hyperemia blood flow) was also considerably reduced (Figure 2B).

Two indexes of the reactive hyperemia re-sponse can be evaluated—peak blood flow re-sponse and total blood flow in excess of resting values.[12,14,22,23] Both of these indexes can be quantitated for various durations of circulatory arrest. Whereas the latter index progressively in-creases as the duration of circulatory arrest is prolonged, the peak blood flow response reach-es a plateau and is not appreciably increased when the ischemic period is increased beyond 5 minutes (Figure 3). The plateau of the peak reactive hyperemia response represents the maximal ability of the arterioles to dilate with a metabolic stimulus. This maximal arteriolar di-lation is relatively uninfluenced by endogenous sympathetic tone, which is effectively antago-nized by local metabolites, a process termed functional sympatholysis.[24,25] Of major sig-nificance is that the maximal ability of the ar-terioles to dilate with this metabolic stimulus is appreciably reduced in congestive heart failure (Figure 3). Likewise, patients with heart failure exhibit a limited arteriolar vasodilator response to exercise, local thermal stress, intraarterial so-dium nitrite and phentolamine.[12] When the pa-tient with heart failure exercises, this arteriolar

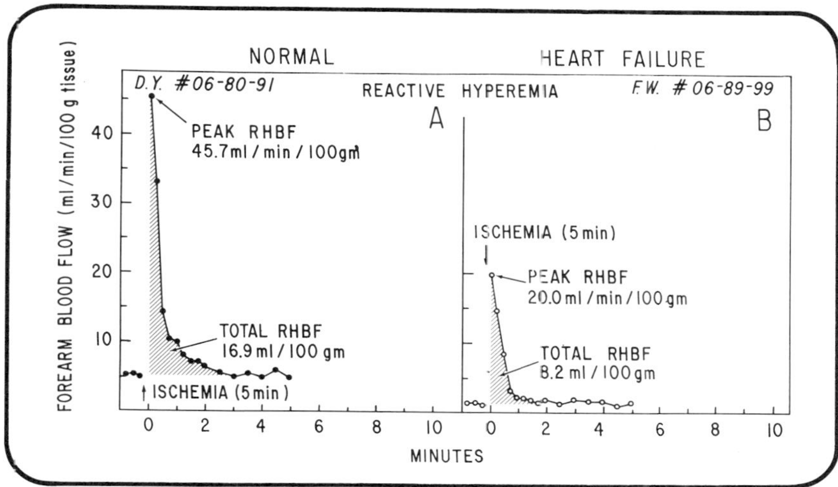

FIGURE 2. The reactive hyperemia response of a normal subject (**A**) and a patient with congestive heart failure (**B**). Forearm blood flow was measured serially with a mercury-in-rubber strain gauge plethysmograph. After determination of basal forearm blood flow, arterial occlusion was produced for 5 minutes. At time zero the circulation was restored, and 5 seconds later the peak reactive hyperemia blood flow (RHBF) was measured. The total RHBF is the total blood flow in excess of control values, the **shaded area** under the curves. Both peak RHBF and total RHBF are reduced in heart failure. (Reprinted by permission from Zelis et al.[12])

stiffness can effectively limit blood flow to active muscle vascular beds and thus helps to maintain arterial pressure in the face of a limited cardiac output response.[10,11]

Causes of Limited Arteriolar Dilator Capacity: The cause of the limited arteriolar dilator capacity in heart failure has not been completely elucidated; however, several possible contributing factors have been investigated. It is unlikely that increased sympathetic tone accounts for the limited vascular response to metabolites. In congestive heart failure the increased arteriolar stiffness was demonstrated despite forearm nerve blockade or alpha adrenergic blockade of a limb with intraarterial injection of phentolamine.[12] Likewise, during systemic infusion of norepinephrine, which increased circulating norepinephrine levels to that normally seen in patients with congestive heart failure during exercise, there was no reduction in the reactive hyperemia response.[12] This is not surprising since effective competition between sympathetic adrenergic tone and local metabolites to determine regional blood flow in skeletal muscle is only evident during submaximal metabolic stimulation.[24,25] During maximal metabolic stimulation, alpha adrenergic tone plays little role in the regulation of skeletal muscle blood flow.

In normal subjects two major factors are thought to contribute to the hyperemia seen after release of temporary arterial occlusion. Part of the response is clearly related to local accumulation of one or a number of vasodilator substances. Also, it has been postulated that the reduction in arterial distending pressure that occurs distal to the site of circulatory arrest as blood collects in the capacitance vessels (Bayliss or myogenic hypothesis) leads to further reduction in smooth muscle tone, especially after brief periods of circulatory arrest.[22,23,26,27] If the venous pressure were abnormally increased, as in heart failure, then the reduction in intraarterial pressure would not be as great and a decrease in reactive hyperemia blood flow would be observed. However, when the forearm was packed with blood by venous congestion before the induction of ischemia, the differences in the reactive hyperemia response between normal subjects and patients with heart failure were still evident. Thus, different venous pressures could not be responsible for the observed differences in reactive hyperemia blood flow between groups.[12] Similarly, if sympathetic tone were in-

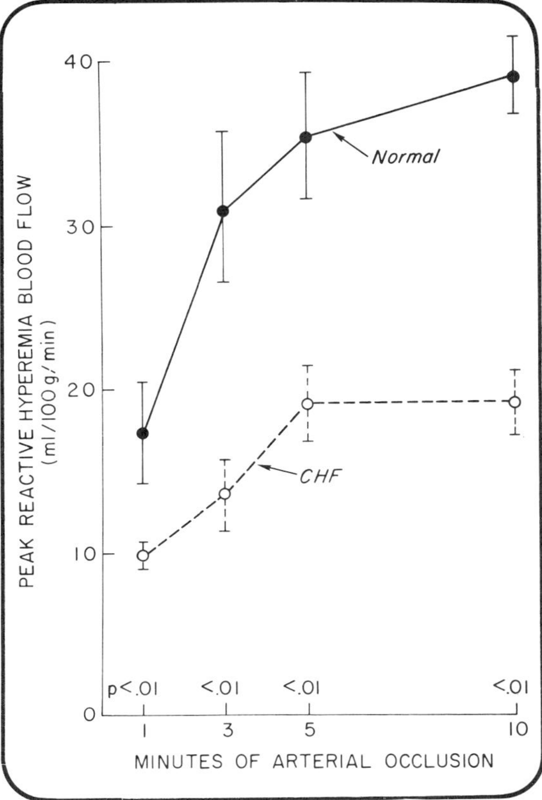

FIGURE 3. Average peak reactive hyperemia blood flow (RHBF) (± standard error of the mean) after release of 1, 3, 5 and 10 minutes of arterial occlusion in normal subjects (**solid circles**) and patients with congestive heart failure (**open circles**). The failure of the peak RHBF to increase significantly more when the duration of ischemia was prolonged beyond 5 minutes suggests that the arterial resistance vessels had achieved maximal dilation. The plateau of peak RHBF was significantly less in congestive heart failure, indicating that in these patients resistance vessels have a limited ability to dilate to a metabolic stimulus. (Reprinted by permission from Zellis et al.[12])

creased, there might be a reduced rate of decline of arterial pressure distal to the occluding cuff and the hyperemia response would be blunted, a phenomenon evoked to explain the inability to hear Korotkoff sounds during indirect blood pressure measurements in shock.[28] Again, this might explain the reduction in reactive hyperemia blood flow after short periods of ischemia but would not be operating during periods of circulatory arrest of 5 to 10 minutes' duration.

Increased Vascular Resistance Due to Increase in Vascular Sodium Content: One factor that might contribute to the arteriolar stiffness seen in congestive heart failure is an increased sodium or water content of the resistance vessels. Initially it was noted that after diuresis there was some restoration of the reactive hyperemia response toward normal.[12] In animals with experimental congestive heart failure, it was also demonstrated that the sodium content of large and small arteries was increased[29] (Figure 4). The observed changes in vascular sodium content are similar to those seen in essential hypertension in which a limited arteriolar dilator capacity has also been demonstrated.[30,31] Lastly, when fluorocortisone and salt were fed to normal volunteers in amounts that produced a significant increase in weight, there was a moderate attenuation of the peak reactive hyperemia response, thereby suggesting that the metabolic responsiveness of resistance vessels can be influenced by sodium retention in man.[32]

Increase in Tissue Pressure in Edematous States: Although an increased sodium content of the resistance vessels could explain part of the arteriolar stiffness in congestive heart failure, another factor was also considered. With maximal arteriolar dilation, two other sites in the vascular tree could serve as resistance vessels. The first is the large and medium size arteries.[14-17] These vessels can be considered resistance vessels during periods of maximal arteriolar dilation in patients with atherosclerotic peripheral vascular disease. It is commonly observed that patients with claudication do have a reduced peak reactive hyperemia response in the affected limbs. In the studies described, the patients with congestive heart failure had rheumatic heart disease, none had atherosclerotic disease and all had evidence of significant sodium retention. Although edema was apparent in the lower limbs of these subjects, none was visible in the upper limbs where the diminished reactive hyperemia response was initially noted. However, some increase in sodium and water retention in the upper limbs might have led to an increase in tissue pressure, especially in skeletal muscles surrounded by poorly compliant fascia. It seemed likely that in the presence of a maximal arteriolar dilator stimulus an

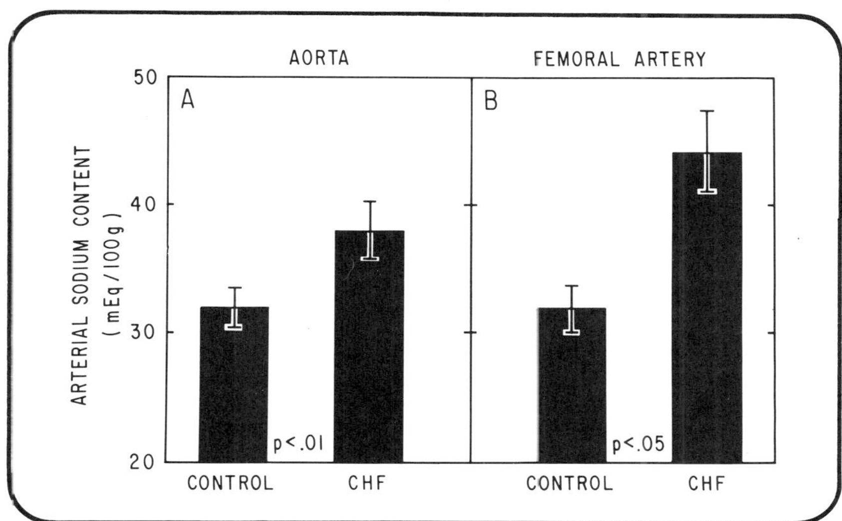

FIGURE 4. Arterial sodium content of the aorta (**A**) and of a tertiary branch of the femoral artery (**B**) in normal dogs and dogs with congestive heart failure (CHF) induced by rapid ventricular stimulation with use of an implanted pacemaker at a fixed rate of 280 beats/min for 11 to 29 days. Animals with heart failure had increased left ventricular filling pressures, depressed contractile indexes and evidence of fluid retention (mean ± standard error of the mean). (Reprinted by permission of the American Heart Association, Inc. from Zelis et al.[29])

increase in tissue pressure might account for some increase in resistance at the level of the small vessels.

Although it has been suggested that changes in tissue pressure could alter resting blood flow and models have been proposed to explain how tissue pressure might regulate reactive hyperemia blood flow,[33–35] it has only been recently demonstrated that such changes could indeed limit maximal metabolic blood flow in experimental animals. In a series of studies designed to evaluate the possible role that tissue pressure might play in regulating reactive hyperemia blood flow, maximal arteriolar dilation was evaluated using both autoperfused and constantly-perfused canine limbs.[36] When the tissue pressure in the limb was increased by venous congestion, there was a marked attenuation of the reactive hyperemia response (Figure 5). The increase in tissue pressure was demonstrated by direct needle measurement and by measurement of pressure within a chronically implanted endothelialized capsule.[37,38] Conversely, infusion of dextran in order to reduce tissue pressure induced directionally opposite changes in metabolic blood flow (Figure 5, C and F). Recently, similar studies in man have also demonstrated that chronic congestion of the forearm can result in attenuation of the peak reactive hyperemia response.[39]

Thus, it seems clear that in congestive heart failure there is a limited ability of the muscle circulation to respond appropriately to an increase in vasodilator metabolites. This is partially accounted for by (1) a reduced arteriolar compliance probably related to an increase in vascular sodium content, and (2) an increase in tissue pressure in edematous states. This increased peripheral vascular stiffness might be expected to reduce resting blood flow minimally but to have its major effect on limiting metabolically determined blood flow as in exercise. The reduction in regional perfusion of active skeletal muscle would therefore be expected to support blood pressure partially during exercise so that flow to the heart and brain could be maintained.

Neurogenic Control of Regional Blood Flow in Congestive Heart Failure

Increased Sympathetic Tone in Heart Failure: Whereas regional arteriolar stiffness may play a minor role in determining muscle blood

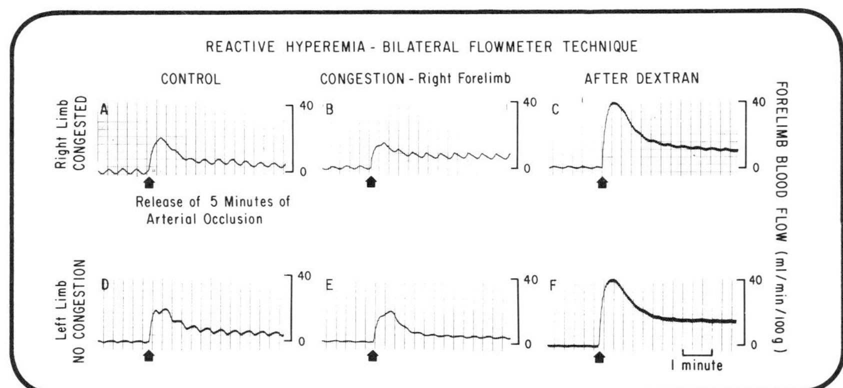

FIGURE 5. Blood flow measured by flowmeters simultaneously, bilaterally on the brachial arteries of a dog following restoration of the circulation (**arrows**) after 5 minutes of arterial occlusion. The reactive hyperemia response was measured before (**control**) and after congestion of the right forelimb at 70 mm Hg for 3 hours, which resulted in an increase in indexes of tissue pressure. The depression in the reactive hyperemia response in the congested limb was markedly lessened following intravenous infusion of dextran, which reduced tissue pressure and increased arterial pressure.

flow during rest in patients with heart failure, an increase in sympathetic nervous system tone may be the more important determinant of blood flow to other regions.[9,13,40] After alpha adrenergic and ganglionic blockade, patients with congestive heart failure have a greater percentage increase in limb blood flow and reduction in venous tone than normal subjects.[12,41,42] This findings has not been consistently observed by all investigators, and some have suggested that sympathetic tone may not be increased under basal conditions in patients with heart failure.[43,44] It seems most likely that during the resting state the degree to which the sympathetic nervous system is activated depends entirely on whether the patient is comfortable and compensated. If the subject is uncomfortable at rest and clearly has functional class IV status (New York Heart Association classification), then one could more easily observe an increase in sympathetic tone and circulating catecholamines.[45]

This hypothesis most readily explains the different circulatory responses to a rapidly acting digitalis preparation in normal subjects and patients with congestive heart failure.[20,46,47] Ouabain normally produces a direct arteriolar constriction that is reflected by an increase in systemic vascular resistance. Conversely, in patients and animals with congestive heart failure, there is a paradoxical reduction in total systemic vascular resistance as well as vascular resistance in the limbs. In severe congestive heart failure when the cardiac output is reduced, the increased sympathoadrenal activity preferentially redirects blood away from the skin and renal circulations toward organs such as the heart and brain whose great metabolic requirements predominate in governing their local blood flow. By augmenting cardiac output in patients with congestive heart failure, digitalis glycosides reduce the need for increased sympathetic tone as a compensatory mechanism. Thus, in heart failure the direct effect of digitalis on the peripheral resistance vessels is also a constriction. However, the indirect effect of digitalis is a reduction in sympathetic adrenergic tone, which occurs as the result of improved myocardial performance. The indirect effect of the glycosides predominates and the net effect is to increase regional blood flow to the limbs.

Vascular Catecholamine Stress in Heart Failure: Whereas it is clear that myocardial norepinephrine stores are depleted in heart failure, results of studies on the catecholamine content of peripheral vessels are conflicting. In man it has been demonstrated that the norepinephrine released by tyramine is increased in the limbs.[48] In these experiments the leg was used as its own bioassay. The increase in vascular resistance that occurred after intraarterial injection of tyramine was compared with the increase in resistance occurring after graded intraarterial injections of norepinephrine. There was a fundamental similarity in the dose response curve to norepinephrine in the patients with and without heart failure. Therefore, there did not appear to be a true hypersensitivity of the resistance vessels to norepinephrine in heart failure. The response to tyramine, however, suggested that more norepinephrine was released in patients with severe congestive heart failure than in those with minimal heart disease.

On the other hand, results of a direct analysis of vascular norepinephrine content in two different animal preparations suggest that vascular catecholamine content is either normal or slightly reduced.[44,49] In one animal experiment direct stimulation of the sympathetic nerves suggested that there was even a reduction in peripheral vascular responsiveness.[44] Although the amount of norepinephrine released by neuronal stimulation and tyramine need not be similar, the differences seen in heart failure are in sharp contrast and have not yet been adequately explained.

Baroreceptor Responsiveness in Heart Failure: There are also paradoxical data on baroreceptor responsiveness in congestive heart failure. Normally, baroreceptor control of heart rate is predominantly parasympathetic.[50] Both in animal and human experiments the heart rate response to baroreceptor stimulation has been shown to be attenuated.[51–53] Similarly, arteriolar constrictor responses to baroreceptor stimulation have also been thought to be reduced in heart failure.[5] This has led to the postulation that both sympathetic and parasympathetic efferent innervation are defective in congestive heart failure. These responses are quite in contrast to the cardiocirculatory responses observed during exercise in which a greatly exaggerated sympathoadrenal discharge apparently occurs in symptomatic subjects with congestive heart failure.[11,13,54,55]

The Regional Circulations during Exercise—A Synthesis

In contrast to the attenuated response of the peripheral circulation to direct stimulation of the sympathetic chain or indirectly by means of

baroreceptor mechanisms, there appears to be a massive sympathetic response when the patient with heart failure exercises. During dynamic exercise a normal person has increased blood pressure, in part due to an increase in the contractile state of the myocardium. The increased blood pressure is necessary for adequate perfusion of the coronary and cerebral circulations. Likewise, the increased systemic arterial pressure facilitates perfusion of exercising muscles, which have greatly dilated resistance vessels. This increased pressure becomes more important as the exercising muscles develop greater tension and sustain it for longer durations. On the other hand, in the nonessential circulations, renal, splanchnic and nonexercising limbs, there is an autoregulatory and sympathetic adrenergic response that prevents blood flow from increasing in the face of an increasing perfusion pressure.[11,13,55–58] In patients with heart failure, blood flow is markedly reduced to the renal, splanchnic and cutaneous circulations, thereby suggesting that there is a greater sympathetic adrenergic activation.

Limb Circulation during Exercise in Normal Subjects: This response is more readily appreciated when one examines blood flow to the nonexercising limbs during exercise. The limbs contain two important circulations with different functions—skin and muscle. By utilizing the technique of epinephrine iontophoresis to suppress skin blood flow temporarily, it has become possible to evaluate independently the differential effect of systemic exercise on these two circulations.[13] In the nonexercising limbs of normal subjects, total blood flow is initially reduced. The magnitude of the reduction in blood flow to both skin and muscle in the nonexercising limbs is in direct proportion to the stress of exercise. The afferent limb of this reflex arc is probably activated by the accumulation of metabolites and perhaps local potassium concentrations in the exercising limbs.[57,58] With moderate exercise there is normally a late increase in cutaneous blood flow as the subject attempts to dissipate heat[13,57–61] (Figure 6). This cutaneous vasodilation is postponed with very severe exercise and is not seen until after the normal subject stops exercising. It would appear that hypothalamic recognition of the increased body temperature during exercise

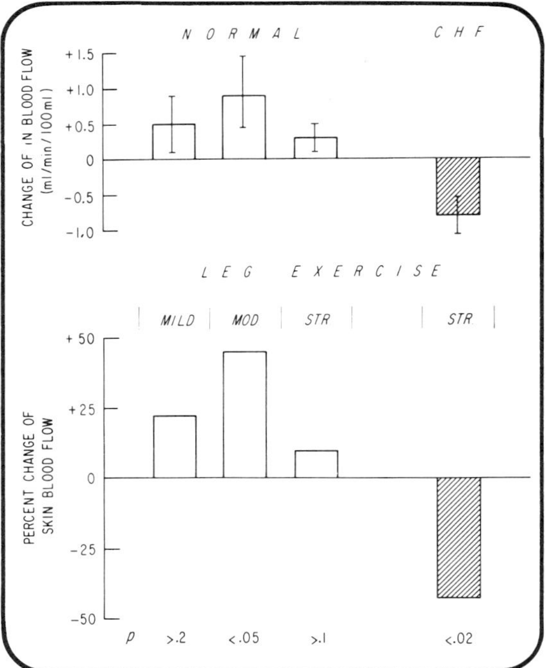

FIGURE 6. Changes in forearm skin blood flow (± standard error of the mean) during the last three minutes of supine leg exercise in normal subjects and patients with congestive heart failure. Normal subjects exercised at three levels of exercise of increasing severity, mild, moderate (MOD) and strenuous (STR) (40,330, and 1,080 to 2,240 ft-lb/min). Subjects with heart failure exercised at a level that was strenuous for them (40 to 330 ft-lb/min). The value for skin blood flow was taken as the difference between blood flow measured in an untreated forearm (skin plus muscle flow) and that measured simultaneously in a forearm that had undergone epinephrine iontophoresis (muscle flow only). The absolute changes in flow are seen in the **top panel** and the percent change in flow in the **bottom panel.** Whereas a cutaneous vasodilation is seen in normal subjects late during the course of moderate exercise, subjects with heart failure maintain a marked cutaneous vasoconstriction. (Reprinted by permission of the American Heart Association, Inc. from Zelis et al.[13])

selectively modulates that part of the sympathetic efferent limb to allow a cutaneous vasodilation during moderate exercise but is unable to overcome the strong afferent impulses that result from very stressful exertion. There is no reason to doubt that sympathetic efferent impulses are just as strong to the exercising as to the nonexercising muscle. However, in the normal subject, the accumulation of metabolites in the exercising muscles can override the effects of

increased sympathetic adrenergic tone and vascular resistance is reduced.[24,25] The combination of increased blood pressure and reduced vascular resistance in the active limbs during rhythmic exercise is an attempt to provide an adequate supply of oxygen and nutrients to the exercising muscles.

Limb Circulation during Exercise in Congestive Heart Failure: In contrast, in congestive heart failure because the muscle resistance vessels have a limited ability to dilate normally, vascular resistance is not appropriately reduced and relative local hypoxia results. This probably causes an exaggerated stimulation of the afferent limb of the reflex arc that originates in the exercising muscle and ultimately leads to the observed massive sympathoadrenal discharge. In these subjects even moderate exercise can be considered extremely strenuous and the efferent sympathetic limb is greatly enhanced. Thus, blood flow to the nonexercising limbs is considerably reduced during exercise. No cutaneous vasodilation is seen either late during exercise or during the postexercise recovery period. These findings would explain why patients with congestive heart failure have a limited ability to tolerate thermal stress and why such patients frequently have low-grade increases in temperature when they are hospitalized with acute heart failure.[62]

Similarly, when patients with congestive heart failure perform dynamic exercise, the blood pressure response is abnormal. Unlike normal subjects who have moderately increased blood pressure, patients with heart failure frequently have little or no increase in blood pressure, and occasionally exercise hypotension results.[10,11] If the resistance vessels in active skeletal muscle dilated normally and there were not excessive arteriolar constriction elsewhere, syncope would occur more commonly during exercise when the cardiac output was inadequate. This can be seen in two clinical situations: (1) when the patient with hypertensive heart disease and congestive heart failure receives drugs that inhibit alpha adrenergic responsiveness; and (2) after prolonged diuresis. In the former instance the increased sympathetic tone to the splanchnic, renal and cutaneous circulations is inhibited and there is no shunting of blood flow away from them to the low resistance vessels in active skeletal muscle. Since the heart cannot maintain an adequate cardiac output during exercise, the lack of alpha adrenergic tone in the nonessential regions allows the reduction in systemic vascular resistance to be more pronounced and blood pressure is inappropriately decreased. Second, after diuresis, which tends to restore normal muscle vascular response to vasodilator metabolites, a greater reduction in the muscle vascular resistance in the exercising limbs occurs. Again, since the cardiac response is limited, blood pressure is reduced and syncope would be expected to occur. This situation is further compounded since total blood volume may be reduced after diuresis and a normal utilization of the Frank-Starling mechanism to maintain cardiac output in heart failure cannot occur.[63] Thus, the combination of an exaggerated sympathoadrenal response and the limited arteriolar muscular dilation to metabolic stimuli work in concert to attempt to maintain an adequate blood pressure to perfuse vital organs during exercise.

At this point it is appropriate to reconsider the role played by the systemic arterial baroreceptors in congestive heart failure. Since heart rate and blood pressure are increased during dynamic exercise, one might expect that the afferent limb of the baroreceptor reflex normally would tend to reduce the magnitude of the sympathetic adrenergic response to exercise.[50] Although the response of heart rate to exercise is normal in heart failure, blood pressure is only minimally increased. The reduced pressor response of cardiac origin, coupled with a blunted baroreflex arc, would tend to facilitate central translation of the reflex originating in exercising muscle into an exaggerated sympathetic efferent discharge.

Metabolic Consequences of Increased Vascular Stiffness in Congestive Heart Failure

Oxygen Extraction and Consumption in Exercising Muscle: Although the increased peripheral vascular stiffness in heart failure might be considered a compensatory mechanism to maintain blood pressure during exercise, it also entails a metabolic cost. The reduced blood flow to exercising muscle might be expected to result in increased oxygen extraction. This has been consistently seen and is one explanation for the widened arteriovenous oxygen difference across the systemic circulation.[9] This increased extraction of oxygen in the muscular circulation, as well as a sympathetically mediated reduction in blood flow to the circulations with lower metabolic requirements (renal, splanchnic and cutaneous), explains why the level of mixed venous oxygen saturation in patients with congestive heart failure may be appreciably lower than that of normal subjects performing maximal exercise.[64] Because red blood cell 2,3-diphosphoglycerate (DPG) is increased in heart failure, a shift in the oxygen dissociation curve takes place to facilitate oxygen transport at the systemic capillary level from blood to tissues.[65-67] The effect of increased DPG, increased tissue acidosis and a slower circulation time all help to facilitate oxygen delivery to the exercising muscles.

The increased extraction of oxygen in the skeletal muscle circulation appears to be adequate to provide for basal metabolic requirements in nonexercising muscle in the face of reduced muscular blood flow in heart failure.[68,69] Although there is an increase in oxygen extraction during exercise, it does not appear to be sufficient to meet the increased oxygen requirements.[69] This was seen in one series of experiments in which intermittent forearm exercise was studied (Figure 7). During these experiments slow intermittent grip exercise was performed. A hand grip was held for 5 seconds four times each minute. During the last 5 seconds of the resting period, forearm blood flow was determined plethysmographically and forearm arteriovenous oxygen differences were evaluated. Since an increase in cardiac output was not necessary to supply the minimal oxygen requirments of one exercising limb, the vascular responses seen in the skeletal muscles of that limb reflected local factors governing oxygen delivery and were not secondary to an impaired cardiac response. In these studies, as the level of exercise increased, there was a growing disparity between the blood flow delivery to the active muscles in the normal subjects and the patients with heart failure. The inability of blood flow to increase appropriately in congestive heart failure was undoubtedly secondary to the

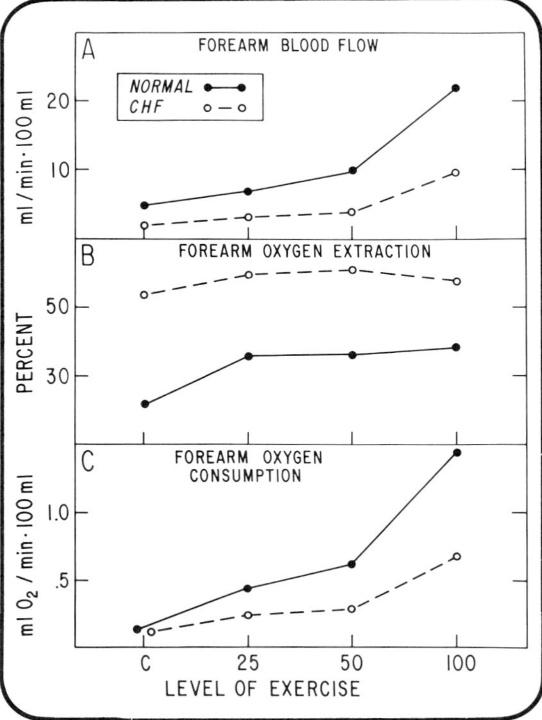

FIGURE 7. Forearm blood flow (**A**), forearm oxygen extraction (**B**) and forearm oxygen consumption (**C**) in a normal subject (**closed circles**) and a patient with congestive heart failure (**open circles**) at rest, c, and during rhythmic grip exercise of progressively increasing severity induced by squeezing a hand dynamometer to 25, 50 or 100 mm Hg for 5 seconds, 4 times/min for 5 minutes. Although forearm blood flow is reduced at rest in the patient with heart failure, the increased oxygen extraction is sufficient to maintain a normal basal forearm oxygen consumption. The higher level of oxygen extraction is not adequate to keep pace with muscle metabolic requirements during exercise and results in a greater shift to anaerobic metabolism, which is reflected in a reduced forearm oxygen consumption.

increased "arteriolar stiffness" described. However, since these were submaximal exercise levels, it is entirely possible that an increased sympathetic adrenergic tone played some role in reducing blood flow during steady state rhythmic exercise. Strikingly, forearm oxygen consumption in subjects with heart failure was considerably less than normal during each level of exercise. This reduced oxygen consumption occured despite increased forearm oxygen extraction. When sympathetic adrenergic block-

ade was performed, the forearm blood flow response increased slightly and there was some increase in forearm oxygen consumption. However, forearm oxygen consumption was still significantly reduced and appeared to reflect an increased anaerobic response to exercise. This might account in part for the pronounced lactic acidemia that can occur in patients with heart failure during exercise.[70,71] Although the limited capacity of the resistance vessels to dilate appropriately to metabolic stimuli might be a short-term compensatory mechanism to maintain blood pressure during exercise, it has an appreciable cost. Thus, the lactic portion of the oxygen debt of exercise is increased with heart failure. Likewise, the inability of the patient with heart failure to dissipate heat appropriately during and after exercise undoubtedly contributes to the lactic portion of the oxygen debt as well.[72,73] It is not known whether there are enzymatic changes in skeletal muscle of patients with heart failure that would tend to facilitate anaerobic metabolism.

Oxygen Diffusion in Exercising Muscles: Although the reduced ability of patients with heart failure to increase blood flow to exercising muscles probably accounts for the diminished forearm oxygen consumption, it is also possible there is a reduced ability of oxygen to diffuse adequately in exercising muscle. Recent studies have suggested that there is an increased thickness of the basal lamina of muscle capillaries similar to that seen in diabetes.[73–75] This alteration may be secondary to tissue injury from local hypoxia; however, the physiologic significance of this finding in heart failure is uncertain. Whereas electrolyte diffusion is enhanced in diabetes secondary to increased basement membrane thickness, oxygen diffusion capabilities have not been studied.[76] It is possible that the increased basement membrane thickness in heart failure might inhibit oxygen transport and be a second factor reducing the ability of forearm oxygen consumption to increase adequately during exercise.

Summary

Two abnormalities occur in the resistance vessels in congestive heart failure. First, there is an increased sympathetic tone to the peripheral resistance vessels. Whether or not sympathetic tone is increased at rest depends on the severity of the heart failure and the symptomatic status of the patient. Conversely, there appears to be a massive sympathoadrenal discharge during exercise which acts to attempt to maintain blood pressure and perfuse essential organs at the expense of nonessential circulations. The afferent limb of this reflex may originate in active skeletal muscle and be supernormally activated by the products of excessive anaerobic metabolism. Reduced baroreceptor activity in heart failure may preferentially facilitate the expression of this response. Second, there appears to be increased "vascular stiffness" of the peripheral arterioles that may be secondary to an increased vascular sodium content or a manifestation of increased tissue pressure seen in edema. During exercise this stiffness reduces the ability of the resistance vessels to dilate. This leads to a higher level of oxygen extraction which is adequate under basal conditions but is insufficient to meet aerobic needs of active muscle and results in a systemic lactic acidemia. Interventions that reduce sympathetic alpha adrenergic tone or restore normal arteriolar dilator capacity might be expected to have the adverse effect of producing exertional syncope.

Acknowledgment: This work was supported in part by American Heart Association Grant 71 888 and National Institutes of Health Grant HL 14780. At the time of these studies, Doctor Capone was supported by National Heart and Lung Institute Research Fellowship HL 52380.

The authors with to thank Robert Kleckner, Alvia Hilliard, Lawrence Baker and Arthur Lewis for their technical assistance and Nancy Carston for her secretarial assistance.

References

1. **Mason DT, Spann JF Jr, Zelis R, et al:** Alterations of hemodynamics and myocardial mechanics in patients with congestive heart failure: pathophysiologic mechanisms and assessment of cardiac function and ventricular contractility. Progr Cardiovasc Dis 12:507, 1970

2. **Mason DT, Zelis R, Amsterdam EA, et al:** Clinical determination of left ventricular contractility by hemodynamics and myocardial mechanics. In, Progress in Cardiology, chap 5 (Yu P, Goodwin J, ed). Philadelphia, Lea & Febiger, 1972, p 121

3. **Mason DT, Zelis R, Amsterdam EA, et al:** Mechanisms of cardiac contraction: structural, biochemical and functional relations in the normal and diseased heart. In, Pathologic Physiology, fifth edition (Sodeman W Jr, Sodeman W, ed). Philadelphia, WB Saunders, 1974, p 206

4. **Zelis R, Salel AF, Capone RJ, et al:** Evaluation of muscle function in the human myocardium by contractility measurements: coronary artery disease. In, Sonderdruck aus Das Chronick Kranke Herz (Roskamm H, Reindell H, ed). Stuttgart, Schattauer Verlag, 1973, p 379

5. **Salel A, Mason DT, Amsterdam EA, et al:** Abnormalities of left ventricular contractility in isolated right ventricular overload (abstr). Amer J Cardiol 29:288, 1972

6. **Salel A, Mason DT, Amsterdam EA, et al:** Marked depression of myocardial contractility in patients with angina pectoris before left ventricular hemodynamic failure (abstr). Clin Res 20:210, 1972

7. **Salel A, Mason DT, Amsterdam EA, et al:** The effect of left ventricular volume and pressure overload on myocardial pump and muscle function in man (abstr). Ninth Interamerican Congress of Cardiology, 1972, p 11

8. **Zelis R, Mason DT:** Compensatory mechanisms in congestive heart failure—the role of the peripheral resistance vessels. New Eng J Med 282:962, 1970

9. **Wade OL, Bishop JM:** Cardiac Output and Regional Blood Flow. Oxford, Blackwell Scientific Publications, 1962, p 134

10. **Epstein SE, Beiser GD, Stampfer M, et al:** Characterization of the circulatory response to maximal upright exercise in normal subjects and patients with heart disease. Circulation 35:1049, 1967

11. **Higgins CB, Vatner SF, Franklin D, et al:** Effects of experimentally produced heart failure on the peripheral vascular response to severe exercise in conscious dogs. Circ Res 31:186, 1972

12. **Zelis R, Mason DT, Braunwald E:** A comparison of the effects of vasodilator stimuli on peripheral resistance vessels in normal subjects and in patients with congestive heart failure. J Clin Invest 47:960, 1968

13. **Zelis R, Mason DT, Braunwald E:** Partition of blood flow to the cutaneous and muscular beds of the forearm at rest and during leg exercise in normal subjects and in patients with heart failure. Circ Res 24:799, 1969

14. **Zelis R, Mason DT, Braunwald E, et al:** Effects of hyperlipoproteinemias and their treatment on the peripheral circulation. J Clin Invest 49:1007, 1970

15. **Holling HE, Boland HC, Russ E:** Investigation of arterial obstruction using a mercury-in-rubber strain gauge. Amer Heart J 62:194, 1961

16. **Winsor T:** Simplified determination of arterial insufficiency. Circulation 3:830, 1951

17. **Shepherd JT:** The blood flow through the calf after exercise in subjects with arteriosclerosis and claudication. Clin Sci 9:49, 1950

18. **Hewlett AW, Van Zwaluwenburg JG:** The rate of blood flow in the arm. Heart 1:87, 1909

19. **Whitney RJ:** The measurement of volume changes in human limbs. J Physiol (London) 121:1, 1953

20. **Mason DT, Braunwald E:** Studies on digitalis. X. Effects of ouabain on forearm vascular resistance and venous tone in normal subjects and in patients in heart failure. J Clin Invest 43:532, 1964

21. **Schweitzer P, Pivonka M, Klvanova H:** The blood flow in the forearm in patients with cardiac failure. I. The relationship between the cardiac output and the blood flow in the forearm. Z Ges Exp Med 143:126, 1967

22. **Patterson GC, Whelan RF:** Reactive hyperemia in the human forearm. Clin Sci 14:197, 1955

23. **Wood JE, Litter J, Wilkins RW:** The mechanism of limb segment reactive hyperemia in man. Circ Res 3:581, 1955

24. **Remensnyder JP, Mitchell JH, Sarnoff SJ:** Functional sympatholysis during muscular activity. Circ Res 11:370, 1962

25. **Strandell T, Shepherd JT:** The effect in humans of increased sympathetic activity on the blood flow to active muscle. Acta Med Scand suppl 472:146, 1967

26. **Bayliss WM:** On the local reactions of the arterial wall to changes of internal pressure. Physiology 28:220, 1902

27. **Genty RM, Johnson PC:** Reactive hyperemia in arterioles and capillaries of frog skeletal muscle following microocclusion. Circ Res 31:953, 1972

28. **Cohn JN:** Blood pressure measurement in shock. Mechanism of inaccuracy in auscultatory and palpatory methods. JAMA 199:972, 1967

29. **Zelis R, Delea CS, Coleman HN, et al:** Arterial sodium content in experimental congestive heart failure. Circulation 41:213, 1970

30. **Conway J:** A vascular abnormality in hypertension: a study of blood flow in the forearm. Circulation 27:520, 1963

31. **Tobian L, Janecek J, Tomboulian A, et al:** Sodium and potassium in the walls of arterioles in experimental renal hypertension. J Clin Invest 40:1922, 1961

32. **Zelis R, Mason DT:** Diminished forearm arteriolar dilator capacity produced by mineralocorticoid-induced salt retention in man. Implications concerning congestive heart failure and vascular stiffness. Circulation 41:589, 1970

33. **Rodbard S, Takeda Y, Takacs L:** Post-occlusion hyperemia: a study on a model. Quart J Exp Physiol 54:346, 1969

34. **Rodbard S:** Capillary control of blood flow and fluid exchange. Circ Res 28 and 29 suppl I:51, 1971

35. **Beer G:** Role of tissue fluid in blood flow regulation. Circ Res 28 and 29 suppl I:154, 1971

36. **Lee G, Barnum J, Mason DT, et al:** The contribution of increased tissue pressure to the "vascular stiffness" of congestive heart failure (abstr). Clin Res 19:115, 1971

37. **Guyton AC:** A concept of negative interstitial pressure based on pressures in implanted perforated capsules. Circ Res 12:339, 1963

38. **Ladegaard-Pedersen HJ:** Measurement of the interstitial pressure in subcutaneous tissue in dogs. Circ Res 26:765, 1970

39. **Mansour E, Capone RJ, Mason DT, et al:** The contribution of edema to the reduced arteriolar dilator response of congestive heart failure (abstr). Circulation 44 suppl II:197, 1971

40. **Mason DT, Zelis R, Amsterdam EA:** Role of the sympathetic nervous system in congestive heart failure. In, Cardiovascular Regulation in Health and Disease (Bartorelli C, Zanchetti A, ed). Milan, Cardiovascular Research Institute, 1971, p 159

41. **Zelis R, Capone RJ, Amsterdam EA, et al:** The mechanism of elevated venous tone in congestive heart failure: the role of local and neurogenic factors (abstr). Ninth Interamerican Congress of Cardiology, 1972, p 10

42. **Wood JE:** The Veins: Normal and Abnormal Function. Boston, Little, Brown, 1965, p 145

43. **Zitnik RS, Lorenz R, Shepherd JT:** Normal venous tone in congestive heart failure (abstr). Circulation 37 and 38 suppl VI: VI-212, 1968

44. **Schmid PG, Nelson LD, Mayer HE, et al:** Neurogenic control of vascular tone in heart failure (abstr). Clin Res 20:396, 1972

45. **Chidsey CA, Braunwald E, Morrow AG:** Catecholamine excretion and cardiac stores of norepinephrine in congestive heart failure. Amer J Med 39:442, 1965

46. **Higgins CB, Vatner SF, Braunwald E:** Regional hemodynamic effects of a digitalis glycoside in the conscious dog with and without experimental heart failure. Circ Res 30:406, 1972

47. **Harvey RM, Ferrer MI, Cathcart RI, et al:** Some effects of digoxin upon the heart and circulation in man: digoxin in left ventricular failure. Amer J Med 7:439, 1949

48. **Kramer RS, Mason DT, Braunwald E:** Augmented sympathetic neurotransmitter activity in the peripheral vascular bed of patients with congestive heart failure and cardiac norepinephrine depletion. Circulation 38:629, 1968

49. **Mayer HE, Mark AL, Schmid PG, et al:** Vascular catecholamines in cardiomyopathic hamsters with heart failure (abstr). Circulation 43 and 44 suppl II:II–112, 1971

50. **Pickering TG, Gribbin B, Petersen ES, et al:** Effects of autonomic blockade on the baroreflex in man at rest and during exercise. Circ Res 30:177, 1972

51. **Higgins CB, Vatner SF, Eckberg DL, et al:** Alterations in the baroreceptor reflex in conscious dogs with heart failure. J Clin Invest 51:715, 1972

52. **Eckberg DL, Drabinsky M, Braunwald E:** Defective cardiac parasympathetic control in patients with heart disease. New Eng J Med 285:877, 1971

53. **Beiser GD, Epstein SE, Stampfer M, et al:** Impaired heart rate response to sympathetic nerve stimulation in patients with cardiac decompensation (abstr). Circulation 38 suppl VI: VI–40, 1968

54. **Wood JE:** The mechanism of the increased venous pressure with exercise in congestive heart failure. J Clin Invest 41:2020, 1962

55. **Chidsey CA, Harrison DC, Braunwald E:** Augmentation of the plasma norepinephrine response to exercise in patients with congestive heart failure. New Eng J Med 267:650, 1962

56. **Millard RW, Higgins CB, Franklin D, et al:** Regulation of the renal circulation during severe exercise in normal dogs and dogs with experimental heart failure. Circ Res 31:881, 1972

57. **Bevegård BS, Shepherd JT:** Reaction in man of resistance and capacity vessels in forearm and hand to leg exercise. J Appl Physiol 21:123, 1966

58. **Bishop JM, Donald KW, Taylor SH, et al:** Blood flow in the human arm during supine leg exercise. J Physiol (London) 137:294, 1957

59. **Clement DL, Pelletier LC, Shepherd JT:** Circulatory reflexes caused by contraction of skeletal muscles in the dog (abstr). Circulation 45 and 46 suppl II:II–80, 1972

60. **Pérez-González JF, Coote JH:** Activity of muscle afferents and reflex circulatory responses to exercise. Amer J Physiol 223:138, 1972

61. **Donald KW, Bishop JM, Wade OL:** Changes in the oxygen content of axillary venous blood during leg exercise in patients with rheumatic heart disease. Clin Sci 14:531, 1955

62. **Burch GE, Giles TD:** The burden of a hot and humid environment on the heart. Mod Conc Cardiovasc Dis 39:115, 1970

63. **Stampfer M, Epstein SE, Beiser GD, et al:** Hemodynamic effects of diuresis at rest and during intense upright exercise in patients with impaired cardiac function. Circulation 37:900, 1968

64. **Epstein SE, Beiser GD, Stampfer M, et al:** Exercise in patients with heart disease: effects of body position and type and intensity of exercise. Amer J Cardiol 23:572, 1969

65. **Benesch R, Benesch RE:** Effect of organic phosphates from human erythrocyte on allosteric properties of hemoglobin. Biochem Biophys Res Commun 26:162, 1967

66. **Eaton JW, Faulkner JA, Brewer GJ:** Response of the human red cell to muscular activity. Proc Soc Exp Biol Med 132:886, 1969

67. **Valeri CR, Fortier NL:** Red-cell 2,3-diphosphoglycerate and creatine levels in patients with red-cell mass deficits or with cardiopulmonary insufficiency. New Eng J Med 281:1452, 1969

68. **Schweitzer P, Pivonka M, Klvanova H:** The blood flow in the forearm in patients with cardiac failure. II. The relationship between the blood flow and oxygen consumption in the muscle of the forearm in patients with low cardiac output. Z Ges Exp Med 143:136, 1967

69. **Longhurst J, Zelis R, Amsterdam EA, et al:** Depressed forearm oxygen consumption in congestive heart failure—physiologic adaptation to impaired metabolic vasodilation? (abstr). Circulation 42 suppl III:72, 1970

70. **Bruce RA, Jones JW, Strait GB:** Anaerobic metabolic responses to acute maximal exercise in male athletes. Amer Heart J 67:643, 1964

71. **Huckabee WE, Judson WE:** The role of anaerobic metabolism in the performance of mild muscular work. 1. Relationship to oxygen consumption and cardiac output, and the effect of congestive heart failure. J Clin Invest 37:1577, 1958

72. **Brooks GA, Hittelman KJ, Faulkner JA, et al:** Temperature, skeletal muscle mitochondrial functions, and oxygen debt. Amer J Physiol 220:1053, 1971

73. **Brooks, GA, Hittelman KJ, Faulkner JA, et al:** Tissue temperatures and whole-animal oxygen consumption after exercise. Amer J Physiol 221:427, 1971

74. **Siperstein MD, Unger RH, Madison LL:** Studies of muscle capillary basement membranes in normal subjects, diabetic, and prediabetic patients. J Clin Invest 47:1973, 1968

75. **Vracko R, Benditt EP:** Capillary basal lamina thickening. Its relationship to endothelial cell death and replacement. J Cell Biol 47:281, 1970

76. **Longhurst J, Capone RJ, Amsterdam EA, et al:** A microcirculatory defect in congestive heart failure—etiology of depressed oxygen consumption during exercise? (abstr). Clin Res 20:208, 1972

77. **Alpert JS, Coffman JD, Balodimos MC, et al:** Capillary permeability and blood flow in skeletal muscle of patients with diabetes mellitus and genetic prediabetes. New Eng J Med 286:454, 1972

Chapter 11

Function of the Hypoxic Myocardium

Experimental and Clinical Aspects

Ezra A. Amsterdam, MD, FACC

Current knowledge of the pathophysiologic consequences of impaired blood flow to the myocardium is the result of scientific inquiry begun almost 300 years ago[2] and sharply accelerated early in this century with the advent of the modern era in cardiovascular medicine and physiology. The past several decades have witnessed an unprecedented proliferation of information on this problem extending from studies at the cellular level to new data on cardiac disease in man, as recently reviewed.[3-11] Progress in this area has resulted in improved understanding of the relation between altered physiology and clinical manifestations in ischemic heart disease, the most prevalent fatal disease in Western society. Increased comprehension of underlying mechanisms has enhanced understanding, evaluation and management of the patient with clinical ischemic heart disease. Further elucidation of this problem is predicated on present knowledge of the pathophysiology of the altered dynamics of heart muscle deprived of adequate oxygen. This discussion will deal with current concepts of the nature of the alterations in myocardial function resulting from inadequate oxygen supply as developed from the study of isolated cardiac muscle, laboratory investigation of the intact organism and clinical evaluation in man.

Relation Between Myocardial Metabolism and Function

The metabolism of the mammalian heart is almost exclusively aerobic, and thus the myocardium is dependent on a continuous high rate of oxygen delivery. In its pivotal metabolic role as the major recipient of the electrons produced during oxidative phosphorylation, oxygen is critical to the function of the myocardial cell, linking intramitochondrial processes to production of high-energy phosphate (Figure 1). Aerobic metabolism, an intramitochondrial process, is an efficient, and thereby the chief, pathway for the high level of energy production required by the myocardium. Anaerobic metabolism, that is, glycolysis, which proceeds in the cytoplasm, can be utilized only to a limited extent by the myocardium for generation of high-energy phosphate[12,13] and is therefore insufficient in itself to maintain cardiac function. This unique metabolic pattern is well adapted to meet the intense energy requirements associated with the omnipresent functional burden of the heart, which is extraordinary compared with that of other organs.[6,7,12,14] However, the extreme dependence of cardiac function on high levels of oxygen supply also is responsible for the vulnerability of cardiac muscle to inadequate availability of oxygen. Thus, a fundamental characteristic of the myocardium is the rapid deterioration of its contractile processes resulting from diminished oxygen delivery.[1,10,15-38] Although it might therefore appear likely that

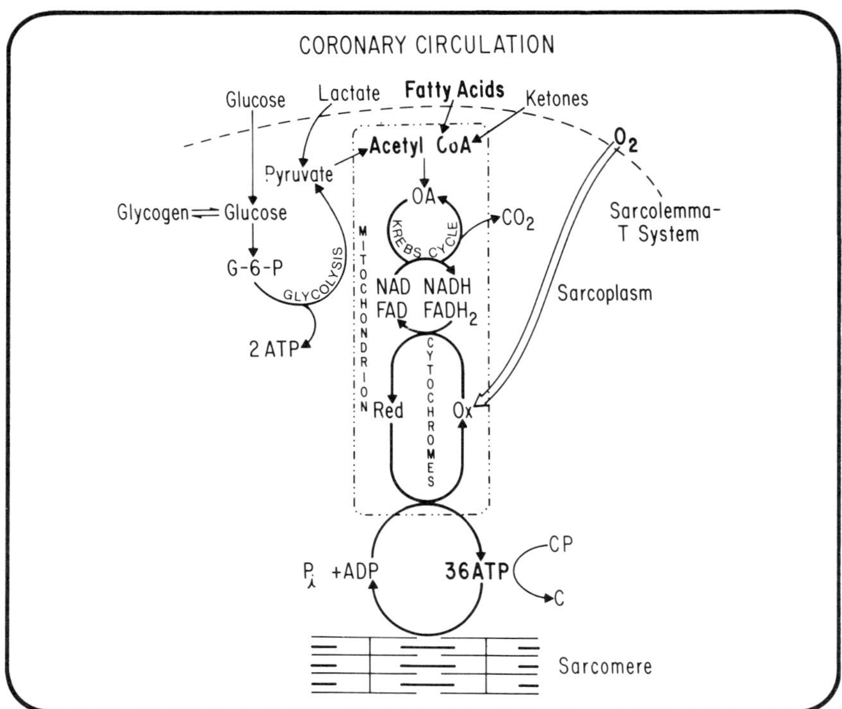

FIGURE 1. Diagram of metabolic pathways of energy (adenosine triphosphate) production within the cardiac cell. Complete oxidation of a substrate such as glucose yields a total of 38 moles of adenosine triphosphate per mole of glucose, whereas glycolysis alone provides only 2 moles of adenosine triphosphate. ADP = adenosine diphosphate; ATP = adenosine triphosphate; C = creatine; CP = creatine phosphate; CoA = coenzyme A; FAD and FADH = flavin adenine dinucleotide and its reduced form, respectively; G-6-P = glucose-6-phosphate; NAD and NADH = nicotinamide adenine dinucleotide and its reduced form, respectively; OA = oxaloacetic acid; Ox = oxidation; P_i = inorganic phosphate; Red = reduction.

the depression of myocardial function associated with oxygen deprivation is the result of failure to generate high-energy phosphate compounds, demonstration of adequate myocardial adenosine triphosphate levels in association with marked reduction in contractile function during the early phase of ischemia suggests that the problem is more complicated.[39]

Impaired oxygen supply to cardiac cells not only results in loss of myocardial functional integrity, but also is manifested by a complex of pathophysiologic events encompassing impaired metabolic activity, deranged mechanical performance, abnormal electrophysiology, altered structural and physical properties and, frequently, clinical signs and symptoms.[1,10,15–38,40–46] These abnormalities can culminate in irreversible structural and functional impairment within minutes if cellular hypoxia is sufficiently

severe.[7,41–43,47] However, even after marked deterioration, there is a limited period during which myocardial structural and functional integrity can be substantially restored by restitution of adequate oxygen supply.[1,7,27,41–43,48–52]

Ischemia vs. Hypoxia: Cellular oxygen delivery may be insufficient because of either (1) inadequate coronary blood flow or (2) reduced oxygen concentration in perfusing blood or other supporting media in which cardiac tissue is immersed. The former condition is referred to as ischemia and the latter as hypoxia. Investigative studies have also employed anoxia, or total absence of oxygen. Both ischemia and hypoxia may be induced experimentally and occur clinically; both produce hypoxia of the myocardial cell. However, there are significant differences in their overall effects. Since ischemia is related to hypoperfusion, it results in a deficiency not only of oxygen, but also of substrates for energy production and an accumulation of metabolic end products and other substances from damaged cells. In the hypoxic heart with normal perfusion, these materials, although released from injured cells, are removed and are of less consequence.

Experimental Studies

Coronary Arterial Ligation: Deterioration of myocardial function is abrupt and profound after deprivation of oxygen supply to the myocardium by interruption of coronary blood flow. The relation between inadequate myocardial oxygenation and compromised function has been amply demonstrated experimentally. Thus, after ligation of a coronary artery, shortening of cardiac muscle ceases in the ischemic area in less than 1 minute, as observed in the classic experiments of Tennant and Wiggers[1] almost 40 years ago. Within 10 seconds the affected area becomes cyanotic,[20] and contraction of ischemic myocardium is impaired. Duration of tension development is diminished,[1] degree of shortening reduced[1] and force of contraction decreased[1,27] (Figure 2). After 30 to 60 seconds, there is passive, systolic expansion of the injured area resulting from the pressure produced by uninvolved myocardium, which distends the ischemic, ineffectively contracting segment.[1,22,27]

If a sufficient quantity of myocardium is involved, the impairment of mechanical function is accompanied by alterations in cardiac pump performance, electrical activity and metabolism. Thus, there are reductions in cardiac output, stroke volume [18,28,29,37,38] and blood pressure;[24] increases in left atrial and left ventricular diastolic pressures;[18,28,29,31–35,37,38] electrocardiographic S-T segment depression;[18,28,29,32,33] and lactate production,[18,28,29,31–34] enhanced glucose extraction[53,54] and decreased free fatty acid extraction by the myocardium.[55] The latter findings only partially reflect the fundamental alterations in intracellular metabolism produced by hypoxia discussed in chapter 6.[39] Typical S-T changes and myocardial lactate production correlate closely as indicators of myocardial ischemia.[18,28,29,32,33]

Hypoxia: The effects of hypoxia on the mechanics of myocardial contraction recently have been investigated in detail in the isolated, supported cat right ventricular papillary muscle.[15-17] Rapid and severe loss of contractile capacity immediately ensues with the onset of hypoxia as reflected by abrupt reduction of tension development (Figure 3). In addition to this decrease in intensity of active state, time to peak tension is markedly reduced, indicating compromise in the duration of active state, during which generation of mechanical energy occurs. During reoxygenation there is an increase in measured time to peak tension, considerably in excess of control levels, which is closely associated with recovery of contractile activity toward normal.[15,16] Further, during recovery from hypoxia, tension development is followed by

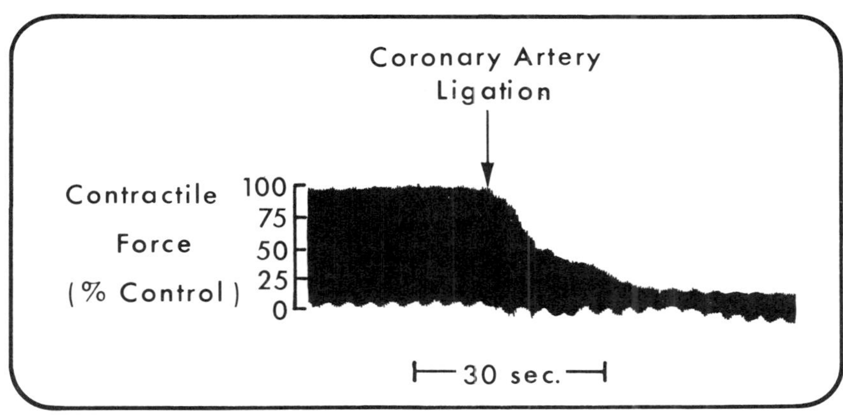

FIGURE 2. Left ventricular contractile force measured by an isometric strain gauge arch sutured into the myocardium of a dog. Note the rapid decline in force after ligation of the left anterior descending coronary artery.

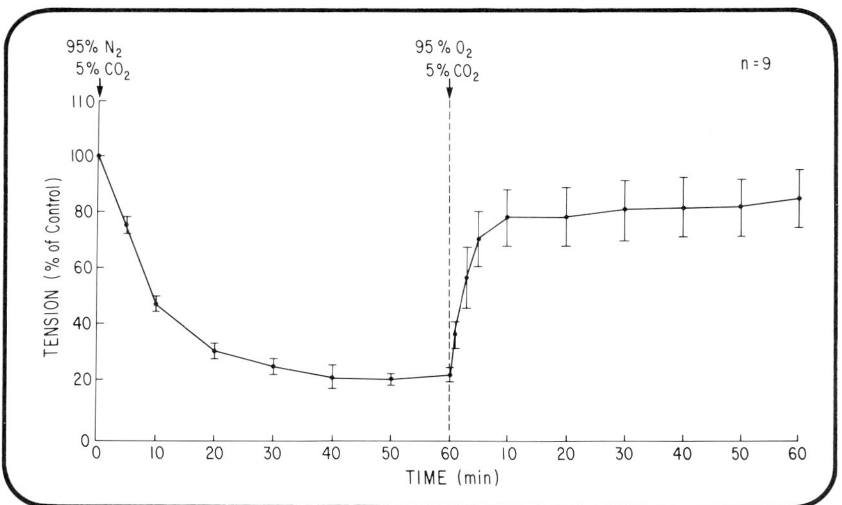

FIGURE 3. Effect of hypoxia on tension (mean ± standard error) developed by isolated cat papillary muscle supported in a Krebs bath. The bath is initially perfused with 95 percent oxygen and 5 percent carbon dioxide. Tension decreases abruptly after substitution of 95 percent nitrogen (N_2) for oxygen, and recovery is rapid after reinstitution of oxygen.

prolongation of relaxation time.[15] It has been suggested that the latter increase—which, together with the increased time to peak tension during recovery from hypoxia, alters the temporal sequence of myocardial contraction—may be related to the phenomenon of dyssynergy in the intact heart with regional ischemia.[56]

Investigations utilizing the isolated, perfused heart have employed anoxia.[19] These studies also demonstrate marked impairment of myocardial mechanical performance as well as abnormal electrical activity and disruption of subcellular architecture by oxygen deprivation. Thus, with onset of anoxia, pulse pressure and maximal rate of rise of left ventricular pressure are reduced, ventricular end-diastolic pressure increases sharply, and structural alterations occur, as manifested by nonalignment of myofilaments, swelling of mitochondrial cristae, loss of transverse tubules and dilatation of longitudinal tubules.[18]

Metabolic Effects of Interrupted Coronary Flow: Although the major consequence of interruption of coronary blood flow is cessation of myocardial oxygen supply, certain other effects merit consideration. The accumulation of products of cellular metabolism and breakdown in the absence of normal perfusion has several po-

tentially detrimental effects. These substances, which include potassium, hydrogen ions and lysosomal enzymes, can depress myocardial metabolic and functional processes and contribute to cellular damage if they are present in sufficiently high concentration. Thus, potassium, in excessive extracellular concentration, can prevent electrical activation of the cell;[7,40] the reduction in intracellular pH resulting from accumulation of hydrogen ions has been implicated in impairment of the contractile process at the level of the interaction between calcium and troponin;[7,39] and the hydrolytic enzymes released from lysosomes are capable of inflicting direct structural injury on the cell.[57-59] In addition, when coronary blood flow is curtailed, the myocardium is deprived of exogenous substrates such as free fatty acids, glucose, amino acids and ketones for energy production. These factors may contribute significantly to depression of myocardial function in states of hypoperfusion. However, experimental studies have indicated that lack of oxygen is the primary deficit in these instances since reduction of oxygen supply by anoxic perfusion, during which other substrate requirements are fulfilled, compromises myocardial mechanical performance to a considerably greater degree than does deprivation of metabolic substrate during conditions of normal oxygenation.[19] Although provision of adequate[19] or augmented glucose[16] during anoxia or hypoxia improves contractile function, the magnitude of this effect is modest relative to the depression of cardiac performance resulting from lack of oxygen per se.[16,19] Conversely, whereas lack of substrate delivery for a brief period has relatively little effect on function during normal oxygenation of the myocardium, it is associated with a greater decrease in contractile performance during anoxia.[19] Attenuation of myocardial energy production in the form of adenosine triphosphate has also been reported as more severe in the absence of oxygen than in that of substrate.[60]

Clinical Studies

Recent investigations have extended the approach discussed to the evaluation of ischemic heart disease in man. Myocardial ischemia occurring clinically may be transient, as in the syndrome of angina pectoris, and reversible in terms of symptoms and associated cardiac functional alterations. Ischemia of sufficient severity and duration results in irreversible loss of structure and function, usually manifested clinically as myocardial infarction. The circulatory dynamics and patterns of ventricular muscle function during ischemia have been clarified to a considerable extent by the recent application of hemodynamic and ventriculographic techniques to this problem.

Angina Pectoris

Among the most consistent findings on cardiac performance during myocardial ischemia is the usually striking evidence of depressed left ventricular function. The frequency and degree of this abnormality have now been well documented in man during both transient ischemia —angina pectoris—and myocardial infarction. The hemodynamic impairment is directly related to the presence of myocardial ischemia and the extent of functional loss is dependent on the quantity of myocardial muscle involved.[8,61–65] The outcome of this deranged functional state is closely associated with the course of the metabolic abnormality since both alterations are intimately related to cellular hypoxia. With subsidence of ischemia, as in angina, ventricular function returns to its pre-ischemic level.[66–68] However, after myocardial infarction, there is usually permanent reduction in cardiac functional capacity.[69–73]

Hemodynamic Effects of Ischemia: The circulatory dynamics associated with angina pectoris have been the subject of recent intensive investigation. The concept that angina is a manifestation of myocardial ischemia and thereby reflects the presence of a disparity between myocardial oxygen supply and demand is affirmed by these studies. Thus, evidence of increased myocardial oxygen requirements, together with inability to commensurately augment coronary blood flow, is typically associated with angina, whether provoked or spontaneous. Indeed, in the clinical evaluation of patients, angina is induced or alleviated by manipulation of those hemodynamic variables that are major determinants of myocardial oxygen needs,[10,11,32–34,66–68,74] that is, heart rate, intramyocardial tension (directly related to blood pressure and ventricular volume) and myocardial contractility.[75] The basis of restricted coronary blood flow is, in all but unusual instances, coronary artery atherosclerosis. It is now also appreciated that spasm of a coronary artery may produce clinical myocardial ischemia, as has recently been documented.[76] The extent to which this phenomenon may be implicated in angina pectoris is unknown. It has been considered chiefly in relation to Prinzmetal or variant angina pectoris.[76,77]

Although functional studies relate to angina induced by a variety of stresses (catecholamine infusion,[74] pacing-induced tachycardia,[32–38,66,68] or exercise[10,38,67]) or occurring spontaneously,[31] the hemodynamic response has been consistent. Thus, as in the experimental studies previously discussed, abnormal cardiac performance indicative of left ventricular failure has been repeatedly demonstrated at the time of angina pectoris.[10,11,31–38,66–68] Left ventricular end-diastolic pressure is increased[31–35,66–68,74] in association with reduced cardiac output, stroke volume and stroke work,[10,11,31–34,66–68,74] and the left ventricular function curve is thereby depressed[37,38,66] (Figure 4). That this evidence of depressed myocardial contractile function during ischemic pain is intrinsic to the anginal state

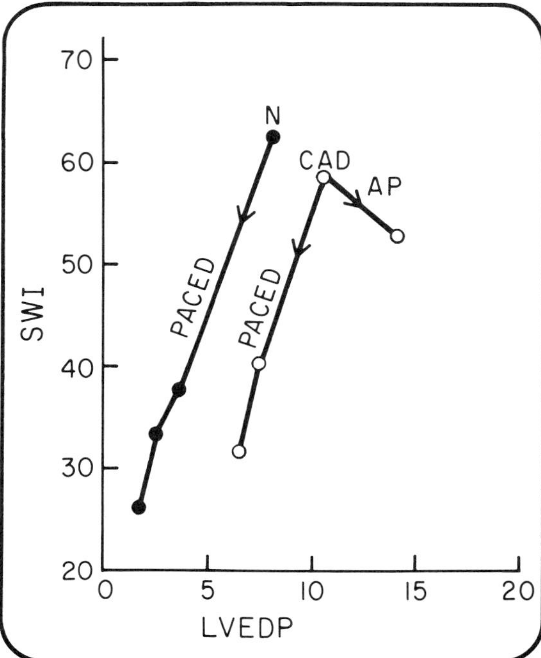

FIGURE 4. Left ventricular function curves produced by atrial pacing in a subject with a normal heart (N, **closed circles**) and a patient with coronary artery disease (CAD, **open circles**). Function is normal in the patient with coronary artery disease until the onset of angina pectoris (AP) at which point the curve becomes depressed. LVEDP = left ventricular end-diastolic pressure (mm Hg); SWI = stroke work index (g-m/m²).

is indicated by lack of these findings in patients with coronary artery disease who do not manifest angina under identical conditions.[32,35,68]

Ventricular Contractility and Wall Motion during Ischemia: The deterioration of cardiac performance accompanying angina is associated with abnormal ventricular wall motion, which has now been documented in man by angiographic studies during angina.[35,36,76] This abnormality of muscle function consists of failure of adequate shortening, which is associated with diminished force development, in one or more areas of ventricular myocardium. These derangements in mechanical performance of cardiac muscle underlie the altered function intrinsic to the ischemic state. Thus, during acute ischemia, the contractile pattern of the ventricle may deteriorate from normal to include one or more areas of inadequate or abnormal motion,

or when the latter is already present, it may become quantitatively greater in the affected area or involve additional regions of myocardium[35,36,78] (Figure 5). Loss of actively contracting muscle deprives the ventricle—for the duration of this defect—of the contribution of involved myocardium to overall cardiac pump function, resulting in decreased stroke volume, cardiac output and ejection fraction with consequent increase in residual ventricular volume and end-diastolic pressure—hemodynamic findings indicative of ventricular failure. A further alteration that recently has been recognized during acute ischemia and which may contribute to the increase in end-diastolic pressure involves the physical properties of the myocardium. Thus, myocardial compliance, or the quantitative relation of passive changes in pressure to changes in volume ($\Delta P/\Delta V$), may decrease during acute, transient ischemia.[9,35]

The impaired ventricular muscle performance in ischemic heart disease is characteristically segmental as determined by the distribution of coronary artery atherosclerosis.[70] Abnormal ventricular wall motion resulting from coronary disease has been categorized into several descriptive patterns under the general term dyssynergy[70] (Figure 6). The degree of hemodynamic impairment is directly related to the quantity of cardiac muscle involved in the dyssynergy process. Thus, when 20 to 25 percent of left ventricular myocardium fails to function adequately, as can be defined by left ventriculography, normal myocardium is unable to compensate completely, overall ventricular function is depressed, and cardiac failure may ensue.[61] Although related to coronary artery disease, dyssynergy is uncommon in the absence of associated permanent loss of myocardium. Thus, we have found that in patients with acute or remote myocardial infarction, as indicated by the electrocardiogram, abnormal ventricular motion is almost a constant finding, whereas even in severe coronary artery disease without electrocardiographic evidence of infarction, left ventricular dyssynergy is unusual in the unstressed ventricle.[73] However, with the onset of acute myocardial ischemia, as in angina, frank dyssynergy can develop in a previously normally contracting ventricle in association with a normal electrocardiogram (Figure 5). In angina

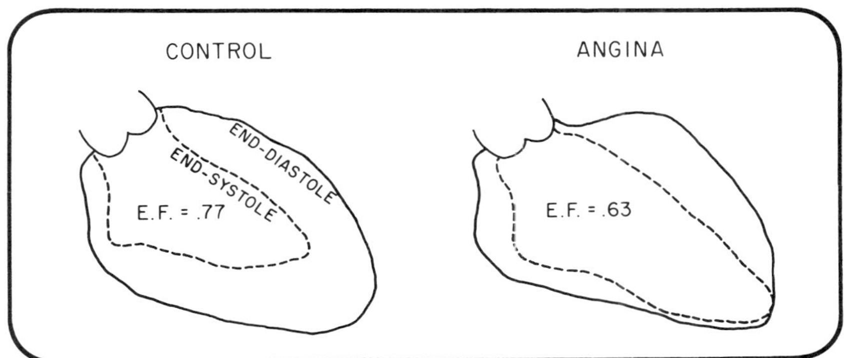

FIGURE 5. Diagrams of left ventricular angiograms from a patient with coronary artery disease. Control angiogram demonstrates a normal contraction pattern. With the onset of angina produced by atrial pacing, there is impairment of myocardial contraction manifested by hypokinesis of the apical-inferior area of the left ventricle which is associated with a fall in ejection fraction (E.F.).

pectoris, this is a transient reversible phenomenon, whereas in the infarcted ventricle the dyssynergy is a permanent manifestation of necrosis and subsequent scarring.

The same complex of altered physiology observed during experimental myocardial ischemia is manifested during this state in man. Thus, in addition to regional abnormalities of cardiac muscle performance and hemodynamic function, there are alterations in myocardial metabolism and the electrocardiogram. These changes are also manifested by myocardial lactate production, enhanced glucose extraction and S-T segment depression.[31–34,54]

The reversible nature of angina is emphasized. The acute myocardial ischemia characteristic of this syndrome is transient and, thus, the entire spectrum of functional manifestations of the metabolic defect, including deranged ventricular contractile pattern and depressed hemodynamic performance, is short-lived, reversion to previous status generally occurring within minutes.[66–68] Support for the absence of myocardial damage during angina is provided by metabolic studies that document myocardial ischemia during acute episodes of pain and simultaneously reveal no evidence of necrosis. In association with symptoms or electrocardiographic indications of ischemia, or both, myocardial lactate production has not been accompanied by evidence of enzyme release from heart muscle, as assessed by coronary sinus sampling.[79]

Congestive Heart Failure

The relation between coronary artery disease and cardiac failure merits further discussion. Although transient episodes of myocardial ischemia can clearly produce temporary depression of left ventricular function, coronary artery disease in the absence of permanent

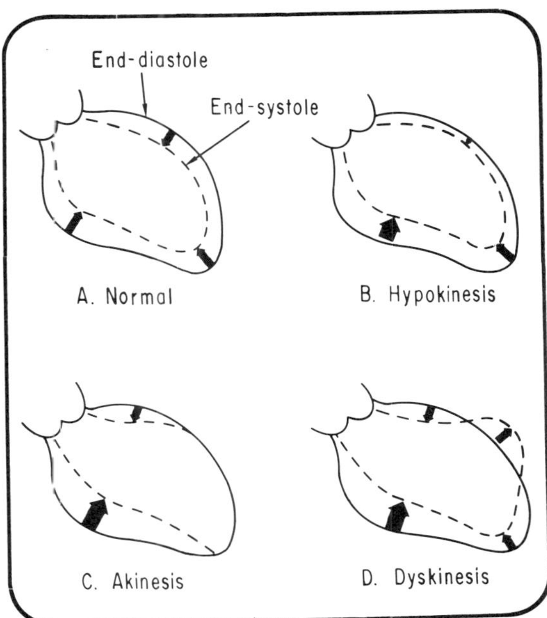

FIGURE 6. Schematic representations of normal and dyssynergic contraction patterns of the left ventricle.

damage to myocardial muscle is uncommonly associated with significant, sustained impairment of cardiac performance under normal conditions. Thus, in the great majority of patients with coronary artery disease without previous myocardial infarction, indexes of ventricular performance such as cardiac output, left ventricular end-diastolic pressure and synergy of contraction are unimpaired. This finding is consistent with the clinical observation that cardiac failure is not usually a significant feature in the patient with angina who has not had a previous myocardial infarction.

Underlying Coronary Artery Disease: In those instances of compromised function without previous infarction, coronary artery disease is usually extensive and involves the left main coronary artery or the proximal portion of the left anterior descending artery. This follows from the relative importance of the individual coronary arteries to ventricular function. Although the latter relation has not been quantitatively assessed, it would be expected, from the extensive distribution of the left anterior descending artery to the free wall of the left ventricle and interventricular septum, that this artery would be of primary importance among the three major coronary trunks, including the right and left circumflex vessels, in the delivery of myocardial blood supply. The left main coronary artery would be even more vital. Conversely, since the right coronary artery supplies a more limited area of the left ventricle, this artery is generally important in maintaining the integrity of ventricular function. Studies thus far have dealt with the relation between the number of diseased coronary vessels—rather than the specific vessels—and impairment of myocardial function. No clear relation is apparent with regard to number of involved vessels.[73] Conversely, the primacy of the left anterior descending artery to left ventricular function is supported by the more serious hemodynamic consequences of anterior myocardial infarction —a result of disease in this vessel—compared with the consequences of inferior infarction— usually the result of involvement of the right coronary artery.

The lack of overt impairment of cardiac hemodynamics at rest in patients with coronary disease without previous myocardial infarction does not imply the presence of a normal ventricle. Indeed, cardiac reserve is diminished, response to an increased work load inadequate and functional impairment manifest when the ventricle is stressed [10,11,31–38,66–68,74] (Figures 4 and 5). Thus, although depressed contractile performance may not be apparent in association with coronary disease in the absence of stress, diminished functional capacity is the rule.

Electrocardiographic Correlation: The relation between the electrocardiogram and ventricular function has been of considerable interest to us. Our studies indicate that within limits the electrocardiogram identifies and localizes[73,80] left ventricular dyssynergy, provides a quantitative estimate of its extent[78] and bears a consistent relation to left ventricular functional status.[73] The presence of pathologic Q waves correlates closely with left ventricular dyssynergy, the site of which is localized by the electrocardiogram.[73,80] Further, other electrocardiographic abnormalities, such as convex S-T segment elevation and T wave inversion, in addition to Q waves, are associated not only with the presence of left ventricular aneurysm, as classically described, but also with dyssynergy of considerably greater extent than that observed when these ST-T wave abnormalities are not present.[80] As noted previously, hemodynamic function in patients with coronary disease is usually not overtly abnormal in the absence of previous myocardial infarction. This relation is most meaningful when infarction is based on electrocardiographic presence of pathologic Q waves. When Q waves of 0.04 second duration are present and are related to involvement of the anterior or combined anterior and inferior regions of the left ventricle, hemodynamics are usually altered.[73] In contrast, prior inferior myocardial infarction is seldom associated with depressed left ventricular function.[73] Previous myocardial infarction, as determined by electrocardiographic diagnosis, is also more closely related to ventricular functional status than is associated coronary artery disease, as indicated by coronary arteriography.[73] Thus, again, overtly depressed function is unusual without associated electrocardiographic evidence of previous myocardial infarction regardless of the extent of coronary artery disease, and function may be seriously altered if there has been an extensive anterior infarction in the past regardless of the number of diseased coronary vessels.[73]

Myocardial Infarction

Myocardial infarction is the result of irreversible ischemic injury to myocardial cells. The consequent loss of functioning cardiac tissue is the primary cause of sustained cardiac failure in patients with coronary artery disease. The pathophysiologic basis of the ischemia that progresses to infarction is, as in angina, a disparity between myocardial oxygen supply and demand. However, in myocardial infarction, this imbalance is more intense and prolonged, persisting beyond the duration for which cell viability can be maintained. Cellular metabolic and electrical activity cease, necrosis of cardiac muscle ensues, and electrocardiographic evidence of transmural loss of myocardium appears and is generally permanent. However, diminution or disappearance of abnormal Q waves may occur, especially in inferior infarction, within months or years.[81,82] When infarction is not transmural the electrocardiographic changes are less specific. The functional derangements observed in the acute transient ischemia of the anginal syndrome are usually present to equal or greater degree in myocardial infarction, but the conditions differ fundamentally in that—with the loss of myocardium in infarction—associated functional impairment is generally irreversible. However, there is some capacity for recovery, as indicated by experimental studies[44,81] demonstrating improved hemodynamic function in the early period post infarction as compared with the acute stage.

Although there is some evidence of impaired cardiac performance in most patients with acute myocardial infarction,[84,85] virtually the entire functional spectrum is present in the group as a whole.[65] Thus, hemodynamic evaluation has revealed myocardial function ranging from normal to the shock state in this syndrome.[65] However, significant depression of ventricular performance is common, as indicated by a 40 to 50 percent incidence of congestive cardiac failure[86] and a 10 to 15 percent incidence of cardiogenic shock.[62,63] The significance of cardiac pump dysfunction in myocardial infarction is emphasized by its role as the leading cause of mortality—accounting for 80 percent—in patients reaching the hospital with infarction.[62] Although the overall hospital mortality rate in acute myocardial infarction is 12 to 20 percent,[87] it rises to 40 percent when congestive failure occurs and is over 80 percent in the presence of shock.[62]

The fundamental pathologic alteration underlying cardiac pump dysfunction in acute myocardial infarction is the loss of functioning myocardium, and the depression of cardiac performance is directly related to the extent of myocardial damage. Relatively small areas of infarction may be associated with little or no discernible impairment of cardiac performance,[65] whereas in myocardial infarction with shock, the loss of functioning myocardium is nearly always extensive, involving at least 40 percent of left ventricular muscle mass as documented by postmortem studies in man.[64,65] These findings are consistent with results of angiographic studies of the left ventricle that we have performed in patients with acute infarction, which demonstrate severe dyssynergy of a massive proportion of left ventricular myocardium when shock is present as opposed to more modest involvement in uncomplicated infarction[88] (Figure 7).

Collateral Circulation

In relation to the quantity of myocardium involved by an infarction, the coronary collateral circulation has classically been assigned an important protective role as a factor limiting infarct size.[39] More recently, the functional significance of coronary collateral vessels in man has received considerable investigative attention, the results of which are largely inconsistent with older views. Angiographically demonstrable coronary collateral arteries have been found only in the presence of severe coronary obstructive disease.[10,90,91] Although their anatomic presence implies a protective effect, and experimental studies indicate enhancement of coronary blood flow in the presence of collateral channels,[90–94] clinical data are at variance with these suggested effects. Recent evaluation of the contribution of collateral arteries to coronary

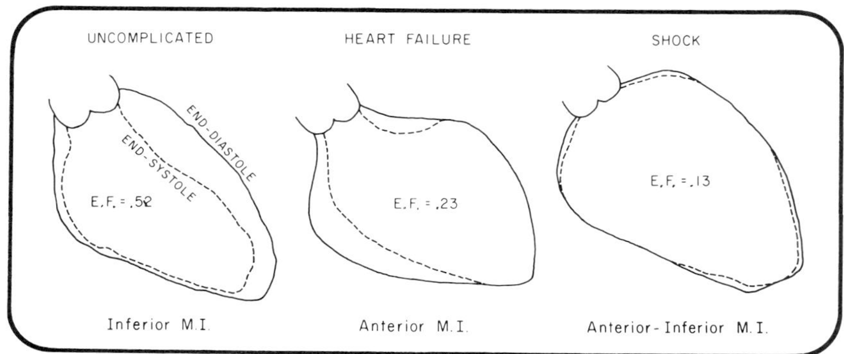

FIGURE 7. Diagrams of left ventricular angiograms of patients with acute myocardial infarction (M.I.). The inferior infarction is associated with inferior wall hypokinesis and is clinically uncomplicated. Heart failure is associated with extensive anterior wall akinesis in the anterior infarction. The anterior-inferior infarction is complicated by shock resulting from the severe, diffuse impairment of contractile function. Ejection fraction (E.F.) is progressively decreased with increasing involvement of left ventricular myocardium.

blood flow in man indicates that they provide minimal augmentation of regional perfusion.[95] Thus, there has been no consistent evidence in man for their beneficial effect on symptoms,[10,90,91] the resting or exercise electrocardiogram,[10,91] hemodynamic function[10,91,96] or regional myocardial performance.[10,90,91] Further, the prevalance of ventricular ectopic beats is not diminished by the presence of collateral vessels,[95] and intitial evidence indicates that survival rates have not been altered by their presence.[90,98]

Correlation with Extent of Myocardial Infarction: Consistent with these findings and directly related to the question of the protective effect of collateral vessels are postmortem studies demonstrating a lack of relation between collateral coronary arteries and the presence and extent of documented myocardial infarction.[99] Thus, although collateral arteries may provide some increase in regional myocardial blood flow, the increment may be insufficient to produce functional clinical benefit. These clinical studies are based largely on angiographic data and retrospective analysis, and their methodologic limitations must be appreciated. It is thus possible that although all collateral vessels in the myocardium are not effective in enchancing coronary blood flow, selected larger ones may be, despite the lack of evidence from present methods of analysis. Conclusions concerning the functional significance of the coronary collateral circulation in man are therefore not justified on the basis of current data and must await further investigation.

Cardiogenic Shock

Since, in the coronary care unit, the chief cause of fatality in myocardial infarction is cardiac pump failure, which in turn is determined by the size of the infarct, prognosis is closely related to the latter. Thus, ability to quantify infarct size would allow rational application of the variety of therapeutic approaches available and systematic evaluation of their efficacy. Degree of functional impairment, which in myocardial infarction is largely a reflection of the quantity of myocardium lost, has been utilized to assess prognosis. Thus, the capacity of the infarcted ventricle to perform hemodynamically, as determined in terms of cardiac work[63,86,102] or stroke work [65,86,100–102] delivered, has provided a useful indication of prognosis. Just as the electrocardiogram relates to cardiac performance in regard to remote infarction, it is also useful in acute myocardial infarction in the prediction of ventricular function and, as a concomitant, prognosis. Thus, cardiac performance, as assessed by catheterization in the acute phase, is most impaired in infarction involving the combined anterior-inferior regions of the left ventricle as localized by electrocardiogram, is depressed with extensive anterior infarction and is commonly within the normal range in inferior infarction,[102–104] thereby suggesting a similar relation of electrocardiographic infarct pattern to quantity of myocardium destroyed. As would be anticipated, the same descending order of frequency in relation to the electrocardiographic location of infarction applies to the incidence of cardiac pump failure and mortality from this syndrome in acute myocardial infarction.[102,103]

Relation to Location and Size of Myocardial Infarct: That the extent of myocardial involvement is greatest in anterior-inferior infarction, least in inferior infarction and intermediate but considerable in anterior infarction is confirmed by angiographic studies of the left ventricle involved with acute or remote infarction.[73,80,88] Thus, in combined anterior-inferior infarction dyssynergy is extensive and left ventricular ejection fraction may be markedly depressed, a condition associated with severe pump dysfunction or shock, whereas only a mild to moderate decrease in ejection fraction without clinical manifestations of cardiac failure often occurs in inferior infarction.[88] A more precise approach has been the recent development of a method for indirect estimation of infarct size, and thereby prognosis, in man that is based on serum enzyme analysis.[105] Favorable prognosis in that study correlated inversely with estimated extent of myocardial damage, the latter differing considerably between survivors and nonsurvivors. Another promising, noninvasive innovation is cardiac scintiphotography, which utilizes intravenously injected radioisotope to image the left ventricle and thereby localize and quantify dyssynergy and determine ejection fraction.[106]

Other Factors Causing Pump Failure: Although cardiac pump dysfunction in acute myocardial infarction is principally related to quantity of damaged myocardium, other factors may also contribute. Mechanical causes of impaired cardiac pump performance are significant in a small proportion of patients with myocardial infarction. Thus, interventricular septum rupture and mitral regurgitation resulting from ischemic dysfunction of a papillary muscle are complications of myocardial infarction that may be superimposed upon the preexisting abnormality of cardiac muscle performance. Their significance lies in the cata-

strophic impairment of cardiac function they may produce and their potential for complete alleviation by surgical correction. In the case of acute ventricular septal defect, in which the high risk of surgery has usually precluded correction before several weeks or, more commonly, months, current techniques have allowed intervention in the acute stages,[107] as exemplified by recent successful long-term correction in two of our patients in the first 24 hours after septal rupture associated with acute myocardial infarction.[108]

Hypovolemia and Reduced Peripheral Vascular Resistance: Extramyocardial factors also appear to contribute to circulatory failure in a small number of patients with myocardial infarction. Thus, hypovolemia[109] and inadequate response of the peripheral vasculature to reduced perfusion pressure[110,111] may be important in the production of low cardiac output and hypotension. Indeed, either of these deficiencies in the presence of reduced contractility resulting from infarction, not in itself sufficient to cause cardiac failure, may lead to cardiocirculatory shock. Hypovolemia in acute myocardial infarction may result from diuretic therapy, low fluid intake, emesis, inadequate fluid replacement and hyperventilation. Impairment of peripheral vascular responsiveness has been attributed to mechanical[112,113] and chemical[110–114] reflexes arising in the injured myocardium. Although hypovolemia and reduced total peripheral vascular resistance apply to a small proportion of patients with myocardial infarction and shock, these physiologic alterations may contribute to a syndrome of severe circulatory failure that, because it is not entirely related to the myocardial insufficiency, usually responds favorably to appropriate medical therapy. By contrast, when the syndrome is the result of a massive destruction of left ventricular muscle, as it is in the great majority of cases observed, it is refractory to medical treatment except in unusual circumstances.

Summary

A fundamental characteristic of cardiac muscle function is rapid deterioration consequent to interruption of myocardial blood supply and oxygen delivery. Experimental and clinical studies have demonstrated, in association with myocardial ischemia or hypoxia, derangements of cardiac mechanical and pump performance, metabolic processes, electrical activity and structure. Deprivation of oxygen is the major factor producing these alterations, but reduced substrate delivery and accumulation of the products of cell metabolism and breakdown are contributing factors. After the onset of myocardial ischemia, there is a period during which the ensuing functional and subcellular structural alterations are reversible with restoration of oxygen supply. After this interval, structural damage is irreversible and there is permanent loss of myocardium. The degree of functional impairment is most closely related to the quantity of myocardium involved. In patients with stable coronary artery disease, clinical cardiac failure is not usually evident in the absence of previous loss of left ventricular myocardium, as occurs with infarction. However, evidence of transient, reversible impairment of ventricular muscle and pump performance is present during episodes of angina pectoris.

Myocardial infarction, or less frequently ischemia, is associated with permanent elimination of normal contractile performance in a localized area of myocardium (dyssynergy). Evidence of cardiac failure is apparent when 20 to 25 percent of left ventricular muscle is dyssynergic. The standard electrocardiogram is useful in estimating location and degree of dyssynergy and also cardiac pump performance by the presence and location of pathologic Q waves and associated electrocardiographic abnormalities. In acute myocardial infarction, the shock syndrome is associated with loss of 40 percent or more of left ventricular myocardium. Since in-hospital prognosis in acute myocardial infarction is closely related to extent of left ventricular damage, estimation of the latter would be helpful in applying the most appropriate forms of therapy in these patients. Recent innovations utilizing serum enzyme analysis and isotopic imaging of left ventricular myocardium have provided promising, noninvasive means of achieving this goal.

Acknowledgment: This study was supported in part by Research Program Project Grant HL 14780 from the National Heart and Lung Institute, National Institutes of Health.

The author wishes to thank Martie Wood, Robbie Brocchini and Robert Kleckner for their technical assistance and Jeri Kemp and Karen Gilmore for their administrative and secretarial assistance.

References

1. **Tennant R, Wiggers CJ:** The effect of coronary occlusion on myocardial contraction. Amer J Physiol 112:351, 1935
2. **Leibowitz JO:** The History of Coronary Heart Disease. Berkeley, University of California Press, 1970, p 49
3. **Harrison TR:** Some unanswered questions concerning enlargement and failure of heart. Amer Heart J 69:100, 1965
4. **Soloff L:** Coronary artery disease and the concept of cardiac failure. Amer J Cardiol 22:43, 1968
5. **Herman MV, Gorlin R:** Implications of left ventricular asynergy. Amer J Cardiol 23:538, 1969
6. **Katz AM:** Effects of interrupted coronary flow upon myocardial metabolism and contractility. Progr Cardiovasc Dis 10:450, 1968
7. **Katz AM:** Effects of ischemia and hypoxia upon the myocardium. In, Coronary Heart Disease (Russek HI, Zohman BL, ed). Philadelphia, Lippincott, 1971, p 45
8. **Hood WB Jr:** Pathophysiology of ischemic heart disease. Progr Cardiovasc Dis 14:297, 1971
9. **Ross RS:** Pathophysiology of coronary circulation. Brit Heart J 33:173, 1971
10. **Amsterdam EA, Miller RR, Hughes JL, et al:** Pathophysiology of angina pectoris. In, Atherosclerosis and Coronary Heart Disease (Likoff W, Segal BL, Insull W Jr, et al, ed). New York, Grune & Stratton, 1972, p 178
11. **Cohn PF, Gorlin R:** Abnormalities of left ventricular function associated with the anginal state. Circulation 46:1065, 1972
12. **Katz AM:** Patterns of energy production and energy utilization in cardiac and skeletal muscle. In, Factors Influencing Myocardial Contractility (Tanz RD, Kavaler F, Roberts J, ed). New York, Academic Press, 1967, p 401
13. **Opie LH:** Metabolism in the heart in health and disease. Part 1. Amer Heart J 76:685, 1968
14. **Gorlin R:** Physiologic studies in coronary atherosclerosis. Fed Proc 21:93, 1962
15. **Tyberg JV, Yeatman LA, Parmley WW, et al:** Effects of hypoxia on mechanics of cardiac contraction. Amer J Physiol 218:1780, 1970
16. **Amsterdam EA, Foley D, Massumi RA, et al:** Enhancement of myocardial function during hypoxia by increased glucose availability (abstr). Amer J Cardiol 29:251, 1972
17. **Nakhjavan R, Parameswaran CY, Srinivasan NV, et**

al: Effects of hypoxia, reoxgenation, and temperature on cat papillary muscle. Amer J Physiol 229:1289, 1971

18. **Scheuer, J:** Myocardial metabolism in cardiac hypoxia. Amer J Cardiol 19:385, 1967

19. **Weissler AM, Kruger FA, Baba N, et al:** Role of anaerobic metabolism in the preservation of functional capacity and structure of anoxic myocardium. J Clin Invest 47:403, 1968

20. **Blumgart HL, Gilligan DR, Schlesinger MJ:** Experimental studies of the effect of temporary occlusion of coronary arteries. II. The production of myocardial infarction. Amer Heart J 22:374, 1941

21. **Wiggers CJ:** The functional consequences of coronary occlusion. Ann Intern Med 23:158, 1945

22. **Prinzmetal M, Schwartz LL, Corday E, et al:** Studies on the coronary circulation. VI. Loss of myocardial contractility after coronary artery occlusion. Ann Intern Med 31:429, 1949

23. **Sayen JJ, Sheldon WF, Pierce F, et al:** Motion picture studies of ventricular muscle dynamics in experimental localized ischemia correlated with myocardial oxygen tension and electrocardiograms. J Clin Invest 33:962, 1954

24. **Wegria R, Frank CW, Misrahy GA, et al:** Immediate hemodynamic effects of acute coronary artery occlusion. Amer J Physiol 177:123, 1954

25. **Bing RJ, Castellanos A, Gredel E, et al:** Experimental myocardial infarction: circulatory, biochemical and pathological changes. Amer J Med Sci 232:533, 1956

26. **Sayen JJ, Sheldon WF, Pierce G, et al:** Polarographic oxygen, the epicardial electrocardiogram and muscle contraction in experimental acute regional ischemia of the left ventricle. Circ Res 6:779, 1958

27. **Tatooles CJ, Randall WC:** Local ventricular bulging after acute coronary occlusion. Amer J Physiol 201:451, 1961

28. **Case RB, Roselle HA, Crampton RS:** Relation of S-T depression to metabolic and hemodynamic events. Cardiolog a 48:32, 1966

29. **Scheuer J, Brachfeld N:** Coronary insufficiency: relations between hemodynamic, electrical and biochemical parameters. Circ Res 18:178, 1966

30. **Bing OHL, Keefe JF, Wolk MJ, et al:** Tension prolongation during recovery from myocardial hypoxia. J Clinn Invest 50:660, 1971

31. **Amsterdam EA, Manchester JH, Kemp HG, et al:** Spontaneous angina pectoris (SAP): hemodynamic and metabolic changes (abstr). Clin Res 17:225, 1969

32. **Parker JO, West RO, Case RB, et al:** Temporal relationships of myocardial lactate metabolism, left ventricular function, and S-T segment depression during angina precipitated by exercise. Circulation 40:97, 1969

33. **Parker JO, Choing MA, West RO, et al:** Sequential alterations in myocardial lactate metabolism, S-T segments, and left ventricular function during angina induced by atrial pacing. Circulation 40:113, 1969

34. **Forrester JS, Hellant RH, Pasternac A, et al:** Atrial pacing in coronary heart disease: effect on hemodynamics, metabolism and coronary circulation. Amer J Cardiol 27:237, 1971

35. **Dwyer EM Jr:** Left ventricular pressure-volume alterations and regional disorders of contraction during myocardial ischemia induced by atrial pacing. Circulation 42:1111, 1970

36. **Pasternac A, Gorlin R, Sonnenblick EH, et al:** Abnormalities of ventricular motion induced by atrial pacing in coronary artery disease. Circulation 45:1195, 1972

37. **Linhart JW:** Myocardial function in coronary artery disease determined by atrial pacing. Circulation 44:203, 1971

38. **Linhart JW, Beller BM, Talley RC:** Coronary artery disease: evaluation by the multistage treadmill exercise test and right atrial pacing. Chest 63:505, 1973

39. **Katz AM:** Effects of ischemia on the contractile processes of heart muscle. In, Congestive Heart Failure (Mason DT, ed). New York, Yorke Medical Books, 1976, p 77

40. **Sommers HM, Jennings RB:** Experimental acute myocardial infarction. Lab Invest 13:1491, 1964

41. **Jennings RB, Baum JH, Herdson PB:** Fine structural changes in myocardial ischemic injury. Arch Path (Chicago) 79:135, 1965

42. **Herdson PB, Sommers HM, Jennings RB:** A comparative study of the fine structure of normal and ischemic dog myocardium with special reference of early changes following temporary occlusion of a coronary artery. Amer J Path 46:367, 1965

43. **Jennings RB:** Early phase of myocardial ischemic injury and infarction. Amer J Cardiol 24:753, 1969

44. **Hood WB Jr, Bianco JA, Kumar R, et al:** Experimental myocardial infarction. IV. Reduction of left ventricular compliance in the healing phase. J Clin Invest 49:1316, 1970

45. **Bristow JD, Van Zee BE, Judkins MP:** Systolic and diastolic abnormalities of the left ventricle in coronary artery disease: studies in patients with little or no enlargement of ventricular volume. Circulation 42:219, 1970

46. **Diamond G. Forrester JS:** Effect of coronary artery disease and acute myocardial infarction on left ventricular compliance in man. Circulation 45:11, 1972

47. **Luchi RJ, Kritcher EM:** Impaired cardiac myosin enzyme activity in acute anoxia (abstr). Circulation 36 suppl II:II-175, 1967

48. **Maroko PR, Libby P, Ginks WR, et al:** Coronary artery reperfusion. I. Early effects on local myocardial function and the extent of myocardial necrosis. J Clin Invest 51:2710, 1972

49. **Ginks WR, Sybers HD, Maroko PR, et al:** Coronary artery reperfusion. II. Reduction of myocardial infarct size at 1 week after the coronary occlusion. J Clin Invest 51:2717, 1972

50. **Amsterdam EA, Miller RR, Mason DT, et al:** Emergency surgical therapy of complicated acute myocardial infarction: indications and results in cardiogenic shock, intractable ventricular tachycardia and extending infarction. In, Cardiovascular Problems: Perspectives and Progress (Russek H, ed). Baltimore, University Park Press. In press

51. **Katz AM, Maxwell JB:** Actin from heart muscle: sulfhydryl groups. Circ Res 14:345, 1964

52. **Ekholm R, Kerstell J, Olsson R, et al:** Morphologic and biochemical studies of dog heart mitochondria after short periods of ischemia. Amer J Cardiol 22:312,

1968

53. **Brachfeld N, Scheuer J:** Metabolism of glucose by the ischemic dog heart. Amer J Physiol 212:603, 1967

54. **Most AS, Gorlin R, Soeldner JS:** Glucose extraction by the human myocardium during pacing stress. Circulation 45:92, 1972

55. **Owen P, Thomas M, Opie L:** Relative changes in serum-free-fatty acid and glucose utilization by ischemic myocardium after coronary-artery occlusion. Lancet 1:1187, 1969

56. **Tyberg JV, Parmley WW, Sonnenblick EH:** In-vitro studies of myocardial asynchrony and regional hypoxia. Circ Res 25:569, 1969

57. **Brachfeld MO:** Maintenance of cell viability (abstr). Circulation 40 suppl IV:202, 1969

58. **Ricciutti M, Scherlag B, Stein E, et al:** Lysosome stability and coronary artery occlusion (abstr). Clin Res 16:245, 1968

59. **Libby P, Maroko PR, Bloor CM, et al:** Reduction of experimental myocardial infarct size by corticosteroid administration. J Clin Invest 52:599, 1973

60. **Regen DM, Davis WW, Morgan HE, et al:** The regulation of hexokinase and phosphofructokinase activity in heart muscle. Effects of alloxan diabetes, growth hormone, cortisol, and anoxia. J Biol Chem 239:43, 1964

61. **Klein MD, Herman MV, Gorlin R:** A hemodynamic study of left ventricular aneurysm. Circulation 35:614, 1967

62. **Swan HJC, Forrester JS, Danzig R, et al:** Power failure in acute myocardial infarction. Progr Cardiovasc Dis 12:568, 1970

63. **Scheidt S, Ascheim R, Killip T III:** Shock after acute myocardial infarction: a clinical and hemodynamic profile. Amer J Cardiol 26:556, 1970

64. **Page DL, Caulfield JB, Kastor JA, et al:** Myocardial changes associated with cardiogenic shock. New Eng J Med 285:133, 1971

65. **Swan HJC, Forrester JS, Diamond G, et al:** Hemodynamic spectrum of myocardial infarction and cardiogenic shock. Circulation 45:1097, 1972

66. **Parker JO, Ledwich JR, West RO, et al:** Reversible cardiac failure during angina pectoris. Hemodynamic effects of atrial pacing in coronary artery disease. Circulation 39:745, 1969

67. **Parker JO, West RO, Ledwich JR, et al:** The effect of acute digitalization on the hemodynamic response to exercise in coronary artery disease. Circulation 40:453, 1969

68. **Helfant RH, Forrester JS, Hampton JR, et al:** Differential hemodynamic, metabolic, and electrocardiographic effects in subjects with and without angina pectoris during atrial pacing. Circulation 42:601, 1970

69. **Ellis LB, Allison RB, Rodriguez FL, et al:** Relation of the degree of coronary-artery disease and of myocardial infarctions to cardiac hypertrophy and chronic congestive heart failure. New Eng J Med 266:525, 1962

70. **Herman MV, Heinle RA, Klein MD, et al:** Localized disorders in myocardial contraction. Asynergy and its role in congestive heart failure. New Eng J Med 277:222, 1967

71. **Baxley WA, Jones WB, Dodge HT:** Left ventricular anatomical and functional abnormalities in chronic postinfarction heart failure. Ann Intern Med 74:499, 1971

72. **Rahimtoola SH, DiGilio MM, Sinno MZ, et al:** Cardiac performance three to eight weeks after acute myocardial infarction. Arch Intern Med (Chicago) 128:220, 1971

73. **Miller RR, Bonanno J, Massumi RA, et al:** Usefulness of the electrocardiogram in assessment of ventricular performance and comparison with coronary arteriography (abstr). Amer J Cardiol 29:281, 1972

74. **Cohen LS, Elliott WC, Rolett EL, et al:** Hemodynamic studies during angina pectoris. Circulation 31:409, 1965

75. **Sonnenblick EH, Ross J Jr, Braunwald E:** Oxygen consumption of the heart. Amer J Cardiol 22:328, 1968

76. **Oliva PB, Potts DE, Pluss RG:** Coronary arterial spasm in Prinzmetal angina. Documentation by coronary arteriography. New Eng J Med 288:745, 1973

77. **MacAlpin R:** Coronary spasm as a cause of angina. New Eng J Med 288:788, 1973

78. **Miller RR, Amsterdam EA, Mason DT, et al:** Electrocardiographic and cineangiocardiographic correlations in assessment of abnormal left ventricular segmental contraction in coronary artery disease. Circulation 49:447, 1974

79. **Amsterdam EA, Zelis R, Bonanno JA, et al:** Relation of cardiac ischemia and necrosis during angina pectoris: comparison of lactate metabolism and enzyme release by the human myocardium (abstr). Circulation 43 and 44 suppl II:130, 1971

80. **Miller RR, Mason DT, Massumi RA, et al:** ECG determination of nature, location and extent of abnormal ventricular segmental contraction in coronary artery disease (abstr). Circulation 45 and 46 suppl II:II–9, 1972

81. **Stokes J III, Dawber TR:** The "silent coronary." The frequency and clinical characteristics of unrecognized myocardial infarction in the Framingham study. Ann Intern Med 50:1359, 1959

82. **Kaplan MB, Berkson DM:** Serial electrocardiograms after myocardial infarction. Ann Intern Med 60:430, 1964

83. **Kumar R, Hood WB Jr, Joison J, et al:** Experimental myocardial infarction. II. Acute depression and subsequent recovery of left ventricular function: serial measurements in intact conscious dogs. J Clin Invest 49:55, 1970

84. **Karliner JS, Ross J Jr:** Left ventricular performance after acute myocardial infarction. Progr Cardiovasc Dis 13:374, 1971

85. **Rackley CE, Russell RO Jr:** Left ventricular function in acute myocardial infarction and its clinical significance. Circulation 45:231, 1972

86. **Wolk MJ, Scheidt S, Killip T:** Heart failure complicating acute myocardial infarction. Circulation 45:1125, 1972

87. **Lown B, Klein LB, Hershberg PI:** Coronary and precoronary care. Amer J Med 46:705, 1969

88. **Amsterdam EA, Choquet Y, Bonanno JA, et al:** Correl-

ative hemodynamics and angiography in acute coronary syndromes (abstr). Clin Res 21:232, 1973

89. **Zoll PM, Wessler S, Schlesinger MJ:** Interarterial coronary anastomoses in the human heart, with particular reference to anemia and relative cardiac anoxia. Circulation 4:797, 1951

90. **Helfant RH, Vokonas PS, Gorlin R:** Functional importance of the human coronary collateral circulation. New Eng J Med 284: 1277, 1971

91. **Miller RR, Mason DT, Salel A, et al:** Determinants and functional significance of the coronary collateral circulation in patients with coronary artery disease (abstr). Amer J Cardiol 29:281, 1972

92. **Chimoskey JE, Szentivanyi M, Zakheim R, et al:** Temporary coronary occlusion in conscious dogs: collateral flow and electrocardiogram. Amer J Physiol 212:1025, 1967

93. **Haft JI, Damato AN:** Measurement of collateral blood flow after myocardial infarction in the closed-chest dog. Amer Heart J 77:641, 1969

94. **Elliot EC, Bloor CM, Jones EL, et al:** Effect of controlled coronary occlusion on collateral circulation in conscious dogs. Amer J Physiol 220:857, 1971

95. **Smith SC, Gorlin R, Herman MV, et al:** Myocardial blood flow in man: effects of coronary collateral circulation and coronary artery bypass surgery. J Clin Invest 10:2556, 1972

96. **Bjork L:** Angiographic demonstration of collaterals to the coronary arteries in patients with angina pectoris. Acta Radiol (Diagn) 8:305, 1969

97. **Amsterdam EA, Vismara L, Miller RR, et al:** Relationship of ventricular ectopic rhythms to angiographically defined coronary artery disease (abstr). Clin Res 21:233, 1973

98. **Amsterdam EA, Most AS, Wolfson S, et al:** Relation of degree of angiographically documented coronary artery disease to mortality. Ann Intern Med 72:780, 1970

99. **Snow PJD, Jones AM, Daber KS:** Coronary disease: a pathological study. Brit Heart J 17:503, 1955

100. **Parmley WW, Diamond G, Tomoda H, et al:** Clinical evaluation of left ventricular pressures in acute myocardial infarction. Circulation 45:358, 1972

101. **Price J, Amsterdam EA, Miller RR, et al:** Prognosis in acute myocardial infarction from quantitative assessment of left ventricular function: relation to hemodynamic and contractile indices. Clin Res 22:150A, 1974

102. **Hughes JL, Salel AF, Massumi RA, et al:** The electrocardiogram as a predictor of ventricular function and cardiogenic shock in acute myocardial infarction (abstr). Circulation 43 and 44 suppl II:179, 1971

103. **Hughes JL, Miller RR, Salel A, et al:** Electrocardiographic localization of injury in acute myocardial infarction: relation to left ventricular function and cardiac pump failure (abstr). Amer J Cardiol 29:271, 1972

104. **Russell RO Jr, Hunt O, Rackley CE:** Left ventricular hemodynamics in anterior and inferior myocardial infarction. Amer J Cardiol 32:8, 1973

105. **Sobel BE, Bresnahan GF, Shell WE, et al:** Estimation of infarct size in man and its relation to prognosis. Circulation 46:640, 1972

106. **Zaret BL, Pitt B, Ross RS:** Determination of the site, extent, and significance of regional ventricular dysfunction during acute myocardial infarction. Circulation 45:441, 1972

107. **Daggett WM, Burwell LR, Lawson DW, et al:** Resection of acute ventricular aneurysm and ruptured interventricular septum after myocardial infarction. New Eng J Med 283:1507, 1970

108. **Miller RR, Amsterdam EA, Iben A, et al:** Successful immediate repair of acquired ventricular septal defect in patients with acute myocardial infarction (abstr). Clin Res 21:439, 1973

109. **Loeb HS, Pietras RJ, Tobin JR Jr, et al:** Hypovolemia in shock due to acute myocardial infarction. Circulation 40:653, 1969

110. **Constantin L:** Extracardiac factors contributing to hypotension during coronary occlusion. Amer J Cardiol 11:205, 1963

111. **Hughes JL, Amsterdam EA, Mason DT, et al:** Abnormal peripheral vascular dynamics in patients with acute myocardial infarction: diminished reflex arteriolar constriction (abstr). Clin Res 19:321, 1971

112. **Aviado DM, Schmidt CF:** Cardiovascular and respiratory reflexes from the left side of the heart. Amer J Physiol 196:726, 1959

113. **Ross J Jr, Frahm CJ, Braunwald E:** The influence of intracardiac baroceptors on venous return, systemic vascular volume and peripheral resistance. J Clin Invest 40:563, 1961

114. **Shillingford J, Thomas M:** Hemodynamic effects of acute myocardial infarction in man. Progr Cardiovasc Dis 10:571, 1968

Chapter 12

Nature and Significance of Alterations in Myocardial Compliance

James W. Covell, MD
John Ross, Jr, MD, FACC

The physical properties of resting cardiac tissue have been the subject of intensive investigation for more than a century. Although it is now clear that the description of active contraction in terms of pure alterations in the viscoelastic properties of muscle is not appropriate,[1] early interest in the stress-strain behavior of muscular tissue centered on the viscoelastic theory of contraction.[1,2] From these studies and more recent information it is now known that muscle in general, and specifically cardiac muscle, displays many elastic and visoelastic properties.[3,4] Moreover, in recent years it has become evident that there are marked alterations in diastolic viscoelastic properties not only with acute interventions, such as changes in frequency of contraction and site of stimulation,[5] but also with rapid volume overloading and chronic interventions, such as myocardial infarction.[6–8] This review discusses the recent knowledge of factors that acutely influence the distensibility of the myocardium in the intact heart and isolated cardiac muscle and reviews the evidence for changes in myocardial compliance in disease states. The terminology involved in describing alterations in compliance or distensibility is, unfortunately, complex and frequently misused in the physiologic literature. Accordingly, we shall first describe or define several commonly used terms. For a more detailed description of terminology, the reader is referred to Remington's excellent monograph on tissue elasticity.[9]

Terminology

Elasticity: The property of a material that determines the tendency of the stressed material to return to its unstressed geometric configuration.

Viscosity: The property of a material that tends to retard deformation of the stressed material.

Plasticity: The property of a material by which it may be subjected to stresses of less than a critical or yield value without undergoing permanent deformation, but which results in flow at stresses above the yield value.

All biological materials have been shown to have these three properties, and a variety of experimental techniques have been utilized to quantitate them.[10] To describe effectively these three basic properties the tissue must be elongated or stressed over a known period of time and then the relation between stress and strain and its time history described. To discuss these relations it is necessary to define several other terms that describe the response of tissue to extension or alterations in stress.

Extensibility of a tissue expresses the ability of

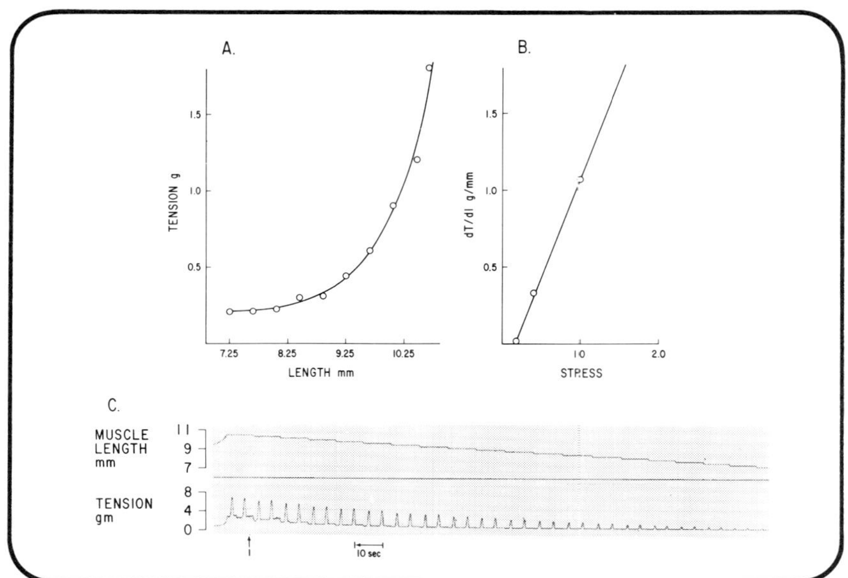

FIGURE 1. The relation between resting tension and muscle length in isolated cardiac muscle. **A,** tension-length relation and its exponentially fitted line ($T = 9 \times 10^{-7}e^{1.31} + 0.199$). **B,** the slope of this line at any level of tension (dT/dl) calcu-lated for this exponential relation. **C,** length-tension data obtained by producing increments in length in an isometri-cally contracting isolated cardiac muscle.

the material to extend (ΔL) with the application of stress ($\Delta L/\Delta T$).

Distensibility refers to the changes in volume of a hollow object induced by a change in internal pressure ($\Delta V/\Delta P$). Distensibility may be expressed by many other terms such as the *cross-sectional distensibility* or the ratio of change in area to change in pressure, *or radial (circumferential) distensibility* expressed as change in radius related to change in pressure.

Stiffness describes the ratio of the increment in stress to the corresponding change in length in isolated muscle ($\Delta T/\Delta L$) or volume stiffness ($\Delta P/\Delta V$) in the intact heart, and *compliance,* the reciprocal of these relations ($\Delta V/\Delta P$ or $\Delta L/\Delta T$). Since all muscle is viscous, the rate of strain affects the measured compliance; thus, for an accurate description the rate of change in stress must be defined.

Creep, hysteresis and stress relaxation are terms that have been used to quantitate the vis-coelastic phenomenon. *Creep* is the increase in deformation that occurs over the course of time under constant stress. *Hysteresis* is the failure of a system to follow identical paths of response upon application of and withdrawal of a forcing

agent. *Stress relaxation* is the decrease in stress that takes place in the course of time under constant strain.

Diastolic Properties of Cardiac Muscle and the Heart

Acute Alterations in Resting Muscle

Most data indicate that in resting cardiac muscle the relation between strain or extension and the change in stress is essentially exponential, and the resulting linear relation between stiffness ($\Delta T/\Delta L$) and stress ($\Delta T/\Delta L = AT + B$) generally has been utilized to describe the resting properties of isolated muscle[10-12] (Figure 1). This type of mathematical relation serves as a resonable framework for discussing induced alterations in the resting stress-strain relation. There is now substantial evidence that the diastolic stress-strain relation of normal isolated mammalian cardiac muscle may be influenced to some degree by several factors.

Perhaps the most easily demonstrated alteration in the resting stress-strain relation is hyster-esis. The stress-strain relation obtained when isolated cardiac muscle is stretched at a given rate over the normal range of lengths is dependent on the rate of stretch[12] and is not the same when the muscle is then shortened at the same rate.[11,13]

Creep in resting cardiac muscle has been frequently documented and may be induced by either diastolic[12] or systolic[14] alterations in force. Little and Wead[12] investigated extensively the reversibility of creep in intact heart muscle and found that the most important factor in predicting the reversibility of creep-induced change is the level of initial stress achieved with rapid stretching of the muscle. Moreover, it has been shown[11–13] that the magnitude of reversible hysteresis and creep is relatively independent of the rate of the initial alteration in muscle length. Creep probably occurs in the intact heart when high levels of end-diastolic pressure are achieved, although quantitative studies on this point are lacking.

A variety of pharmacologic agents described under the general categories of positive and negative inotropic influences do not appear to alter the resting stress-strain relation of isolated cardiac muscle,[14] except as they may influence active force, as mentioned. However, there is some evidence to the contrary.[15] It is generally agreed that alterations in muscle temperature, osmolarity, previous stress-strain history and hypoxic damage[14,16–19] do influence the resting stress-strain relation in isolated cardiac muscle. Increases in osmolarity and decreases in temperature increase the stiffness of muscle, whereas hypoxia and tissue damage substantially decrease the resting value for stiffness of isolated cardiac muscle.

Chronic Alterations in Resting Muscle

Until recently, chronic alterations in compliance in resting isolated muscle have received relatively little experimental attention. In isolated cardiac muscle, chronic alterations in resting and active compliance have been examined in muscles from hypertrophied hearts, after depletion of norepinephrine by administration of reserpine and in the hyperthyroid state. Possible age-related changes in resting compliance also have been examined. Utilizing right ventricular papillary muscles removed from cats, hearts de-

pleted of norepinephrine or hypertrophied cat hearts, Parmley et al.[20] found no alteration in the resting length-tension curve induced by these factors. The effects of rapidly induced experimental myocardial hypertrophy on resting compliance remain unclear. Spann et al.,[21] studying right ventricular papillary muscles from cats subjected to chronic pulmonary arterial constriction, found no changes, whereas Bing et al.[22] documented an increased resting value for stiffness of such papillary muscles, when the data were normalized for muscle cross-sectional area.

Recent experimental evidence suggests that there are age-dependent alterations in diastolic compliance. Studies have shown that fetal heart muscle, when considered in terms of normalized stress and strain, is stiffer than either newborn or adult muscle;[23] however, Romero et al.[24] found no significant alterations in left ventricular diastolic compliance after the first weeks of life.

Acute Changes in Diastolic Properties of the Whole Heart

Diastolic stress-strain relations in the intact heart have important implications relative to filling pressures in the pulmonary and systemic veins and have been of interest to physiologists and cardiologists for many years. However, several factors continue to limit ability to describe adequately the full range of the passive properties of the muscle of the whole heart. In the intact heart it is difficult to measure directly diastolic myocardial wall stress and strain simultaneously. Thus, it is usually necessary to assume a geometric reference figure for the ventricle in question and to utilize ventricular volume, pressure and wall thickness to calculate the diastolic stress-strain relation at one or more points in diastole.[25]

Several simplified experimental approaches recently have been employed. The arrested ventricle can be removed from the circulation and filled directly with increments of volume[26,27] (Figure 2). Under these circumstances, the whole range of diastolic pressures and volumes was examined and an exponential relation was found between pressure and volume.[27] This has been expressed mathematically as a linear rela-

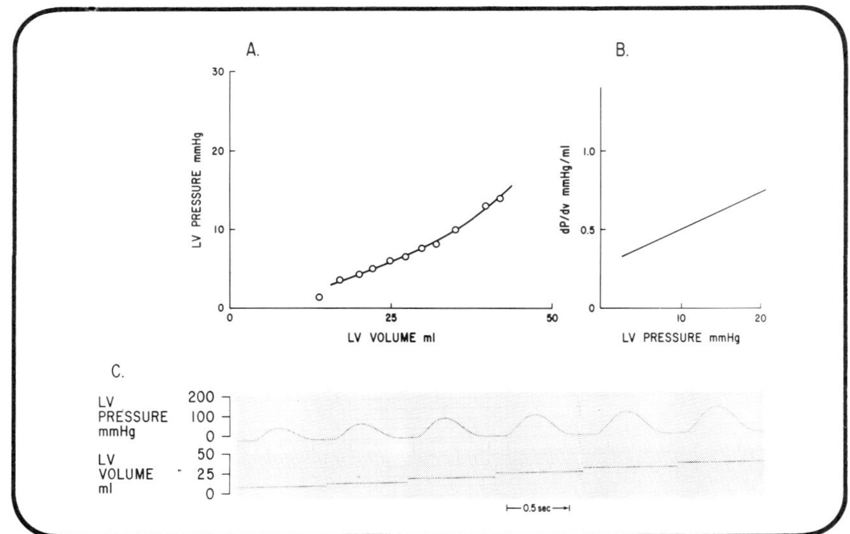

FIGURE 2. A, relation between left ventricular diastolic pressure and left ventricular volume, expressed as the exponential relation: $P = 8.75e^{0.02V} - 9.95$. **B,** the slope—stiffness ($\Delta P/\Delta V$)—of this line at any left ventricular pressure. **C,** original data determined by incrementing left ventricular volume in an isovolumically contracting canine left ventricular preparation.

tion between stiffness ($\Delta P/\Delta V$) and intracavitary pressure.[26] The isolated supported heart preparation, in which end-diastolic volume can be measured in the beating heart, also has provided substantial information on the normal resting stress-strain relations in the intact heart.[28,29] These results have yielded a similar exponential relation between pressure and volume. Although hysteresis and creep have been demonstrated in such studies, no quantitative information is available on the magnitude of such creep or the factors that influence it or produce hysteresis.

Alterations in systolic stress can produce diastolic stress relaxation, and inadequate diastolic relaxation time may result in increased left ventricular stiffness.[14,28-33] The effects of a variety of positive and negative inotropic influences on the compliance of the isolated supported heart, or in more intact heart preparations, also have been investigated. Although there is some evidence to the contrary,[15,32] most recent data indicate that no appreciable alterations in the diastolic properties of the intact heart are induced by altering the contractility of the ventricle.[28,29,34,35] In addition, Nobel et al.[30] found that infusions of saline solution, isoproterenol, cal-

cium or methoxamine caused no change in diastolic properties during the slow phase of ventricular filling, but compliance during the rapid phases of filling was sometimes significantly affected.

Chronic Changes in Diastolic Properties

There is much clinical evidence that diastolic compliance in the diseased human left ventricle is altered.[36-38] However, the rate of development of these alterations and their reversibility have only recently been considered. In the clinical setting or in the awake animal, the entire pressure-volume relation for a particular heart is generally not known, and the relation at end-diastole alone does not neccessarily reflect compliance over the filling cycle for the ventricle in question. Since compliance decreases in the normal heart as cardiac filling increases, the detection of significant chronic alterations in compliance in the dilated or hypertrophied heart, or both, as compared with findings in a normal chamber, may be difficult unless the relation between pressure and volume is a single exponential one. This has not yet been clearly documented in patients with a wide variety of cardiac diseases. Major alterations in ventricular volume and wall thickness make comparisons of muscle compliance even more complicated.

Some investigators[39,40] have attempted to calculate compliance and to normalize for differences in cardiac volume by expressing the compliance of the ventricle per milliliter of end-diastolic volume $(\Delta V/\Delta PV_{ED})$. However, division by the operating end-diastolic volume may result in questionable conclusions under some circumstances. Moreover, difficulties may arise if a nonexponential relation with the same pressure intercept for $\Delta P/\Delta V$ (stiffness) versus pressure in different hearts is assumed.[40] For example, the data shown in Figure 3 were measured early and late after the creation of a large arteriovenous fistula, the points on the curve being obtained at end-diastole by infusions and bleeding. Left ventricular end-diastolic diameter was measured utilizing radiographic techniques developed by Mitchell et al.,[41] and end-diastolic pressure was measured with a chronically implanted left ventricular tube.[7] Stiffness $(\Delta P/\Delta D)$ is clearly increased when the curve on the left is compared with that on the right (Figure 3) over the normal range of filling. However, selecting an end-diastolic pressure of 11 mm Hg (end-diastolic volume 85 ml early post shunt and 123 ml late post shunt) and assuming a constant pressure intercept on the pressure scale, the calculated K constant or

stiffness is decreased, but when normalized for end-diastolic volume the value for compliance $(\Delta V/\Delta PV_{E})$ calculates as unchanged by this method.[40]

The term functional compliance was introduced in our recent study to indicate compliance over a range of filling up to the operating end-diastolic pressure,[7] "functional compliance" equaling $\Delta D/\Delta P$ with ΔP being the range of pressure between left ventricular end-diastolic pressure ± 5 mm Hg. This approach is somewhat similar to that recently employed by Diamond and Forrester,[6] in which ΔV was considered equal to the stroke volume and ΔP the pressure range from end-systole to end-diastole; the slope of the relation $\Delta P/\Delta V$ versus $\bar{P}$ (mean filling pressure) was then calculated.

An alternative approach has been to analyze single cardiac filling cycles using high fidelity micromanometers and angiography or, in experimental studies, by use of multiple implanted tantalum screws in the left ventricular myocardium;[30] ultrasonic techniques also may prove suitable for this purpose. In clinical studies, Dodge et al.,[38] using angiographic methods to construct pressure-volume loops (left ventricular contraction cycles) in patients with a variety of cardiac lesions, showed differences in the slopes of these curves at comparable diastolic volumes or pressures. Gault et al.,[42] studying patients with chronic volume overloading due to free aortic regurgitation, found that the left ven-

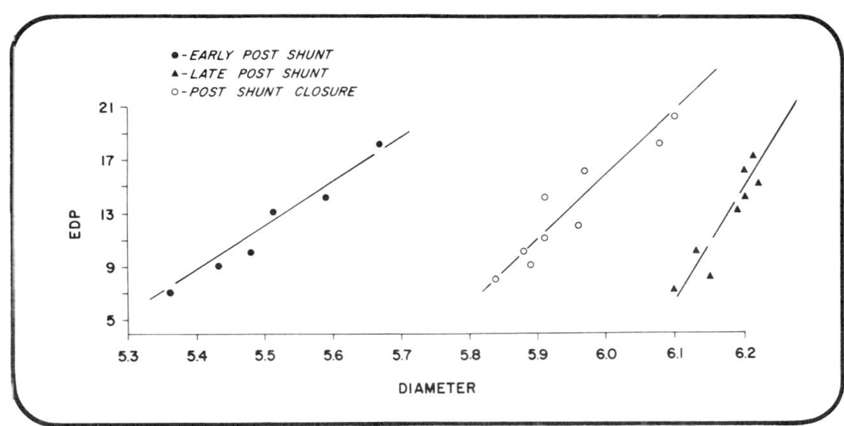

FIGURE 3. Relation between end-diastolic pressure and end-diastolic diameter determined immediately after production of an arteriovenous shunt in a conscious animal, several weeks after arteriovenous shunt, and 1 week after shunt closure.

tricular diastolic pressure-circumference relation (internal circumference at the minor equator) frequently was shifted to the right from normal. Six months to a year after aortic valve replacement, patients with evidence of depressed myocardial inotropic state preoperatively had lower left ventricular end-diastolic pressure values due to slightly reduced ventricular diameter but appeared to have the same steep and rightwardly displaced pressure-volume curve that existed before operation. However, when myocardial inotropic state was normal preoperatively, the diastolic pressure-circumference curve shifted leftward into the normal range after operation, thus suggesting reversibility of the altered diastolic properties in these patients.[42] Other investigators[43] have demonstrated directionally similar changes in pressure-volume relations after corrective operations in children with ventricular septal defect.

Recent experiments indicate that the left ventricle becomes markedly stiffer after the chronic and healing phases of myocardial infarction,[39,44-46] and similar observations recently have been made in man.[6] Although it is difficult to evaluate quantitatively the effects of graded amounts of scar tissue on left ventricular compliance, there is evidence that end-diastolic ventricular compliance in man and in experimental animals is decreased at each level of end-diastolic volume, even after a small myocardial infarction.

Cardiac enlargement and changes in compliance induced by chronic volume overload may be reversible with time in some patients in the absence of chronic cardiac failure.[7,42,42] Whether or not changes in compliance resulting from pressure-induced hypertrophy, or those due to myocardial ischemic damage, will regress after corrective operations or other therapy remains unanswered at present. The mechanisms of the changes in compliance also are unexplored. In the chronically volume-overloaded heart, left ventricular wall thickness is not markedly increased[7] and sarcomere lengths in these hearts are not appreciably greater than in the overfilled normal heart, although there may be some loss of register of the sarcomeres.[47] New sarcomeres are unquestionably introduced during dilatation or hypertrophy, or both, but it is not certain whether alterations in sarcomere of cell struc-

ture, connective tissue changes or other factors are involved in observed changes in compliance. Finally, although it would appear that passive compliance of the whole ventricle can now be estimated by several methods, better approaches must be devised to assess stress-strain relations of the myocardium itself

Active Stiffness of Cardiac Muscle and the Heart

The nature and significance of active stress-strain relation in isolated cardiac muscle have been investigated extensively over the past 20 years. There is now substantial evidence that cardiac muscle may be described as containing undamped elastic elements that are in the series with a force-generating site commonly called the contractile element.[48,50,51] During the past several years, considerable controversy has centered about the description of the active elastic properties of isolated cardiac muscle by a variety of mechanical analogs.[52,53] Series elasticity probably remains unchanged throughout active contraction,[49,50] although this hypothesis has recently been questioned.[51,52] This general area of endeavor has provided much useful information about function of the cardiac muscle, but its significance to the clinician or to the physiologist working in the whole heart is not yet entirely clear. Moreover, it has recently been shown that most mechanical analogs for muscle may be reduced to a single mathematical expression.[53] Although this review does not consider the relative merits of the various analog treatments of cardiac muscle, it is of interest that a wide variety of positive and negative inotropic agents have been examined for their potential influence on the measured active compliance of isolated cardiac muscle. There is now general agreement that alterations in inotropic state acutely induced by pharmacologic agents do not influence active compliance in isolated muscle.[50,54]

The examination of active stiffness in the intact heart is difficult; nevertheless, several techniques have recently been applied, and there is now some evidence that the intact heart functions as if it contains passive elements in series with the contractile elements.[54-58] Figure 4

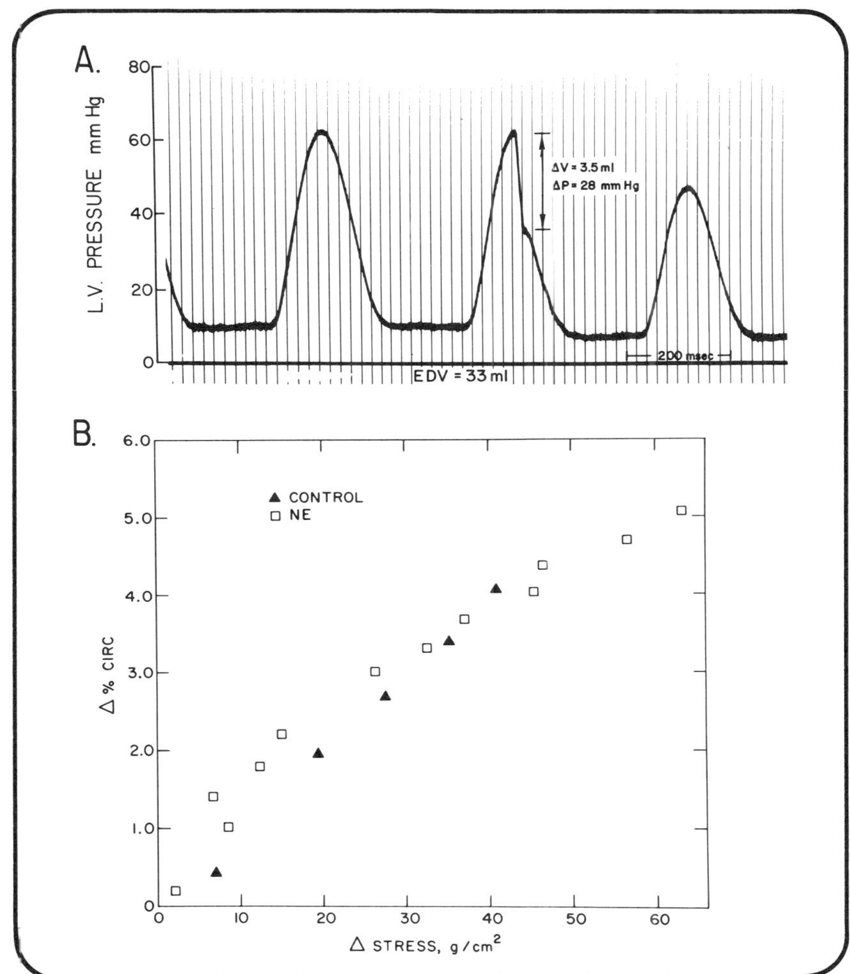

FIGURE 4. Active stiffness of the left ventricle determined by quick release. **B,** rapid withdrawal of an increment of volume in the isovolumically contracting left ventricle. The relation between change in volume and change in pressure may then be used to calculate the percent extension of passive elements in the left ventricle at peak systole as expressed in **A** (see text).

shows a representative example of studies obtained by rapid volume withdrawals from the dog left ventricle.[55,57] Scatter in data derived with these techniques is substantial, but it has been shown that series elasticity can be described by an exponential relation. Templeton et al.[58] recently described an ingenious technique for examining the frequency dependency of the stress-strain relation during active contraction. These investigators produced small sinusoidal volume changes in the isovolumically contracting left ventricle and examined the frequency dependence of the relation between volume and pressure changes throughout systole and diastole. At frequencies of more than 30 Hz, a linear relation between volume stiffness ($\Delta P/\Delta V$) and pressure in the intact heart during systole was shown.[58] Further studies with this type of approach should allow quantitative investigation of the viscous and inertial properties of muscle.

Summary

There is evidence that most alterations in inotropic state occurring under normal circumstances do not substantially influence diastolic compliance, except perhaps in the rapid phases of cardiac filling. Nevertheless, recent studies have clearly shown that left ventricular compliance can be markedly altered in chronic disease states, acute myocardial infarction, chronic ventricular hypertrophy and failure and chronic dilatation influencing diastolic compliance in an important manner. The large shift to the right of the pressure-volume relation observed in the chronically dilated left ventricle allows the ventricle to operate from a large radius and to deliver a normal or increased stroke volume without a great increase in end-diastolic pressure. In contrast, the decrease in compliance without a shift to the right that appears to occur in acute myocardial infarction may increase filling pressure without this mechanical advantage and be detrimental. The question of when and by what mechanism changes in heart size and compliance appear to become irreversible seems to be amenable to experimental study and could have important clinical implications. It is suggested that one appropriate way to evaluate chronic changes in cardiac compliance is to assess the diastolic pressure-volume relation or the pressure-circumference relation over a range of pressures up to end-diastolic pressure, or over the range of volume accompanying the stroke volume. This approach, encompassing a normal cardiac filling cycle and defined as "functional compliance," should offer useful clinical information on the filling characteristics of the ventricle relative to pressures transmitted in retrograde manner to the lungs or the systemic venous circulation. The assessment of the passive stress-strain relation of the myocardium itself in the whole heart remains a difficult and challenging problem.

Acknowledgment: This study was supported in part by National Heart and Lung Institute Grant HK-12373 and National Heart and Lung Institute Contract PH-43-NHLI-68-1332. Doctor Covell is the recipient of National Heart and Lung Institute Research Career Development Award HL-21132.

References

1. **Hill AV:** The heat of shortening and the dynamic constants of muscle. Proc Roy Soc (Biol) 126:136, 1938
2. **Fenn WO:** A quantitative comparison between the energy liberated and the work performed by the isolated sartorius muscle of the frog. J Physiol (London) 58:175, 1923
3. **Buchthal F, Rosenfalck P:** Elastic properties of striated muscle. In, Tissue Elasticity (Remington JW, ed). Baltimore, Waverly Press, 1957, p 73
4. **Alexander RS:** Viscoelastic determinants of muscle contractility and "cardiac tone." Fed Proc 21:1001, 1962
5. **Gilmore JP, Cingolani HE, Taylor RR, et al:** Influence of ventricular activation on ventricular compliance. Amer J Physiol 211:1227, 1966
6. **Diamond G, Forrester JS:** Effects of coronary artery disease and acute myocardial infarction on left ventricular compliance in man. Circulation 45:11, 1972
7. **McCullagh WH, Covell JW, Ross J Jr:** Left ventricular dilatation and diastolic compliance changes during chronic volume overloading. Circ Res 40:943, 1972
8. **Bristow JD, Van Zee BE, Judkins MP:** Systolic and diastolic abnormalities of the left ventricle in coronary artery disease. Studies in patients with little or no enlargement of ventricular volume. Circulation 42:219, 1970
9. **Landowne M, Stacy RW:** A glossary of terms. In Ref 3, p 191
10. **Fung YCB:** Elasticity of soft tissues in simple elongation. Amer J Physiol 213:1532, 1967
11. **Levin A, Wyman J:** The viscous elastic properties of muscle. Proc Roy Soc (Biol) 101:218, 1927
12. **Little RC, Wead WB:** Diastolic viscoelastic properties of active and quiescent cardiac muscle. Amer J Physiol 221:1120, 1971
13. **Abbott BC, Lowy J:** Stress relaxation in muscle. Proc Roy Soc (Biol) 146:281, 1956
14. **Sonnenblick EH, Ross J Jr, Covell JW, et al:** Alterations in resting length-tension relations of cardiac muscle induced by changes in contractile force. Circ Res 11:980, 1966
15. **Bartelstone HJ, Scherlag BJ, Hoffman BF, et al:** Demonstration of variable diastolic compliance associated with paired stimulation of the dog heart. Bull NY Acad Med 41:616, 1965
16. **Yeatman LA, Parmely WW, Sonnenblick EH:** Effects of temperature on series elasticity and contractile element motion in heart muscle. Amer J Physiol 217:1030, 1969
17. **Parmley WW, Sonnenblick EH:** Mechanical effects of increased series elasticity: an in vitro model of mitral regurgitation and ventricular aneurysm. Amer J Cardiol 27:376, 1971
18. **Parmley WW, Sonnenblick EH:** Series elasticity in cat papillary muscle: increased stiffness after segmental damage. Proc Soc Exp Biol Med 124:1182, 1967

19. **Pinto JG:** Mechanical Properties of the Papillary Muscle in the Passive and Active State. PhD thesis, University of California, San Diego, 1972, p 123

20. **Parmley WW, Spann JF Jr, Taylor RR, et al:** The series elasticity of cardiac muscle in hyperthyroidism, ventricular hypertrophy and heart failure. Proc Soc Exp Biol Med 127:606, 1968

21. **Spann JF Jr, Buccino RA, Sonnenblick EH, et al:** Contractile state of cardiac muscle obtained from cats with experimentally produced ventricular hypertrophy and heart failure. Circ Res 21:341, 1967

22. **Bing OHL, Matsushita S, Fanburg BL, et al:** Mechanical properties of rat cardiac muscle during experimental hypertrophy. Circ Res 28:234, 1971

23. **Friedman WF:** The intrinsic physiologic properties of the developing heart. Progr Cardiovasc Dis 15:87, 1972

24. **Romero T, Covell JW, Friedman WF:** A comparison of pressure-volume relations of the fetal, newborn, and adult heart. Amer J Physiol 222:1285, 1972

25. **Ross J Jr, Sonnenblick EH, Taylor RR, et al:** Diastolic geometry and sarcomere lengths in the chronically dilated canine left ventricle. Circ Res 28:49, 1971

26. **Diamond G, Forrester JS, Hargis J, et al:** The diastolic pressure-volume relationships of the canine left ventricle. Cir Res 29:267, 1971

27. **Ross J Jr, Covell JW, Sonnenblick EH, et al:** Contractile state of the heart characterized by force-velocity relations in variably afterloaded and isovolumic beats. Circ Res 18:149, 1966

28. **Monroe RG, LaFarge CG, Gamble WJ, et al:** Left ventricular pressure-volume relations and performance as affected by sudden increases in developed pressure. Circ Res 22:333, 1968

29. **Templeton GH, Ecker RR, Mitchell JH:** Left ventricular stiffness during diastole and systole: the influence of changes in volume and inotropic state. Cardiovasc Res 6:95, 1972

30. **Noble MIM, Milne EN, Goerke RJ, et al:** Left ventricular filling and diastolic pressure-volume relations in the conscious dog. Circ Res 24:269, 1969

31. **Bianco JA, Freedberg LE, Powell WJ Jr, et al:** Influence of vagal stimulation on ventricular compliance. Amer J Physiol 218:264, 1970

32. **Goldberg AH, Phear WPC:** Halothane and paired stimulation: effects on myocardial compliance and contractility. J Appl Physiol 28:391, 1970

33. **Clancy RL, Graham TP Jr, Ross J Jr, et al:** Influence of aortic pressure-induced homeometric autoregulation on myocardial performance. Amer J Physiol 214:1186, 1968

34. **Wildenthal K, Mierzwiak DS, Mitchell JH:** Influence of vagal stimulation on left ventricular end-diastolic distensibility. Amer J Physiol 217:1446, 1969

35. **Widenthal K, Mullins CB, Harris MD, et al:** Left ventricular end-diastolic distensibility after norepinephrine and propranolol. Amer J Physiol 217:812, 1969

36. **Jones JW, Rackley CE, Bruce RA, et al:** Left ventricular volumes in valvular heart diease. Circulation 29:887, 1964

37. **Dodge HT:** Functional characteristics of the left ventricle in heart disease. Ann Intern Med 69:941, 1968

38. **Dodge HT, Hay RE, Sandler H:** Pressure-volume characteristics of the diastolic left ventricle of man with heart disease. Amer Heart J 64:503, 1962

39. **Hood WB Jr, Bianco JA, Kumar R, et al:** Experimental myocardial infarction. IV. Reduction of left ventricular compliance in the healing phase. J Clin Invest 49:1316, 1970

40. **Gaasch WH, Battle WE, Oboler AA, et al:** Left ventricular stress and compliance in man. With special reference to normalized ventricular function curves. Circulation 45:746, 1972

41. **Mitchell JH, Wildenthal K, Mullins CB:** Geometrical studies of the left ventricle utilizing biplane cinefluorography. Fed Proc 28:1334, 1969

42. **Gault JH, Covell JW, Braunwald E, et al:** Left ventricular performance following correction of free aortic regurgitation. Circulation 42:773, 1970

43. **Jarmakani JMM, Graham TP Jr, Canent RV Jr, et al:** The effect of corrective surgery on left heart volume and mass in children with ventricular septal defect. Amer J Cardiol 27:254, 1971

44. **Russ RO Jr, Rackley CE, Pombo J, et al:** Effects of increasing left ventricular filling pressures in patients with acute myocardial infarction. J Clin Invest 49:1539, 1970

45. **Levine HJ:** Compliance of the left ventricle. Circulation 46:423, 1972

46. **Weiss AB, Saffa RS, Levinson GE, et al:** Left ventricular function during the early and late stages of scar formation following experimental myocardial infarction. Amer Heart J 79:370, 1970

47. **Yoran C, Covell JW, Ross J Jr:** Structural basis for the ascending limb of left ventricular function. Circ Res 32:297, 1973

48. **Brady AJ:** The three element model of muscle mechanics: its applicability to cardiac muscle. Physiologist 10:75, 1967

49. **Hefner LL, Bowen TE Jr:** Elastic components of cat papillary muscle. Amer J Physiol 212:1221, 1967

50. **Parmley WW, Sonnenblick EH:** Series elasticity in heart muscle. Its relation to contractile elment velocity and proposed muscle models. Circ Res 20:112, 1967

51. **Noble MIM, Else W:** Reexamination of the Hill model of muscle to cat myocardium. Circ Res 31:580, 1972

52. **Pollack GH, Huntsman LL, Verdugo P:** Cardiac muscle models: an overextension of series elasticity. Circ Res 31:569, 1972

53. **Fung YC:** Comparison of different models of the heart muscle. J Biomech 4:289, 1971

54. **Sonnenblick EH:** Series elastic and contractile elements in heart muscle: changes in muscle length. Amer J Physiol 207:1330, 1964

55. **Covell JW, Taylor RR, Ross J Jr:** Series elasticity in the intact left ventricle determined by a quick release technique (abstr). Fed Proc 26:382, 1967

56. **Forwand SA, McIntyre KM, Lipana JG, et al:** Active stiffness of the intact canine left ventricle: with observations on the effect of acute and chronic myocardial infarction. Circ Res 19:970, 1966

57. **Covell JW:** Mechanics of contraction in the intact heart. In, Biomechanics: Its Foundations and Objectives (Fung YC, Perrone N, Anliker M, ed). Englewood Cliffs, New Jersey, Prentice-Hall, 1972, p 289

58. **Templeton GH, Mitchell JH, Ecker RR, et al:** A method for measurement of dynamic compliance of the left ventricle in dogs. J Appl Physiol 29:742, 1970

Chapter 13

Renal Function and Edema Formation in Congestive Heart Failure

Melvin J. Tonkon, MD
Stanley M. Rosen, MD
Dean T. Mason, MD, FACC

Although it is now clearly recognized that abnormal cardiac performance initiates the events leading to organ congestion in the heart failure state, alterations in renal function play a central role in the fluid retention and electrolyte imbalances characteristic of this condition. Thus, the fundamental cause of congestive heart failure is disturbance in hemodynamics; retention of body salt and, subsequently, water results principally from the response of the kidneys to the reduced renal perfusion accompanying lowered cardiac output. Pulmonary and systemic edema ensues as a consequence of interstitial fluid accumulation, coupled with increased venous pressure behind the failing ventricles.

The predominate feature involved in the electrolyte and water imbalance in congestive heart failure is renal conservation of sodium. It appears that the kidneys, through their complex tubular and hormonal functions, operate as a compensatory mechanism to restore normal renal blood flow by promoting increased retention of sodium and, thus, water in an effort to improve cardiac output by augmenting circulatory blood volume and thereby enhancing ventricular filling and cardiac function.[1] However, this renal adaptive mechanism is ineffective hemodynamically, and the improvement in cardiac output and renal perfusion is slight compared with the edematous state that develops. Furthermore, patients with congestive heart failure have difficulty excreting sodium loads. Although normal subjects can ingest several grams of sodium per day without edema formation, small amounts of sodium in patients with cardiac dysfunction provoke water retention.[2] Therefore, the kidney-induced increase in total body sodium in congestive heart failure causes expansion of the extracellular fluid compartment and contraction of the intracellular space.[3]

Concerning the integrated mechanisms of salt and water retention in congestive heart failure, three factors are considered the major determinants in sodium preservation (Figure 1). Factor I relates to the mechanical reduction of glomerular filtration rate and is of particular importance in initiating considerable fluid retention in congestive heart failure. Factor II is concerned with stimulation of the renin-angiotensin-aldosterone hormonal axis, which is of substantial significance in maintaining and amplifying fluid accumulation in chronic heart failure. Factor III appears to involve the absence of an incompletely identified hormonal substance that normally causes proximal renal tubular sodium rejection.

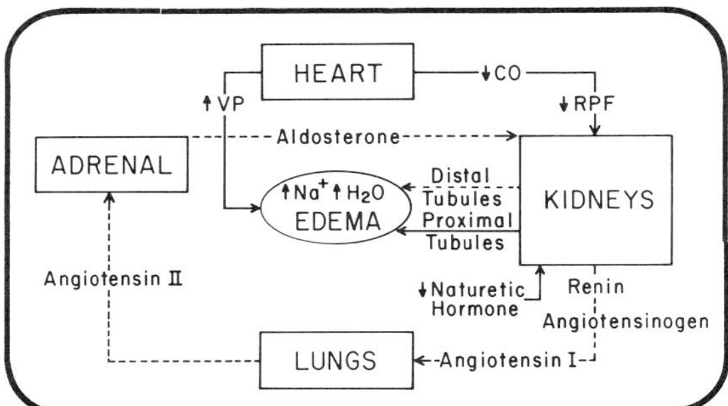

FIGURE 1. Schematic representation of factors producing sodium and water retention in congestive heart failure. Cardiac dysfunction leads to lowered cardiac output (CO) with concomitant reduction in renal plasma flow (RPF), thereby causing increased reabsorption of sodium (Na⁺) and water (H₂O) from the proximal renal tubules. These events focused on ↓RPF (Factor I) are shown by the **solid clockwise arrows.** Reduced RPF and related influences activate the renal secretion of renin, which ultimately results in increased adrenal secretion of aldosterone, thus producing increased Na⁺ and H₂O reabsorption from the distal renal tubules. These events centered on the elaboration of aldosterone (Factor II) are demonstrated by the **broken clockwise arrows.** In addition, deficiency of a humoral natriuretic substance (Factor III) is shown influencing the kidneys to allow greater Na⁺ and H₂O reabsorption from the proximal tubules. Finally, the hemodynamic effect of elevated venous pressure (VP) on edema formation is depicted by the **solid counterclockwise arrow.**

Glomerular Filtration Rate

Normally, 20 percent of the cardiac output is partitioned into the renal circulation[4] (Figure 2). Thus, 1 liter of blood per minute is delivered by the afferent arterioles to the glomeruli, with approximately 10 percent of this plasma filtered through the glomeruli into the proximal tubules and the remaining 90 percent retained within the diffuse efferent arteriolar network of the kidneys. Therefore, the normal glomerular filtrate rate is 100 ml/min with the protein-free filtrate containing concentrations of sodium and other electrolytes equal to those in plasma. In the proximal tubule, sodium is pumped into the interstitium, which is followed by passive isosmotic reabsorption of water (Figure 3). The transmembrane movement of sodium is accomplished by two active processes, one accompanied by chloride and the other in exchange for hydrogen, into the tubular fluid generated by carbonic anhydrase in the proximal tubular cells. Normally, only 1 percent of the total glomerular filtrate is finally excreted in the urine, and the other 99 percent is returned to the circulation by intrarenal tubular transport mechanisms; the majority (70 percent) of this reabsorption takes place in the proximal tubules as described, with isotonic sodium and water reaching the peritubular capillaries of the efferent arteriolar system.

With the decline in cardiac output in heart failure, there is disproportionate regional distribution of total blood flow away from the kidneys to organs with higher metabolic oxygen requirements[4] (Figure 2). Furthermore, renal blood flow may be diminished in cardiac dysfunction—even prior to reduction of cardiac output—due to increased adrenergic activity that results in relatively greater vasoconstriction in the renal arteriolar bed.[5] Accompanying the decrease in renal plasma flow is a decline in the glomerular filtration rate;[6,7] consequently, with the ability of the proximal tubules to reabsorb sodium remaining at least constant, there is increased net retention of sodium and water[8] (Figure 1). Since the decrease in renal plasma flow is greater than that in the glomerular filtration rate, the fraction of plasma filtered at the glomerular membrane is thus increased. Therefore, it has been suggested that proximal tubular reabsorption of sodium also is enhanced in congestive heart failure. The postulated mechanism is the elevation of oncotic pressure in the efferent arterioles and the downstream peritubular capillaries by increased filtration of protein-free fluid into the proximal tubules.[9,10] This increased peritubular colloid osmotic pressure provides augmented uptake of interstitial fluid that may, in turn, accelerate proximal renal tubular sodium reabsorption.

An additional mechanism contributing to increased proximal tubular reabsorption of sodium and water appears to be related to the relative redistribution of intrarenal blood flow away from the cortex toward the medulla that occurs in heart failure. Less reabsorptive capacity in the short outer cortical nephrons compared with that in the longer juxtamedullary nephrons in the outer medulla of the kidney has been indicated.[11] Further, a washout technique employing inert gas has been used in human subjects to separate four different blood flow components within the kidney.[12] Comparable flow components in the normal canine kidney have been named components I, II, III and IV[13] (Figure 4) and have been demonstrated by radioautography to represent blood flow through the cortex, outer medulla, inner medulla and peripheral fat, respectively[14] (Figure 5). Changes in these washout curves have been demonstrated to be similar in both human and canine subjects during renal homotransplant rejection,[12,13] the percentage of total renal blood flow represented by component I serially decreasing as renal function deteriorates. Eventually components I and II fuse into a single component. Radioautography in the dog demonstrated that these changes in the components represented decreasing rates of blood flow to the cortex and that fusion of components I and II represented similar rates of blood flow in the cortex and outer medulla.[13]

The same washout technique using inert gas has been applied clinically to investigate renal hemodynamics in congestive heart failure.[15] Two groups of patients were categorized. In the first group the washout curve could be separated into four exponential components, whereas in the second group only three exponential components could be recognized. In the latter group fusion of components I and II had occurred. Cardiac output was significantly higher in the first group. There was a correlation between cardiac output and glomerular filtration rate in the first group, but no correlation could be found in the second group. There was no significant difference between the glomerular filtration rates in the two groups. A correlation existed between cardiac output and percentage of total renal blood flow supplied to the combined components I and II in both groups. These observations demonstrated that filtration rate and cardiac output are not necessarily interrelated. This observation was also inferred by other workers who noted that recovery from congestive heart failure was not necessarily accompanied by improved filtration.[16,17] The progressive redistribution of blood flow within the kidney at lower levels of cardiac output without substantial changes in filtration rate implies that changes in net proximal tubular reabsorption may be a more dominant feature in the sodium retention of congestive heart failure than is reduced glomerular filtration rate per se.

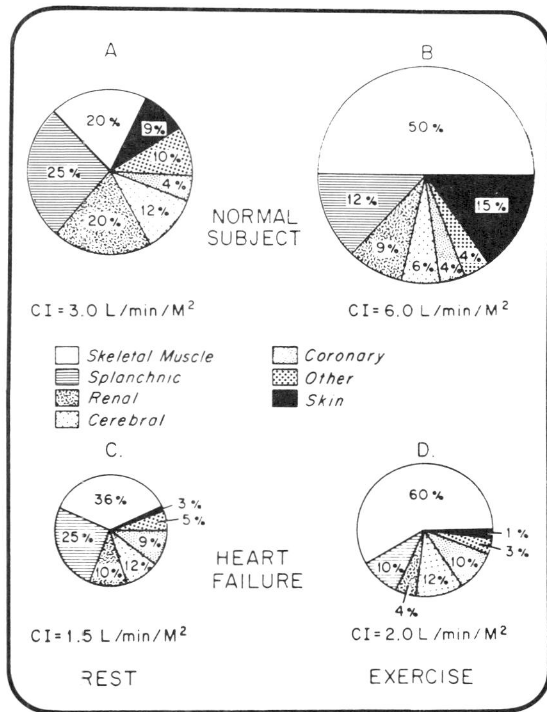

FIGURE 2. Regional distribution of blood flow at rest and during exercise in normal subjects and in patients with congestive heart failure. CI = cardiac index. (Reproduced by permission from Mason.[4])

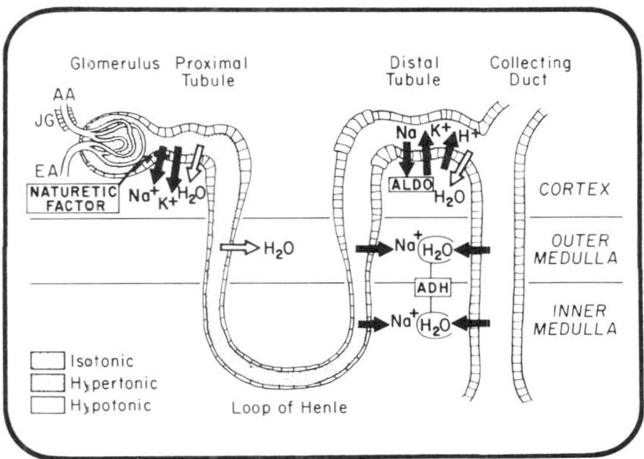

FIGURE 3. Schematic representation of the movement of salt and water in the nephron. AA = afferent arteriole; aldo = aldosterone; ADH = antidiuretic hormone; EA = efferent arteriole; JG = juxtaglomerular apparatus. **Solid arrows** indicate active transport of sodium, potassium hydrogen and water; **open arrows** denote passive movement of water.

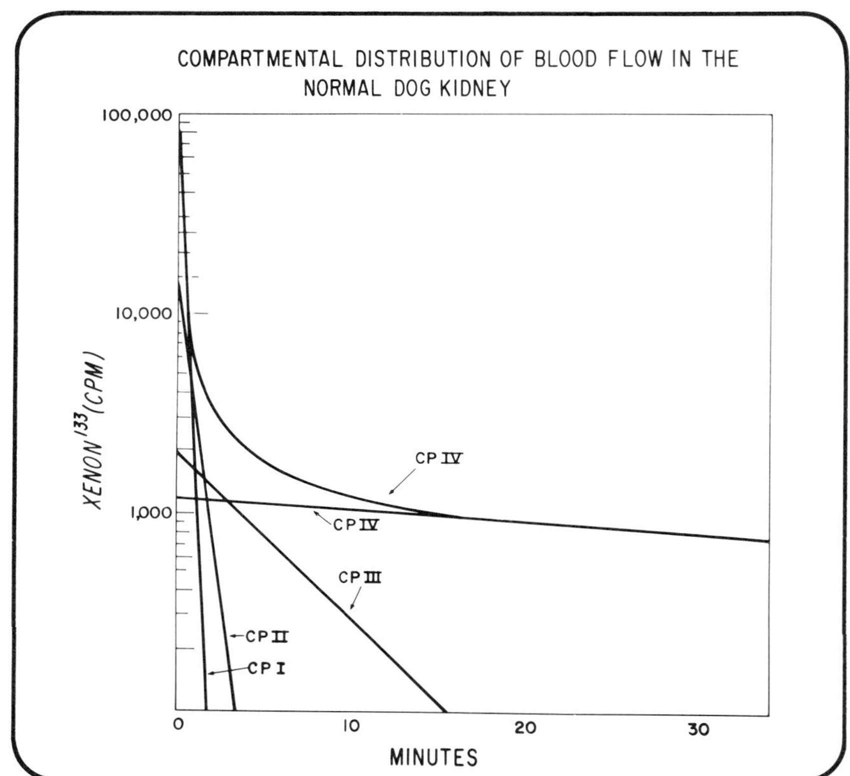

FIGURE 4. Washout curve from the renal parenchyma recorded on an external scintillation counter after injection of a bolus of ^{133}Xe into the renal artery. Counts per minute (CPM) are plotted on a logarithmic scale on the ordinate, and time is plotted on an arithmetic scale. The curve was analyzed as the sum of four exponential components represented by lines. The fasted component I represents blood flow through the cortex. Components II, III and IV represent blood flow through outer medulla, inner medulla and perirenal fat, respectively. (Reproduced by permission from Rosen et al.[13])

Renin-Angiotensin-Aldosterone

Humoral control of sodium and water by aldosterone in the kidneys is effected in the distal renal tubule (Figure 3). The stimulus for increased aldosterone secretion from the zona glomerulosa of the adrenal cortex by circulating angiotensin II initially involves renal secretion of renin[18] (Figure 1). Renin is elaborated into the circulation from the juxtaglomerular cells surrounding the afferent renal arterioles (Figure 3). The trigger for renin release in congestive heart failure is believed to be multifactorial:[19] (1) stimulation of baroreceptors in the afferent arterioles sensitive to diminished stretch caused by reduction of renal perfusion pressure secondary to decreased renal blood flow; (2) stimulation of the macula densa in the first portion of the distal tubule (Figure 3), located adjacent to the juxtaglomerular apparatus, by a diminished tubular sodium load reaching this structure after selective sodium reabsorption in the ascending loop of Henle; and (3) stimulation of the juxtaglomerular cells by sympathetic nerves and increased circulating norepinephrine.

Renin is a proteolyte enzyme that is synthesized, stored and released by the juxtaglomerular cells. The circulating substrate for renin is an alpha-2 globulin—angiotensinogen—that is synthesized by the liver.[18,19] In the plasma, renin acts on angiotensinogen, to produce angiotensin I, a decapeptide. During circulation through the lungs, a converting enzyme cleaves two amino acids from angiotensin I to form angiotensin II, an octapeptide (Figure 1). This potent vasoconstrictive substance serves as the principal stimulus for release of aldosterone from the adrenal gland. Angiotensin II is also an important component for feedback control of renin release.[19] Decreased hepatic breakdown also contributes to the increased quantities of circulating aldosterone present in congestive heart failure, since the liver is the principal site of aldosterone metabolism, which is suppressed by diminished hepatic blood flow. In patients with severe congestive heart failure, aldosterone secretion may be increased to 4 to 5 mg daily, in contrast to secretion of 50 to 200 μg per day in normal subjects.[20]

Aldosterone acts on the distal renal tubule to enhance the active reabsorption of sodium[21] (Figure 3). In the distal tubule, sodium passively diffuses from the tubular lumen into the interior of the tubular cells. Osmotic gradients must be overcome for sodium to pass into the interstitium, and it is postulated that aldosterone catalyzes a set of reactions that liberate adenosine triphosphate (ATP) for the energy required for

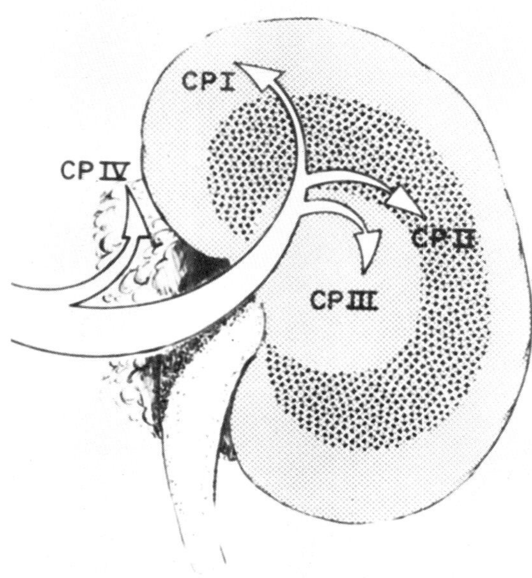

FIGURE 5. Components I, II, III and IV represent that portion of total nutrient renal blood flow supplied to cortex, outer medulla, inner medulla and perihilar fat, respectively.

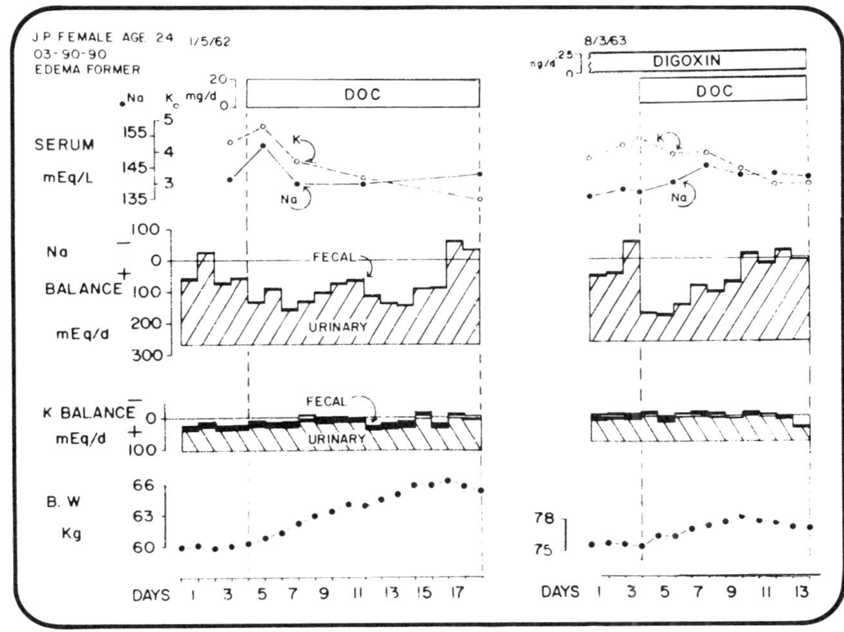

FIGURE 6. Effects of desoxycorticosterone (DOC) on serum sodium and potassium levels, sodium and potassium balance and body weight in a patient with congestive heart failure before and during treatment with digoxin. Note the smaller amounts of sodium retained and weight gained before escape from the sodium-retaining effects of DOC during treatment with digoxin. (Reproduced by permission from Gill et al.[31])

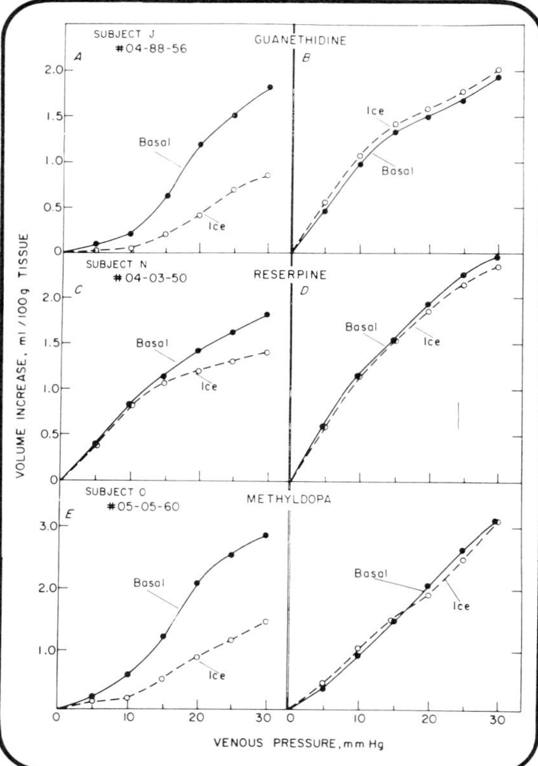

FIGURE 7. Effects of the antiadrenergic drugs guanethidine, reserpine and methyldopa on the response of venous pressure-volume curves to immersion of the hand in ice water. Venous tone was determined by the progressive, stepwise occlusion of venous outflow from the forearm, and the volume of the venous bed at equilibrium was measured at each level of venous pressure by a plethysmographic technique. Control studies are on the **left;** drug studies are on the **right.** Prior to adrenergic blockade, ice water provoked a reflex increase in venous tone, thereby indicating a sympathetically induced redistribution of blood volume from the systemic venous reservoir centrally with resultant increase in cardiac filling. At the time of the drug studies, venomotor reactivity was abolished. (Reproduced by permission from Mason et al.[43])

this active transport of sodium. Another suggestion is that aldosterone increases sodium permeability of the membrane on the luminal side of the distal tubular cells. With the passage of sodium into the interstitium, this movement is passively accompanied by water.

Natriuretic Hormone

An additional factor, about which there is considerable controversy, is a postulated hormonal substance believed to be important in the proximal tubular handling of sodium and referred to as a salt-losing factor or natriuretic hormone[22,23] (Figure 3). Several experiments have pointed to the existence of a salt-losing factor that functions at the proximal tubule independent of changes in the glomerular filtration rate and mineralocorticoid activity.[22–25] Normal subjects escape the sodium-retaining action of aldosterone,[26–28] whereas this escape phenomenon does not occur in those with cardiac dysfunction[29–31] (Figure 6); this has been explained by the lack of production of some factor or group of factors that reject sodium and water retention in congestive heart failure. Further, cross-circulation experiments in dogs, designed to eliminate the role of glomerular filtration and aldosterone in the recipient animal, have shown enhanced excretion of sodium when a saline load was administered to the donor of the pair.[32]

In normal subjects with sodium loading, but not in those with sodium depletion, a natriuretic hormonal protein has been isolated with biologic activity lasting for a few hours after an initial lag period.[22] Other studies have suggested that this natriuretic substance originates in the kidneys and that it might be a renal medullary prostaglandin or involve the renal kallikrien system.[33] In summary, there is evidence to suggest that when the extracellular fluid volume is expanded in normal subjects a humoral substance is elaborated that facilitates proximal renal tubular excretion of sodium, and that an insufficiency of this natriuretic hormone may contribute to edema formation in heart failure (Figure 1).

Antidiuretic Hormone

Another humoral participant in water and electrolyte balance is arginine vasopressin, antidiuretic hormone (ADH). This polypeptide is formed in the supraoptic nuclei of the hypothalamus and migrates to the posterior pituitary. As a physiologic regulatory mechanism, ADH release is stimulated by extracellular fluid hyper-

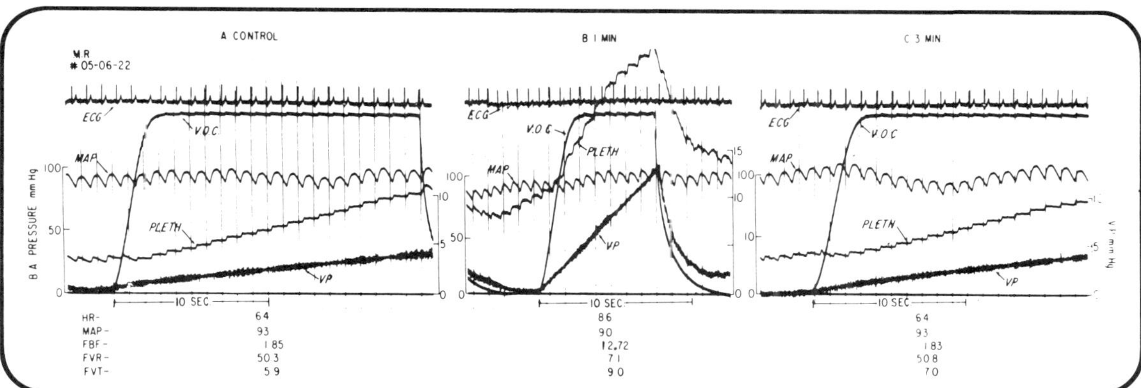

FIGURE 8. Three segments of records obtained from a normal subject illustrating the effects of epinephrine on the vascular bed of the forearm. The tracing on the left (**A**) was obtained during the control period; that in the middle (**B**), 1 minute after the intravenous injection of $5\,\mu$g of epinephrine into the opposite forearm; and that on the right (**C**), 3 minutes after epinephrine. MAP = mean arterial pressure; PLETH = forearm plethysmograph tracing; VOC = pressure within the venous occluding cuff on the upper arm; VP = forearm venous pressure. The numbers below the tracings indicate the variables which were measured or calculated: HR = heart rate; FBF = forearm blood flow; FVR = forearm vascular resistance; FVT = forearm venous tone. Note that in panel **B** the increase in venous pressure is considerably more rapid relative to the increase in forearm venous volume, as shown by the slope of VP indicating marked venoconstriction produced by epinephrine. The greater rate of rise of PLETH in **B** shows that forearm blood flow was increased after epinephrine. Since MAP remained essentially unchanged, forearm vascular resistance was reduced. Such an increase in the ratio of systemic postcapillary resistance to precapillary resistance, when sustained for a prolonged period of time, may result in loss of plasma volume into the extravascular space. (Reproduced by permission from Mason et al.[43])

osmolality and decreased extracellular fluid volume.[34] Current evidence is unconvincing that atrial receptors play an important role in ADH secretion.[35] ADH acts on the nephron to increase the water permeability of the collecting ducts, so that free water can be reabsorbed from the ductal fluid into the hypertonic medullary interstitium (Figure 3). Increased ADH secretion does not appear to be a principal feature of congestive heart failure,[36] although it may contribute to the syndrome of inappropriate ADH secretion with dilutional hyponatremia[37] and impairs the ability of patients with heart failure to excrete an ingested water load. However, decreased free water clearance can occur in heart failure, without increased ADH secretion, due to inadequate delivery of sodium and water to the distal nephron.

Sympathetic Nervous System

Increased activity of the sympathetic nervous system plays a prominent role in the support of cardiac and peripheral circulatory dynamics in the heart failure state,[1,5] as discussed in chapter 9 on the regulation of cardiac performance in heart disease. In terms of alterations in renal function, heightened adrenergic activity contributes to the reduction of renal blood flow and participates in the redistribution of intrarenal blood flow already delineated.[4] In addition, increased sympathetic discharge contributes to edema formation by increasing systemic venous tone and thereby elevating venous pressure. Adrenergic stimulation may magnify renin release by direct renal nerve traffic and by humoral beta receptor stimulation.[38,39]

The overall effects of increased sympathetic activity on extracellular fluid and electrolyte balance include: (1) immediate effects of redistribution of effective blood volume by systemic venoconstriction (Figure 7), shifting peripheral intravascular volume centrally for enhanced filling of the cardiac chambers;[40] (2) early effects resulting from peripheral transcapillary loss of intravascular fluid to the interstitial space by endogenous catecholamine-induced increase in the ratio of systemic postcapillary resistance to

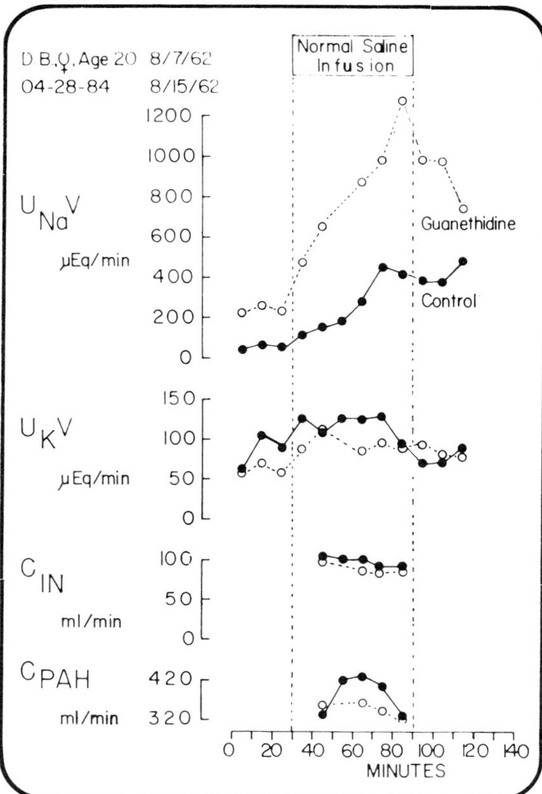

FIGURE 9. Changes in renal sodium excretion ($U_{Na}V$), potassium excretion (U_KV), insulin clearance (C_{IN}) and para-aminohippuric acid clearance (C_{PAH}) with infusion of 2 l of physiologic saline solution before (**dots** and **solid lines**) and during (**open circles** and **broken lines**) treatment with guanethidine in a normal subject. Adrenergic blockade resulted in a much greater excretion of the sodium load compared with the control infusion of saline without guanethidine. Therefore, adrenergic blockade in normal subjects results in enhanced diuresis with increased sodium excretion. (Reproduced by permission from Gill et al.[28])

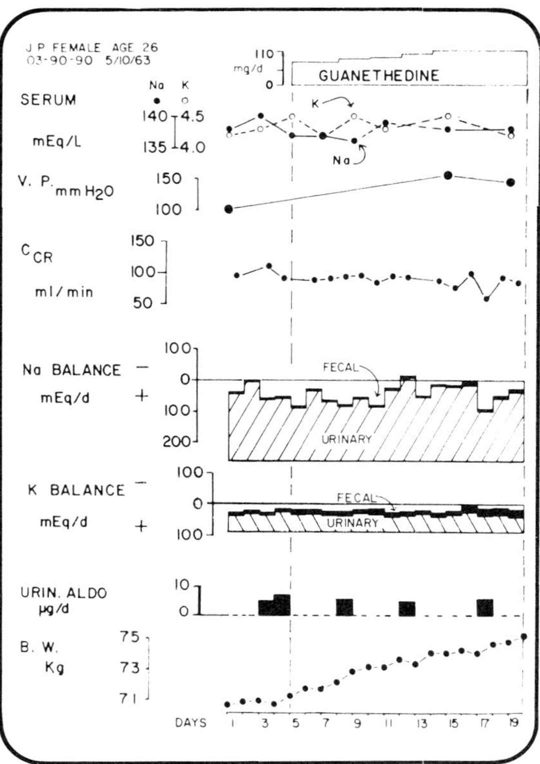

FIGURE 10. Effect of treatment with guanethidine on serum sodium and potassium, venous pressure (VP), creatine clearance (C_{CR}), sodium and potassium balance, urinary aldosterone and body weight in a patient with congestive heart failure. The antiadrenergic drug resulted in sustained retention of sodium, which persisted during all but 1 of the 15 days of administration. (Reproduced by permission from Gill et al.[31])

precapillary resistance (Figure 8);[41,42] and (3) late effects resulting in renal salt and water retention by stimulation of the renin-aldosterone system.[43] Finally, unlike normal subjects who exhibit diuresis with adrenergic blockade[28] (Figure 9), in patients with congestive heart failure any tendency for an antiadrenergic effect to enhance sodium excretion is overcome by worsening of the depressed cardiocirculatory status, which produces further retention of sodium and water[31,44] (Figure 10).

Potassium Balance

Although potassium is readily filtered through the glomeruli, the cation is essentially totally reabsorbed in the proximal tubules. The potassium excreted in the urine is largely that secreted into the distal tubules in exchange for sodium (Figure 3). Therefore, the excretion rate of potassium depends upon the amount of sodium delivered to the distal tubules for exchange with potassium. Further, urinary potassium is also dependent upon the quantity of aldosterone present. In addition, the acid-base balance influences potassium excretion; with deficit of chloride, there is a concomitant loss of potassium in the distal tubules in exchange for sodium. Since hypochloremia presents an inadequate potassium exchange mechanism in the distal tubules, concomitant chloride replacement should accompany potassium supplementation in the correction of hypokalemia.[45]

Potassium depletion is often present in congestive heart failure. Thus, the secondary aldosteronism that frequently occurs in cardiac failure tends to augment sodium-potassium exchange at the distal site with associated potassium depletion. In addition, the thiazide diuretics—by their accelerated sodium delivery to the distal tubules—increase distal tubular exchange of sodium for potassium and thereby produce potassium loss. Further, the contraction alkalosis common with too vigorous diuretic therapy tends to force potassium into the intracellular space and results in hypokalemia. Conversely, there are circumstances in which hyperkalemia may occur in congestive heart failure. Thus, with markedly increased sodium reabsorption in the proximal tubules in severe heart failure, very little sodium may be delivered to the distal tubules, resulting in minimal sodium-potassium exchange and the possibility of hyperkalemia.

Several studies have pointed out the regulatory effect of potassium on the secretion of both renin and aldosterone. An increase in the potassium content of the perfusate of adrenal tissues accelerates aldosterone production.[46] Renin secretion is also affected by potassium, since plasma renin decreases when dietary potassium is increased.[22] Direct potassium infusion into the renal artery also causes a decline in renin activity.[47]

Summary

The fluid and electrolyte derangements in congestive heart failure are multifactorial. Decreased cardiac output is translated into diminished renal perfusion resulting in outer cortical ischemia with an increased percentage of total renal blood flow supplied to the inner cortex and medulla. Glomerular filtration is reduced, the filtration fraction is increased, and reabsorption of sodium and water in the proximal renal tubules is enhanced. In addition, lack of a postulated natriuretic hormone that normally rejects proximal renal tubular sodium reabsorption may play a role in the formation of the edematous state. The renin-angiotensin-aldosterone humoral system is also activated in congestive heart failure. Increased renin activity and the consequent augmentation of aldosterone secretion serve to increase sodium reabsorption in the distal tubules at the expense of potassium loss. Inappropriate secretion of antidiuretic hormone may occur in some patients with heart failure and contributes to dilutional hyponatremia. Increased activity of the sympathetic nervous system partitions regional blood flow away from the kidneys, redistributes intrarenal blood flow from cortical to medullary areas, and stimulates the renin-aldosterone humoral system. In the early stages of congestive heart failure, increased net proximal renal tubular reabsorption of sodium is the predominant feature in fluid retention; however, in the chronic edematous state, the renin-aldosterone humoral mechanism exerts a critical influence.

Acknowledgment: This work was supported in part by Research Program Project Grant HL 14780 from the National Heart and Lung Institute, National Institutes of Health.

The authors wish to thank Leslie J. Silvernail for her administrative and technical assistance.

References

1. **Mason DT, Spann JF, Zelis R, et al:** Alterations of hemodynamics and myocardial mechanics in patients with congestive heart failure: pathophysiologic mechanisms and assessment of cardiac function and ventricular contractility. Progr Cardiovasc Dis 12:507, 1970

2. **Braunwald E, Plauth WH, Morrow AG:** A method for the detection and quantifications of impaired sodium excretion: results of an oral sodium tolerance test in normal subjects and in patients with heart disease. Circulation 32:223, 1965

3. **Pacifico AD, Digerness S, Kirklin JW:** Regression of body composition abnormalities after intracardiac op-

erations. Circulation 42:999, 1970

4. **Mason DT:** Control of the peripheral circulation in health and disease. Mod Conc Cardiovasc Dis 36:25, 1967

5. **Mason DT:** Autonomic nervous system and regulation of cardiovascular performance. Anesthesiology 29:670, 1968

6. **Merrill AJ:** Edema and decreased renal blood flow in patients with chronic congestive heart failure: evidence of "forward failure" as the primary cause of edema. J Clin Invest 25:389, 1946

7. **Mokotoff R, Ross G, Leiter L:** Renal plasma flow and sodium reabsorption and excretion in congestive heart failure. J Clin Invest 27:1, 1948

8. **Fritcher PH, Schroeder HA:** Studies on congestive heart failure; impaired renal excretion of sodium chloride. Amer J Med Sci 204:52, 1942

9. **Earley LE, Friedler RM:** Effects of combined renal vasodilation and pressor agents on renal hemodynamics and tubular reabsorption of sodium. J Clin Invest 45:542, 1966

10. **Brenner BM, Falcheik KH, Keinowitz RL, et al:** Relation between peritubular capillary protein concentration and fluid reabsorption by renal proximal tubule. J Clin Invest 48:1519, 1969

11. **Barger AC:** Renal hemodynamics in congestive heart failure. Ann NY Acad Sci 139:276, 1966

12. **Rosen SM, Hollenberg NK, Dealy JB, et al:** Measurement of the distribution of blood flow in the human kidney using the intra-arterial injection of ^{133}Xe. Relationship to function in normal and transplanted kidney. Clin Sci 34:287, 1968

13. **Rosen SM, Touniger BP, Krek HR, et al:** Intrarenal distribution of blood flow in the normal and transplanted dog kidney: effect of denervation and rejection. J Clin Invest 46:1239, 1967

14. **Thorburn GD, Kopald HH, Herd JA, et al:** Intrarenal distribution of nutrient blood flow, determined with krypton 85 in the unanesthetized dog. Circ Res 13:290, 1963

15. **Fluck DC, Evans TR, Siggers DC, et al:** Distribution of renal blood flow in patients with heart disease. Clin Sci 42:627, 1972

16. **Seymour WB, Pritchard WH, Langley LP, et al:** Cardiac output, blood and interstitial fluid volumes, total circulating serum protein, and kidney function during cardiac failure and after improvement. J Clin Invest 21:229, 1942

17. **Heller BI, Jacobson WE:** Renal hemodynamics in heart disease. Amer Heart J 39:188, 1950

18. **Peart WS:** Renin-angiotensin system. New Eng J Med 292:302, 1975

19. **Oparil S, Haber E:** The renin-angiotensin system. New Eng J Med 291:389, 1974

20. **Davis JO:** The role of the adrenal cortex and kidney in the pathogenesis of cardiac edema. Yale J Biol Med 35:402, 1963

21. **Wolff HP, Bette L, Blaise H, et al:** Role of aldosterone in edema formation. Ann NY Acad Sci 139:285, 1966

22. **Sealey JE, Kirshman JD, Laragh JH:** Natriuretic activity in plasma and urine of salt-loaded man and sheep. J Clin Invest 48:2210, 1969

23. **Bricker NS:** The control of sodium excretion with normal and reduced nephron populations. Amer J Med 43:313, 1967

24. **Blythe WB, Weit LG:** Dissociation between filtered load of sodium and its rate of excretion in urine. J Clin Invest 42:1491, 1963

25. **Martinez-Maldonado M, Kurtzman NA, Rector FC, et al:** Evidence for a hormonal inhibitor of proximal tubular reabsorption. J Clin Invest 46:1091, 1967

26. **Relman AS, Schwartz WB:** The effect of DOCA on electrolyte balance in normal man and its relation to sodium chloride intake. Yale J Biol Med 24:540, 1952

27. **August JT, Nelson DH, Thorn GW:** Response of normal subjects to large amounts of aldosterone. J Clin Invest 37:1549, 1958

28. **Gill JR, Mason DT, Bartter, FC:** Adrenergic nervous system in sodium metabolism: effects of guanethidine and sodium-retaining steroids in normal man. J Clin Invest 43:177, 1964

29. **Nelson DH, August JT:** Abnormal response of oedematous patients to aldosterone or deoxycortone. Lancet 2:883, 1959

30. **Urquhart J, Davis JO, Higgins JT:** Simulation of spontaneous secondary hyperaldosteronism by intravenous infusion of angiotensin II in dogs with an arteriovenous fistula. J Clin Invest 43:1355, 1964

31. **Gill JR, Mason DT, Bartter FC:** Idiopathic edema resulting from occult cardiomyopathy. Amer J Med 38:475, 1965

32. **Johnson C, Davis JO, Howards SS, et al:** Cross-circulation experiments on the mechanism of the natriuresis during saline loading in the dog. Circ Res 21:1, 1967

33. **Muirhead EE:** The role of the renal medulla in hypertension. In, Advances in Internal Medicine (Stollerman GH, ed). Chicago, Year Book Medical, 1974, p 81

34. **Berliner RW, Levinsky NG, Davidson DG, et al:** Dilution and concentration of the urine and the action of antidiuretic hormone. Amer J Med 24:730, 1958

35. **Goetz KL, Bond GC, Bloxham DD:** Atrial receptors and renal function. Physiol Rev 55:157, 1975

36. **Laragh JH:** Hormones and the pathogenesis of congestive heart failure: vasopressin, aldosterone and angiotensin II. Further evidence for renal-adrenal interaction from studies in hypertension and in cirrhosis. Circulation 25:1015, 1962

37. **Bartter FC, Schwartz WB:** The syndrome of inappropriate secretion of antidiuretic hormone. Amer J Med 42:790, 1967

38. **Reid IA, Schrier RW, Earley LE:** An effect of extrarenal beta adrenergic stimulation on the release of renin. J Clin Invest 51:1861, 1972

39. **Vandongen R, Pert WS, Boyd GW:** Adrenergic stimulation of renin secretion in the isolated perfused rat kidney. Circ Res 32:290, 1973

40. **Mason DT, Braunwald E:** Effects of guanethidine, reserpine and methyldopa on reflex venous and arterial constriction in man. J Clin Invest 43:1449, 1964

41. **Cohn JN:** Relationship of plasma volume changes to resistance and capacitance vessel effects of sympathomimetic amines and angiotensin in man. Clin Sci 30:267, 1966

42. **Mason DT, Melmon KL:** Abnormal forearm vascular

responses in the carcinoid syndrome: the role of kinins and kinin-generating system. J Clin Invest 45:1685, 1966

43. **Mason DT, Bartter FC:** Autonomic regulation of blood volume. Anesthesiology 29:681, 1968

44. **Gaffney TE, Braunwald E:** Importance of the adrenergic nervous system in support of circulatory function in patients with congestive heart failure. Amer J Med 34:320, 1963

45. **Daxsier JP, Schwartz WB:** Correction of metabolic alkalosis in man without repair of potassium deficiency. Reevaluation of the role of potassium. Amer J Med 40:19, 1966

46. **Dluhy RG, Axelrod L, Underwood RH:** Studies on the control of plasma aldosterone concentration in normal man. Effect of dietary potassium and potassium infusion. J Clin Invest 51:1950, 1972

47. **Davis JO:** The regulation of aldosterone secretion. In, The Adrenal Cortex (Eisenstein AB, ed). Boston, Little, Brown, 1967, p 203

PART II: EVALUATION

Chapter 14

Physical Findings in Heart Failure and Their Physiologic Basis

Robert A. O'Rourke, MD, FACC
Michael H. Crawford, MD

Recent advances in cardiac diagnostic techniques have strengthened the role of bedside cardiac examination in the detection of heart failure by elucidating the physiologic principles underlying certain abnormal physical findings. Thus, a careful physical examination remains one of the best noninvasive methods for the early detection of left and right heart failure. This chapter presents first the physical findings related to reduced myocardial function and subsequently the signs resulting from the operation of compensatory reserve mechanisms. Many of the physical findings in patients with heart failure are caused by a combination of myocardial dysfunction and the action of certain reserve mechanisms. Therefore, each physical finding will be discussed in the section that describes what we believe to be the major underlying mechanism.

Signs of Myocardial Dysfunction

Pulsus Alternans: One of the most frequently overlooked signs of abnormal left ventricular function is an alternation in the amplitude of the arterial pulse despite a regular rhythm. Often, pulsus alternans is noted first after a premature contraction. The degree of difference in the systolic pressure in alternating beats then diminishes for several cycles until the pulse amplitude

is again constant. The initiation of postextrasystolic pulsus alternans probably is related to the increased duration of left ventricular diastolic filling after the extrasystole resulting in a greater end-diastolic volume and hence increased contractile force due to the Frank-Starling mechanism. The enhanced left ventricular postextrasystolic contraction empties the ventricle more completely and the subsequent end-diastolic volume is lower than usual. This sequence then results in a diminished contraction that incompletely empties the ventricle, so that the subsequent beat starts from a higher end-diastolic volume and the arterial pulse strength alternates in a diminishing fashion until the control end-diastolic volume is reestablished.[1-3] This phenomenon usually does not occur in the normal left ventricle because contractile force is much less dependent on end-diastolic volume.[4]

Severe depression of left ventricular function often results in sustained pulsus alternans (Figure 1). There is alternation of aortic flow, systolic left ventricular pressure, aortic systolic pressure and the rate of rise of left ventricular pressure during systole in patients with pulsus alternans due to left ventricular failure. However, studies in animals and man with persistent pulsus alternans have failed to demonstrate consistently significant changes in left ventricular end-diastolic volume during alternate beats,

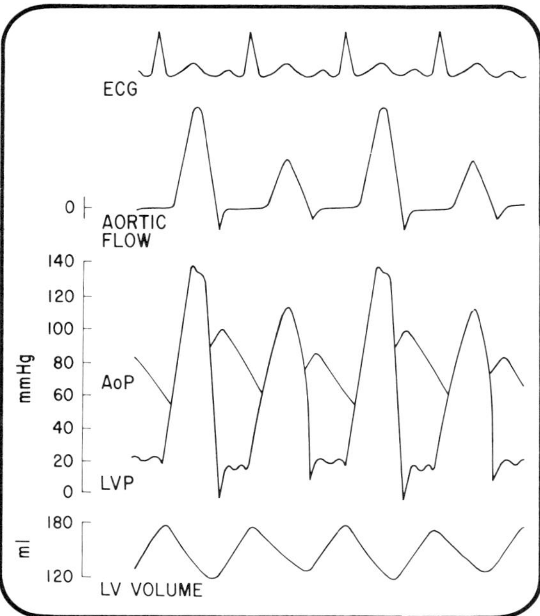

FIGURE 1. In this schematic presentation, the ECG, aortic flow velocity curve, aortic pressure pulse (AoP), left ventricular pressure curve (LVP) and left ventricular volume curve are shown in a patient with pulsus alternans. There is a decrease in the aortic flow velocity and stroke volume (end-diastolic minus end-systolic volume) in the beats with a diminished arterial pulse amplitude.

which may be due to the insensitivity of the techniques used for measuring small changes in ventricular volumes.[3,5] It has been postulated that sustained pulsus alternans is due to alternation of the contractile state of at least part of the left ventricular myocardium, which may be caused by a failure of electromechanical coupling in some cells during the diminished contraction. The subsequent enhanced contraction would then represent contraction of all cells, some of which were potentiated.[5] A premature contraction almost always transiently accentuates persistent pulsus alternans, and therefore alterations in excitation-contraction coupling and end-diastolic fiber length may be operant in the same patient.[3]

Pulsus alternans often is appreciated best by palpating a distal artery (for example, the radial) that has a slightly wider pulse pressure than that of more central arteries (for instance, the carotid). The patient should hold his breath, since the small changes in arterial pressure caused by normal respiration may lead to a false impression of pulsus alternans or obscure its recognition. The presence of pulsus alternans can be documented further using the sphygmomanometer to detect alternating Korotkov sounds at one level of systolic pressure and Korotkov sounds with every beat at a lower systolic pressure. The difference between the two pressure readings is the amount of alternans in millimeters of mercury. Pulsus alternans is often associated with a third heart sound (discussed later).

Dicrotic Pulse: Although this sign was originally described in patients with febrile illnesses such as typhoid, a palpable dicrotic carotid pulse is often associated with left ventricular failure.[6] The normal carotid pulse (Figure 2A) consists of an initial rapid rise to the anacrotic shoulder, which is coincident with peak carotid blood flow (percussion wave). The subsequent more slowly rising tidal wave is interrupted on its descending limb by the dicrotic notch, which closely follows aortic valve closure. The dicrotic notch is followed by a small diastolic wave, which usually is not palpable. Left ventricular failure may result in a diminished tidal wave and an accentuated diastolic wave that becomes palpable, producing the dicrotic pulse (Figure 2B). The dicrotic pulse is commonly observed in young patients with primary myocardial disease and advanced left ventricular failure, but it has also been described in low output states after open heart surgery, with pericardial tamponade and rarely in heart failure associated with atherosclerotic heart disease.[6–8]

Reduced stroke volume, a shortened ejection period and elevated peripheral vascular resistance appear to be the most significant factors producing the dicrotic pulse. Accordingly, the diastolic wave often is accentuated in beats that follow shorter diastoles during arrhythmias and during the low amplitude beats of pulsus alternans when stroke volume is smaller and left ventricular ejection time is shorter. Conversely, the diastolic wave is diminished during the beat after a premature contraction and during the high amplitude beats of pulsus alternans because of the augmented stroke volume and the longer left ventricular ejection time in these beats. The importance of peripheral vascular resistance can be demonstrated by the augmentation of the diastolic wave produced by arterial compression distal to the site of palpation and by local intraarterial infusion of vasoconstricting agents. Furthermore, lowering of peripheral vascular resistance with amyl nitrite inhalation decreases the diastolic wave.[6,7]

Chest Examination: Left ventricular failure leads to a rise in left atrial pressure that is transmitted to the pulmonary capillaries. When pulmonary capillary hydrostatic pressure exceeds colloid osmotic pressure, transudation of fluid into the interstitial spaces leads to increased pulmonary extravascular fluid content.[9] This interstitial edema may result in bronchiolar edema and the audible wheezes of "cardiac asthma." When the capability of the lymphatic system to drain the interstitial fluid is compromised by increased systemic venous pressure or by fibrosis or when the hydrostatic pressure is excessive (usually greater than 25 mm Hg), transudation of fluid into the alveoli results. Alveolar fluid produces audible inspiratory rales first in the most dependent parts of the lungs and finally throughout all lung fields. Pulmonary rales are not specific for heart disease and can be found in primary lung disease and certain systemic diseases. Rales due to lung disease represent the most difficult diagnostic problem, but they often can be differentiated by their failure to migrate to the most dependent part of the lungs with changes in body position as the rales of heart failure usually do. For example, inspiratory rales due to heart disease may only be heard over the right lung when the patient has been in the right lateral decubitus position for 30 minutes or longer.

Pleural effusions are common in chronic congestive heart failure and although they most often occur on the right, they may also be left-sided or bilateral. Starling's law of capillary exchange indicates that there should be transudation of fluid from the systemic capillaries of the parietal pleura and reabsorption by the pulmonary capillaries of the visceral pleura.[10] Theoretically, therefore, increases in systemic venous or pulmonary capillary pressure could lead to pleural effusions. However, animal experiments suggest that increases in the former are more important than are those in the latter.[11] This apparently necessary elevation of systemic venous

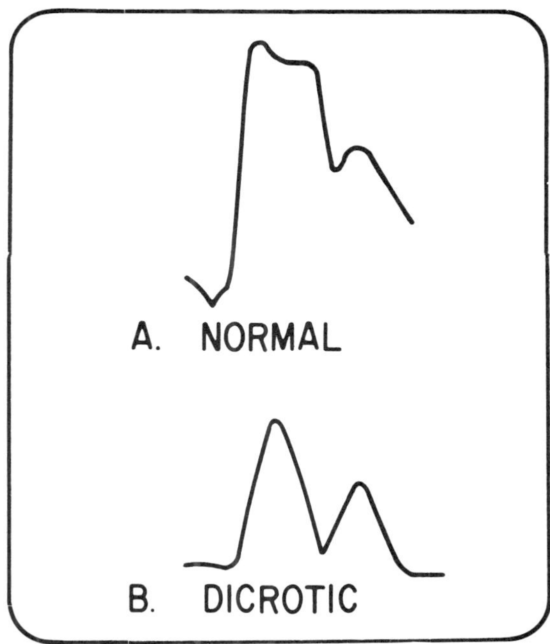

FIGURE 2. The normal carotid arterial pulse (**A**) is compared with the abnormal dicrotic pulse (**B**). The dicrotic pulse results from a decrease in the amplitude of the systolic wave and an increase in the amplitude of the dicrotic wave, which becomes palpable (see text).

pressure is consistent with the clinical observation that hydrothorax most often occurs with right ventricular or biventricular failure. Pneumonia and pulmonary emboli can also cause pleural effusions, and since these disorders are often associated with heart failure, determination of the cause of hydrothorax may be difficult using the physical examination alone.

Jugular Venous Pulse: The normal jugular venous pulse represents the phasic pressure changes in the right atrium. Right ventricular diastolic pressure rises with right heart failure and this leads to an elevation of right atrial pressure, which is reflected in the jugular venous pulse. Salt and water retention and increased adrenergic tone (discussed later) also contribute to the elevated central venous pressure in right heart failure. This elevated pressure is best observed in the right internal jugular vein, with the head of the patient elevated so that the top of the oscillating column of blood can easily be seen. The height of this column is estimated using the sternal angle as the reference point, since in the average patient the center of the right atrium is approximately 5 cm below the sternal angle, regardless of body position.[12] The vertical distance between the level of the sternal angle and the top of the oscillating column of blood is normally less than 3 cm (3 cm + 5 cm = 8 cm of blood).

The normal jugular venous pulse exhibits two prominent waves during each cardiac cycle. The dominant wave is the presystolic "a" wave, which is generated by right atrial contraction. The second wave is the late systolic "v" wave, which results from the increasing volume of blood flowing into the right atrium during right ventricular systole when the tricuspid valve is closed. When tricuspid regurgitation results from right ventricular dilatation secondary to right heart failure, the "v" wave of the jugular venous pulse will occur earlier and be accentuated. The "a" wave of the jugular venous pulse may be accentuated when right heart failure accompanies severe right ventricular hypertension and diminished right ventricular compliance, but a large "a" wave in the jugular venous pulse is not a sign of right heart failure per se.

The careful observer can distinguish between these two waves of jugular venous pulse by simultaneous palpation of the opposite carotid artery, since the systolic arterial pulse occurs between the "a" and "v" waves of the jugular venous pulse. Occasionally, prominent carotid pulsations may cause confusion in interpreting the jugular venous pulse. However, light pressure above the clavicle obliterates venous waves so that the carotid pulsations can be separated from the internal jugular pulsations, which reappear when the pressure is released.

Abdominal Examination: Elevated right atrial pressure also increases venous pressure in the abdomen, which causes engorgement of the abdominal organs. Hepatomegaly is the usual finding, and further elevation of venous pressure also produces splenomegaly. When these organs are also tender, acute congestion is suggested. Severe tricuspid regurgitation may lead to palpable systolic pulsations in the liver. Ascites may occur in severe chronic heart failure and will be discussed later.

In patients with a normal jugular venous

pulse who are suspected of having right ventricular failure, an abnormal rise in central venous pressure often can be elicited by gradually applying pressure to the right upper quadrant of the abdomen with the open hand for 30 to 60 seconds. Presumably, the increased abdominal pressure greatly enhances venous return to the failing right heart, which cannot accept the increased blood volume, causing a persistent rise in right atrial pressure and the jugular venous pulse. This abnormal rise in the jugular venous pulse is also dependent on increased venous tone.[13] This "hepatojugular reflux" maneuver may also accentuate the "v" wave of tricuspid regurgitation.

Cardiac Auscultation: Ventricular failure almost always is accompanied by a low frequency early diastolic sound which is audible when the bell of the stethoscope is placed lightly over the apex of the left ventricle in patients with left ventricular failure or over the right ventricle in patients with right ventricular failure. This early diastolic gallop or third heart sound is coincident with rapid filling of the ventricle and is sometimes accompanied by a palpable rapid filling wave in mid-diastole. The third heart sound is one of the early signs of ventricular failure. A presystolic or fourth heart sound may be heard in patients with heart failure but it is not by itself a sign of ventricular decompensation. It usually is associated with decreased diastolic compliance of the ventricle. When tachycardia is present, the third and fourth sounds may merge during diastole to produce a loud summation gallop.[14] The third heart sound may be heard in normal young persons, in patients with high output states and in patients who have mitral or tricuspid valve regurgitation but not heart failure.

The depressed rate of rise of left ventricular pressure in the failing heart leads to a decrease in the intensity of the first heart sound. Heart sounds also may alternate in intensity if pulsus alternans is present. Left ventricular ejection is often delayed when the myocardium fails. If the delay is long enough relative to right ventricular ejection, the pulmonic component of the second sound may precede the aortic component, causing a split second sound during expiration. During inspiration when the pulmonic second sound is delayed, the split will close, resulting in reversed splitting of the second sound. In the absence of left bundle branch block, such reversed splitting in patients with left heart failure suggests severe impairment of left ventricular function.[15]

Detection of Compensatory Mechanisms

Increased Sympathetic Tone: One of the earliest occurring compensatory mechanisms in myocardial decompensation is increased sympathetic tone. Sympathetic stimulation augments cardiac output and causes selective peripheral vasoconstriction, which increases blood pressure and directs blood flow to vital organs. The most easily detected sign of increased sympathetic tone is an increase in the resting heart rate. More specific, perhaps, is the excessive rise in pulse rate that persists after minimal exertion—such as changing position in bed to facilitate the physical examination. The sympathetic discharge in acute heart failure may elevate the blood pressure to abnormal levels, but this effect is usually transient. Venoconstriction due to increased sympathetic tone may contribute to the increased jugular venous pressure mentioned previously.

A subtle sign of increased sympathetic tone is a diminished or absent circulatory response to the Valsalva maneuver. The maneuver consists of forceful expiration of air against the closed glottis. Initially (Figure 3A) there is a small rise in systemic arterial pressure, which probably results from the sudden emptying of blood from the pulmonary bed into the left atrium and from augmentation of left ventricular ejection due to increased intrathoracic pressure. Right ventricular inflow is impeded, however, and there is a subsequent fall in cardiac output and systemic blood pressure, which in a normal person causes the baroreceptors to stimulate sympathetically mediated vasoconstriction and cardiac acceleration. After 10 seconds or more the maneuver is halted and there is a sudden augmentation of right and then left ventricular filling and hence systemic stroke output. This causes an overshoot in the systemic blood pressure that results in a reflex bradycardia. The patient with increased sympathetic tone secondary to mild left ventricular failure may not display the char-

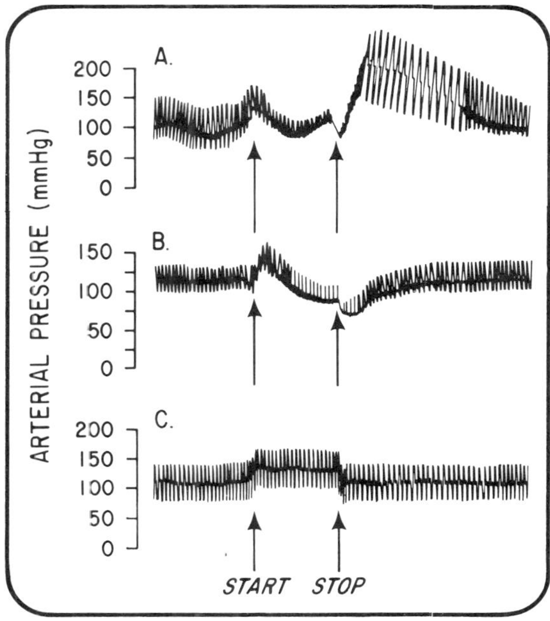

FIGURE 3. The effect of the Valsalva maneuver on the systemic arterial pressure pulse is shown in a normal subject (**A**), in a patient with mild left ventricular failure (**B**) and in a patient with overt congestive heart failure (**C**). The duration of the Valsalva maneuver is indicated by the vertical arrows (see text).

acteristic normal blood pressure overshoot and diminution of heart rate (Figure 3B). These changes usually can be appreciated by carefully palpating the brachial artery. However, the abnormal response to the Valsalva maneuver is not specific for heart failure and may be seen with various diseases affecting the autonomic nervous system.[16] Furthermore, this maneuver should be performed cautiously in patients with myocardial ischemia or recent infarction because of transiently decreased coronary blood flow.[17]

In overt congestive heart failure, pulmonary venous congestion serves as a reservoir that tends to maintain left ventricular filling during the Valsalva maneuver. Consequently, left ventricular ejection is sustained and systemic blood pressure remains elevated with the increase in intrathoracic pressure.[18] Thus, baroreceptor stimulation remains constant and there is no overshoot in systemic blood pressure or reflex bradycardia when the maneuver is halted (Figure 3C). This abnormal response to the Valsalva maneuver also is seen in other conditions involving increased pulmonary blood volume, such as large atrial septal defects.

As heart failure progresses, sympathetic vasoconstriction causes a decrease in skin temperature, especially in the distal extremities, and an increase in sweating, which result in the cool, clammy hands of the patient with severe heart failure. As the blood flow to the skin decreases in an attempt to shunt blood to vital organs, a mottled or reticulated cyanosis often appears initially in the distal extremities and later progresses to the knees and elbows and finally, the trunk.

Ventricular Dilatation: As left ventricular failure progresses, ventricular dilatation ensues in an attempt to maintain cardiac output by the Frank-Starling mechanism. Left ventricular enlargement can be detected by palpation of the precordium. Percussion of the extent of cardiac dullness occasionally can be useful but is not a reliable indicator of cardiac size. The normal left ventricular impulse in the supine position is a brief tap in the fourth or fifth intercostal space medial to the mid-clavicular line that occurs when the cardiac apex contacts the chest wall in early systole. An apical impulse that is lateral to the mid-clavicular line or increased in size (greater than 3 cm in diameter) is indicative of an enlarged left ventricle in the absence of apical dyskinesis or massive right ventricular enlargement (discussed later). Rarely, the heart may be so enlarged that it compresses the posterior left lung, causing signs of consolidation at the left posterior lung base (Ewart's sign).

Left ventricular dilatation often leads to concomitant dilatation of the mitral valve ring, which may result in systolic regurgitant murmurs. The dilated ventricle also changes its shape and the subsequent altered alignment of the papillary muscles and chordae tendineae may also contribute to incompetence of the mitral valve leaflets.[19] Such altered geometry of the mitral valve and it's supporting apparatus may occur during certain parts of systole, resulting in late, mid or even early systolic murmurs. The absence of the classic pansystolic blowing murmur of mitral valve regurgitation may lead to the false impression that the murmur is due to flow across the aortic or pulmonic valve. Usually the murmur of mitral regurgitation can be intensified by augmenting peripheral resistance during handgrip exercise, and it does not change in intensity during the cardiac cycle after a premature contraction as does the usual outflow tract murmur, which becomes much louder.[20] The murmur of mitral regurgitation is best heard over the left ventricular apex with the patient in the left lateral decubitus position but may radiate anteriorly to the aortic area or posteriorly to the back depending upon the direction of the regurgitant jet in the atrium.

Tricuspid regurgitation can result from right ventricular failure and dilatation. It is best detected at the lower left sternal border where the murmur increases in intensity during the inspiratory augmentation of right heart blood flow. When pulmonary hypertension is present the murmur of tricuspid regurgitation is pansystolic, but when right ventricular pressure is lower the murmur often is heard only in early systole when the gradient between the right ventricle and right atrium is the highest.

Salt and Water Retention: Heart failure leads to a gradual retention of salt and water by the kidneys through multiple mechanisms. These mechanisms can be divided into three discrete factors for convenience. First, diminished cardiac output from the failing heart leads to a reduction in renal blood flow and in the glomerular filtration rate and therefore decreases salt and water excretion acutely. Second, and more important, is the increased secretion of aldosterone by the adrenal glands secondary to the activation of the renin-angiotensin system by the reduced renal blood flow in patients with heart failure. Also, aldosterone levels often are elevated in severe heart failure because of a decreased hepatic clearance caused by the reduced hepatic blood flow. Third, there appears to be a so-called extra-adrenal sodium-retaining factor operant in heart failure that has not been fully characterized.[21] Fluid retention is often manifested only by an increase in the patient's weight.

As heart failure worsens, the combination of increased capillary hydrostatic pressure and decreased lymph flow due to elevated venous pressure and excessive salt and water retention lead to the transudation of fluid into the interstitial spaces of the dependent parts of the body.

Edema may appear first in the left ankle because of the slightly increased venous pressure in the left leg, which is a result of the compression of the left common iliac vein against the spine by the crossing of the right common iliac artery at its origin from the aorta. In bedridden patients, dependent edema first appears in the sacral area or the inner aspects of the thighs. Severe long-standing heart failure can lead to anasarca and ascites. The latter usually occurs when excessive venous pressure and fluid retention are accompanied by a low serum albumin concentration.

Ventricular Hypertrophy: Chronic heart failure eventually results in progressive ventricular hypertrophy, and palpation of the precordium is probably a more sensitive method for detecting ventricular hypertrophy than is the electrocardiogram. Furthermore, concentric hypertrophy without dilatation may not enlarge the cardiac silhouette on the chest x-ray film.[22] Left ventricular hypertrophy results in an increase in the amplitude and duration of the apical impulse, often without modification of its location. In emphysematous or thick-chested patients, abnormalities in the character of the apical left ventricular impulse are best appreciated with the patient in the left lateral decubitus position. Normally, the decreasing right ventricular volume during systole produces a slight inward movement of the chest wall along the left sternal border. As the right ventricle undergoes hypertrophy, the normal inward motion is replaced by an abnormal outward motion with an amplitude and duration roughly proportional to the degree of right ventricular hypertrophy.[23] In patients with right ventricular hypertrophy due to pulmonary hypertension resulting from chronic obstructive lung disease, the right ventricular impulse may only be felt below the xiphoid process during inspiration as an inferiorly directed systolic impulse.

Summary

The value of certain physical findings in heart failure has been strenthened by an increased understanding of underlying physiologic principles. On examination of the peripheral arterial pulses, the resting heart rate and blood pressure should be assessed and also their response to the Valsalva maneuver. Also, the peripheral arteries should be palpated carefully for pulsus alternans and a dicrotic pulse. Examination of the chest may reveal audible rales and wheezes and signs of hydrothorax. The jugular venous pressure may be elevated and the configuration of its pressure waves altered. Cardiac palpation often demonstrates abnormal pulsations due to ventricular dilatation or hypertrophy. Cardiac auscultation may uncover abnormal heart sounds and regurgitant murmurs. Examination of the abdomen may reveal signs of organomegaly and fluid retention. Finally, heart failure causes a decrease in skin temperature, an increase in perspiration and dependent edema.

References

1. **Gleason WL, Braunwald E:** Studies on Starling's law of the heart. VI. Relationships between left ventricular end-diastolic volume and stroke volume in man with observations on the mechanism of pulsus alternans. Circulation 25:841, 1962
2. **Mitchell JH, Sarnoff SJ, Sonnenblick EH:** The dynamics of pulsus alternans: alternating end-diastolic fiber length as a causative factor. J Clin Invest 42:55, 1963
3. **Cohn KE, Sandler H, Hancock EW:** Mechanisms of pulsus alternans. Circulation 36:372, 1967
4. **Ross J Jr, Sobel BE:** Regulation of cardiac contraction. Ann Rev Phys ol 34:47, 1972
5. **Guntheroth WG, Morgan BC, McGough GA, et al:** Alternate deletion and potentiation as the cause of pulsus alternans. Amer Heart J 78:669, 1969
6. **Meadows WR, Draur RA, Osadjan CE:** Dicrotism in heart disease, correlations with cardiomyopathy, pericard al tamponade, youth, tachycardia, and normotension. Amer Heart J 82:596, 1971
7. **Ewy GA, Rios JC, Marcus FI:** The dicrotic arterial pulse. Circulation 39:655, 1969
8. **Barner HB, Willman VL, Kaiser GC:** Dicrotic pulse after open heart operation. Circulation 42:993, 1970
9. **Yu PN:** Lung water in congestive heart failure. Mod Conc Cardiovasc Dis 40:27, 1971
10. **Agostoni E, Mead J:** Statics of the respiratory system. In, Handbook of Physiology, sect 3, vol I (Fenn WO, Hermann R, ed). Washington, American Physiological Society, 1964, p 401
11. **Mellins RB, Levine OR, Fishman AP:** Effect of systemic

and pulmonary venous hypertension on pleural and pericardial fluid accumulation. J Appl Physiol 29:564, 1970

12. **Wood P:** Diseases of the Heart and Circulation. Philadelphia, JB Lippincott, 1956, p 45

13. **Constant J, Lippschutz EJ:** The one-minute abdominal compression test or "the hepatojugular reflux," a useful bedside test. Amer Heart J 67:701, 1964

14. **Shah PM, Gramiak R, Kramer DH, et al:** Determinants of atrial (S_4) and ventricular (S_3) gallop sounds in primary myocardial disease. New Eng J Med 278:753, 1968

15. **O'Rourke RA, Braunwald E:** Physical examination of the heart. In, Principles of Internal Medicine (Wintrobe MM, Thorn GW, Adams RD, et al, ed). New York, McGraw-Hill, 1974, p 1078

16. **Thomson PD, Melmon KL:** Clinical assessment of autonomic function. Anaesthesia 29:724, 1968

17. **Benchimol A, Wang TF, Desser KB, et al:** The Valsalva maneuver and coronary arterial blood flow velocity. Ann Intern Med 77:357, 1972

18. **Judson WE, Hatcher JD, Wilkins RW:** Blood pressure responses to the Valsalva maneuver in cardiac patients with and without congestive failure. Circulation 11:889, 1955

19. **Perloff JK, Roberts WC:** The mitral apparatus, functional anatomy of mitral regurgitation. Circulation 46:227, 1972

20. **Dohan MC, Criscitiello MG:** Physiological and pharmacological manipulatons of heart sounds and murmurs. Mod Conc Cardiovasc Dis 39:121, 1970

21. **Davis JO:** Mechanisms of salt and water retention in cardiac failure. In, The Myocardium: Failure and Infarction (Braunwald E, ed). New York, HP Publishing, 1972, p 80

22. **Toutouzas P, Shillingford J:** Impulse cardiogram in early diagnosis of left ventricular dysfunction in hypertension. Brit Heart J 31:97, 1969

23. **Eddleman EE Jr:** Examination of the precordial movements. In, The Heart (Hurst JW, Logue RB, Schlant RC, et al, ed). New York, McGraw-Hill, 1966, p 189

Chapter 15

Echographic Evaluation of Cardiac Function

Anthony N. DeMaria, MD, FACC
Alexander L. Neumann, BS
Dean T. Mason, MD, FACC

The most important diagnostic tool in cardiovascular medicine developed within the past decade is echocardiography. This noninvasive technique is based upon the utilization of pulsed, reflected ultrasound to obtain a graphic representation of dynamic cardiac anatomy.[1] A large number of recent studies have clearly documented the value of ultrasonography in the detection and management of a multiplicity of cardiovascular disorders and the method has now become an integral component of the clinical diagnostic armamentarium of the modern cardiologist. The purpose of this chapter is to consider the advantages and limitations of echocardiography in the assessment of cardiac function.

Ultrasonic Principles

To provide proper perspective for this discussion, the technical principles underlying the utilization of ultrasound to record intracardiac structures are briefly reviewed. By definition, ultrasound includes any sounds of frequencies above 20 thousand cycles per second, thereby exceeding human audibility. However, clinical echocardiography utilizes sonic waves of considerably greater frequency—2 to 3 million cycles per second—since such waves may readily be directed as a beam that will closely obey the natural laws of reflection and refraction.[2] The

sound beam usually is generated by a piezo-electrode crystal, which alternately expands and is compressed when it is subjected to an intermittent electrical current. This same piezoelectrode also acts to receive the returning sound waves reflected from tissue interfaces during cyclic periods of nonactivation and converts them into electrical signals that can then be recorded.

In actual practice, the echograph transducer is positioned on the chest wall along the left sternal border and is directed posteriorly. The ultrasonic beam generated travels in a straight line until an interface of differential acoustic impendance—between muscle and blood or between muscle and air—is encountered. At this interface, some sound waves are transmitted, others are refracted, and certain sound waves are reflected back to the piezoelectrode transducer, which converts them into electrical signals. The percentage of reflected sound waves (echoes) depends upon how nearly perpendicular to the interface is the transmitted sonic beam.

Sound travels at relatively constant velocity through soft tissues. Thus, the distance of any interface from the transducer can be calculated from the knowledge of the time required for transmission and return of a sound wave from the structure; such electrical circuitry is stan-

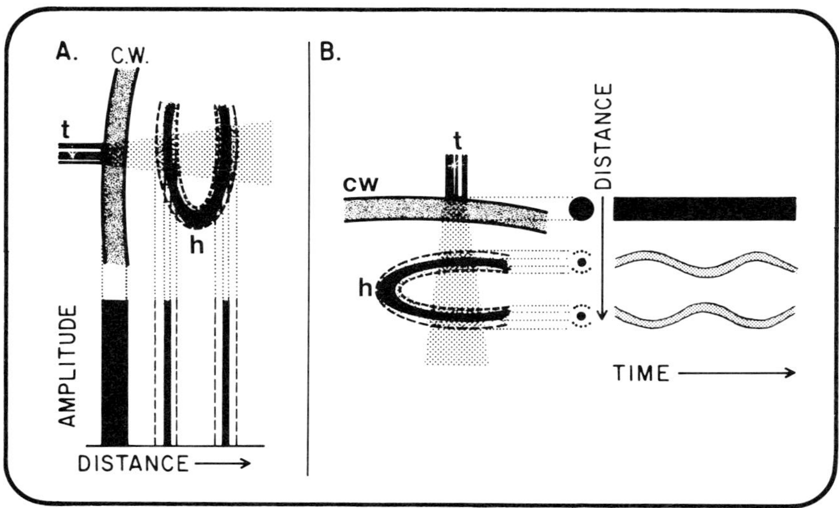

FIGURE 1. Schematic illustrations of the two major modes of presentation of the ultrasound signals obtained from an echocardiographic examination. **A,** the A mode presentation of these data wherein the amplitude of the echo signals returning from the various cardiovascular structures is plotted along the vertical axis, while the distance of these structures from the echographic transducer (t) is recorded on the horizontal axis. As shown in the diagram, since the heart (h) moves throughout the cardiac cycle (**dotted lines**), the echo signals are observed to move toward (to the left) or away (to the right) during the various phases of systole and diastole. **B,** the time-motion (M mode), in which the echo signals are represented by dots whose amplitude is related to brightness and size. The distance from the origin of the various echo signals to the transducer is plotted along the vertical axis. The dot signals so obtained are then swept from left to right as a function of time, so that the motion of the corresponding anatomic structures toward and away from the transducer during the various phases of the cardiac cycle are represented by alterations in the position of the dots according to time. CW=chest wall.

dard equipment on commercial echographs. This ability to measure the depth of an ultrasound interface is utilized in displaying the echographic signals, which are both depicted and recorded as electrical signals at a given distance from the transducer. In one modality of presentation, termed "A" (for amplitude) mode, the ultrasonic signals are arranged relative to distance from the transducer along the horizontal axis and according to amplitude on the vertical axis (Figure 1A). In the most commonly used modality of clinical echo presentation, called "M" (for motion) mode, the echo from a given structure is represented as a dot in which amplitude is expressed by its intensity and size. This dot is displayed on a horizontal axis relative to its distance from the transducer and then swept along the vertical axis with time (Figure 1B). Thus M mode provides an opportunity to record the motion of the various cardiac structures as they alter their position in relation to the transducer during the phases of the cardiac cycle.

Normal Echocardiographic Features

Figure 2 is a schematic illustration of the cardiovascular structures from which echoes can be obtained and a typical graphic M mode record that such signals produce. With the echo transducer angled inferiorly and to the patient's left, the ultrasound beam traverses the plane through the cardiac apex as indicated by Sector 1. Thus, in Sector 1, the initial echo-producing structures traversed are the chest wall and the anterior right ventricular wall, the echoes from which are recorded at the top of the tracing immediately below the crystal artifact produced by the transducer. Subsequently, the sound beam traverses the right ventricular cavity, which appears as a sonolucent area; the interventricular septum, with accentuation of endocardial surfaces; the left ventricular cavity, which again is echo-free; and the left ventricular posterior wall, which is the most posterior echo-producing cardiovascular structure, as

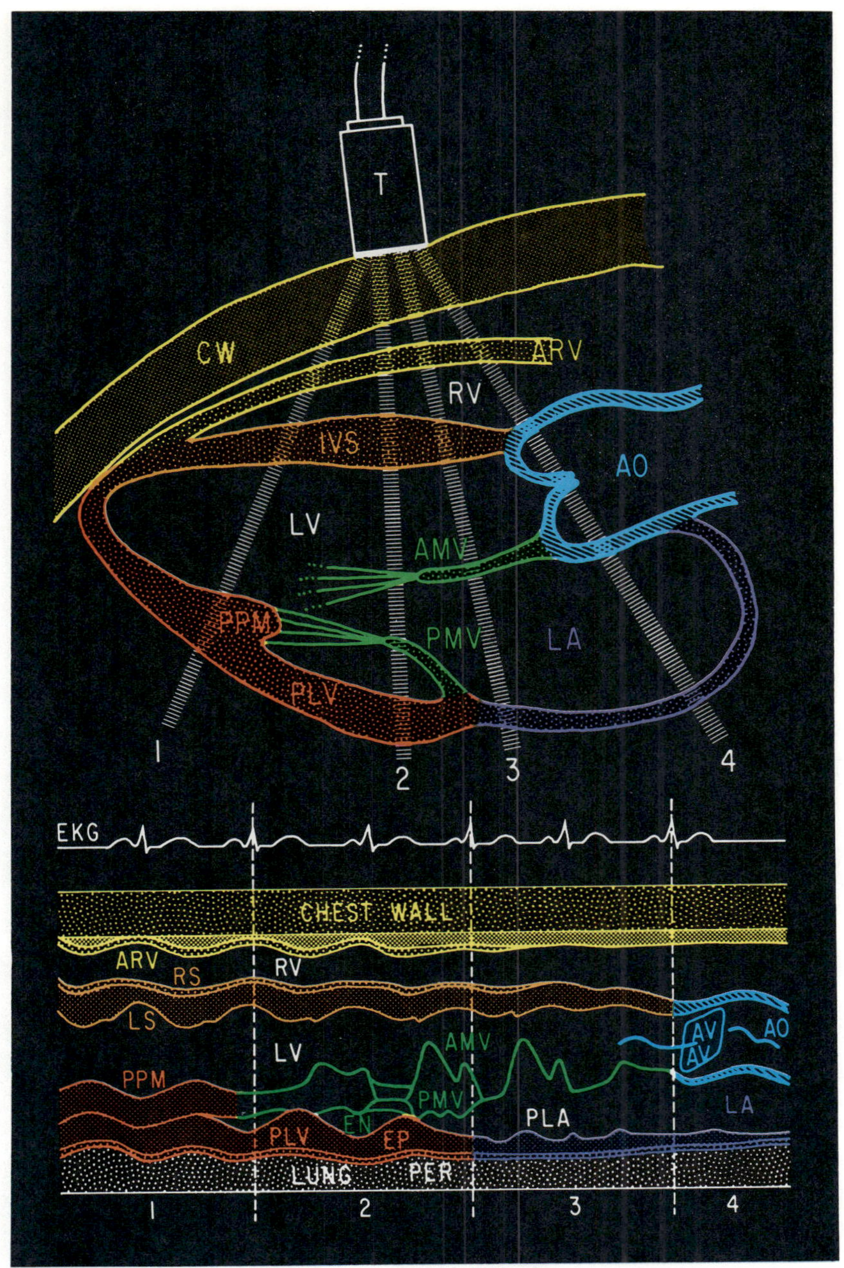

FIGURE 2. Schematic representation of the cardiovascular structures from which echo signals can be obtained and a typical M mode record that such signals produce. Four sectors are illustrated as the transducer is arched from apex to base. AMV = anterior mitral valve; AO = ascending aorta; ARV = anterior right ventricular wall; AV = aortic valve leaflets; CW = chest wall; EN = endocardium; EP = epicardium; IVS = interventricular septum; LA = left atrium; LS = left IVS endocardium; LV = left ventricle; PER = pericardium; PLA = posterior left atrial wall; PLV = posterior left ventricular wall; PMV = posterior mitral valve; PPM = posterior papillary muscle; RS = right IVS endocardium; RV = right ventricle; T = transducer. (Adapted by permission from Feigenbaum.[103])

shown on the ultrasound tracing from above to below. During the cardiac cycle, these heart structures alter their position with reference to the transducer as contraction and relaxation occur, and this motion is exemplified by the movement of the interventricular septum and the left ventricular posterior wall during the cardiac cycle contained between the designated QRS complexes in Sector 1 on Figure 2. When the position of the transducer is then progressively arced superiorly and to the patient's right, the echo beam transects the mitral leaflets, the aorta, the aortic leaflets, and the left atrium as observed in Sectors 2, 3 and 4, respectively (Figure 2).

The mitral valve presents the most dramatic and easily recognizable echographic pattern and is the most commonly utilized landmark from which to locate the other cardiovascular structures. Thus, the mitral leaflets coapt at the onset of systole, designated as the C point, and exhibit one to three echoes, which pursue a gradual straight-line anterior movement attributed to gradual forward motion of the mitral annulus as the left ventricle empties and the left atrium fills. At the onset of diastole (D point), the mitral valve opens and the anterior mitral leaflet echo is recorded as a brisk forward motion to full excursion towards the transducer at the E point (Figure 2). The anterior leaflet then floats posteriorly towards a closed position in response to rapid ventricular filling to reach the F point during the first third of diastole. In response to atrial contraction during late diastole, the anterior leaflet again moves abruptly forward (A point) and then returns posterior to a closed position at the onset of systole. The com-

posite diastolic motion of the anterior mitral leaflet therefore describes an "M" configuration, whereas the posterior mitral leaflet demonstrates a mirror image "W" contour (Figure 2).

In contrast to mitral valve motion, the opening movements of the aortic cusps occur during left ventricular ejection (Figure 2). Thus, the temporal echographic configuration of the aortic valve leaflets is comprised of single opening and closing motions, which manifest a box-type appearance during systole. Echoes may also be recorded from the tricuspid and pulmonic valves and resemble the mitral and aortic valve motions, respectively.

Figure 3 is an actual echographic scan obtained in a normal subject in our laboratory, demonstrating the dynamic behavior of the cardiac structures just described. Thus, an echocardiographic scan noninvasively provides accurate information regarding right ventricular, left ventricular, left atrial and aortic size, as well as the movements of the interventricular septum and left ventricular posterior wall and the cardiac valves.

Echocardiography in Cardiac Diagnosis

Numerous investigations have clearly established the role of echocardiography in the diagnosis of a variety of cardiovascular disorders. The mitral valve echogram reveals pathognomonic alterations in mitral stenosis[3-5] (Figure 4), mitral prolapse[6-9] (Figure 5), idiopathic hypertrophic subaortic stenosis[10-16] (Figure 6) and left atrial myxoma[17-21] (Figure 7). Further, the echoes of the mitral leaflets provide important diagnostic information regarding aortic regurgi-

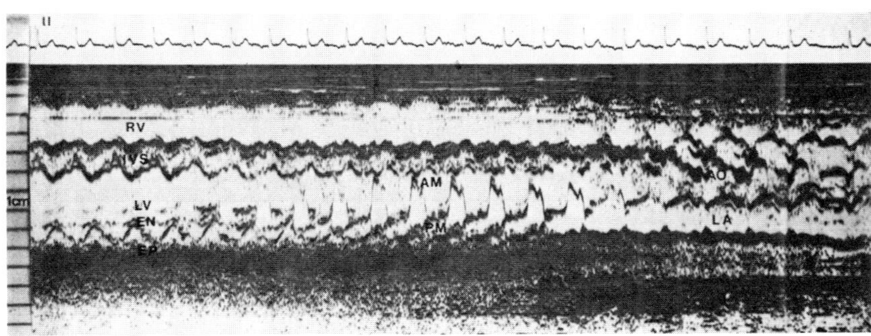

FIGURE 3. Echocardiographic scan from cardiac apex (**left**) to base (**right**) in a normal subject. AM=AMV; PM=PMV.

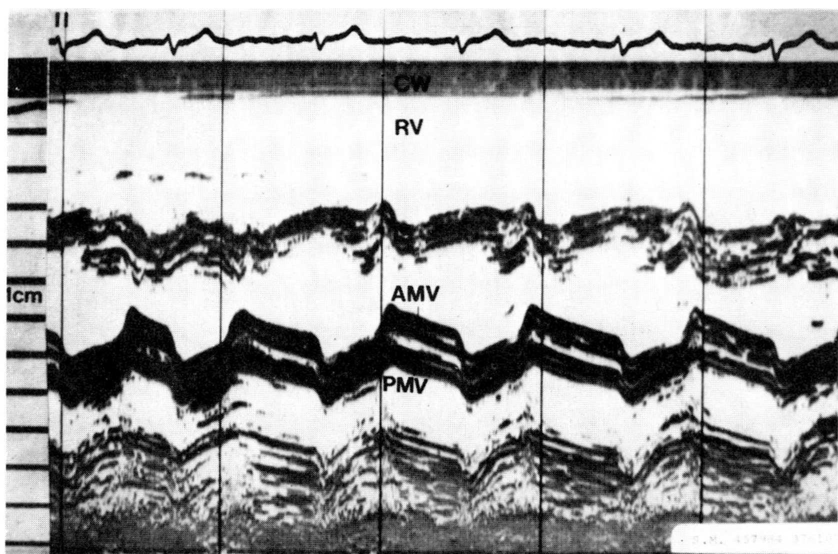

FIGURE 4. Echocardiogram obtained in a patient with severe mitral stenosis showing thickened leaflets, diminished opening amplitude of AMV, reduced AMV diastolic closing velocity and forward diastolic motion of PMV. In this and subsequent figures, the major vertical time lines denote 1 second intervals.

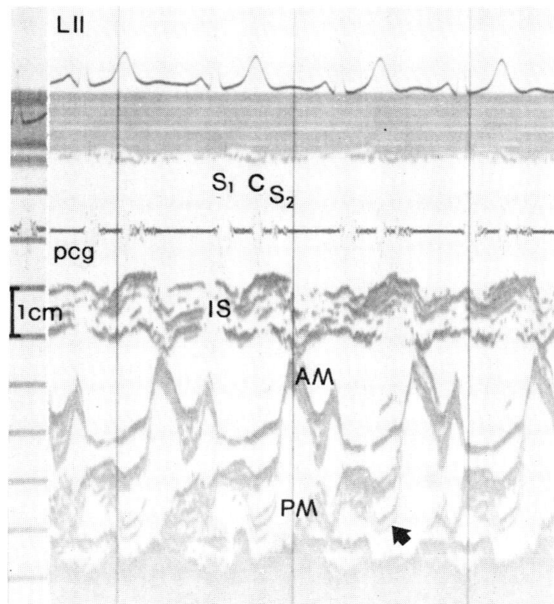

FIGURE 5. Echocardiogram and phonocardiogram (PCG) in a patient with mitral valve prolapse syndrome. C = midsystolic click; IS = IVS; S_1 = first heart sound; S_2 = second heart sound. **Arrow** indicates the posterior systolic buckling motion of the mitral leaflets.

tation[22-24] (Figure 8) and mitral regurgitation secondary to torn chordae tendineae[9,25,26] (Figure 9). In addition, the echogram of the aortic leaflets has proved valuable in the identification of aortic stenosis[27] (Figure 10) and also in aortic regurgitation, especially that secondary to bacterial endocarditis[24] (Figure 11). Ultrasound has also been demonstrated to be a highly sensitive and specific method for the detection of pericardial effusion[28-32] (Figure 12). Although the tricuspid valves (Figure 13) and pulmonic valves (Figure 14) have received less attention, recent studies have documented the ability to detect pulmonic stenosis and pulmonary hypertension by alterations of the pulmonary echogram[33-35] (Figure 15, A and B). In regard to quantitative evaluation of cardiac diseases, the mitral valve echogram has been utilized to provide an estimate of the severity of obstruction in patients with mitral stenosis[36,37] and in idiopathic hypertrophic subaortic stenosis.[13]

However, echograms of the cardiac valves would not be anticipated to be as useful in the evaluation of cardiac function as they have been in the diagnosis and evaluation of cardiovascular diseases. Therefore, additional echo-

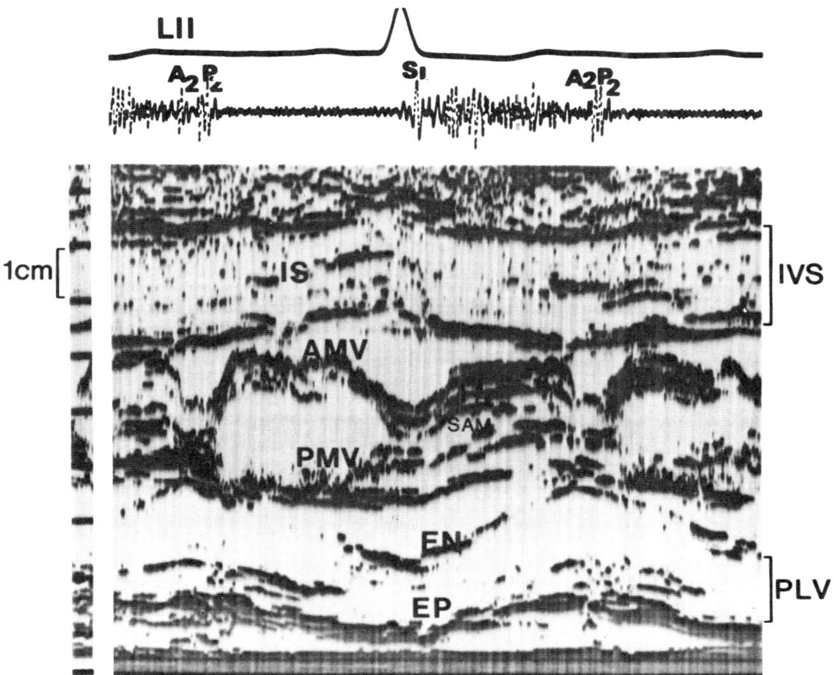

FIGURE 6. Echocardiogram and PCG obtained from a patient with idiopathic hypertrophic subaortic stenosis (IHSS). SAM = systolic anterior motion of the anterior mitral leaflet (AMV) characteristic of IHSS. A₂ (aortic) and P₂ (pulmonic) valve c osure sounds are indicated. (Reproduced by permission from King et al.[16])

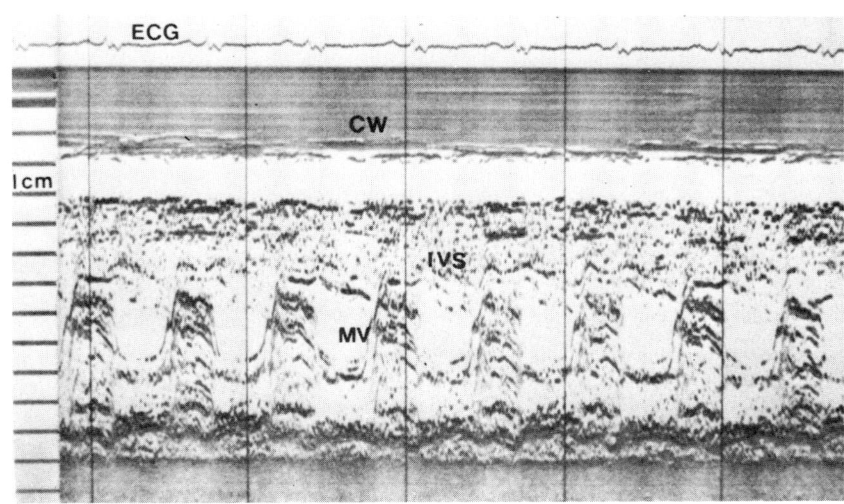

FIGURE 7. Echocardiogram obtained from a patient with left atrial myxoma. The tumor appears as a cloud of echoes posterior to the anterior mitral leaflet (MV) in diastole.

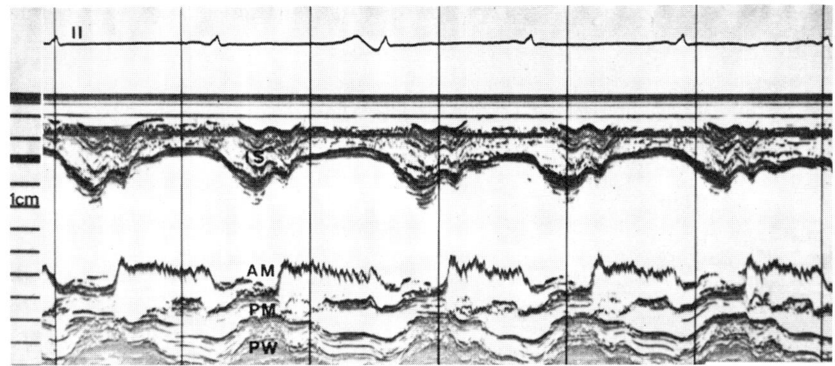

FIGURE 8. Echocardiogram demonstrating fine diastolic flutter of the mitral valve leaflets, particularly the AM, in a patient with severe aortic regurgitation.

graphic modalities have been utilized to assess: (1) cardiac chamber size and wall thickness; (2) derived left ventricular volume; (3) left ventricular wall motion; (4) velocity of circumferential fiber shortening; and (5) alterations of mitral valve motion. Since impairment in the performance of the heart is frequently accompanied by alterations in cardiac chamber size and wall motion, the basis for the detection of cardiac dysfunction by ultrasound is provided. The remaining discussion, therefore, primarily focuses upon the utilization of echocardiographic measurements of intracavitary chamber dimensions and wall motion in the assessment of cardiac function.

Echocardiographic Determination of Left Ventricular Volume

The first attempt to quantify cardiac function by ultrasound was made by Feigenbaum and associates[38] in 1967. Believing that the ultra-

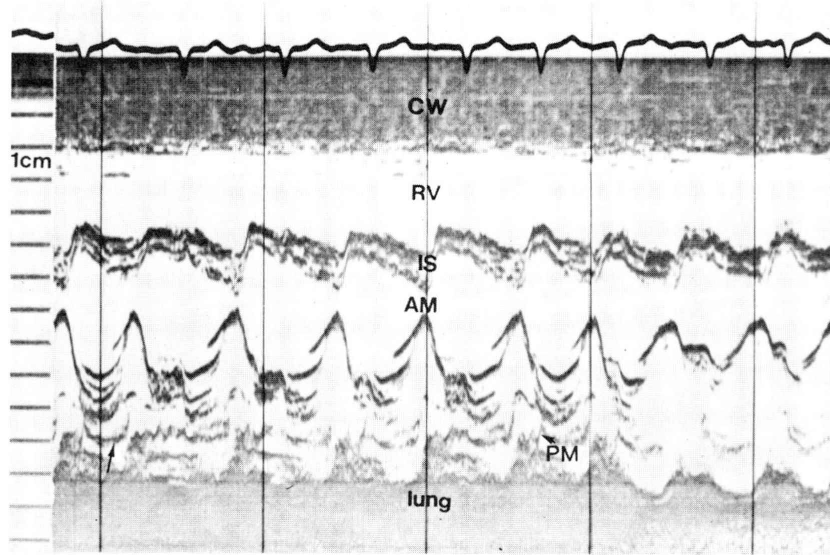

FIGURE 9. Ultrasound recording from a patient with torn chordae tendineae demonstrating pansystolic prolapse of the mitral leaflets (**left two thirds**). **Arrow** indicates a portion of the prolapsed posterior mitral leaflet (PM) in systole that moves anteriorly (flail) during diastole. As the echo beam is directed in the left atrium toward the aorta (**right third**), echoes from the prolapsed mitral leaflets continue to be recorded. (Reproduced by permission from DeMaria et al.[9])

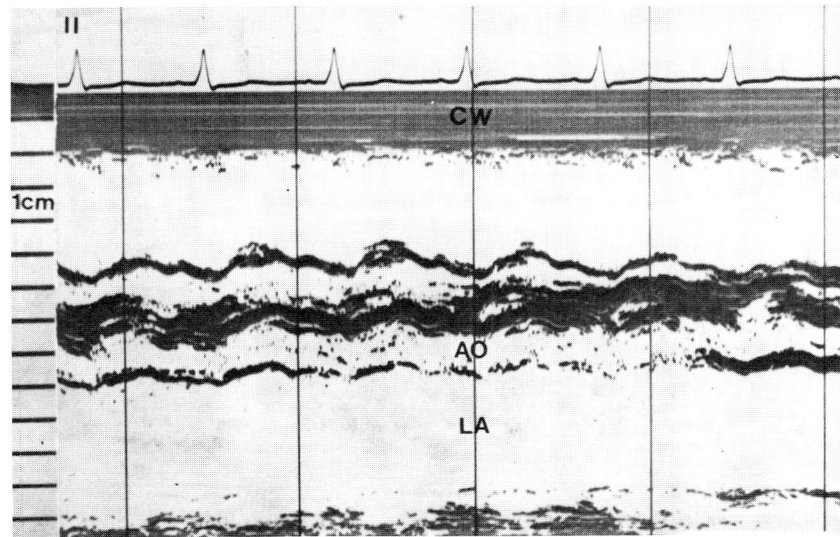

FIGURE 10. Echocardiogram obtained in a patient with calcific aortic stenosis demonstrating thickened immobile aortic leaflets. (Reproduced by permission from DeMaria al.[24])

sonic beam traversed only the left ventricle, these workers utilized a total cardiac echo dimension—inclusive of both right and left ventricular chambers—and the mitral valve echo in an attempt to determine stroke volume. Surprisingly, this method provided a relatively close estimation of actual stroke volume and was the first of many empiric attempts to evaluate cardiac volumes and output by ultrasound.

Two years later the Indiana group described the identification of the interventricular septum on echocardiogram[39] and confirmed their anatomic findings with intracardiac injections of indocyanine green.[40] In this manner, these pioneer investigators were readily able to detect abnormalities in cardiac chamber size, distinguishing right ventricular volume overload states from those involving left ventricular volume overload. The pathway was thereby opened for the attempt to quantify actual left ventricular volumes by means of echocardiography.

Feigenbaum and co-workers[41] initially compared left ventricular systolic and diastolic dimensions determined by echography to the corresponding left ventricular volumes obtained by cineangiography. Although there was a correlation between the echographic and angiographic measurements, it was found empirically that the relation could be enhanced substantially by cubing the echographic dimension.[41] Subsequently, a number of other investigators evaluated the ability of echocardiography to determine left ventricular volumes by internal chamber dimensions.[42-52]

The explanation for the good correlation between the cube of the ultrasonically determined

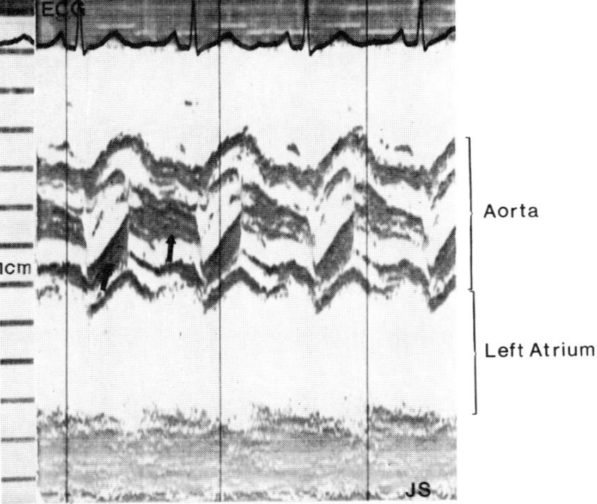

FIGURE 11. Echocardiogram of the aortic valve in a patient with acute aortic regurgitation and bacterial endocarditis demonstrating irregular thickened echoes in both systole (**left arrow**) and diastole (**right arrow**) of fully mobile leaflets. (Reproduced by permission from DeMaria et al.[24])

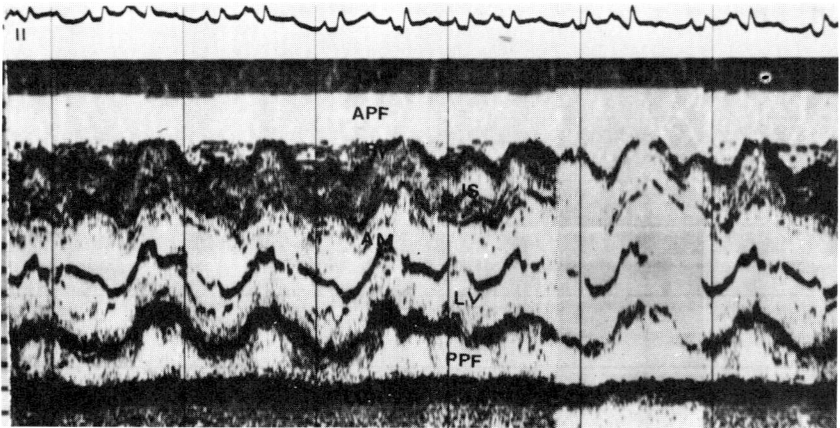

FIGURE 12. Echocardiogram obtained in a patient with massive pericardial effusion secondary to malignant disease. APF = anterior pericardial effusion; PPF = posterior pericardial effusion. The heart is seen to rock freely anteriorly and posteriorly in the pericardial sac with each cardiac cycle. The ultrasonic energy is abruptly reduced in the latter third of the recording, clearly identifying both right ventricular and left ventricular surfaces, as well as a thickened pericardium interposed between pericardial and pleural fluid.

left ventricular dimensions and cineangiographically determined left ventricular volumes has been provided by several investigators.[42,43] A number of angiographic studies have indicated that the left ventricle geometrically conforms to the shape of a prolate ellipse (ellipsoid of revolution about the major axis), in which the short anteroposterior and lateral diameters are considered equal.[53,54] Moreover, angiographic data are also available to document that the major diameter of the left ventricle is approximately twice the minor diameter in both systole and diastole.[55] Therefore, the volume of the left ventricle as determined by echocardiography was derived in the following manner. The volume of a prolate ellipse is expressed as:

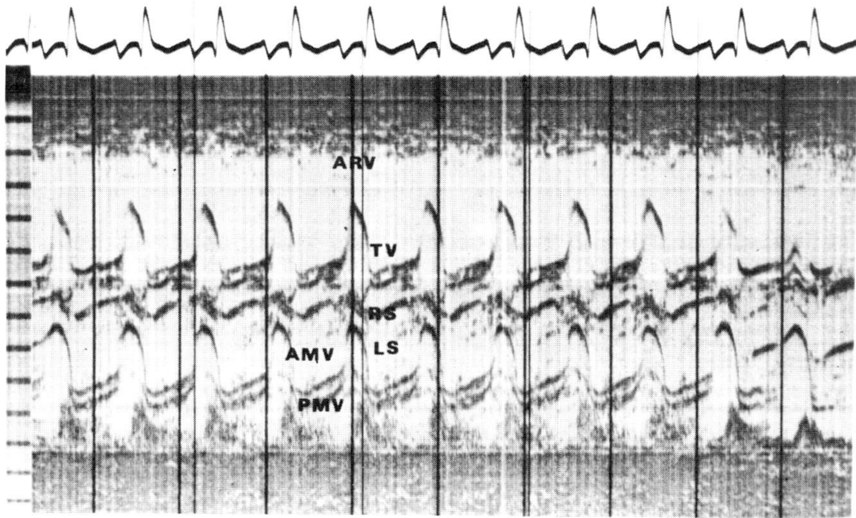

FIGURE 13. Echocardiogram demonstrating simultaneous recording of the tricuspid valve (TV) and mitral valve in a patient with an atrial septal defect.

(1) $V = \frac{\pi}{6} D_{AP} \cdot D_L \cdot D_M$

where D_{AP} and D_L represent the anteroposterior and lateral minor diameters and D_M, the major longitudinal axis. Since D_{AP} equals D_L (henceforth expressed as D),[56] equation 1 may be reformulated as:

(2) $V = \frac{\pi}{6} D^2 \cdot D_M$

Since the major diameter is twice the minor axis, equation 2 may be rewritten as:

(3) $V = \frac{\pi}{6} D^2 \cdot 2D$ or

(4) $V = \frac{2\pi}{6} \cdot D^3$

Since it can be assumed that $\frac{2\pi}{6}$ is equal to unity, then equation 4 may be rewritten as:

(5) $V = D^3$

Both left ventricular end-diastolic and end-systolic volumes can be calculated by this approach. Thus, stroke volume may be determined as the difference between end-diastolic and end-systolic volumes, and ejection fraction, as stroke volume related to end-diastolic volume (Figure 16).

Since a variety of ventricular diameters may be recorded on the echogram, it is important to utilize a standardized technique that will yield the echographic dimension bearing optimal relation to ventricular volume. Thus, previous studies have demonstrated the necessity to record an echo that traverses the interventricular septum and left ventricular posterior wall simul-

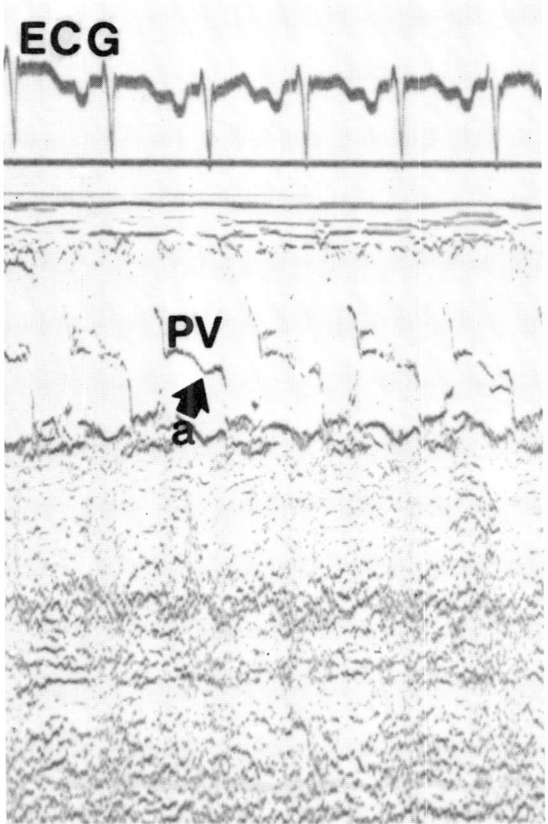

FIGURE 14. Echogram showing two cusps of the pulmonic valve (PV) in a normal subject. The PV deflection caused by right atrial contraction is indicated by **arrow a.** Normal posterior movement of the PV in ventricular diastole is observed.

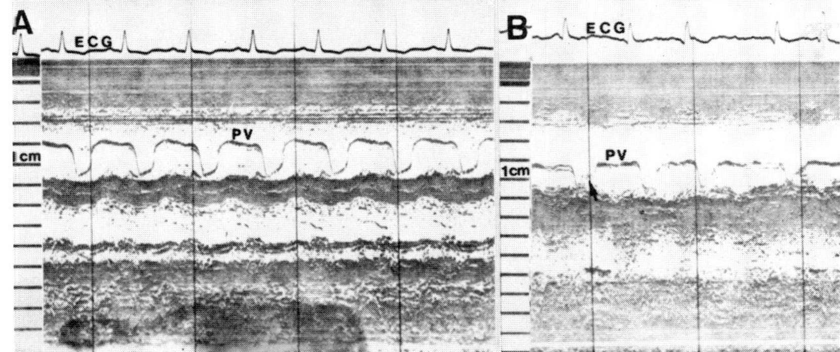

FIGURE 15. A, pulmonic echogram in a patient with pulmonary hypertension due to mitral stenosis. Note the absence of an a deflection and also the absence of anterior-to- posterior slope in diastole. **B,** echogram from PV in patient with Eisenmenger's syndrome and ventricular septal defect. Note the notching of the PV in systole (**arrow**).

$$EDV = EDD^3$$

$$ESV = ESD^3$$

$$SV = EDV - ESV$$

$$EF = \frac{SV}{EDV}$$

$$VC_F = \frac{EDD - ESD}{ET \cdot EDD}$$

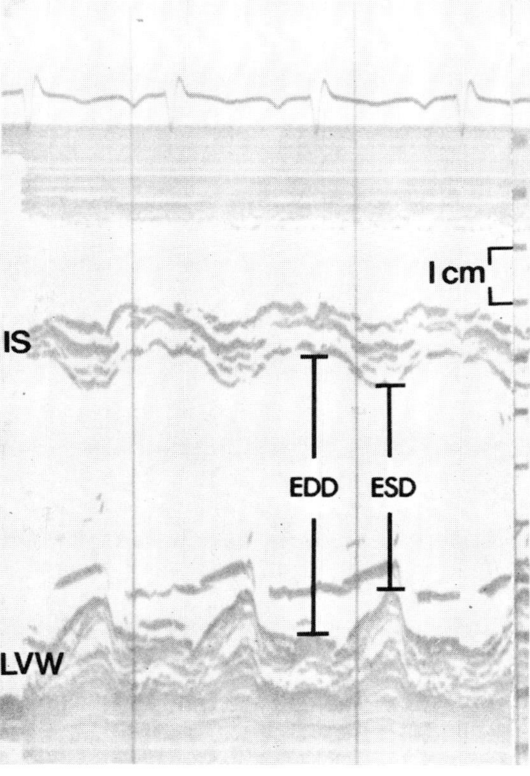

FIGURE 16. Echocardiogram demonstrating left ventricular dimensions obtained from a normal subject, as well as parameters of cardiac function derived from these measurements. EDD = end-diastolic dimension; EDV = end-diastolic volume; EF = ejection fraction; ESD = end-systolic dimension; ESV = end-systolic volume; ET = ejection time; LWV = PLV; SV = stroke volume; V_{CF} = mean velocity of circumferential fiber shortening.

taneously, in an area just below the major deflection of the mitral leaflets.[41,42] The dimension obtained in this manner has been shown to possess the optimal relation to the left ventricular minor axis dimension as measured angiographically. In addition, although the left ventricular posterior wall is concave in respect to the echo transducer and thus may be recorded by a variety of transducer positions and angulations, the interventricular septum is convex in respect to the transducer and thereby will be perpendicular to the echo beam in only a limited area. Therefore, the requirement of simultaneous recording of both the interventricular septum and left ventricular posterior wall results in a standardized measurement that is readily reproducible at various times by different echocardiographers. In some patients, satisfactory echographic recordings that simultaneously display the interventricular septum and left ventricular posterior wall in the sector just below the mitral leaflets may be recorded from several interspaces. In such cases the echogram obtained from the interspace in which the transducer is most perpendicular to the chest wall should be the tracing selected for analysis. It should be pointed out, however, that in a certain percentage of subjects satisfactory echographic dimensions for calculation of left ventricular volume will be impossible for technical reasons.

The importance of obtaining careful left ventricular endocardial measurements in the calculation of ventricular volume has also been emphasized.[42] Although the recognition of the left ventricular septal surface is usually not difficult, the identification of the endocardium of the left ventricular posterior wall may be quite confusing. Alteration of echographic gain usually permits distinction of the endocardium from the epicardium, and scanning from apex to base usually permits distinction between chordae tendineae and endocardium.

Although the end-diastolic measurement is taken 0.04 seconds after the onset of the QRS complex of the ECG in our laboratory,[57] many workers prefer to utilize the peak of the R wave.[42,43,46] Further, the interventricular septum and left ventricular posterior wall both move anteriorly in the latter part of systole due to forward motion of the entire heart, so that contraction of the left ventricular posterior wall appears to peak after that of the interventricular septum.[58] For this reason, the end-systolic dimension should be measured as the nearest approximation of these two walls regardless of timing. It should be pointed out that precise echo measurements of end-systolic volumes are difficult in the presence of conditions in which there is inappropriate or anterior motion of the interventricular septum.

Numerous investigators have correlated left ventricular volumes obtained by echocardiography in the manner just described with those obtained by cineangiography.[41-52] The majority of these studies have demonstrated a close relation of end-diastolic and end-systolic left ventricular volumes, stroke volume and ejection fraction obtained by echography with those obtained by the invasive radiologic technique, with the correlation coefficients usually being above 0.80.[41,43,46,47] In addition, Pombo and associates[44] have been able to demonstrate a close correlation between echographic stroke volume and stroke volume obtained by the dye dilution method in acute myocardial infarction. Moreover, these investigators have shown that ultrasound measurements were subject to only minor variations when obtained by different technicians or on different days. In addition, Redwood and co-workers,[48] have documented the ability of echocardiography to detect even minor alterations in left ventricular volume. Although some workers have proposed utilization of either the amplitude of mitral annulus motion or a variety of regression equations to enhance the predicability of echographic left ventricular volumes,[46,49] the cube echo dimension has generally proved as reliable as any of these modified calculations. Thus, the majority of available literature attests to the feasibility of assessing left ventricular volumes by echocardiography. Nevertheless, it should be recognized that a technique that utilizes only a single-plane measurement to calculate the volume of a three-dimensional object is susceptible to many sources of error. Thus, as has been demonstrated by Popp et al.[50] and Teichholz et al.,[49] in the presence of ventricular dilation, the ratio of the major to the minor axis approaches 1:1, resulting in a significant overestimation of left ventricular volume. Moreover, in the presence of segmental myocardial dysfunction such as

might be found in patients with coronary atherosclerosis, the echographic beam may traverse a segment of myocardium that is not representative of the entire ventricle because of either hyperkinetic or hypokinetic motion.[59] As anticipated, these discrepancies are exaggerated in systole as compared with diastole. Despite this problem, however, Ratshin and co-workers[52] correlated left ventricular volumes determined echographically with those obtained angiographically in a group of patients with ventricular dyssynergy. Using large-frame angiographic cut-film, these workers were able to show a significant discrepancy in echographic volumes only during systole in patients with major dyskinesis involving a substantial portion of the anterior or inferior wall. In addition, they noted adequate correlations of end-diastolic echographic and angiographic volumes regardless of the extent of ventricular dyssynergy. Thus, it appears that echographic volumes are unreliable in the presence of extreme left ventricular dilation or substantial areas of left ventricular dyskinesis.

From these observations, the application of echocardiography to the measurement of left ventricular volumes can be summarized as follows.

(1) There appears to be close correlation between the cube function of the transverse echocardiographic ventricular dimensions recorded just below the major deflection of the mitral leaflets and left ventricular volumes when high quality ultrasound tracings are obtained in patients with normal left ventricular geometry.

(2) Left ventricular volumes determined by echocardiography are unreliable in the presence of major distortion of ventricular geometry by virtue of dilation or dyskinetic segments.

(3) In general, left ventricular end-diastolic volume determined by echocardiography remains relatively accurate and correlates well with that determined by angiography even in the presence of left ventricular dyssynergy.

(4) Ventricular volumes obtained by echogram are particularly useful in assessing directional changes resulting from interventions when the patient serves as his own control or in making serial determinations in the same patient.

(5) Because of the substantial standard error

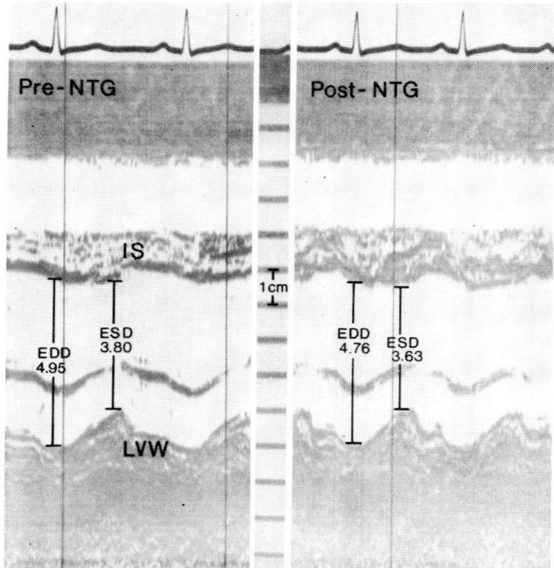

FIGURE 17. Echocardiogram of the left ventricle before (pre-) and after (post-) sublingual nitroglycerin (NTG). After nitroglycerin, the left ventricular dimensions were reduced. (Reproduced by permission from DeMaria et al.[57])

ate cardiovascular function in a variety of settings. Echocardiography has been valuable in determining total left ventricular stroke volume as an adjunct in the evaluation of the severity of mitral or aortic valvular regurgitation.[42] In addition, echocardiographic ventricular measurements have been utilized in the serial evaluation of patients with myocardial infarction[60,61] as well as in the assessment of prognosis for individual patients with infarction.[62] Echocardiographic volumes have also been utilized for noninvasive determination of systemic vascular resistance[63] and for investigation of the cardiocirculatory alterations induced by isometric handgrip exercise.[64] Ultrasound also has been applied in the evaluation of the effects of aortocoronary bypass surgery on cardiac function[65] and to analyze left ventricular preload, afterload and compliance.[66] Further, echocardiographic volumes have been used in our laboratories to evaluate the effects of nitroglycerin[57] (Figure 17) and direct current cardioversion[67] (Figure 18) on cardiac chamber size and ventricular function.

of the estimate of echographic volumes observed in many studies, left ventricular volumes determined by ultrasound may correlate well with those obtained by angiogram in a group of patients but may be misleading in an individual patient.

In view of these values and limitations, left ventricular volumes determined by echocardiography have already been utilized to evalu-

Echocardiographic Determination of Left Artrial Size

Alterations in left atrial size frequently accompany disturbances in cardiac function. Thus, the accurate estimation of left atrial size by echogram may be utilized as an important reflection of cardiac performance[67] (Figure 19).

Hirata and associates[68] demonstrated the abil-

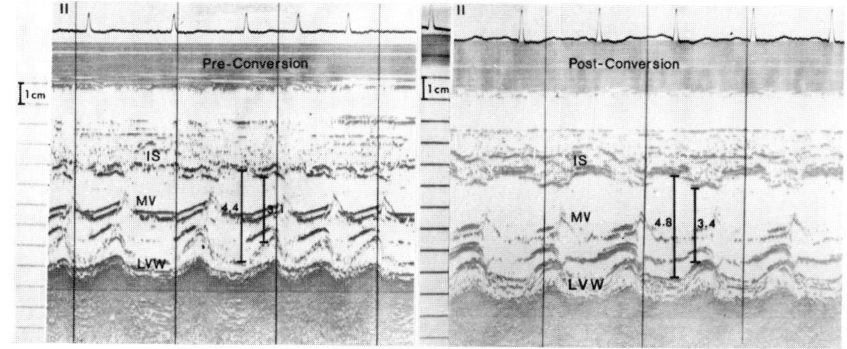

FIGURE 18. Echocardiogram before (pre-) and after (post-) direct current cardioversion of atrial fibrillation to normal sinus rhythm in a patient with coronary disease, showing increases in left ventricular end-diastolic and end-systolic dimensions after conversion. (Reproduced by permission from DeMaria et al.[67])

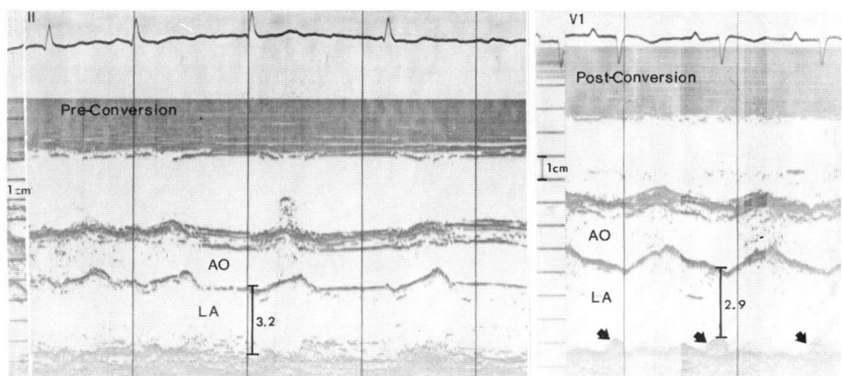

FIGURE 19. Echocardiogram of the left atrium (LA) before (pre-) and after (post-) direct current cardioversion of atrial fibrillation to normal sinus rhythm in a patient with coronary disease. **Arrows** point to atrial contraction of the posterior left atrial wall with restoration of normal sinus rhythm resulting in decrease in LA end-diastolic dimension. (Reproduced by permission from DeMaria et al.[67])

ity of ultrasound to provide a left atrial dimension that bears a high degree of correlation to that obtained by cineangiography. These investigators utilized an echographic left atrial dimension that was obtained posterior to the aorta in an area of minimal motion of the left atrial wall, and the dimension was taken from the intimal surface of the posterior aortic wall to the endocardium of the posterior atrial wall at end-systole. Subsequently, Brown and co-workers[69] proposed that the ratio of the left atrial dimension to the aortic root dimension provides a more sensitive indication of left atrial enlargement. Regardless of which criterion is chosen, echocardiography appears to afford an accurate estimate of left atrial size.

Echocardiographic Evaluation of Left Ventricular Wall Thickness

The ability of ultrasound to evaluate left ventricular wall thickness provides an important facet in the assessment of cardiac function. Recent studies have correlated left ventricular wall thickness found on echography with values obtained at operation,[70] at necropsy[70] and by left ventricular angiography.[71,72] Good correlation between ultrasonic and direct measurement of posterior wall thickness has been reported.[70–72] Moreover, echocardiography accurately predicted the presence of left ventricular hypertrophy in nearly all patients with this abnormality. Thus, left ventricular posterior wall thickness on

echogram (Figure 20) provides a reliable index of left ventricular hypertrophy and has been utilized in the calculation of left ventricular mass.[72]

In addition to measurement of the left ventricular posterior wall thickness, echocardiography allows quantitative estimation of the width of the interventricular septum[12,14,16,71,73] (Figure 20). The comparison of the width of the left ventricular posterior wall and interventricular septum has proved to be of major importance in

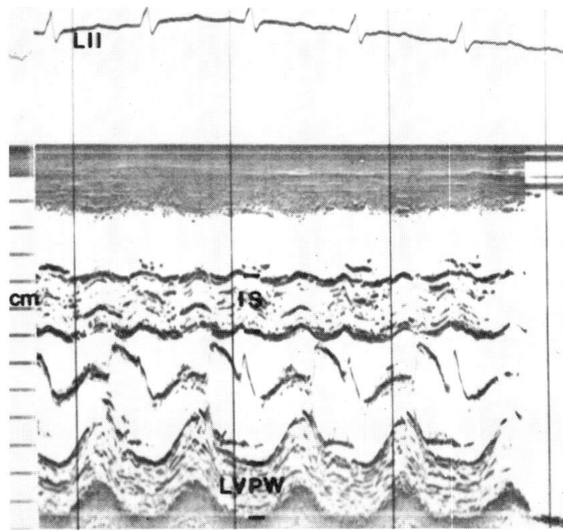

FIGURE 20. Echocardiogram demonstrating concentric left ventricular hypertrophy in a patient with hypertensive cardiovascular disease.

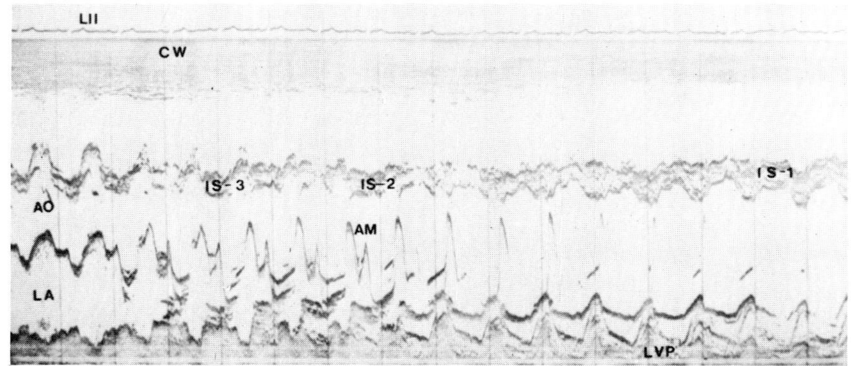

FIGURE 21. Echocardiographic scan from cardiac base (**left**) to apex (**right**) showing the heterogeneity of interventricular septal (IS) motion in a normal subject.

distinguishing ventricular hypertrophy due to hypertensive cardiovascular disease from that produced by hypertrophic cardiomyopathy. Several investigators have demonstrated that hypertensive cardiovascular disease results in concentric left ventricular hypertrophy, whereas hypertrophic cardiomyopathy presents with asymmetric septal hypertrophy primarily involving the interventricular septum.[12,14]

Echocardiographic Evaluation of Left Ventricular Wall Motion

The pattern of left ventricular wall motion on the cineangiogram has been recognized as a valuable parameter of cardiac function. Thus, examination of the extent and velocity of circumferential fiber shortening[74,75] and of the temporal sequence of segmental left ventricular contraction[76,77] have been utilized in the assessment of ventricular performance in patients with a variety of cardiac disorders. Echocardiography, by virtue of its ability to record intracardiac anatomy, provides a unique noninvasive method for the recording of the velocity and amplitude of left ventricular wall motion, as well as the sequence of contraction and the extent of wall thickening during systole. It is not surprising, therefore, that many investigators have applied the assessment of left ventricular wall motion by echogram in the evaluation of cardiac function.[58,73,78-92]

Posterior Wall Motion: The contractile characteristics of the portions of the left ventricular wall accessible to ultrasound examination—the interventricular septum and the left ventricular posterior wall—have been examined in normal hearts by several workers.[58,73,78,91,92] The ultrasonic tracing of the normal left ventricular posterior wall during the cardiac cycle has the appearance of an inverted ventricular volume curve (Figure 16). At the onset of ventricular ejection, the left ventricular posterior wall moves anteriorly toward the ultrasound transducer. The velocity of anterior motion is rapid at first, but then it is progressively reduced until the termination of systole. Subsequently, during diastole, the left ventricular posterior wall moves posteriorly, again displaying a greater velocity of motion in early diastole than in late diastole. In contrast to the uniform contractile pattern of the posterior wall, the normal motion of the interventricular septum has been found to be heterogeneous (Figure 21). The most superior portion of the interventricular septum, representing the membraneous septum, typically exhibits a slight anterior motion (Figure 21, IS–3) during systole similar to—and probably influenced by—the movement of the aorta. In contrast, the apical portion of the septum characteristically reveals a substantial posterior systolic motion approximating the posterior wall as ejection occurs (Figure 21, IS–2). The middle portion of the interventricular septum—that segment recorded in the area of the mitral leaflets —represents a transition zone in which septal motion is usually notched or flat but may be either slightly wholly anterior or posterior

(Figure 21, IS-1). It is important to note that in young children the mitral leaflets occupy a greater portion of the left ventricle, and thus the appropriate motion of the lower portion of the septum in the echo plane traversing the mitral valve may be posterior in direction. In addition to heterogeneous motion, the echo from the entire interventricular septum displays a prominent notch at the end of ejection and the beginning of diastole (Figure 21). Careful analysis by McDonald and colleagues[58] has revealed this notch to be a function of displacement of the entire heart with consequent simultaneous movement of both the interventricular septum and left ventricular posterior wall in the same direction, first anterior at end-systole and then posterior at the onset of diastole. This total heart displacement serves to increase the amplitude of upward movement of the posterior wall, while decreasing the downward motion of the interventricular septum at this time in the cardiac cycle.

Since it is technically easier to record the left ventricular posterior wall than the interventricular septum, initial investigative efforts were directed toward the study of the former (Figure 16). Kraunz and associates[78,79] demonstrated the ability of echo to detect changes in both the velocity and extent of posterior wall contraction induced by exercise and vasoactive drugs.[78,79] Subsequently, Smithen and co-workers[83] confirmed that the movement of the posterior wall was enhanced in response to exercise and determined that this improvement was related to sympathetic stimulation, since they found decreases in both velocity and extent of contraction in response to increased heart rate alone. Abnormalities of posterior wall motion on the echogram have been reported in the presence of myocardial infarction[80,81,85,86] and congestive heart failure due to left ventricular dysfunction of other causes,[82] and it has been proposed that these values of left ventricular posterior wall contraction represent indexes of ventricular function. Subsequent studies, however, have not confirmed this postulation. Fogelman et al.[84] evaluated changes in posterior wall contraction occurring during exercise-induced angina pectoris and found no significant changes in velocity or extent of systolic motion of the left ventricular posterior wall, although marked alter-

ations in both maximal and mean diastolic relaxation velocities were observed.[84] Further, although Kerber and Abboud,[86] utilizing an experimental canine preparation, were able to demonstrate that abnormalities of posterior wall motion could be detected by ultrasound during acute myocardial infarction, such disturbances in contractile pattern could be recorded only when the echo beam traversed the area of posterior wall that was infarcted. In addition, Ludbrook and associates[87,88] found poor correlation between the velocity of posterior wall motion determined by ultrasound and ejection fractions and mean velocity of circumferential fiber shortening obtained both echographically and cineangiographically.[87,88]

In our laboratories we also have found that posterior wall motion does not provide an accurate reflection of overall left ventricular performance, but rather that the pattern of motion indicates the status of segmental contraction when this area of myocardium is examined.[92] Indeed, we frequently have observed compensatory hyperkinesis—increased velocity and extent of contraction—of the posterior wall on the echogram in the presence of extensive dyskinesis of the remaining ventricular perimeter when the posterior wall was spared from the ischemic process (Figure 22). An additional reason for the conflicting data regarding the value and limitation of left ventricular posterior wall motion in the assessment of cardiac function may be attributable to the fact that the epicardium rather than the endocardium was examined in the earlier studies in this area. Although it is technically more difficult to record endocardium by ultrasound, motion of this structure is of much greater physiologic significance than is that of the epicardium.

In summary, concerning motion of the left ventricular posterior wall, measurements of posterior wall contraction on echography reflect the performance only of that myocardial segment. However, echocardiography is capable of accurately detecting alterations in the contractile pattern of the posterior wall, such as those induced by pharmacologic agents or exercise, and thus provides a sensitive method for assessment of the effects of interventions upon posterior wall motion or for the serial evaluation of cardiac performance in individual patients.

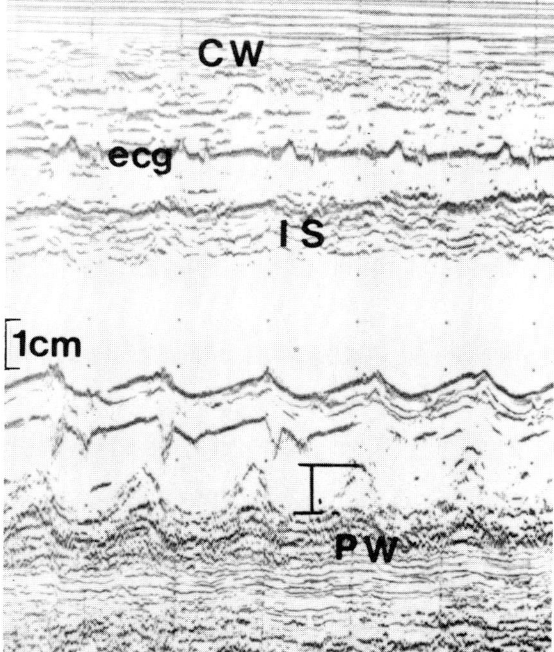

FIGURE 22. Echocardiogram in a patient with anterior septal myocardial infarction in whom the left ventricular posterior wall manifests exaggerated contractions (**vertical marker,** PW).

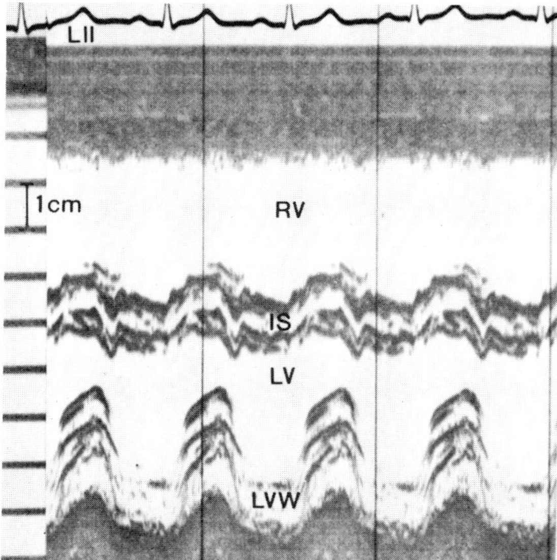

FIGURE 23. Echocardiogram demonstrating a dilated right ventricle and inappropriate anterior movement of the interventricular septum (IS) during systole in a patient with right ventricular volume overload secondary to an atrial septal defect.

Finally, changes during diastolic relaxation of the posterior wall on echography may be a more sensitive indicator of ischemia of this segment than are alterations in systolic motion.

Interventricular Septal Motion: Despite its heterogeneity and greater technical difficulty in ultrasonic recording, the contractile pattern of the interventricular septum on the echogram has provided important information regarding the status of cardiac performance. Thus, the finding of inappropriate or paradoxical anterior systolic motion of the interventricular septum in patients with right ventricular volume overload represents one of the earliest diagnostic abnormalities described by echocardiographers[93] (Figure 23) and established the utility of the contractile pattern of the interventricular septum for detection of disorders of cardiac function. Although it was initially thought that inappropriate septal motion was a highly sensitive indicator of right ventricular volume overloading, increased experience[91,94] and greater appreciation of the variable contractile pattern of different segments of the interventricular septum have revealed that a significant minority of such patients may have normal septal movement.

More recently it has become recognized that the contractile pattern of the septum undergoes a characteristic alteration on the echogram in patients with left bundle branch block.[95-98] In the presence of this conduction abnormality, on ultrasound study the interventricular septum exhibits a rapid, sharp, posterior peak that occurs within 100 msec of the onset of the QRS complex and is followed by a sustained paradoxical anterior motion (Figure 24). Although this typical motion is not invariable, it has been observed in almost all patients with left bundle branch block. No definitive explanation for the mechanism of this abnormal pattern has yet been established, nor is it understood why an occasional patient with this conduction disorder has normal motion.

As experience with echocardiography has increased, additional cardiac disorders have been added to the number of conditions that may manifest inappropriate septal motion. Thus, septal dyssynergy—either akinesis or dyskinesis—has recently been reported in primary cardiomyopathies,[99] idiopathic hypertrophic subaortic stenosis,[100] constrictive pericarditis[101,102] and the postoperative state after sternotomy.[103]

However, due to the high prevalence of coronary atherosclerosis, major attention has been focused upon the effects of coronary artery disease on the contractile pattern of both the interventricular septum and posterior wall.

Jacobs and associates[104] reported the initial observation that in coronary patients left ventricular dyssynergy of the interventricular septum and left ventricular posterior wall noted on echocardiography could be correlated with contraction abnormalities in these regions determined by cineangiography. Using values for amplitude of interventricular septal and posterior wall contraction determined in normal subjects, these workers evaluated 48 patients with both echocardiographic and cineangiographic studies and were able to detect abnormal wall motion by ultrasound in 24 of 25 patients found to have dyssynergy by angiography. In addition, the echocardiogram detected abnormalities of interventricular septal motion in 8 patients with obstruction of the left anterior descending coronary artery who had normal findings on left ventricular cineangiography. Moreover, it was found that the segmental echocardiographic abnormalities correlated with areas of infarction on the electrocardiogram. Thus, echocardiography was found to be a valuable method for the detection of segmental dyssynergy in the presence of ischemic heart disease.

Subsequently, Brown et al.[99] evaluated the ability of the echographic recordings of interventricular septal motion to identify obstruction of the left anterior descending coronary artery. Using criteria including the amplitude of both systolic and diastolic motion as well as systolic thickening of the interventricular septum, these investigators were able to detect abnormalities of the contractile pattern of the interventricular septum in 30 of 32 patients with flow-limiting stenosis in this major coronary vessel. In addition, abnormal septal motion has been noted by other workers in the presence of interventricular septal ischemia.[92]

The echographic detection of left ventricular dyssynergy due to coronary artery disease has also been a subject of major interest in our laboratories.[92] Studies of ischemia of the interventricular septum must take into account the heterogeneity of its normal contraction pattern, the difficulties in recording both interventricular septal surfaces and the endocardium of the pos-

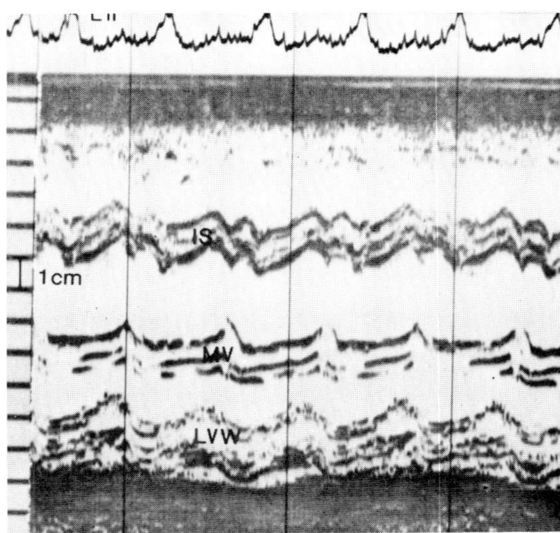

FIGURE 24. Echocardiogram obtained in a patient with left bundle branch block. The IS shows sharp early posterior contraction followed by sustained paradoxic anterior movement later in systole. The posterior LVW exhibits normal temporal anterior motion during systole.

terior wall and the segmental nature of ischemic heart disease itself. Thus, high quality echographic records of the endocardial surfaces of both the interventricular septum and left ventricular posterior wall throughout the majority of the left ventricle are necessary for assessment of the presence of dyssynergy. This frequently requires echographic scans from more than one precordial area. Moreover, interpretation of such records demands knowledge of the heterogeneity of normal wall motion in the different areas of the interventricular septum and, in the case of ultrasonic scans, the ability of the echocardiographer to separate echo alterations due to true dyssynergy from those that are only the result of technique. Nevertheless, utilizing careful technique and the combination of amplitude and thickening of the interventricular septum and left ventricular posterior wall during systole, we have been able to detect abnormal contractile patterns on the echogram in 75 percent of patients found to have ventricular dyssynergy on angiography.[92]

Included in our group of patients with wall motion disorders noted on echography were 10 without electrocardiographic evidence of myocardial infarction. Therefore, echocardiographic

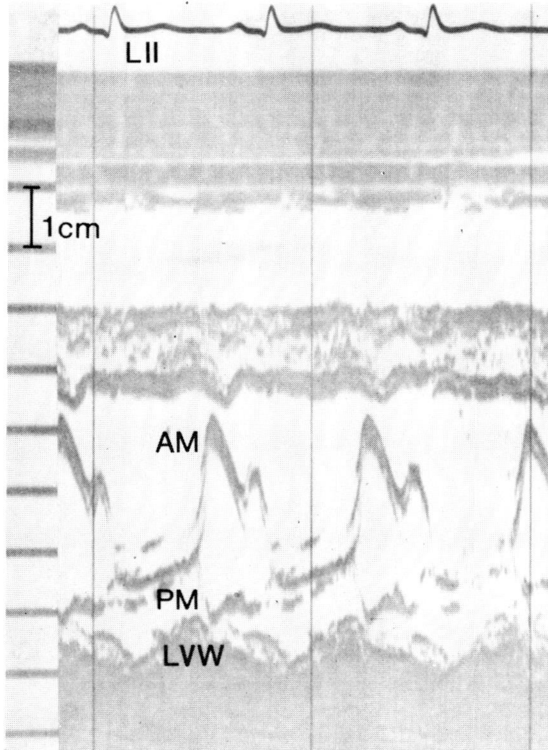

FIGURE 25. Echogram of interventricular septum (**middle**) in a patient with proximal left anterior descending coronary artery stenosis and normal ECG. IVS ischemia is noted by absence of posterior systolic contraction with abnormal abrupt early diastolic posterior motion of IVS.

analysis enabled the prediction of significant coronary obstruction (more than 75 percent stenosis) of the left anterior descending coronary artery by the detection of interventricular septal dyssynergy in some of these patients even with a normal electrocardiogram (Figure 25). Of additional importance was the fact that echographic hyperkinesis, manifested by increased amplitude of motion of either wall or marked posterior motion of the septum in the superior interventricular septal segment, was noted in patients with significant apical septal dyssynergy on angiography in whom the superior septal segment was uninvolved in the ischemic process (Figures 26 and 27). Thus, an individual patient might exhibit both akinesis and hyperkinesis in different areas of the ventricle (Figures 26 and 27), again emphasizing the importance of examining the entire longitudinal cardiac axis. Therefore, echocardiographic evaluation of left ventricular wall motion requires careful technique and is of substantial benefit in the assessment of left ventricular dyssynergy. In addition, the ability to detect left ventricular segmental dyssynergy on the echogram may permit the discovery of significant coronary obstruction even in the absence of electrocardiographic abnormalities at rest and during exercise.

Velocity of Circumferential Fiber Shortening

The velocity of circumferential fiber shortening (V_{CF}), as determined from the left ventricular cineangiogram, has been found to be a useful indicator of left ventricular performance and also has been proposed as a measure of left ventricular contractility.[75] It was therefore logical to attempt to determine V_{CF} by echocardiography for assessment of cardiac function. Paraskos and co-workers[105] found that echographically measured midwall V_{CF} correlated well with endocardial V_{CF} and that mean V_{CF} values correlated well with maximal V_{CF} values obtained by the analysis of serial V_{CF} measurements taken throughout systole at 50 msec intervals. In addition, these investigators demonstrated that V_{CF} determined by ultrasound allowed distinction of patients with normal ventricular function from those with abnormal function. Furthermore, Cooper and colleagues[106] were able to show a high degree of correlation between echographically and cineangiographically obtained V_{CF} and again confirmed the ability of ultrasound to separate normal from disordered ventricular function. These investigators quantitated mean V_{CF} as $(Dd-Ds)/(ET \times Dd)$, where Dd is end-diastolic dimension, Ds is end-systolic dimension, and ET is ejection time (measured as the time from onset of QRS on the electrocardiogram to the peak posterior wall contraction, minus 50 msec for isovolumic contraction). Subsequently, Ludbrook and associates[87,88] reported that mean V_{CF} determined by echocardiography was superior to the echographic evaluation of posterior wall motion in the assessment of overall cardiac performance.

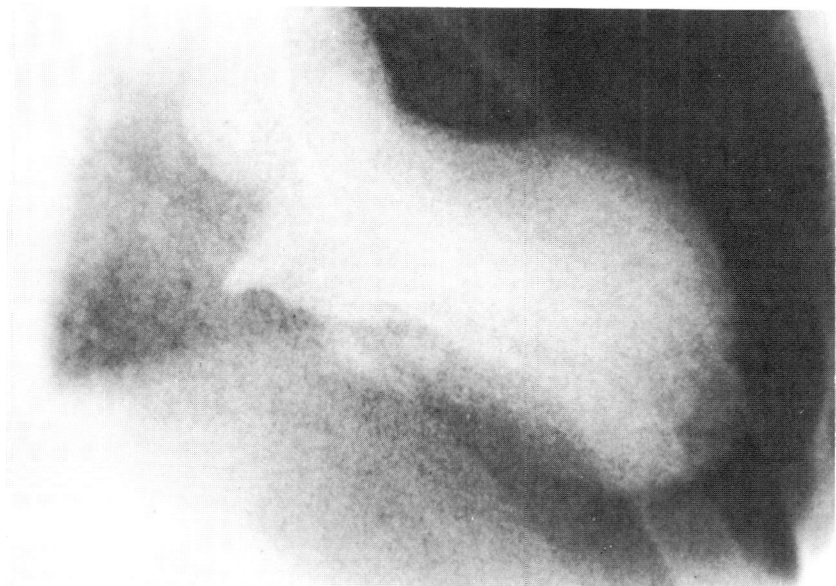

FIGURE 26. Left ventricular cineangiogram (right anterior oblique view) at end-systole demonstrating a large anterior apical left ventricular aneurysm.

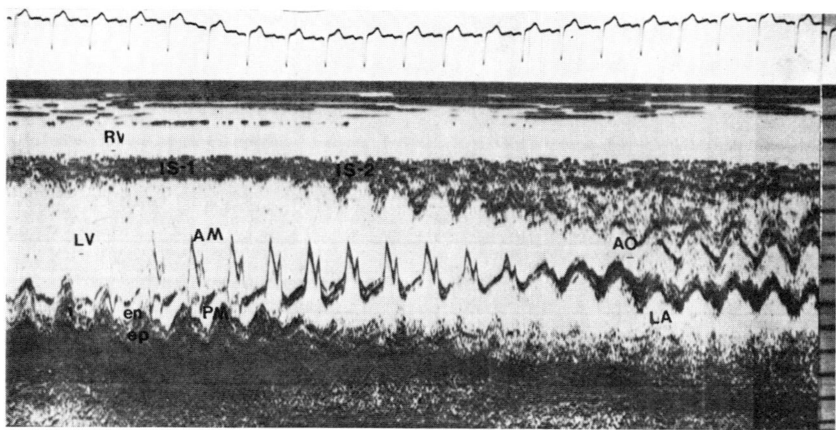

FIGURE 27. Echocardiographic scan from apex (**left**) to base (**right**) in the patient whose left ventriculogram is shown in Figure 27. IS–1, dense akinetic echoes from the aneurysm; IS–2, the hyperkinetic contractions of the uninvolved portion of the interventricular septum.

Quinones and co-workers[107] have also found echographic V_{CF} measurements to be of value in the assessment of ventricular performance.

Experience in our laboratory with echographic V_{CF} has been in general accord with the results of other workers. Thus, we have found that echographic V_{CF} provides a reliable index of ventricular performance, especially in the presence of valvular heart disease or cardiomyopathy (Figure 28). The good correlation of echographic V_{CF} with ventricular function in some patients with segmental wall abnormalities due to coronary disease may be related to the hyperkinesis of the uninvolved myocardium, as described in the section on interventricular septal wall motion. In this regard, Corya et al.[108] have

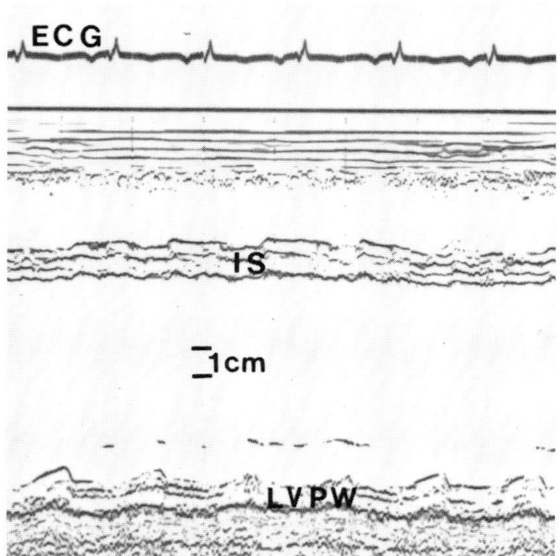

FIGURE 28. Left ventricular echogram obtained in a patient with congestive cardiomyopathy. Illustrated is left ventricular dilation and generalized hypokinesis involving both IS and left ventricular posterior wall (LVPW).

recently found that the preservation of a normal or increased amplitude of contraction of one ventricular wall was the principal echographic feature that distinguished coronary patients with congestive heart failure from those with congestive cardiomyopathy in whom wall motion was characteristically diffusely depressed. Studies in our laboratories and those of others have suggested that echographic V_{CF} is affected by alterations in ventricular afterload[57,109] and, to a lesser extent, ventricular preload. Thus, it appears that V_{CF} measured by ultrasound reflects overall cardiac pump performance rather than myocardial contractility specifically.

Mitral Valve Motion

Since mitral valve motion is primarily a function of intracardiac blood flow and pressures, several investigators have attempted to utilize the mitral echogram to evaluate cardiac function. Fischer and associates[110] analyzed the area between the anterior and posterior mitral leaflets on the echogram and demonstrated a good correlation between this measurement and stroke volume determined by the Fick method

in patients without mitral valve disease. Subsequently, Konecke and colleagues[111] studied the effects of elevated left ventricular diastolic pressures upon mitral valve motion on the echogram. These workers demonstrated that the slope of the D-E segment (velocity of opening of the anterior mitral leaflet on echogram) was reduced below 25 mm/sec in the presence of an increase in left ventricular initial diastolic pressure greater than 14 mm Hg. In addition, they found that the period from the A point (peak anterior mitral leaflet opening after atrial contraction) to the C point (point of mitral leaflet closure) adjusted for atrioventricular conduction by subtracting this time period from the PR interval on electrocardiogram—a measure designated the PR-AC interval—was reduced in the presence of left ventricular end-diastolic pressure greater than 20 mm Hg with a concomitant atrial pressure wave of 8 mm Hg on the ventricular pressure pulse. Moreover, in the presence of such alterations in end-diastolic pressure, the A-C segment was frequently interrupted by a plateau. Although these observations were largely empiric, they have provided evidence that quantitative assessment of the mitral echogram may be utilized in the evaluation of cardiac function.

It has been speculated by several investigators that the diastolic closing velocity on the echogram—the E-F slope—is related to left ventricular diastolic compliance. Quinones and associates[112] have demonstrated a general relationship between a reduced E-F slope and decreased ventricular compliance. Results in our laboratories have also been in general agreement with this observation. However, we have not found a good correlation between the mitral E-F slope and various indexes of left ventricular diastolic compliance in individual patients.[112] Therefore, we explored the relation between the mitral E-F slope and left ventricular sequential diastolic flow in each third of diastole as measured by cineangiography. An excellent correlation was observed between transmitral flow in the first third of diastole and the E-F slope, with a correlation coefficient of 0.87.[113] In addition, a difference in the relation of atrioventricular flow to diastolic closing velocity was noted between patients with hypertrophic cardiomyopathy and those with coronary disease;

patients with hypertrophic cardiomyopathy exhibited a less steep E-F slope for the reduction of flow in the first third of diastole. We have interpreted this observation to suggest an alteration in the mitral valve apparatus induced by hypertrophic disease as opposed to ischemic heart disease. In the former condition, hypertrophy of the interventricular septum may produce anteromedial displacement of the anterior papillary muscle, thereby causing the chordae tendineae to be taut during diastole. Therefore, it appears that the mitral E-F slope on the echogram is primarily related to the amount of atrioventricular flow in the first third of diastole. Reduction of left ventricular compliance in patients with either hypertrophic cardiomyopathy or coronary disease usually results in diminution of transmitral flow in the first third of diastole and thereby is generally accompanied by decreased E-F slope on the echogram.

Multidimensional Echocardiography

The major limitation of conventional echocardiography in the evaluation of cardiac performance is that the standard method utilizes only a one-dimensional view to evaluate a three-dimensional object. Thus, the traditional icepick view of the heart provided by an echogram has been likened to shining a flashlight into a dark room from the outside, so that only those areas in the path of the light beam may be examined at any given time.[114] The determination of left ventricular volumes and ejection fraction and the assessment of segmental wall motion has, therefore, been limited by the restricted area of cardiac anatomy that can be examined at one time.

Several investigators have therefore attempted to develop multidimensional echographs that provide either a superior to inferior or lateral dimension in addition to the usual anteroposterior dimension. Cardiac ultrasonography is a technique proposed by King[115] that utilizes conventional B mode cardiac scanning gated to the electrocardiogram so that echograms may be obtained in a single phase during the cardiac cycle. Figure 29, A and B, shows such a B mode scan obtained from a patient in our laboratory utilizing a commercially available echograph. In this procedure the orientation of the transducer in space is recorded electrically while the transducer is rocked through an arc of 30 to 60 degrees, and the ultrasonic signals are then displayed in the appropriate distribution on the oscilloscope. Thus, when the transducer is angled superiorly, the ultrasound signals are displayed on the upper portion of the oscilloscope. The advantages of this type of multidimensional technique are that

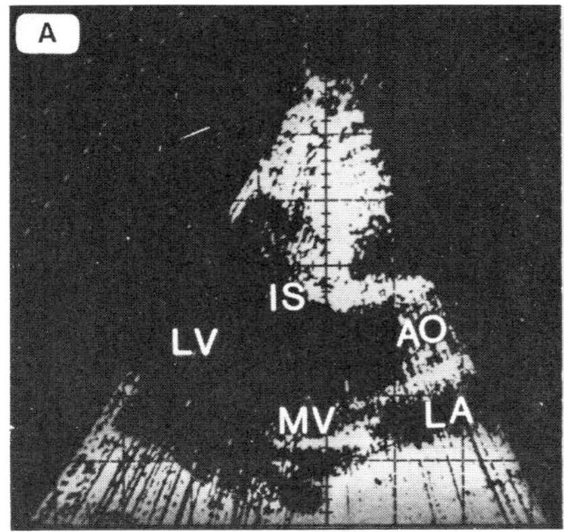

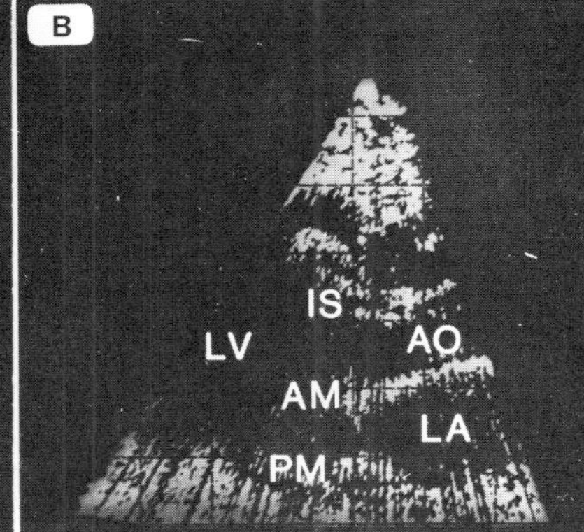

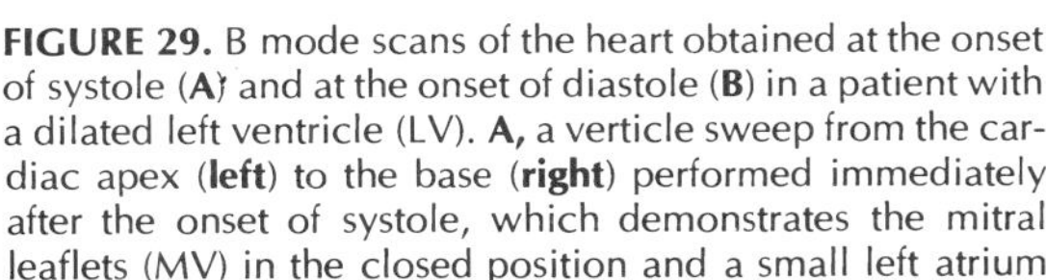

FIGURE 29. B mode scans of the heart obtained at the onset of systole (**A**) and at the onset of diastole (**B**) in a patient with a dilated left ventricle (LV). **A,** a verticle sweep from the cardiac apex (**left**) to the base (**right**) performed immediately after the onset of systole, which demonstrates the mitral leaflets (MV) in the closed position and a small left atrium (LA) after atrial contraction. **B,** a similar B mode tracing obtained immediately after the onset of diastole, which illustrates widely separated anterior (AM) and posterior (PM) mitral valve leaflets and a dilated left atrium. AO = ascending aorta; IS = intraventricular septum.

it requires minimal sophisticated electronic equipment and enables the examiner to retain manual control of transducer angulation. The disadvantage is that it requires many beats to obtain an adequate scan, necessitating extra time and the absence of arrhythmias.

Subsequently, Bom and co-workers[116,117] developed the technique of multiscan echocardiography that involves a multielement transducer composed of 20 adjacent piezoelectric crystals in a linear array. Each element is activated in sequence and the ultrasound signals are displayed in a B mode fashion, with the signal from the most superior element at the uppermost portion of the oscilloscope. In addition to the ability to add a superior-to-inferior dimension to standard echocardiography, this technique includes the option of a transverse dimension. The technique is rapid and offers potential inclusion of all cardiovascular structures in a single echogram if the structures are of small size. These attributes have proved most advantageous in pediatric cardiology. The disadvantages of the system are that it requires a generous cardiac window through which the sound beam may gain access to the cardiovascular structures and that the transducer cannot easily be rocked in an arc. Since the ventricular walls are either concave or convex with respect to the chest wall, this difficulty in adjusting the transducer arc can prevent the perpendicular orientation of the ultrasound beam to all portions of the left ventricular wall, especially the apical segment. Nevertheless, recent work has shown this method to provide technically adequate echograms in most children and in a majority of adults.[116,117]

Several additional types of two-dimensional echographs have recently been developed utilizing the principle of an arc scanner.[118,119] These ultrasound systems have in common the fact that they maintain a single piezoelectric transducer that can be rocked through a 30, 60 or even 90 degree arc and thus remain perpendicular to the left ventricular posterior wall throughout virtually its entire longitudinal extent. Arc scanners employ a motor connected to the transducer that serves to oscillate the transducer rapidly through the 30 to 90 degree arc at rates of approximately 30 to 60 rev/sec and thus display a complete arc in a B mode fashion at a

similar rate. Arc scanners also can be employed for a horizontal section. Although the vibrations that arc scanners provide may prove irritating to some patients, this method requires no greater window than that required by conventional echocardiography while retaining a high degree of digital control of the transducer.

Recently a two-dimensional echographic system has been developed that utilizes a multielement transducer of smaller size interfaced to a computer.[120] Although this system has provided excellent two-dimensional studies, the technical sophistication of the equipment required may limit its widespread application.

It appears likely that a multidimensional echograph will become generally commercially available in the near future. Although this technique may not add substantially to standard echocardiography in the evaluation of segmental wall motion, it should significantly enhance the ability to evaluate cardiac volumes and ejection fraction by ultrasound. Therefore, multidimensional echography promises to increase the role of ultrasound in the evaluation of cardiac function.

Echographic Approach to the Patient with Cardiomegaly and Congestive Heart Failure of Unknown Etiology

One of the most common problems encountered in clinical cardiology occurs in the patient with an enlarged heart and congestive heart failure. Although the etiology of the cardiac dysfunction is often indicated by murmurs or other abnormalities detected on standard clinical evaluation, the diagnosis may remain uncertain in a substantial proportion of such patients even after routine diagnostic measures have been employed. Thus, the advent of echocardiography has provided an important new approach to the evaluation of patients with congestive heart failure of uncertain etiology.

The types of heart disease that may present as congestive heart failure of unknown cause include:

I. Pericardial effusion
II. Intrinsic cardiac enlargement
  A. Silent valvular heart disease
  B. Congenital heart disease
  C. Pulmonary vascular disease

D. Hypertensive cardiovascular disease
E. Coronary artery disease
F. Cardiomyopathy

Thus, an enlarged heart and the picture of congestive heart failure may be due to the presence of pericardial effusion in the absence of any myocardial abnormality. More often, however, intrinsic cardiac disease is responsible for the congestive heart failure state, and cardiac enlargement is present. Although six categories of cardiac disease that may account for cardiomegaly and congestive heart failure are enumerated, the majority of these disorders do not usually constitute a diagnostic dilemma to the examining physician. In our experience it is extremely uncommon for valvular heart disease to be silent, although heart murmurs may be misleading concerning the severity of valvular disease present. Similarly, congenital heart disease with heart failure and cardiomegaly only occasionally presents in the absence of diagnostic cardiac murmurs. In addition, congestive failure with cardiac enlargement due to pulmonary disease or hypertensive cardiovascular disease is usually readily manifest on bedside examination, and coronary heart disease is usually detectable by electrocardiographic abnormalities. Although a large heart and congestive heart failure without cardiac murmurs usually signifies a cardiomyopathy, such a combination represents a diagnostic challenge in the exclusion of atypical presentations of other types of heart disease.

Pericardial Effusion: An enlarged cardiac silhouette and congestive heart failure secondary to pericardial effusion frequently may be difficult to distinguish from intrinsic ventricular dysfunction. Thus, the ability of echocardiography to definitively discern between these two entities played a major role in the development of this noninvasive technique. Figures 2 and 3 illustrate normal echocardiograms demonstrating the pericardial cavity to be only a potential space that is not visualized by ultrasound in normal subjects. In the normal echocardiogram, echoes from the anterior right ventricular wall are directly opposed to the chest wall echoes, and the left ventricular posterior wall is normally positioned directly in contact with the lung.

Figure 30A illustrates the echocardiogram obtained from a patient with carcinoma of the breast who was referred for cardiac ultrasound examination because of an enlarged heart and congestive heart failure. It is evident that a large space representing a massive pericardial effusion exists both anteriorly—between the chest wall and the anterior right ventricular wall—and posteriorly—between the lung and the posterior left ventricular wall. This patient was subsequently subjected to pericardiocentesis with the removal of 800 cc of sanguineous fluid. Figure 30B was obtained after removal of all fluid. This figure illustrates the absence of the previously noted anterior and posterior spaces between the heart and pericardium, and in addition, a solitary echo is recorded when the echocardiograph damp control is utilized to reduce the ultrasound energy so that only the strongest ultrasonic interface remains. This damping maneuver may prove crucial in the detection of small pericardial effusions.

The majority of pericardial effusions that are detected by echocardiography, however, are not of major degree but rather are minor accumulations of fluid secondary to the presence of congestive heart failure. Inasmuch as echograms are normally made with the patient in the supine position, posterior fluid accumulation characteristically is found prior to anterior accumulation. Figure 31 shows the echocardiogram obtained in a patient who was found to have pericardial effusion secondary to congestive heart failure. In this echogram, the small amount of pericardial fluid was not obvious before the reduction of ultrasound energy by means of the damping device. Thus, midway through the echogram the ultrasonic energy was decreased so that the left ventricular epicardium and the immobile pericardium were seen to be separated by a minor degree of pericardial fluid.

In addition, echocardiography also provides data regarding the quantity of pericardial effusion;[121] Horowitz and co-workers conducted a study comparing the amount of pericardial fluid revealed by an echogram obtained just prior to cardiac surgery with that removed at the time of operation. These authors found that echocardiograms indicating a clear separation of the left ventricular epicardium from an immobile pericardium throughout the entire cardiac cycle represented the most reliable ultrasonic mani-

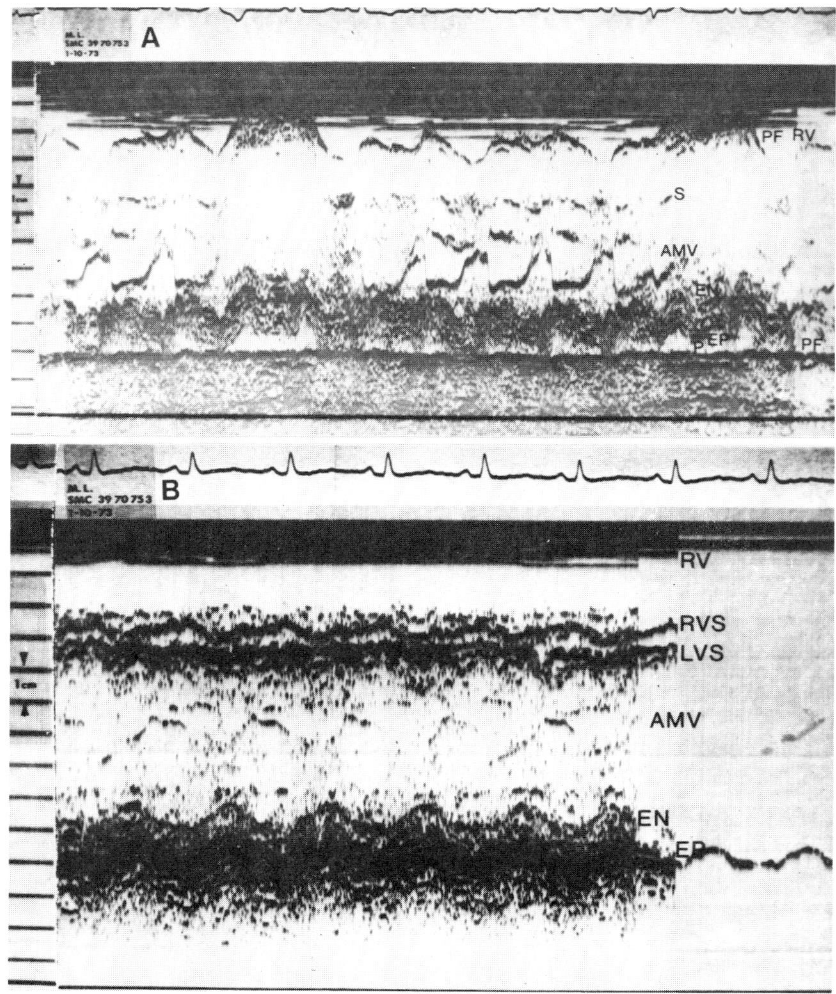

FIGURE 30. Echocardiograms in a patient with a large pericardial effusion. **A,** before and **B,** after removal of the pericardial fluid by needle aspiration. EN = LV endocardium; EP = LV epicardium; P = pericardium; PF = pericardial fluid; S = IVS.

festation of pericardial fluid. Further, these workers attempted to quantify pericardial effusion by correlating the cube of the size of the left ventricle with the cube of the pericardial cavity as measured by echocardiogram. Although this method provided a satisfactory general relation between the amount of pericardial fluid predicted by echogram and that found on pericardiocentesis, it must be remembered that pericardial fluid normally collects in the most dependent portion of the pericardium. Thus, an echocardiographic scan from the apex to base of the heart is the most useful technique for quantifying the amount of effusion by ultrasound (Figure 32).

Intrinsic Cardiac Disorders: When pericardial effusion is absent in a patient with an enlarged heart and congestive heart failure, a cardiac abnormality is present. As stated previously, silent valvular heart disease of substantial degree is rare in our experience, although the magnitude of the cardiac murmur may frequently be misleading in terms of the severity of valvular disorder, especially in the presence of reduced cardiac output. However, occasionally a patient presents with cardiomegaly and congestive heart failure in the absence of any readily detectable auscultatory cardiac abnormalities. Figure 33 illustrates the echocardiogram obtained in such a patient who was referred for ultrasound examination because of congestive heart failure of unknown etiology. The echocardiogram revealed massive left ventricular enlargement with an end-diastolic dimension of 8 cm but with relatively normal wall motion. Further, the anterior leaflet of the mitral valve was noted to undergo the fine fluttering movements characteristic of aortic regurgitation, and this diagnosis was subsequently confirmed by cardiac catheterization. Thus, in this patient with confusing auscultatory findings, echocardiography documented the valvular disorder.

Congenital heart disease may also present as cardiomegaly and congestive heart failure without cardiac murmurs. Such may be the case when previous left-to-right intracardiac shunting is prevented by elevated pulmonary vascular resistance. In these situations, the right ventricle is usually found to be enlarged to a greater degree than is the left ventricle. Figure 23 illustrates the echocardiogram in a patient with cardiomegaly, paroxysmal atrial fibrillation and congestive heart failure who was subsequently documented to have an atrial septal defect. This echogram shows that the right ventricle has undergone dilation so that it approximates the left ventricle in dimension. In addition, the interventricular septum manifests marked paradoxi-

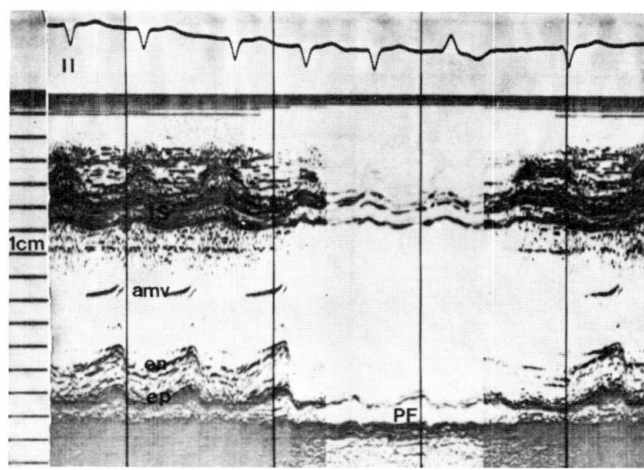

FIGURE 31. Echocardiogram demonstrating a small posterior pericardial effusion (PF) obtained in a patient with congestive heart failure. Ultrasonic energy was abruptly reduced in the **midportion** of the recording.

cal or inappropriate anterior septal motion. Specific echocardiographic findings may be noted in a variety of other congenital heart diseases. Thus, echocardiography serves as a valuable noninvasive method in the recognition of congenital heart disorders when these entities present as congestive failure in the absence of diagnostic auscultatory abnormalities.

Athough cor pulmonale is usually readily evident by the presence of severe pulmonary disease, on occasion the cause of right heart enlargement may be obscure. Echocardiography may provide evidence that right heart failure is due to parenchymal or vascular pulmonary disease by the detection of a predominant right ventricle. Figure 34 illustrates an echocar-

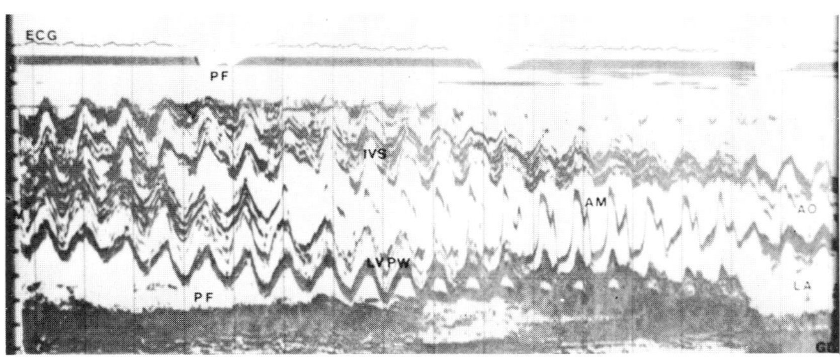

FIGURE 32. Echocardiographic scan from apex (**left**) to base (**right**) in a patient with pericardial effusion (PF). Since the patient's bed was elevated 30 degrees, a greater fluid accumulation occurred at the cardiac apex.

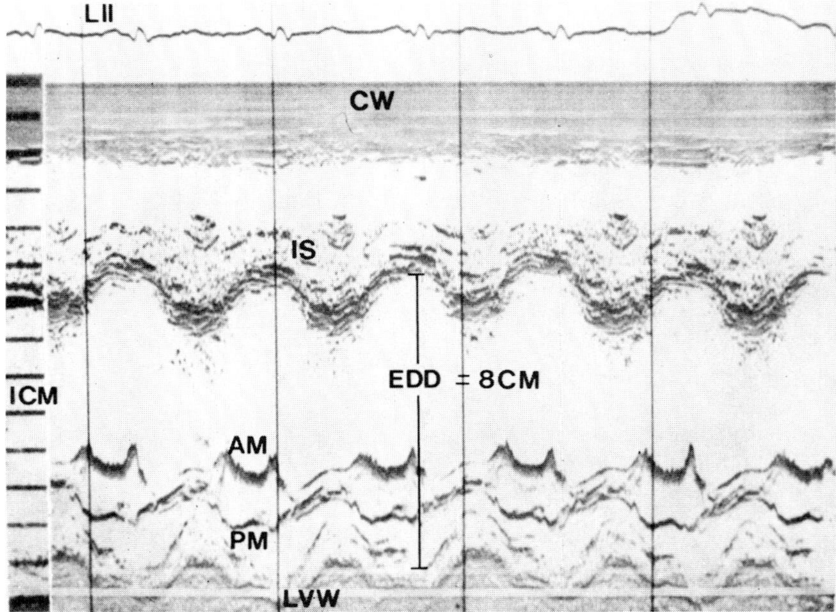

FIGURE 33. Echocardiogram obtained in a patient with massive left ventricular dilation secondary to severe silent aortic regurgitation.

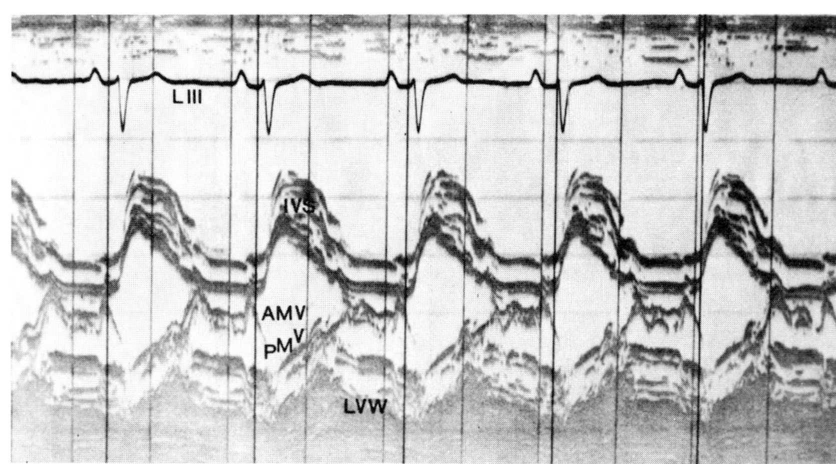

FIGURE 34. Echocardiogram obtained in a patient with severe tricuspid regurgitation secondary to primary pulmonary hypertension. Illustrated is marked right ventricular enlargement and inappropriate septal motion.

diogram that was obtained from a patient who had cardiomegaly and congestive failure subsequently determined by cardiac catheterization to be the result of primary pulmonary hypertension with secondary tricuspid regurgitation. As is evident, the right ventricle is enormously enlarged and the motion of the interventricular septum is markedly paradoxical. Thus, echocardiography may be of considerable utility in unusual patients with cardiac disorders referable to pulmonary diseases.

The majority of patients with cardiomegaly

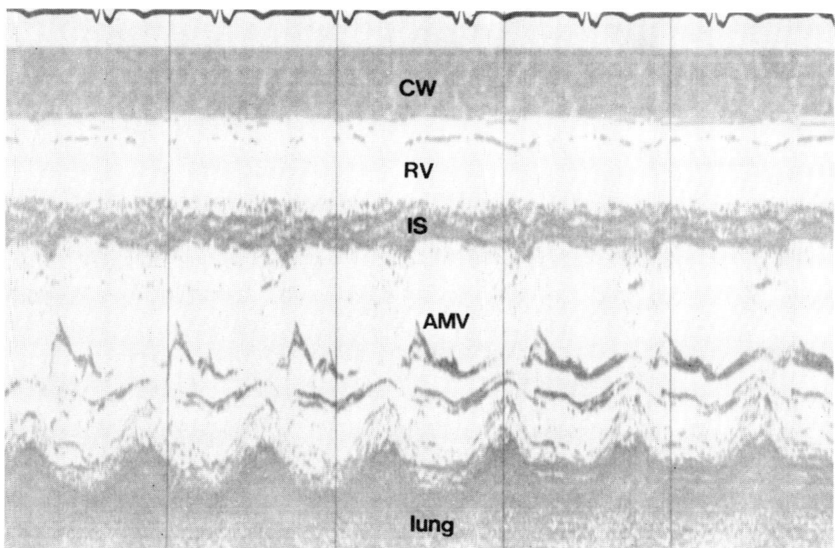

FIGURE 35. Echogram in a patient with an old anterior myocardial infarction with interventricular septum (IS) akinesis and abnormal passive diastolic recoil, and compensatory hyperkinesis of the left ventricular posterior wall (**bottom**).

and congestive heart faliure have disease predominating in the left ventricle. Echocardiography may provide the initial diagnostic clue in this setting by determining whether the underlying process is one of left ventricular hypertrophy or dilation. Cardiac hypertrophy may be due to hypertensive cardiovascular disease, in which the echogram reveals a symmetric or concentric increase in left ventricular wall thickness. In contrast, hypertrophy may be the result of a hypertrophic cardiomyopathy or idiopathic hypertrophic subaortic stenosis, in which the echogram in the majority of patients shows asymmetric septal hypertrophy. Figure 20 demonstrates the echogram in a patient with ventricular hypertrophy due to hypertensive cardiovascular disease. The interventricular septum and left ventricular posterior wall are hypertrophied to approximately the same extent. In contrast, Figure 6 reveals the selective hypertrophy of the interventricular septum in a patient with idiopathic hypertrophic subaortic stenosis. Thus, echocardiography may provide evidence of ventricular hypertrophy as the cause of cardiac enlargement and failure, as well as distinguish between hypertensive cardiovascular disease and hypertrophic cardiomyopathy.

Congestive Cardiomyopathy vs. Coronary Heart Disease: Most patients with congestive heart failure of uncertain etiology encountered by the clinical cardiologist present the vexing problem of differentiating idiopathic cardiomyopathy from coronary artery disease. Echocardiography has recently been documented to be of substantial value in this differentiation by virtue of its ability to detect segmental abnormalities of wall motion in patients with coronary atherosclerosis, as opposed to diffuse or generalized abnormalities of wall motion in patients with congestive cardiomyopathy. Figure 27 illustrates the echocardiogram in a patient with previous anterior-septal myocardial infarction and an aneurysm involving the anterior-apical third of the left ventricle. Note that interventricular septal motion is akinetic in the area of the cardiac apex, whereas left ventricular posterior wall motion is hyperkinetic and the interventricular septum is unaffected by the ischemic process in the area of the cardiac base. Figure 35 illustrates findings in another patient with an anterior myocardial infarction in whom the interventricular septum revealed dyskinesis during systole, although the left ventricular posterior wall was somewhat hyperkinetic.

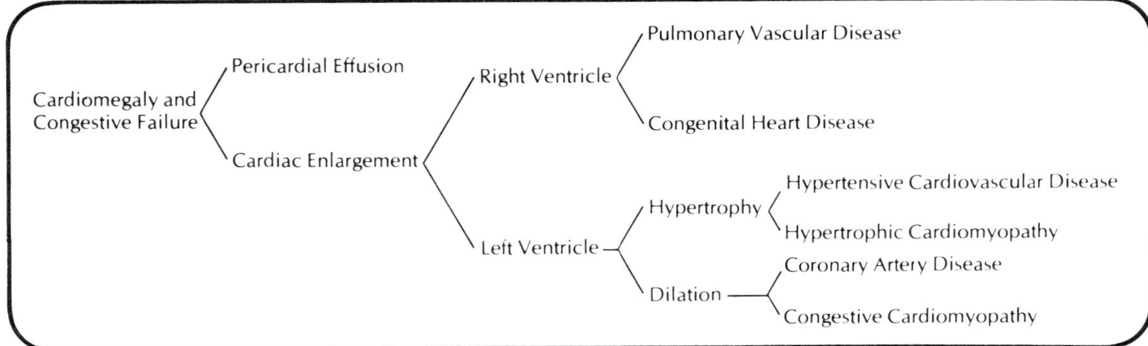

FIGURE 36. Echographic evaluation of cardiomegaly.

In contrast, Figure 28 presents the echocardiogram obtained from a patient with congestive cardiomyopathy. Note that in addition to the marked ventricular dilation, there is severe hypokinesis with reduction in both velocity and extent of contraction involving the interventricular septum as well as the left ventricular posterior wall. Corya and co-workers[108] have found the most valuable echographic parameter in distinguishing congestive cardiomyopathy from coronary heart disease with congestive failure to be the sum of the amplitudes of systolic motion of the left interventricular septum and left ventricular posterior wall. In patients with coronary artery disease, contraction of one wall was typically maintained so that the sum of the amplitudes was usually greater than that in patients with congestive cardiomyopathies in whom the amplitude of both ventricular surfaces was markedly reduced. Thus, echocardiography may be invaluable in achieving the difficult differentiation between congestive cardiomyopathy and coronary artery disease with congestive heart failure.

In summary, these observations have led to the evolution of an echocardiographic approach to the patient with an enlarged heart and congestive heart failure at our institution. Thus, as delineated in Figure 36, the patient is approached from an anatomic standpoint, with etiologic deductions being drawn from morphologic data. As shown, the first step in this procedure involves the determination of the presence or absence of pericardial effusion. When pericardial effusion is found absent and cardiomegaly is present, we then focus attention upon whether the pathologic process principally affects the right or left ventricle. When echographic abnormalities of the right ventricle predominate, the presence of congenital or pulmonary heart disease is strongly suggested. In contrast, when the left ventricle is primarily involved, we attempt to distinguish between left ventricular hypertrophy or dilation. When left ventricular hypertrophy is present, a determination is made as to whether the process most closely conforms to hypertrophic cardiomyopathy with asymmetric septal hypertrophy or hypertensive cardiovascular disease. The typical patient, however, will be found to have left ventricular dilation rather than hypertrophy. An attempt is made to distinguish congestive cardiomyopathy from coronary artery disease with congestive failure by the presence of diffuse abnormalities of ventricular wall motion in the former, as opposed to segmental abnormalities of ventricular wall motion in the latter. Thus, the utilization of echocardiography in this format may contribute considerably to the evaluation of patients with cardiac enlargement and congestive heart failure.

Summary

Echocardiography has rapidly become an invaluable examining technique that utilizes pulsed, reflected ultrasound to obtain noninvasively a graphic representation of dynamic cardiac anatomy. In addition to the ability of ultrasound to identify a variety of cardiac diseases, this method provides a practical and reliable means for the assessment of cardiac function in terms of both hemodynamic and mechanical properties of performance. Thus, by giving absolute dimensions of cardiac chambers and structures, echocardiography allows the determination of the volume, wall thickness, segmental motion, and velocity of circumferential fiber shortening of the left ventricle, as well as the size of the left atrium. In addition, study of mitral valve movement affords evaluation of left ventricular sequential diastolic inflow. It is emphasized that important advantages and limitations pertain to these measurements, and considerable experience is necessary to obtain satisfactory cardiac ultrasound recordings. The recent advent of multidimensional echocardiography provides a technique for extending the standard one-dimensional echographic view to three-dimensional analysis of the heart. Finally, this chapter delineates the echographic approach to the diagnostic examination of cardiomegaly and congestive heart failure of unknown etiology.

Acknowledgment: This work was supported in part by Research Program Project Grant HL 14780 from the National Heart and Lung Institute, National Institutes of Health.

The authors gratefully acknowledge the technical assistance of Lillian Reese, Marilyn McChesney and Leslie J. Silvernail.

References

1. **Edler I, Hertz CH:** Use of ultrasonic reflectoscope for continuous recording of movements of heart walls. Kurgle Fysicgr Sallad i Fund Forhandl 24:5, 1954

2. **Kossof G:** Diagnostic applications of ultrasound in cardiology. Aust Radiol 10:101, 1966

3. **Edler I, Gustafson A:** Ultrasonic cardiogram in mitral stenosis. Acta Med Scand 159:85, 1957

4. **Segal BL, Lehoff W, Kingsley B:** Echocardiography: clinical application in mitral stenosis. JAMA 193:161, 1966

5. **Effert S:** Pre- and postoperative evaluation of mitral stenosis by ultrasound. Amer J Cardiol 19:59, 1967

6. **Dillon JC, Haine CL, Chang S, et al:** Use of echocardiography in patients with prolapsed mitral valve. Circulation 43:503, 1971

7. **Kerber RE, Isaeff DM, Hancock EW:** Echocardiographic patterns in patients with the syndrome of systolic click and late systolic murmur. New Eng J Med 284:691, 1971

8. **Popp RL, Brown OR, Silverman JF, et al:** Echocardiographic abnormalities in the mitral valve prolapse syndrome. Circulation 49:428, 1974

9. **DeMaria AN, King JF, Bogren H, et al:** The variable spectrum of echographic manifestations of the mitral valve prolapse syndrome. Circulation 50:33, 1974

10. **Shah PM, Gramiak R, Kramer DH:** Ultrasound localization of left ventricular outflow obstruction in hypertrophic obstructive cardiomyopathy. Circulation 40:3, 1969

11. **Popp RL, Harrison DC:** Ultrasound in the diagnosis and evaluation of therapy of idiopathic hypertrophic subaortic stenosis. Circulation 45:905, 1969

12. **Abbasi AS, MacAlpin RN, Eber LM, et al:** Echocardiographic diagnosis of idiopathic hypertrophic cardiomyopathy without outflow obstruction. Circulation 46:897, 1972

13. **Henry WI, Clark CE, Glancy DL, et al:** Echocardiographic measurement of the left ventricular outflow gradient in idiopathic hypertrophic subaortic stenosis. New Eng J Med 288:989, 1973

14. **Henry WL, Clark CE, Epstein SE:** Asymmetric septal hypertrophy: the unifying link in the IHSS disease spectrum. Circulation 47:827, 1973

15. **King JF, DeMaria AN, Reis RL, et al:** Echocardiographic assessment of idiopathic hypertrophic subaortic stenosis. Chest 64:723, 1973

16. **King JF, DeMaria AN, Miller RR, et al:** Markedly abnormal mitral valve motion without simultaneous intraventricular pressure gradient due to uneven mitral-septal contact in idiopathic hypertrophic subaortic stenosis. Amer J Cardiol 34:360, 1974

17. **Effert S, Domanig E:** The diagnosis of intra-atrial tumors and thrombi by the ultrasonic echo method. German Med Monthly 4:1, 1959

18. **Wolfe SB, Popp RL, Feigenbaum H:** Diagnosis of atrial tumors by ultrasound. Circulation 39:615, 1969

19. **Schattenberg TT, Tajik AJ, Gan GT:** Echocardiogram in left atrial myxoma. Chest 63:423, 1973

20. **Waxler EB, Kawai N, Kasparian H:** Right atrial myxoma: echocardiographic, phonocardiographic, and hemodynamic signs. Amer Heart J 83:251, 1972

21. **DeMaria AN, Vismara LA, Miller RR, et al:** Unusual echographic manifestations of cardiac myxomas. Amer J Med 59:713, 1975

22. **Pridie RB, Benham R, Oakley CA:** Echocardiography of the mitral valve in aortic valve disease. Brit Heart J 33:296, 1971

23. **Winsberg F, Gabor GE, Hernberg JG, et al:** Fluttering of mitral valve in aortic insufficiency. Circulation 41:225, 1970

24. **DeMaria AN, King JF, Salel AF, et al:** Echography and phonography of acute aortic regurgitation in bacterial endocarditis. Ann Intern Med 82:329, 1975

25. **Sweatman T, Selzer A, Kamagaki M, et al:** Echocardiographic diagnosis of mitral regurgitation due to ruptured chordae tendineae. Circulation 46:580, 1972

26. **Duchak JM, Chang S, Feigenbaum H:** Echocardiographic features of torn chordae tendineae. Amer J Cardiol 29:260, 1972

27. **Gramiak R, Shah PM:** Echocardiography of the nor-

mal and diseased aortic valve. Radiology 96:1, 1970

28. **Feigenbaum H:** Echocardiographic diagnosis of pericardial effusion. Amer J Cardiol 26:475, 1970

29. **Klein JJ, Segal BL:** Pericardial effusion diagnosed by reflected ultrasound. Amer J Cardiol 22:57, 1968

30. **Pridie RB, Turnbull TA:** Diagnosis of pericardial effusion by ultrasound. Brit Med J 3:356, 1968

31. **Goldberg BB, Olstrum BJ, Isara HJ:** Ultrasonic determination of pericardial effusion. JAMA 202:927, 1967

32. **Horowitz MS, Schultz CS, Stinson EB, et al:** Sensitivity and specificity of echocardiographic diagnosis of pericardial effusion. Circulation 50:239, 1974

33. **Weyman AE, Dillon JC, Feigenbaum H, et al:** Echocardiographic patterns of pulmonic valve motion in pulmonic stenosis. Amer J Cardiol 33:178, 1974

34. **Nanda NC, Gramiak R, Robinson TI, et al:** Echocardiographic evaluation of pulmonary hypertension. Circulation 50:575, 1974

35. **Weyman AE, Dillon JC, Feigenbaum H, et al:** Echocardiographic patterns of pulmonary valve motion in valvular pulmonary stenosis. Amer J Cardiol 34:644, 1974

36. **Gustafson A:** Correlation between ultrasound cardiography hemodynamic and surgical findings in mitral stenosis. Acta Med Scand suppl 461:1, 1966

37. **Joyner CR, Reid JM, Bond JP:** Reflected ultrasound in the asssessment of mitral valve disease. Circulation 27:503, 1963

38. **Feigenbaum H, Zaky A, Nasser WK:** Use of ultrasound to measure left ventricular stroke volume. Circulation 35:1092, 1967

39. **Popp RL, Wolfe SB, Hirata T, et al:** Estimation of right and left ventricular size by ultrasound. A study of echoes from the interventricular septum. Amer J Cardiol 24:523, 1969

40. **Feigenbaum H, Stone JM, Lee DA, et al:** Identification of ultrasound echoes from the left ventricle using intracardiac injections of indocyanin green. Circulation 41:615, 1970

41. **Feigenbaum H, Popp RL, Wolfe SB, et al:** Ultrasound measurements of the left ventricle: a correlative study with angiocardiography. Arch Intern Med 129:461, 1972

42. **Popp RL, Harrison DC:** Ultrasonic cardiac echography for determing stroke volume and valvular regurgitation. Circulation 41:493, 1970

43. **Pombo JF, Troy BL, Russell RO Jr:** Left ventricular volumes and ejection fraction by echocardiography. Circulation 43:480, 1971

44. **Pombo JF, Russell RO, Rackley CE, et al:** Comparison of stroke volume and cardiac output determination by ultrasound and dye dilution in acute myocardial infarction. Amer J Cardiol 27:630, 1971

45. **Gibson DG:** Measurement of left ventricular volumes in man using echocardiography. Comparison with biplane angiographs. Brit Heart J 33:614, 1971

46. **Fortuin NJ, Hood WP, Sherman E, et al:** Determinations of left ventricular volumes by ultrasound. Circulation 44:575, 1971

47. **Murray JA, Johnston W, Reid JM:** Echocardiographic determination of left ventricular dimensions, volumes, and performance. Amer J Cardiol 30:252, 1972

48. **Redwood DR, Henry WL, Epstein SE:** Evaluation of the ability of echocardiography to measure acute alterations in left ventricular volume. Circulation 50:901, 1974

49. **Teichholz LE, Kruclen TH, Herman MV, et al:** Problems in echocardiographic volume determinations: echo-angiographic correlations. Circulation 46 suppl II: II–275, 1972

50. **Popp RL, Alderman EL, Brown OR, et al:** Sources of error in calculation of left ventricular volumes by echography. Amer J Cardiol 31:152, 1973

51. **Belenkie I, Nutter DO, Clark DW, et al:** Assessment of left ventricular dimensions and function by echocardiography. Amer J Cardiol 31:755, 1973

52. **Ratshin RA, Boyd CN, Rackley CE, et al:** The accuracy of ventricular volume analysis by quantitative echocardiography in patients with coronary artery disease with and without wall motion abnormalities. Amer J Cardiol 33:164, 1974

53. **Davila JC, Sanmarco ME:** An analysis of the fit of mathematical models applicable to the measurement of left ventricular volume. Amer J Cardiol 18:31, 1966

54. **Ross J, Sonnenblick EH, Covell JW, et al:** The architecture of the heart in systole and diastole. Circ Res 21:409, 1967

55. **Gault JH, Ross J, Braunwald E:** Contractile state of the left ventricle in man: instantaneous tension-velocity-length relations in patients with and without disease of the left ventricular myocardium. Circ Res 22:451, 1968

56. **Sandler H, Dodge HT:** The use of single plane angiocardiograms for the calculation of left ventricular volume in man. Amer Heart J 75:325, 1968

57. **DeMaria AN, Vismara L, Auditore K, et al:** Effects of nitroglycerin upon left ventricular cavitary size and cardiac performance determined by ultrasound in man. Amer J Med 57:754, 1974

58. **McDonald IG, Feigenbaum H, Chang S:** Analysis of left ventricular wall motion by reflected ultrasound. Circulation 46:14, 1972

59. **Feigenbaum H:** Echocardiographic examination of the left ventricle. Circulation 51:1, 1975

60. **Ratshin RA, Rackley GE, Russell RO:** Serial evaluation of left ventricular volumes and posterior wall movement in the acute phase of myocardial infarction using diagnostic ultrasound. Amer J Cardiol 29:286, 1972

61. **Broder MI, Cohn JN:** Evolution of abnormalities in left ventricular function after acute myocardial infarction. Circulation 46:731, 1972

62. **Corya BC, Feigenbaum H, Rasmussen S, et al:** Echocardiographic findings predicting mortality in acute myocardial infarction. Circulation 50 suppl III:29, 1974

63. **Stefadouros MA, Dougherty MJ, Grossman W, et al:** Determination of systemic vascular resistance by a noninvasive technique. Circulation 47:101, 1973

64. **Stefadouros MA, Grossman W, El Shahawy M, et al:** The effect of isometric exercise on the volume of the left ventricle in normal man. Circulation 49:1185, 1974

65. **Kisslo J, Wolfson S, Ross A, et al:** Ultrasound assessment of left ventricular function following aortocoro-

nary saphenous vein bypass grafting. Circulation 48 suppl III:156, 1973

66. **Ratshin RA, Rackley CE, Russell RO:** Determination of left ventricular preload and afterload by quantitative echocardiography in man. Circ Res 34:711, 1974

67. **DeMaria AN, Lies JE, King JF, et al:** Echographic assessment of atrial transport, mitral movement, and ventricular performance following electroversion of supraventricular arrhythmias. Circulation 51:273, 1975

68. **Hirata T, Wolfe SB, Popp RL, et al:** Estimation of left atrial size using ultrasound. Amer Heart J 78:43, 1969

69. **Brown OR, Harrison DC, Popp RL:** An improved method for echographic detection of left atrial enlargement. Circulation 50:58, 1974

70. **Feigenbaum H, Popp RL, Chip JN, et al:** Left ventricular wall thickness measured by ultrasound. Arch Intern Med 121:391, 1968

71. **Sjogren AC, Hytonen I, Frick MH:** Ultrasonic measurements of left ventricular wall thickness. Chest 57:37, 1970

72. **Troy BL, Pombo J, Rackley CE:** Measurement of left ventricular wall thickness and mass by echocardiography. Circulation 45:602, 1972

73. **Sawaya J, Tongo MR, Schlant RC:** Echocardiographic interventricular septal wall motion and thickness: a study in health and disease. Amer Heart J 87:681, 1974

74. **Herman MV, Hermle RA, Klein MD, et al:** Localized disorders in myocardial contraction: asynergy and its role in congestive heart failure. New Eng J Med 277:222, 1967

75. **Karliner JS, Gault JH, Echberg D, et al:** Mean velocity of fiber shortening. Circulation 44:323, 1971

76. **Abildskov JA, Erik RH, Harmins K, et al:** Observations on the relation between ventricular activation sequence and hemodynamic state. Circ Res 17:236, 1965

77. **Tyberg JV, Parmley WW, Sonnenblick EH:** In-vitro studies of myocardial asynchrony and regional hypoxia. Circ Res 25:569, 1969

78. **Kraunz RF, Kennedy JW:** Ultrasonic determination of left ventricular wall motion in normal man: studies at rest and after exercise. Amer Heart J 79:36, 1970

79. **Kraunz RF, Ryan TJ:** Ultrasound measurements of ventricular wall motion following administration of vasoactive drugs. Amer J Cardiol 27:464, 1971

80. **Inoue K, Smulyan H, Mookherjee S, et al:** Ultrasonic measurement of left ventricular wall motion in acute myocardial infarction. Circulation 43:778, 1971

81. **Wharton CF, Smithen CS, Sowton E:** Changes in left ventricular wall movement after acute myocardial infarction measured by reflected ultrasound. Brit Med J 4:75, 1971

82. **Carson P, Kanter L:** Left ventricular wall movement in heart failure. Brit Med J 4:77, 1971

83. **Smithen CS, Wharton CF, Sowton E:** Independent effects of heart rate and exercise on left ventricular wall movement measured by reflected ultrasound. Amer J Cardiol 30:43, 1972

84. **Fogelman AM, Abbasi AS, Pearce ML, et al:** Echocardiographic study of the abnormal motion of the posterior or left ventricular wall during angina pectoris. Circulation 46:905, 1972

85. **Stefan G, Bing RJ:** Echocardiographic findings in experimental myocardial infarction of the posterior left ventricular wall. Amer J Cardiol 30:629, 1972

86. **Kerber RE, Abboud FM,:** Echocardiographic detection of regional myocardial infarction. Circulation 47:997, 1973

87. **Ludbrook P, Karliner JS, Peterson K, et al:** Comparison of ultrasound and cineangiographic measurements of left ventricular performance in patients with and without wall motion abnormalities. Brit Heart J 35:1026, 1973

88. **Ludbrook P, Karliner J, London A, et al:** Posterior wall velocity: an unreliable index of total left ventricular performance in patients with coronary artery disease. Amer J Cardiol 33:475, 1974

89. **Burch GE, Giles TG, Martinez E:** Echocardiographic detection of abnormal motion of the interventricular septum in ischemic cardiomyopathy. Amer J Med 57:293, 1974

90. **Quinones MA, Gaasch WH, Alexander JK:** Echocardiographic assessment of left ventricular function with special reference to normalized velocities. Circulation 50:42, 1974

91. **Hagan AD, Francis GS, Sahn DJ, et al:** Ultrasound evaluation of systolic anterior motion in patients with and without right ventricular volume overload. Circulation 50:248, 1974

92. **DeMaria AN, Lies J, Neumann A, et al:** Abnormalities of left ventricular segmental contraction of echogram in coronary disease: correlation with cineangiography and electrocardiography. Clin Res 23:78, 1975

93. **Diamond MA, Dillon JC, Haine CL, et al:** Echocardiographic features of atrial septal defect. Circulation 43:129, 1971

94. **Tajik AJ, Gau GT, Schattenberg TT, et al:** Echocardiogram in atrial septal defect with small left to right shunt. Chest 63:95, 1973

95. **McDonald IG:** Echocardiographic demonstration of abnormal motion of the interventricular septum in left bundle branch block. Circulation 58:272, 1973

96. **Abbasi AS, Eber LM, MacAlpin RN, et al:** Paradoxical motion of interventricular septum in left bundle branch block. Circulation 49:423, 1974

97. **Dillon JC, Chang S, Feigenbaum H:** Echocardiographic manifestations of left bundle branch block. Circulation 49:876, 1974

98. **King JF, DeMaria AN, Bonanno JA, et al:** The temporal sequence of myocardial contraction in bundle branch block determined by echocardiography. Circulation 48 suppl IV:127, 1973

99. **Brown DR, Popp RL, Harrison DC:** Abnormal interventricular septal motion in patients with significant disease of the left anterior descending coronary artery or other conditions of septal failure. Amer J Cardiol 31:123, 1973

100. **Rossen RM, Goodman DJ, Ingham RE, et al:** Hypertrophic subaortic stenosis: ventricular septal thickening and excursion. New Eng J Med 291:1317, 1974

101. **Gibson TC, Grossman W, McLaurin LP, et al:** Echocardiography in patients with constrictive pericarditis.

Circulation 50 suppl III:86,1974

102. **Pool PE, Seagren SE, Abbasi AS, et al:** Echocardiographic manifestations of constrictive pericarditis: abnormal septal motion. Circulation 50 suppl III:240, 1974

103. **Feigenbaum H:** Echocardiography. Philadelphia, Lea & Febiger, 1972, p 123

104. **Jacobs JJ, Feigenbaum H, Corya B, et al:** Detection of left ventricular asynergy by echocardiography. Circulation 48:263, 1973

105. **Paraskos JA, Grossman W, Saltz S, et al:** A noninvasive technique for the determination of velocity of circumfirential fiber shortening in man. Cir Res 29:610, 1971

106. **Cooper RH, O'Rourke RA, Karliner JS, et al:** Comparison of ultrasound and cineangiographic measurements of mean rate of circumfirential fiber shortening in man. Circulation 46:914, 1972

107. **Quinones MA, Gaasch WH, Alexander JK:** Echocardiographic assessment of left ventricular function. Circulation 50:42, 1974

108. **Corya BC, Feigenbaum H, Rasmussen S, et al:** Echocardiographic features of congestive cardiomyopathy compared with normal subjects and patients with coronary artery disease. Circulation 49:1153, 1974

109. **Quinones MA, Gaasch JH, Cole JS, et al:** Instantaneous left ventricular stress—velocity relations during ejection in man: with reference to the acute changes in loading and contractility. Clin Res 22:297, 1974

110. **Fischer JC, Chang S, Konecke LL, et al:** Echocardiographic determinations of mitral valve flow. Amer J Cardiol 29:262, 1972

111. **Konecke LL, Feigenbaum H, Chang S, et al:** Abnormal mitral valve motion in patients with elevated left ventricular diastolic pressures. Circulation 47:989, 1973

112. **Quinones MA, Gaasch WH, Waisser E, et al:** Reduction in the rate of diastolic descent of the mitral valve echogram in patients with altered left ventricular diastolic pressure-volume relations. Circulation 49:246, 1974

113. **DeMaria AN, Miller RR, Amsterdam EA, et al:** Mitral valve early diastolic closing velocity on echogram: relation to sequential diastolic flow and ventricular compliance. Circulation 50 suppl III:144, 1974

114. **Popp RL:** The noninvasive left ventriculogram. New Eng J Med 291:1254, 1974

115. **King DL:** Cardiac ultrasonography: cross-sectional ultrasonic imaging of the heart. Circulation 47:843, 1973

116. **Bom N, Lancee CT, VanZwieten G, et al:** Multiscan echocardiography. I. Technical description. Circulation 48:1066, 1973

117. **Kloster FE, Roelandt J, Ten Cate FJ, et al:** Multiscan echocardiography. II. Technique and initial clinical results. Circulation 48:1075, 1973

118. **Griffith JM, Henry WL:** A sector scanner for real time two-dimensional echocardiography. Circulation 49:1147, 1974

119. **Eggleton RC, Dillon JC, Feigenbaum H, et al:** Visualization of cardiac dynamics with real time B-mode ultrasonic scanner. Circulation 50 suppl III:27, 1974

120. **VonRamm O, Kisslo J, Thurstone FL, et al:** A new high resolution, real-time, two-dimensional, ultrasound sector scanner. Circulation 50 suppl III:27, 1974

121. **Horowitz MS, Schultz CS, Stinson EB, et al:** Sensitivity and specificity of echocardiographic diagnosis of pericardial effusion. Circulation 50:239, 1974

Cardiac Catheterization in the Clinical Assessment of Heart Disease and Ventricular Performance

Dean T. Mason, MD, FACC

Richard R. Miller, MD, FACC

Daniel S. Berman, MD

Louis A. Vismara, MD, FACC

David O. Williams, MD

Antone F. Salel, MD, FACC

Anthony N. DeMaria, MD, FACC

Hugo G. Bogren, MD

Gerald L. DeNardo, MD

Ezra A. Amsterdam, MD, FACC

The most important advancement in cardiovascular medicine and research in the past quarter century has been the development of methods for catheterization of the human heart that can be carried out with relative ease and safety. Application of these techniques has provided an appreciation of the pathophysiologic mechanisms in heart disease and has established cardiovascular diagnosis and evaluation on a scientific basis. The ability to define precisely and to quantify even the most complex cardiac disorders has spearheaded innovative medical therapy, successful surgical treatment and investigative interest in heart disease in general. In this chapter, major emphasis is placed on the proper application of the methods that permit an assessment of human cardiovascular function, as well as on the interpretation of the physiologic information obtained from these studies.

Right Heart Catheterization

Catheterization of the right side of the heart consists of introducing a radiopaque plastic catheter into an antecubital, axillary, saphenous or femoral vein and, under fluoroscopic control, passing the tube to the chambers of the right side of the heart and pulmonary artery. Pressures are recorded, blood samples are drawn from these sites, and indicator or radiopaque dyes may be injected.[1,2] The recognition of an abnormal catheter course in the heart and great vessels may be helpful in the diagnosis of certain congenital anomalies such as atrial and ventricular septal defects, patent ductus arteriosus, aorticopulmonary window, left superior vena cava, anomalous pulmonary venous drainage and transposition of the great arteries. When the catheter cannot be passed across the tricuspid or pulmonic valves, the presence of valvular stenosis or atresia should be suspected.

Left Heart Catheterization

Although right heart catheterization permits the definition of many congenital cardiac malformations, this technique provides only indirect information concerning physiologic events on the left side of the heart, which is primarily involved in most patients with acquired heart disease. Several methods have been developed to provide direct access to the left atrium and left ventricle. The retrograde arterial, transseptal and anterior percutaneous techniques have proved to be the most suitable. In addition, when an interatrial septal defect or patent foramen ovale is present, the catheter may be passed from the right to the left atrium and then into the left ventricle.

The retrograde arterial technique is the most widely employed approach for left heart catheterization, which is often combined with selective coronary arteriography.[3] This technique is carried out by insertion of a catheter into the arterial tree, either through a right brachial arteriotomy or through the right femoral artery percutaneously, with passage of the catheter across the aortic valve into the left ventricle and sometimes into the left atrium as well. This method, when combined with aortography and left ventricular angiocardiography, is particularly helpful in precisely localizing obstruction to left ventricular outflow and in assessing the severity of aortic stenosis and regurgitation and mitral regurgitation.

The transseptal technique consists of puncture of the atrial septum from the right atrium[4] and thus may be performed simultaneously with right heart catheterization. The principal advantage of transseptal catheterization is that both the left atrial and left ventricular chambers may be entered easily, and thus it is especially useful for the study of patients with mitral valve disease. Contrast material may be injected into the left atrium or left ventricle.

The insertion of a needle through the anterior chest wall directly into the left ventricle constitutes the anterior percutaneous approach.[5] Direct puncture of the left ventricle is technically simple and permits the rapid measurement of the intracavitary pressure, as well as determination of cardiac output by Cardio-Green® dye injected into this chamber. Modification of this technique by passage of a short plastic catheter over the needle into the chamber allows left ventriculography as well.[6] Percutaneous puncture of the left ventricle has been particularly useful in the study of aortic stenosis when the retrograde approach is unsuccessful and in the postoperative evaluation of a patient with an aortic valve prosthesis.

Atrial Pressure Pulses

The normal atrial pressure pulse has a characteristic configuration composed of three positive waves (a, c and v) and the corresponding descent of these waves (x, x_1 and y) (Figure 1A). The a wave results from atrial contraction and commences 0.06 to 0.09 seconds after the onset of the P wave of the electrocardiogram. During atrial relaxation, atrial pressure declines (x descent). The z point of the atrial pressure tracing occurs 0.05 to 0.07 seconds after the beginning of the QRS complex at the time when ventricular contraction commences. Isovolumic ventricular systole results first in closure and then in an upward bulging of the atrioventricular valves toward the atria, producing the c wave. During ventricular ejection, the atrioventricular ring descends into the ventricle, thereby increasing atrial capacity and resulting in a decrease in atrial pressure, termed the x_1 descent.

As ventricular systole progresses, the atria continue to fill from the venae cavae and pulmonary veins. Since this occurs in the presence of closed atrioventricular valves, atrial volume and pressure both increase, producing the v wave. The y descent begins at the peak of the v wave, at the end of isovolumic relaxation of the ventricles and at the time of the opening of the atrioventricular valves. During the early or rapid phase of ventricular filling, the atrial and ventricular pressures decline rapidly. However, when blood continues to enter the well filled ventricle in mid-diastole, the ventricular pressure rises slightly. This increase in pressure is

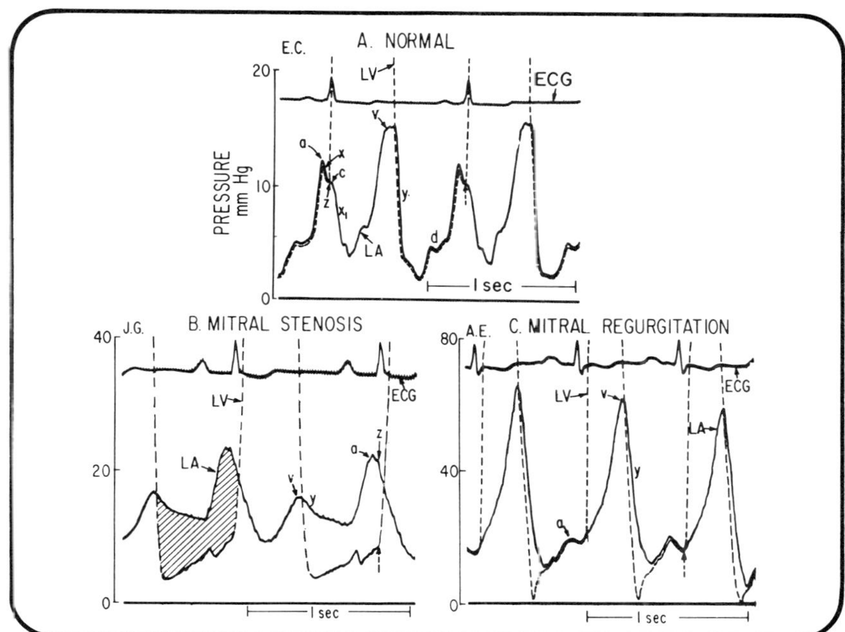

FIGURE 1. Simultaneously recorded left atrial (LA, **solid lines**) and left ventricular (LV, **broken lines**) pressure pulses in a normal subject (**A**), in a patient with mitral stenosis (**B**) and in a patient with mitral regurgitation (**C**). The A, C and V waves, the x, x₁ and y descents, the z point and the diastasis rise (d) of the left atrial pressure tracings are shown and discussed in the text. The **vertical broken arrows** indicate the left ventricular end-diastolic pressure. In **B** the diastolic pressure gradient across the mitral valve is shown by the shaded area. (Reproduced by permission from Mason et al.[2])

transmitted to the atria and results in a fourth elevation of atrial pressure during diastasis, the slow phase of ventricular filling.

Normally, there are only minor differences in the pressure pulses in the two atria (Table I). The dominant wave in the right atrial tracing is generally the a wave, whereas the v wave ordinarily is the tallest wave in the normal left atrial tracing. Mean left atrial pressure normally exceeds mean right atrial pressure.

Certain modifications of the contour of the atrial pressure pulse are of considerable physiologic and diagnostic significance. In atrial fibrillation, the a wave is absent; in nodal rhythm or atrioventricular dissociation, the atria may contract against closed atrioventricular valves resulting in giant a waves. The atrial a wave is particularly prominent in patients with ventricular hypertrophy and reduced ventricular compliance. In patients with atrial septal defect, the height of the right atrial v wave exceeds that of the a wave since the shunting of blood

into the right atrium during ventricular systole results in augmented filling of the atrium when the tricuspid valve is closed. For a similar reason, the left atrial v wave is prominent in patients with ventricular septal defect or patent ductus arteriosus and large left-to-right shunts. When a cardiac catheter is passed across an interatrial communication, sequential pressure recordings of both atrial mean pressures are of value in the differentiation of a large atrial septal defect from a small defect or a nonshunting patent foramen ovale; in the first condition, there is little or no interatrial pressure gradient, whereas a relatively large gradient (greater than 2 mm Hg) usually occurs in the latter two conditions. It is important to remember that many of the characteristics of the right atrial pulse may also be detected in the vena caval or jugular venous pulse, and that information concerning the left atrial pressure pulse may be obtained from analysis of pulmonary arterial wedge pressure tracings.

TABLE I
Normal Hemodynamic Values

Location	Upper Limits of Normal (mm Hg)
Right atrium	
a	7
v	5
mean	5
Right ventricle	
S	30
ED	5
Pulmonary artery	
S	30
D	20
mean	24
Pulmonary arterial wedge	
a	7
v	15
mean	12
Left atrium	
a	16
v	21
mean	12
Left ventricle	
S	145
ED	12

Cardiac index: 2.50 to 3.60 L/min/M^2 BSA. Pulmonary arteriolar resistance: less than 250 dynes sec cm^{-5}. S = systolic pressure; D = diastolic pressure; ED = ventricular end-diastolic pressure.

When stenosis of the mitral or tricuspid valves is present, the atrial pressure is also altered in a characteristic manner[2] (Figure 1B). The obstruction to atrial emptying results in an elevation of the mean pressure in the atrium above the valve. Patients with tricuspid stenosis may exhibit enormous atrial *a* waves with peaks that approach or even exceed the magnitude of the right ventricular systolic pressure. Prominence of the left atrial *a* wave is marked in patients with mitral stenosis. The relative height of the *a* wave varies inversely with the hemodynamic severity of mitral obstruction, indicating that left atrial contraction may become weaker and make a smaller contribution to left ventricular filling as the disease progresses.[7] The most characteristic modification of the atrial pressure pulse in patients with mitral and tricuspid stenosis, however, occurs during ventricular dias-

tole. Since the normal rapid emptying of the atria and filling of the ventricles that occur after the opening of the atrioventricular valves and the peak of the *v* wave are prevented, the atrial pressure declines slowly during early diastole, resulting in a gradual and prolonged *y* descent. The presence of obstruction to atrial emptying prevents adequate ventricular filling, and atrial pressure continues to fall slowly throughout diastole until the next atrial contraction; diastasis is thus eliminated.

In the presence of atrioventricular regurgitation, blood enters the atrium not only from its tributary veins during ventricular systole, but also from the ventricle, and results in a prominent *v* wave (Figure 1C). With extreme degrees of regurgitation of the atrioventricular valve, "ventricularization" of the atrial pressure pulse occurs, that is, the pressure pulses in the atrium and corresponding ventricles are similar.[8] After ventricular relaxation, the distended atrium empties rapidly, resulting in a steep *y* descent; diastasis is present. These alterations of the pressure pulse induced by valvular regurgitation are more prominent in the left than in the right atrium.[9] Since the volume of the left atrial/pulmonary venous compartment is much smaller than that of the corresponding right atrial/vena caval compartment, the regurgitation of a given volume of blood results in a larger pressure change and a greater elevation of the *v* wave in the left than in the right atrium. Thus, analysis of the atrial pressure pulse is of greater value in the detection of mitral than in that of tricuspid regurgitation. The compliance or pressure-volume relationship of the left atrium is a major determinant of the pressure pulse within this chamber.[10] Therefore, patients with severe, long-standing mitral regurgitation with large, thin-walled atria may have relatively normal left atrial pressures, whereas patients with small, thick-walled atria and diminished compliance of this chamber may have striking elevations of this pressure with smaller degrees of regurgitation.

Although detailed analysis of the left atrial pressure pulse usually permits separation of patients with isolated mitral stenosis from those with pure mitral regurgitation, it is of little value in determining the severity of mitral regurgitation when both lesions coexist.[11] The most useful methods of left atrial pulse pressure exami-

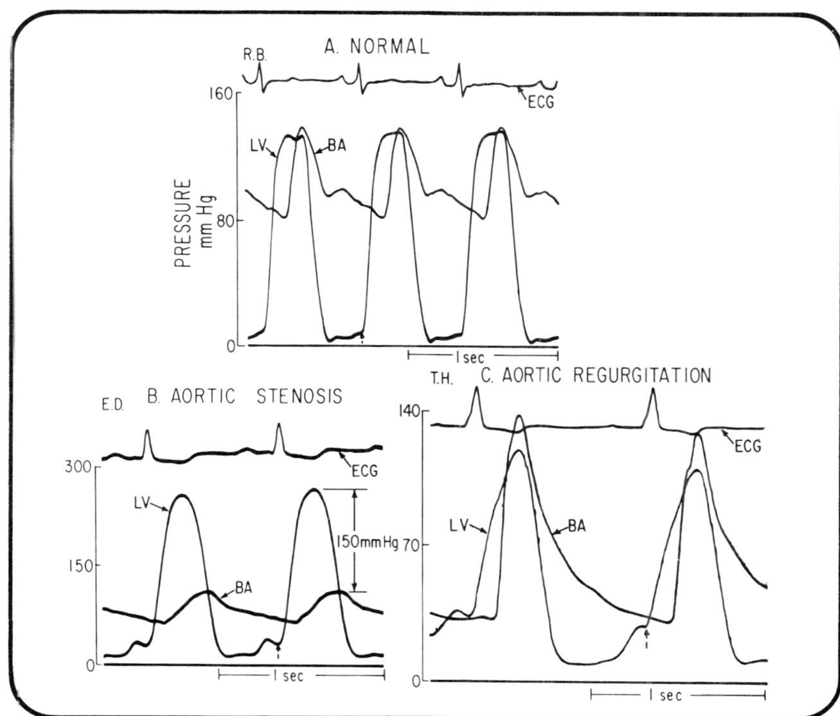

FIGURE 2. Simultaneously recorded brachial arterial (BA) and left ventricular (LV) pressure pulses in a normal subject (**A**), in a patient with valvular aortic stenosis (**B**) and in a patient with aortic regurgitation (**C**). The **vertical broken arrows** indicate the left ventricular end-diastolic pressure. In **B** the transaortic peak systolic pressure gradient is shown by **vertical solid arrows.** (Reproduced by permission from Mason et al.[2])

nation are the ratio of the rate of the y descent to the mean left atrial pressure, the ratio of the y descent in 0.1 second to the mean left atrial pressure and the presence or absence of diastasis. With predominant, severe mitral regurgitation, these ratios exceed 4.0 and 0.50, respectively, and diastasis is present.

Ventricular Pressure Pulses

The normal intraventricular pressures are given in Table I and a normal left ventricular pressure pulse is shown in Figure 2A. The ventricular pressure pulse is modified in a characteristic manner by severe stenosis of the semilunar valves (Figure 2B). In this circumstance, the affected ventricle contracts in a more nearly isometric manner than normal, and the pressure tracing exhibits a peaked summit during mid-systole instead of the normal plateau.[12] The duration of ventricular systole is prolonged by severe obstruction to ventricular outflow. In patients with severe mitral regurgitation, an abnormal abrupt decline in left ventricular pressure takes place at the termination of ventricular systole (Figure 1C). In conditions in which ventricular diastolic distensibility is diminished, such as constrictive pericarditis (Figure 3), endocardial fibroelastosis, amyloid disease and severe concentric hypertrophy of any etiology, a characteristic modification of the ventricular pressure pulse also takes place.[13] The early, rapid phase of ventricular filling is abruptly terminated as ventricular filling is slowed by the restriction to ventricular expansion. Ventricular pressure remains elevated during mid- and late diastole. The ventricular pressure pulse during diastole thus exhibits an early dip followed by a plateau.

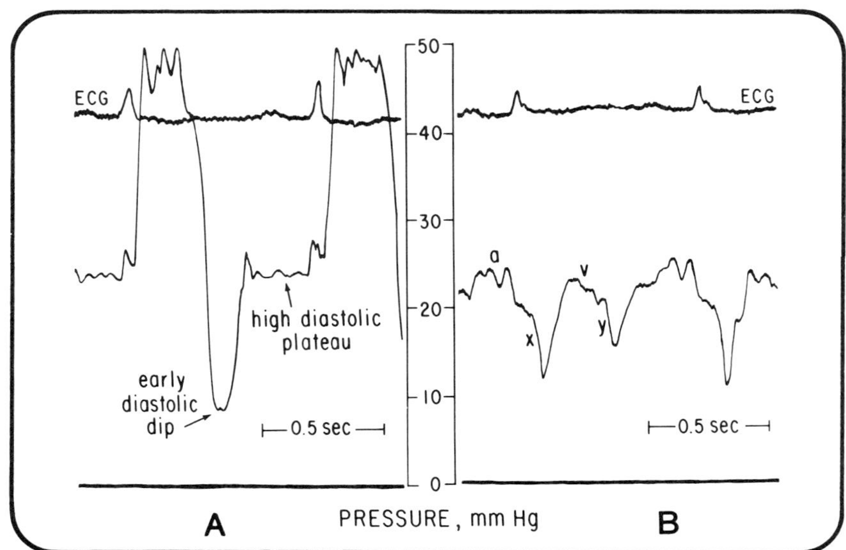

FIGURE 3. Characteristic pressure tracings from the right ventricle (**A**) and right atrium (**B**) in constrictive pericarditis caused by tuberculosis. (Reproduced by permission from Bonanno et al.[180])

An early response to depressed myocardial contractility and to systolic mechanical ventricular overloading is dilation of the ventricle during diastole, a compensatory mechanism that tends to maintain the force of ventricular contraction through operation of the Frank-Starling mechanism. Since the elevation of ventricular end-diastolic volume is often accompanied by an elevation of ventricular end-diastolic pressure, the level of the ventricular end-diastolic pressure may serve as an index of ventricular function in the absence of pericardial or endocardial disease. An elevated ventricular end-diastolic pressure in turn increases the corresponding atrial and venous pressures, which ultimately may be responsible for many of the symptoms of congestive heart failure.

Arterial Pressure Pulses

During the first week of life a gradual decrease in the pulmonary arterial pressure occurs; by one month of age this pressure has declined to the level normally present in adults (Table I). Pulmonary arterial pressure is often abnormally low in patients with severe obstruction to right ventricular outflow and is elevated as a result of left heart disease or lesions that restrict the lumen of the pulmonary vascular bed.

The contours of the central aortic and peripheral arterial pressure pulses are modified in a characteristic manner by aortic valve deformities.[14] In patients with severe aortic stenosis, the velocity of left ventricular ejection is diminished and the central and peripheral arterial pressure pulse rise is abnormally slow (Figure 2B). The central aortic pressure pulse is characterized by several prominent oscillations on the anacrotic limb and by a delayed peak. In the brachial artery pressure pulse, the anacrotic shoulder is abnormally prominent and lower on the ascending limb. Both the peak systolic pressure and the dicrotic notch are delayed. In contrast to the fixed types of aortic stenosis in which the obstruction remains constant throughout systole, in idiopathic hypertrophic subaortic stenosis, the arterial pressure pulse rises more rapidly than normal, since the left ventricle ejects a disproportionately large fraction of its stroke volume during early systole.[15]

In aortic regurgitation, the upstroke in both the central and peripheral pulses is quite steep, the descending limb is collapsing, and the incisural pressure is usually quite low in relation to the peak systolic pressure (Figure 2C). In the peripheral arterial pulse, the dicrotic notch is inconspicuous or absent. In the presence of combined aortic stenosis and regurgitation, the central and peripheral arterial pressure tracings present a combination of the features described for each individual lesion and frequently exhibit two distinct peaks during systole—a phenomenon termed pulsus bisferiens.

Cardiac Output

Fick Principle: Two methods, the Fick method and the indicator-dilution technique, are generally used for the measurement of cardiac output—the quantity of blood ejected by the heart per unit of time. The Fick principle may be applied for the determination of blood flow to a variety of organs since the total uptake or release of a substance by an organ is the product of the blood flow to the organ and the arteriovenous concentration of the substance.[16] This principle may be applied to the measurement of pulmonary blood flow—the total effective cardiac output—in patients without circulatory shunts by determining simultaneously the oxgen uptake by the lungs and the difference in oxygen content between the pulmonary arterial and pulmonary venous blood. For example, if the difference in oxygen content between the pulmonary arterial and pulmonary venous blood is 4 ml per 100 ml of blood, then each 25 ml of blood must have acquired 1 ml of oxygen in its transit through the lungs. If the simultaneously determined oxygen intake during a 1 minute period is 250 ml, then this amount of oxygen must have been transported by 6,250 ml (250 × 25) of blood during that 1 minute period; this value represents the cardiac output. In practice, the value for pulmonary venous oxygen content is generally taken from the systemic arterial blood. The diffusion of oxygen across the pulmonary alveolar-capillary membrane is assumed to be equal to the oxygen uptake at the mouth and, in an equilibrium state, to the oxygen consumption of the peripheral tissues during the period of measurement. Since various tissues utilize different proportions of the oxygen delivered to them, it is essential to sample mixed venous blood in order to determine the overall arteriovenous oxygen difference of the body. Venous blood is well mixed in the pul-

monary artery and sometimes in the right ventricular outflow tract as well.

Total oxygen consumption should be determined with the patient in a steady or equilibrium state, and ventilation and oxygen consumption must remain constant during the entire period of measurement. In addition to the heart rate, minute ventilation and oxygen consumption for the verification of the basal state, the respiratory quotient (RQ, the ratio of carbon dioxide production to oxygen utilization) should be between 0.70 to 0.90 in the postabsorptive state. During transient hypoventilation or hyperventilation, the oxygen utilization of peripheral tissue is unequal to the uptake of oxygen at the mouth, thereby invalidating application of the Fick principle. Furthermore, if the respiratory midposition is altered significantly during the course of the cardiac output determination, the oxygen uptake at the mouth is not equal to that across the alveolar-capillary membrane, again introducing an error. In the presence of a left-to-right intracardiac shunt, the quotient of oxygen consumption and pulmonary arteriovenous oxygen difference provides an estimate of the pulmonary blood flow; however, in the presence of a large shunt, the arteriovenous oxygen difference is small and even small inaccuracies in the determination of blood oxygen content produce large errors in cardiac output determination. Also, it should be appreciated that in patients with right-to-left shunts, the oxygen content of arterial blood cannot be used to estimate pulmonary venous oxygen content; instead, the latter may ordinarily be assumed to approximate 95 percent of the oxygen-carrying capacity of the blood.

Indicator-Dilution Technique: This method for the measurement of cardiac output is based on the principle that after injection of an indicator into the circulation, its particles are dispersed and a smooth time-concentration curve results when it is sampled at an appropriate point in the circulation beyond the injection site[17] (Figure 4A). In practice, a known quantity of an indicator substance, such as indocyanine dye, is rapidly injected into the cardiovascular system, usually the venous system or lesser circulation; the resultant changing concentration of dye in the peripheral arterial blood is determined by drawing blood through a densitome-

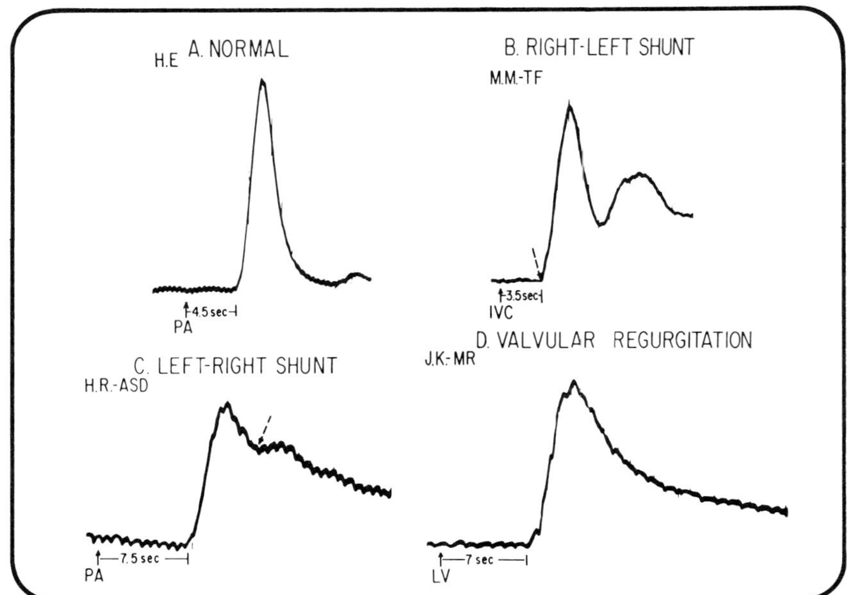

FIGURE 4. Indicator-dilution curves recorded from the brachial artery after injection of indocyanine dye into the pulmonary artery (PA) in a normal subject (**A**), into the inferior vena cava (IVC) in a patient with tetralogy of Fallot (TF) (**B**), into the pulmonary artery in a patient with an uncomplicated atrial septal defect (ASD) (**C**) and into the left ventricle (LV) in a patient with mitral regurgitation (MR) (**D**). The **vertical solid arrows** indicate the time of injection, and the appearance time of the indicator is shown. The **oblique broken arrows** indicate the appearance of dye that had passed across the ventricular septal defect (**B**) and across the ASD (**C**). (Reoroduced by permission from Mason et al.[2])

ter or oximeter sensitive to the changes in light transmission of whole blood produced by the dye. Calculation of the average concentration of the indicator during the inscription of the curve yields the total volume of blood in which the indicator has been diluted during its passage from the site of injection to the site of sampling. The time-concentration curve also indicates the time required for this volume of blood to pass the site of sampling, thus permitting calculation of the cardiac output. For example, if 2.0 mg of indocyanine dye is injected into the pulmonary artery and the mean concentration in the curve sampled from the femoral artery equals 1.0 mg/L, then the dye must have been diluted in 2.0 L of blood. If the dye appeared at the sampling site 10 seconds after injection and disappeared 30 seconds after injection, then the flow rate equals 2.0 L in 20 seconds, or 6.0 L per minute. The blood volume between the injection and sampling sites can also be calculated as the product of the cardiac output and the mean transit time between the two sites.

The principle of the indicator-dilution technique is based on the time-concentration characteristics of the indicator during its first passage from the site of injection to the site of sampling. Since the circulatory paths vary widely in length, it is possible for some particles of the indicator to pass the site of sampling twice before other particles have passed once. If the recirculating indicator is not recognized, the indicator dilution curve encompasses an inappropriately large area and therefore yields a falsely low cardiac output. The indicator mixes completely in the central circulation, and its rate of washout at any moment is directly proportional to the quantity remaining in the central circulatory bed. Therefore, the descending limb forms a straight line when the time-concentration curve is plotted on semilogarithmic paper. A significant departure from this straight line generally results from recirculation of the indicator. The disturbing influence of this recirculating indicator may be eliminated by assuming a logarithmic washout of the dye for the entire descending limb of the indicator-dilution curve and extrapolating the last few seconds of the curve. Distortion of the primary dilution curve by recirculating indicator occurs most commonly when the volume of blood between the injection and sampling sites is augmented as in congestive heart failure, when the circulation is slowed as in heart failure or shock, or when a central right-to-left or left-to-right shunt or valvular regurgitation is present. Determination of cardiac output by the indicator-dilution method is useful for evaluating the functional state of the cardiovascular system at rest and particularly during exercise, since a prolonged steady state is not essential, as it is with the Fick technique.

Cardiac output also can be measured by noninvasive radioisotopic techniques, which offer the advantage of external scintillation counting, thereby obviating arterial sampling. The standard radioisotopic cardiac output technique is analogous to the indocyanine dye-dilution technique just described. Rapid injection is made preferably into the central circulation to maintain a compact bolus of a radionuclide that disappears slowly from the intravascular compartment—radioiodinated human serum albumin or indium 113m (^{113m}In) chloride, which binds instantaneously in vivo to transferrin. Scintigraphic data are obtained by precordial probe with strip-chart recorder or scintillation camera with video-tape storage and playback system and area-of-interest capabilities. Blood volume is calculated using the standard radioisotopic technique of determining the count in a venous blood aliquot after equilibration and comparing it with the total count injected. The area under the isotope time-activity curve inscribed during the initial transit of radioactivity through the heart is planimetered after logarithmic extrapolation of the descending limb, as in the indocyanine dye technique. Cardiac output is calculated as the product of the amplitude of the curve at equilibrium, blood volume and speed of recording paper, divided by the planimetered area under the initial transit curve. The accuracy of this technique has been documented clinically by comparison with cardiac output obtained by the Fick principle.[18,19]

Radioisotopic cardiac output determinations also can be carried out by the constant peripheral venous infusion technique, in which ^{113m}In is detected by a single external probe and the resultant time-activity curve is analyzed by computer model. This method is atraumatic, requiring neither injection into the central circulation nor intraarterial cannulation. We recently have documented the reliability of this procedure in a large group of patients by comparison with simultaneous dye-dilution and Fick cardiac output measurements.[20] In addition, the constant infusion radioisotopic technique affords a means for the accurate determination of cardiac output in the presence of valvular regurgitation or intracardiac shunts. Thus, this method is applicable in a variety of clinical settings in which the standard invasive techniques for the measurement of cardiac output are either impractical, invalid or unavailable.

Since cardiac function can be assessed by consideration of the adequacy with which the heart supplies the peripheral tissues with oxygen, the systemic arteriovenous mixed oxygen difference becomes an important and meaningful index. Regardless of the absolute level of cardiac output, an abnormally wide arteriovenous mixed oxygen difference—above 5.5 volumes/100 ml at rest—signifies that the heart fails to make adequate quantities of blood available to the peripheral tissues.

It has now become possible to study noninvasively phasic arterial blood flow and velocity in the central aorta and the peripheral arteries in unanesthetized patients. An initial approach to the determination of instantaneous velocity of blood flow was its continuous computation from the pressure difference recorded through a double-lumen catheter.[21] Improvements in the design of electromagnetic flowmeter circuits and the miniaturization of flow transducers have produced suitable perivascular flowmeters for the measurement of pulsatile brachial arterial blood flow in man.[22] More recently, the catheter-tip blood velocity meters have provided a means for recording with precision and relative ease the dynamics of ventricular ejection and the flow characteristics in the vessels of the central circulation[23] (Figure 5).

Pulmonary Vascular Resistance

Because of the frequency of pulmonary vascular disease in patients with diseases involving the left side of the heart or the pulmonary parenchyma, the determination of the pulmonary vas-

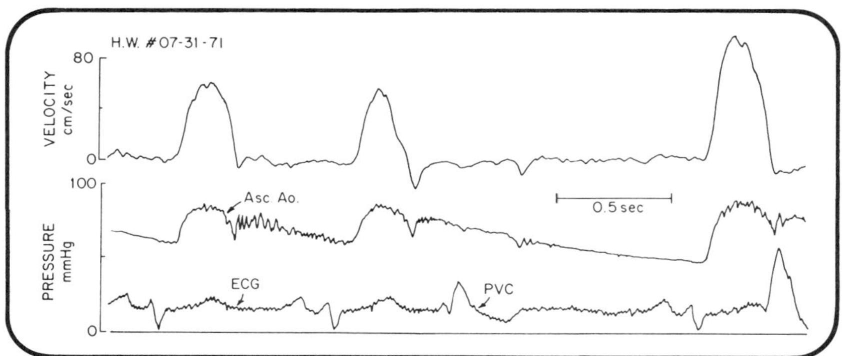

FIGURE 5. Phasic blood flow velocity and pressure in the ascending aorta (asc. ao.) before and after a premature ventricular contraction in a patient with rheumatic mitral valvular disease and normal sinus rhythm. Velocity is the top tracing recorded by the catheter-tip electromagnetic velocity flow probe. (Reproduced by permission from Mason et al.[23])

cular resistance is often of importance. The pressure drop across the pulmonary vascular bed is assumed to be dependent not only upon the cross-sectional area of the pulmonary vessels, but also upon the flow rate, and the resistance is calculated by dividing the mean pressure drop—mean pulmonary arterial pressure minus mean left atrial or pulmonary arterial wedge pressure—by the cardiac output. Under ordinary circumstances, the resistance offered by the pulmonary vascular bed is about one-sixth that of the systemic vascular bed. With primary or secondary pulmonary vascular disease, the resistance to flow offered by the pulmonary vasculature is higher and may even exceed that of the systemic circuit, placing an extreme work load on the right ventricle.

Intravascular Shunts

Indicator-Dilution Technique: Continuously recorded indicator-dilution curves are of considerable value in the recognition and localization of a variety of inter- and extracardiac shunts as well as in the detection of valvular regurgitation.[24] After injection into the right side of the heart proximal to the origin of a right-to-left shunt, an indicator follows two circulatory paths (Figure 4B). A portion takes the normal route through the pulmonary circulation, and then through the left side of the heart and into the systemic arterial bed, producing the normal component of the resultant dilution curve. The remainder of the indicator follows the blood through its abnormal circulatory path and is shunted from the right to the left side of the heart, bypassing the pulmonary circulation and resulting in the abnormal component of the dilution curve, represented by an abnormal early appearance time and an early peak preceding the normal component of the dilution curve. Selective injection of indicator into the right atrium, right ventricle and pulmonary artery makes possible the precise localization of the origin of a right-to-left shunt. For example, in a patient with pulmonic stenosis and a right-to-left shunt through a patent foramen ovale, injection into the right atrium results in an abnormal dilution curve, whereas a normal curve follows injection into the right ventricle. In contrast, in a patient with tetralogy of Fallot, injections into the right atrium and into the right ventricle both result in abnormal curves with early appearance times, whereas injection into the pulmonary artery yields a curve with normal appearance time and contour. The injection of an indicator into a peripheral vein serves as a valuable screening test in the study of patients with cyanosis of central origin. Abnormal curves are obtained in patients in whom cyanosis is secondary to a right-to-left shunt originating in the heart or main pulmonary artery. However, a normal dilution curve is found in patients with cyanosis secondary to intrapulmonary shunting through small vessels or to perfusion of areas of the lung that are inadequately ventilated.

When indicator is injected into a peripheral vein, the right side of the heart or pulmonary artery in a patient with a left-to-right cardiac shunt, it is dispersed into the abnormally large volume of blood that traverses the pulmonary vascular bed and a fraction continues to circulate through the defect (Figure 4C). Consequently, the resultant dilution curve obtained by sampling from a systemic artery has a low peak concentration and an abnormally prolonged descending limb after a distinct interruption of this limb by dye that has recirculated through the shunt. The indicator-dilution method, with injection into the right side of the heart and arterial sampling, is of considerable value in detecting—but not in localizing—left-to-right shunts that exceed approximately 25 percent of the pulmonary blood flow. However, precise localization of such shunts can be accomplished by serial injections of the indicator into the chambers of the left side of the heart and into the aorta. For example, the indicator-dilution technique is particularly useful in the study of patients with interatrial septal defects. Injection of indicator into the left ventricle with sampling from the femoral artery yields a normal curve. However, when the indicator is injected into the left atrium, only a fraction proceeds to the left ventricle and into the aorta, producing the first peak of the curve; the remainder is shunted across the interatrial defect and then follows the normal path of the circulation through the pulmonary vascular bed and left side of the heart, ultimately producing a second peak. An abnormal dilution curve after left ventricular injection in such patients indicates the presence of a complicating lesion—mitral regurgitation or an additional downstream left-to-right shunt, such as a ventricular septal defect or patent ductus arteriosus.

Indicator-dilution curves are of considerable value in determining the drainage path of pulmonary veins entered during the course of right heart catheterization.[25] If the pulmonary vein in question drains normally into the left atrium, the dilution curve obtained from a systemic artery after injection into such a vein is characterized by an early appearance time and a contour that resembles that after left atrial injection. Con-

versely, after injection of indicator into a pulmonary vein that drains into the right atrium, the dilution curve has an appearance time that is prolonged and a contour resembling one after right atrial injection. The site of entry of left-to-right shunts can also be determined by using the double-catheter upstream sampling technique in which indicator is injected into the distal pulmonary artery and is sampled at a variety of sites upstream to the pulmonary artery,[24] as well as by injecting indicator into a peripheral vein and sampling from various positions in the right side of the heart.

Although indocyanine dye is the most commonly employed indicator in clinical practice, other substances such as sodium ascorbate or cold saline also may be used.[26] With these agents, the detecting thermistor or electrodes are introduced directly into the vascular system, obviating the withdrawal of blood, which makes these substances particularly appropriate for use in infants and young children.

Radioisotopic Screening Techniques: Several noninvasive radioisotopic techniques employing external scintillation counting are sensitive screening tests for detection, localization and even quantification of left-to-right or right-to-left intracardiac shunts. These methods require neither cardiac catherterization nor arterial blood sampling. Left-to-right shunts may be detected by simple externally obtained pulmonary vascular dilution curves.[27] In this method a scintillation probe placed over a peripheral lung field records the continuous curve of scintigraphic data after intravenous injection of a gamma-emitting isotope, most commonly technetium 99m (^{99m}Tc) pertechnetate. In patients with left-to-right shunts, the recirculating radioisotope causes a prolongation of the downslope of the curve. Mathematic evaluation of the curve is performed by defining two points on the curve, C_1 and C_2. C_1 is the peak of the curve, and C_2 is a point on the downslope occurring at the time from the peak (T_2) equal to the time from the initial upslope of the curve to the peak (T_1). The heights of the curve at C_1 and C_2 are measured, and the ratio of C_2 to C_1 is determined. In the presence of a left-to-right intracardiac shunt, this ratio is elevated above normal values.

A refinement of the technique employs the scintillation camera equipped with video-tape

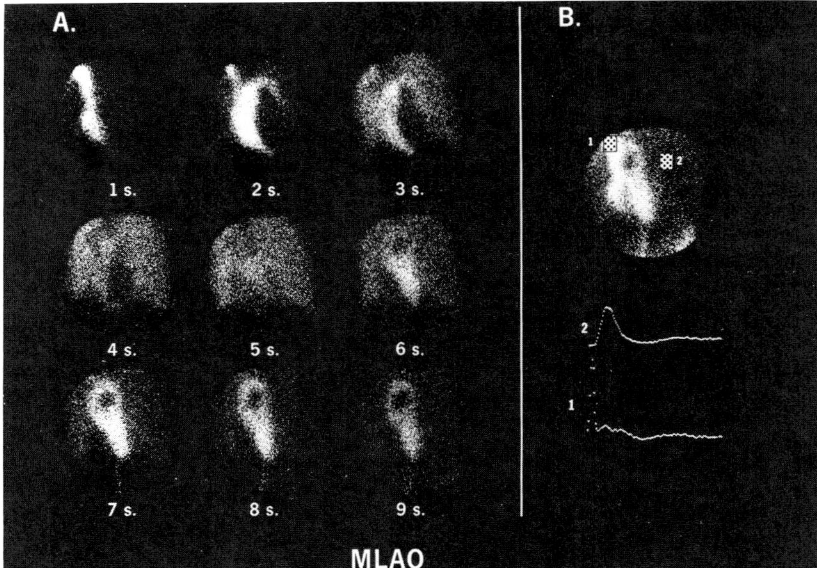

FIGURE 6. A, sequential 1 second (s) images obtained in the modified left anterior oblique view (MLAO) after intravenous bolus injection of ^{99m}Tc in a normal subject. In the first 4 seconds the right heart chambers and lungs are visualized. During this time period, no radioactivity is present in the region of the left ventricle, thereby excluding a right-to-left shunt. At second 5, the left atrium is seen. In seconds 6 through 9, the left ventricle and aorta are evident. During this latter interval, decreased radioactivity is noted in the region of the right atrium and right ventricle, thereby ruling out a left-to-right shunt. **B,** the radionuclidic image is a composite of seconds 1–2 and 7–8 from the normal flow study shown in **A.** The time-activity curves were obtained from the indicated areas of the image: **area 1,** the superior vena cava; **area 2,** the left lung. The rapid rise and fall of the pulmonary curve (**2**) excludes the presence of a left-to-right intracardiac shunt.

data storage and playback system and area-of-interest capabilities[28] (Figure 6). When this improved method is performed with the detector in a modified left anterior oblique position, activity curves can be generated from a variety of sites, such as the superior vena cava, right heart chambers, lung and left ventricle, using the scintigraphic data collected from a single intravenous injection (Figure 6B). Analysis of the superior vena caval curve allows confirmation of the compactness of the bolus injection and thus eliminates false-positive results, which may occur from splaying of the bolus before activity reaches the heart. Analysis of pulmonary time-activity curves can be used to accurately separate normal subjects from patients with left-to-right intracardiac shunts.[28] Curves generated from the various regions can be used to localize the shunt. For example, a normal right atrial C_2/C_1 ratio accompanied by an abnormal right ventricular C_2/C_1 ratio implies the presence of a left-to-right shunt at the ventricular level. Similarly, normal right atrial and right ventricular curves associated with abnormally high C_2/C_1 ratio from the pulmonary curve indicates a left-to-right shunt beyond the right ventricle, such as with a patent ductus arteriosus. An additional advantage of this scintillation camera technique is that serial rapid-sequence images of passage of radioactivity through the heart can be obtained. These images demonstrate the flow pattern through the individual cardiac chambers and the lungs. The diagnosis of a right-to-left or left-to-right shunt usually can be established or excluded with a high degree of certainty by inspection of these images alone.

By use of the scintillation camera combined with a mini-computer, data from initial transit of radioactivity through the cardiac chambers and lungs can be processed to provide quantification of left-to-right shunts.[29,30] These techniques have been shown to be accurate with ratios of pulmonic to systemic flow as low as 1.2:1.0 and as high as 3.0:1.0.[29]

Right-to-left intracardiac shunts also can be detected easily and sensitively by noninvasive radioisotopic techniques. Through the use of the scintillation camera, serial rapid-sequence images can be inspected for evidence of early arrival of activity in the left ventricle or aorta signifying a right-to-left shunt[31] (Figure 6A). By using area-of-interest capabilities, histograms obtained from the left ventricular area of interest can be evaluated for an early peak corresponding to the timing of right ventricular filling, thereby indicating a right-to-left shunt. Through computer processing, the right-to-left shunt can be quantified.[29]

Another scintillation camera method employs the injection of two radioisotopes.[32] With this technique, in addition to the initial transit of ^{99m}Tc pertechnetate through the cardiac chambers, the transit of xenon 133 (^{133}Xe) after intravenous injection is also evaluated. Normally, area-of-interest curves generated from the left ventricular region are flat with ^{133}Xe, due to efficient extraction of the noble gas in the lungs. In the presence of right-to-left shunting, however, some ^{133}Xe bypasses the lungs and reaches the left ventricle. The consequent detection of ^{133}Xe activity within the left ventricular area of interest signifies a right-to-left intracardiac shunt.

Finally, right-to-left shunting can be evaluated by observing the fraction of intravenously injected particles of ^{99m}Tc-labeled human serum albumin that reach the systemic vascular tree. These are the same particles that are used for conventional lung perfusion scanning. Normally, virtually all of the radioactive particles lodge within the pulmonary vascular bed during the initial circulation. In right-to-left intracardiac shunting, a fraction of the injected particles reach the systemic circulation; by calculation of this fraction, the shunt can be quantified.[33] Since this method carries the potential risk of microembolization to the systemic organs, the number of particles injected must be carefully controlled to maintain a range of safety. With the possible exception of this last technique, these radioisotopic techniques offer the advantage of extreme safety as well as accuracy in the noninvasive detection of intracardiac shunts. The hazards are essentially only those of veni-

puncture and radiation exposure approximately equivalent to one chest roentgenogram. These features allow sensitive screening for intracardiac shunts, which is of particular value in evaluating pediatric patients.

Oxygen Analysis: The sampling of blood from the venae cavae, right heart and pulmonary artery and the demonstration of an oxygen increase as the catheter is advanced from one chamber to the next has been the standard method for the detection, localization and quantification of left-to-right cardiac shunts. When the average right atrial oxygen content exceeds the average vena caval content by more than 1.5 volumes/100 ml, a left-to-right shunt entering the right atrium is usually present. An increase of 1.0 volume/100 ml from the right atrium to right ventricle or from the right ventricle to pulmonary artery is generally sufficient evidence for the diagnosis of shunts into these areas. The value of the oxygen method for the detection of left-to-right shunts is limited by the changes in the patient's metabolic state during the time required for positioning the catheter and obtaining blood samples, as well as by incomplete mixing of blood in the venae cavae and right atrium. The use of a cuvette oximeter for the immediate analysis of blood withdrawn from the catheter makes it possible to analyze multiple samples in rapid succession, increasing the accuracy of the method.

The development of a fiberoptic catheter system now permits the direct and continuous measurement of intravascular oxygen saturations[34] (Figure 7). In addition, the introduction of the cinetrace method for the simultaneous recording of oscillographic and radiologic events on radiographic film permits precise correlations between the anatomic position of the catheter tip and the intracardiac oxygen saturation and pressure and intracardiac electrocardiogram[35] (Figure 8).

Foreign Gas Techniques: The foreign gas method for characterizing left-to-right shunts employs the inhalation of physiologically inert gases and thereby avoids the limitations of the oxygen method.[36] Thus, when nitrous oxide or radioactive krypton 85 is inhaled for 30 sec, the arterial level of the gas rises abruptly; however, because of the solubility of the gas in the tissues,

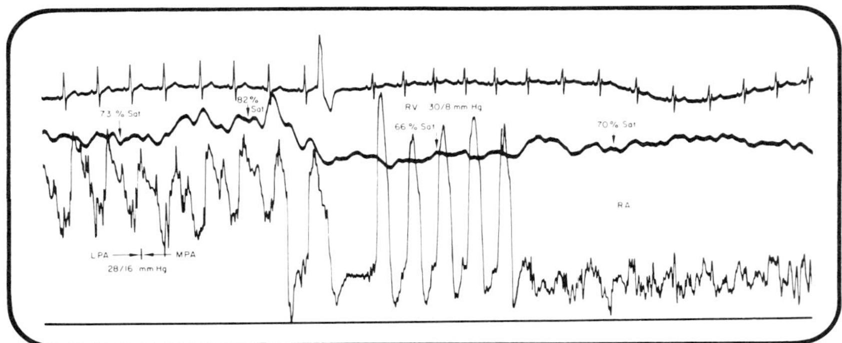

FIGURE 7. Application of the catheter-tip oximeter allowed continuous, simultaneous recordings of intracardiac oxygen saturations and pressures in a patient with anomalous origin of the left coronary artery from the pulmonary artery. The oxygen saturation was 73 percent in the left pulmonary artery (LPA), rose to an average of 82 percent in the main pulmonary artery (MPA), fell to 66 percent in the right ventricle (RV) and then rose slightly to 70 percent in the right atrium (RA). The electrocardiogram (lead II) displays sinus rhythm with a premature ventricular contraction initiating a temporary period of aberrant intraventricular conduction. (Reproduced by permission from Cohen et al.[42])

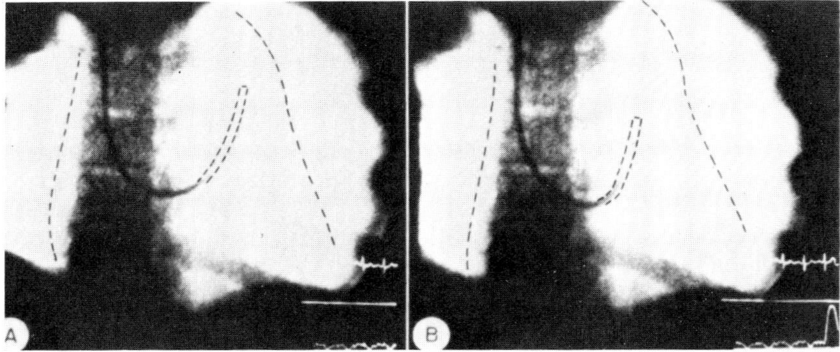

FIGURE 8. Application of the cinetrace system during cardiac catheterization in a patient with congenital valvular pulmonic stenosis, showing the position of the catheter tip and the simultaneously recorded pressure pulses (**lower right** in both panels) from the catheter tip as it was drawn from the main pulmonary artery (**A**) into the right ventricle just proximal to the stenotic pulmonic valve (**B**). (Reproduced by permission from Rockoff et al.[35])

the concentration in the right side of the heart rises very slowly and, in the absence of a left-to-right shunt, is less than 13 percent of the concentration in the systemic arterial vascular bed. In contrast, in the presence of a left-to-right shunt, blood from the left side of the heart—rich in foreign gas content—enters the right side of the heart through the defect, elevating the concentration of gas and consequently the ratio of the concentration of gas in the right side of the heart to that in systemic arterial blood. The advantages of the ^{85}Kr foreign gas method are that an immediate answer is provided, the results are not greatly influenced by changes in the pa-tient's metabolic state, and the accurate localization and precise quantification of the shunt are achieved with the withdrawal of only small volumes of blood.

Hydrogen gas may also be inhaled in the detection and localization of left-to-right shunts.[37] Based on the principle that a platinum electrode develops a potential when exposed to hydrogen, this technique employs a catheter with sensing electrodes at its tip positioned sequentially in various locations in the right side of the heart after inhalation of the gas. In the absence of a left-to-right shunt, the time-concentration curves for hydrogen in the right side of the heart have delayed appearance times and low peak concentrations. However, when the catheter tip is positioned at or distal to the entry of a left-to-right shunt, the gas appears in the right heart shortly after the onset of inhalation. Although this technique is extremely sensitive, it is more difficult to adapt for quantification of the shunt than is the [85]Kr method.

Valvular Stenosis

The presence of functionally significant obstruction to blood flow—whether it be at the level of the cardiac valves or at some other point in the circulation—is represented by a pressure gradient at the stenotic orifice during that portion of the cardiac cycle in which blood flows across it. Since blood flow across stenotic heart valves is turbulent and not laminar, the flow rate across such valves is not a linear function of the flow but is more closely proportional to the square root of the pressure gradient. Thus, the transvalvular pressure gradient is related to the square of the flow rate, and a doubling of blood flow across a stenotic valve produces a quadrupling of the gradient across the orifice. Estimation of the severity of valvular stenosis by the determination of pressure gradients alone is therefore not possible, since the gradient is dependent on the flow as well as on the size of the orifice. However, since normally there is no measurable transvalvular pressure gradient, the detection of transvalvular pressures alone is of value in determining the presence or absence of stenosis.

The application of hydraulic principles to the hemodynamics of valvular stenosis by Gorlin has provided clinically useful formulas for the estimation of effective orifice size.[38,39] When valvular regurgitation coexists with stenosis, the flow rate across the valve is the sum of the forward cardiac output and the regurgitant flow; therefore, if a large amount of regurgitant flow is neglected in the calculations, the size of the orifice may be falsely underestimated. Since there are no routine clinical techniques available for the precise measurement of regurgitant flow, the effective orifice size of a stenotic valve cannot be determined with accuracy in the presence of regurgitation. In addition, changes in heart rate modify the time during which blood flows across cardiac valves; an increase in heart rate shortens diastole relatively more than systole. Thus, at any level of cardiac output, tachycardia tends to augment the pressure gradient across the atrioventricular valves and to diminish the pressure gradient across the semilunar valves.

In general, a reduction of approximately 50 percent of the normal cross-sectional area of a heart valve must occur in the presence of normal blood flow before a transvalvular pressure gradient is detectable. This implies that the heart valves have a large functional reserve, and that audible murmurs produced by turbulent flow across mildly stenotic valves are not necessarily accompanied by measurable pressure gradients. As the stenosis increases in severity, however, a pressure gradient develops when cardiac output and, thus, transvalvular flow are elevated, as during exercise or in the presence of anxiety, fever, anemia, pregnancy or tachycardia. With more advanced stenosis, significant pressure gradients may be recorded at rest. However, a marked increase in the gradient during exercise may not occur, since the cardiac output in response to exercise may be subnormal. In addition, with very severe valvular obstruction the cardiac output may be reduced even at rest, limiting the transvalvular gradient.

Valvular Regurgitation

In contrast to valvular stenosis, the precise definition of the severity of valvular regurgitation is difficult. Indicator-dilution curves afford a means for the recognition of valvular regurgitation (Figure 4D). When a valve that regurgitates a significant volume of blood is interposed between the sites of injection and sampling of the indicator, the curve characteristically exhibits depression of the peak, slight prolongation of the ascending limb, more striking prolongation of the descending limb and disappearance of the normal recirculation peak. When the injection is made in the chamber just beyond the regurgitant valve, the descending limb is also relatively prolonged in comparison with the ascending limb. However, a normal contour is obtained when the indicator is injected into a site distal to the chamber associated with the regurgitant valve, such as injection into the pulmonary artery in a patient with tricuspid regurgitation. By varying the site of injection, the valvular regurgitation may be localized. Detailed analysis of such curves, however, has not provided an accurate and reliable method for the measurement of regurgitant flow.

Regurgitation also can be recognized by the detection of dye in the chamber proximal to the injection site. For example, when dye injected into the pulmonary artery through the distal lumen of a cardiac catheter appears immediately in blood sampled from the right ventricle through the proximal lumen of the catheter, the diagnosis of pulmonary regurgitation is confirmed. Utilizing simultaneous left ventricular catheterization and left atrial puncture, mitral regurgitation may be detected in a similar manner. Although some investigators have used this approach for the quantification of mitral regurgitation, the validity of such methods remains to be demonstrated.

The technique most widely applied currently for the assessment of valvular regurgitation is selective cineangiography performed by injecting contrast material into the chamber immediately beyond the incompetent valve.[40] Visual grading of the relative amount of contrast dye retrogradely opacifying the upstream cardiac chamber provides a semi-quantitative means for evaluation of valvular regurgitation that is sufficiently accurate for the majority of clinical situations. More precise determination of valvular reguritation can be obtained by use of the biplane angiographic technique for the measurement of left ventricular volume.[41] Left ventricular stroke volume may be calculated angiographically by subtraction of end-systolic volume from end-diastolic volume and, in the absence of mitral or aortic regurgitation, correlates closely with the stroke volume determined by the Fick or indicator-dilution technique. This ventricular volume technique is suited for the accurate measurement of the volume of regurgitant flow, since the volume of reflux is equal to the difference between the total left ventricular stroke volume, calculated angiographically, and the effective stroke volume determined by the Fick or indicator-dilution technique.

Intracardiac Phonocardiography

The recording of sounds from within the heart has permitted the precise localization of the origin of murmurs [35] (Figure 9). The intracardiac

microphones most commonly employed are barium titanate crystals and inductance-type transducers. Some investigators simply employ a specially filtered external strain gauge to pick up sound waves transmitted by the column of fluid within the catheter. Not only is this technique a valuable ancillary diagnostic tool, but also it provides a physiologic basis for the study of the origin of cardiovascular sounds. Murmurs characteristically follow the stream of blood flow. Therefore, the systolic ejection murmurs in pulmonic stenosis or atrial septal defect, as well as the continuous murmur in uncomplicated patent ductus arteriosus are recorded in the pulmonary artery. In contrast, the murmurs of ventricular septal defect and left ventricular/right atrial communication are localized to the right ventricle and right atrium, respectively.

Intracardiac Electrocardiography

The intracardiac electrocardiogram may be obtained from an exploring electrode attached to the tip of a cardiac catheter and has been a helpful diagnostic tool in certain types of congenital heart disease. The diagnosis of Ebstein's anomaly may be confirmed by the demonstration of right ventricular intracardiac potential within an area from which a right atrial pressure pulse is recorded.[35] In addition, the intracardiac electrocardiogram may be used to record P waves in the diagnosis of obscure arrhythmias. The application of both the intracardiac electrocardiographic and phonocardiographic techniques has been extended by combining them with the simultaneous recording of intracardiac pressure pulses on cineradiographic film.[42] Most importantly, the development of His bundle electrography has provided an improved method for the detection, localization and analysis of disorders of cardiac conduction and rhythm.[43]

Ventricular Function

As delineated in chapter 9, ventricular function and cardiac performance are terms used in the general sense to express the combined action of the four major determinants of cardiac output,[44–47] which consist of the three factors regulating stroke volume: (1) preload—ven-

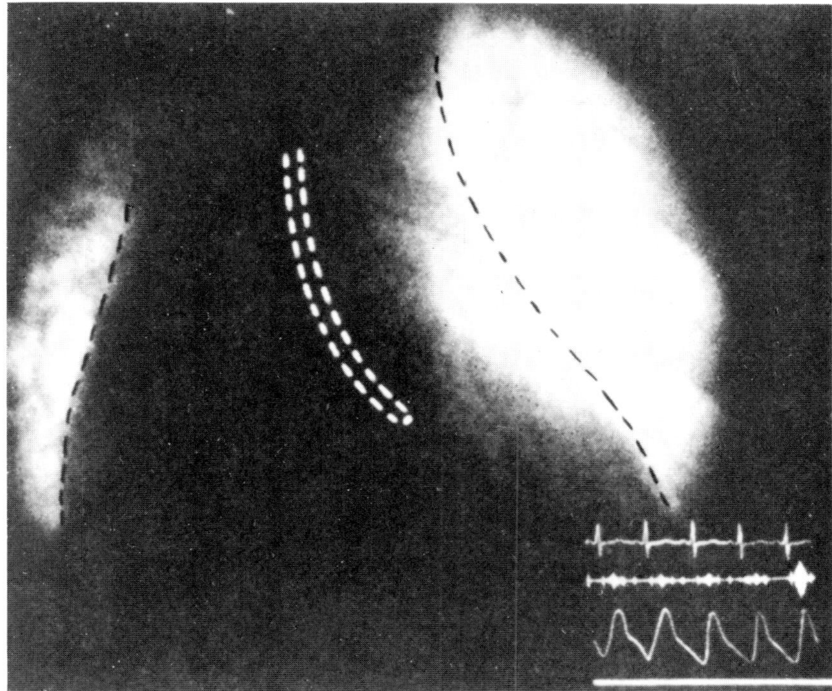

FIGURE 9. Application of the cinetrace in determining the location of the systolic ejection murmur in a patient with idiopathic hypertrophic subaortic stenosis, showing the position of the retrograde intracardiac phonocatheter at the instant when the maximal murmur was recorded within the left ventricular cavity as the catheter was slowly pulled antegrade from the body of the chamber. The electrocardiogram, brachial arterial pressures and the intracardiac sound are recorded simultaneously (**lower right**). By superimposing this catheter-tip point onto the left ventricular cineangiogram, it was possible to show that the ejection murmur originated at the site of the systolic anterior mitral leaflet abutment against the hypertrophied septum. (Reproduced by permission from Rockoff et al.[35])

tricular end-diastolic fiber length; (2) afterload—intraventricular systolic tension during ejection; and (3) contractility—variable force of ventricular contraction independent of loading; and (4) heart rate. When considering cardiac function in segmental disorders of the ventricle as in coronary heart disease, it is important to add a fifth determinant, one that adversely affects forward stroke volume: dyssynergy or abnormal temporal sequence of ventricular wall contraction. In the evaluation of the principal determinants of cardiac performance in heart disease, it has been possible to measure precisely ventricular preload (end-diastolic pressure, volume and tension) and afterload (Laplace relation, in which systolic tension is directly equated with the product of ventricular systolic pressure and radius) and to characterize the nature and extent of dyssynergy. However, it has been considerably more difficult to assess accurately contractility (inotropic or contractile state) of the intact human heart. There are two general approaches to the evaluation of contractility and function of the heart—its pump (hemodynamics) and muscle (mechanics) performance characteristics.[44–48]

Cardiac Pump Function

Ventricular End-Diastolic Pressure

Inadequate systolic emptying of the ventricle leads to an increased end-systolic residual volume in this chamber and thereby an augmentation of ventricular end-diastolic volume. Since the elevation of ventricular end-diastolic volume is usually accompanied by an elevation of ventricular end-diastolic pressure, the level of ventricular end-diastolic pressure may serve as a measure of ventricular function. The upper limit of normal of left ventricular end-diastolic pressure (LVEDP) is 12 mm Hg. However, LVEDP may be elevated without increased end-diastolic volume due to diminished ventricular compliance in hypertrophy, fibrosis and infiltrative disease of the ventricle and in pericardial disease.[49-52] Conversely, ventricular end-diastolic volume may be increased without elevation of LVEDP when ventricular compliance is increased, such as in some instances of ventricular systolic volume overloading.

Although acute hypervolemia due to fluid accumulation in the absence of heart disease results in an increase in LVEDP, this variable should remain within normal limits in the absence of an abnormality of myocardial compliance or contractility. Thus, although acute systolic mechanical overloading of the left ventricle may cause LVEDP elevation due to increased left ventricular end-diastolic volume, an LVEDP above 12 to 15 mm Hg indicates at least a certain component of depressed ventricular contractility when the compliance of this chamber is normal.

Elevation of LVEDP in turn increases mean left atrial and pulmonary venous pressures and, consequently, pulmonary and right ventricular systolic and diastolic pressures. In the absence of mitral valve obstruction or increased left atrial contraction with diminished left ventricular compliance, mean left atrial pressure and the pulmonary capillary wedge pressure closely reflect LVEDP. Similarly, without increased pulmonary vascular resistance and mitral obstruction, the pulmonary arterial diastolic pressure provides an estimation of LVEDP. The pulmonary arterial diastolic pressure correlates more closely with the left atrial mean pressure and the left ventricular diastolic pressure immediately before the onset of atrial contraction.[53] The recent development of catheters that can be placed easily in the pulmonary artery has allowed the monitoring of pulmonary arterial diastolic pressure as an indicator of left ventricular function in patients with acute myocardial infarction.[54] Although central venous pressure provides a useful estimation of total blood volume and evaluation of right ventricular function, this variable does not necessarily reflect the level of left ventricular function.[55]

Cardiac Output

The determination of the cardiac output by the Fick principle or indicator-dilution technique provides a useful measure of overall cardiac performance. The lower limit of normal of this variable is 2.50 L/min per square meter of body surface area, and the upper limit usually is not above 3.60 L/min/M^2. However, the cardiac index may not be diminished except with advanced abnormalities of ventricular contractility or with severe mechanical overloading or underloading of the ventricle.[56] Thus, in lesser degrees of heart disease, operation of the ventricular compensatory mechanisms of elevation of LVEDP, ventricular hypertrophy and enhanced activity of the sympathetic nervous system usually maintain the basal cardiac index at a normal level, despite impaired contractility and excessive loading of the ventricle.

Stroke Volume and Systolic Ejection Rate

The stroke volume indirectly reflects the extent of ventricular fiber shortening. However, this variable—like the cardiac output—is influenced by ventricular loading in addition to contractility. Further, the stroke volume may be reduced when the cardiac output is normal due to a tachyarrhythmia and increased in the presence of a bradycardia.

The mean systolic ejection rate (MSER) is indirectly related to the velocity of ventricular shortening.[57] However, the MSER index—normally 159 ± 39 standard deviation (SD) ml/sec/M^2—is directly related to the loading conditions of the heart, as well as to contractility.[58]

Exercise and Oxygen Consumption

Exercise Factor: Since impairment of cardiac function often does not result in distinct hemodynamic abnormalities at rest, dysfunction of the heart may be revealed by the cardiocirculatory response to muscular exercise. One approach has been the measurement of cardiac output at rest and during submaximal supine exercise and the calculation of the exercise factor—ratio of the increase in cardiac output to the increase in total body oxygen consumption.[59] In normal persons the cardiac output rises by more than 600 ml/min for each 100 ml increase in oxygen consumption. However, only relatively light external work can be performed in the supine position, and thus this technique is a relatively insensitive test of cardiac performance.

Cardiac Output Relative to Pulmonary Arterial Oxygen Saturation: Cardiac function can be evaluated more precisely by employing maximal levels of upright exercise. Although the determination of maximal oxygen intake has provided useful information concerning overall cardiac performance,[60] this measurement cannot be obtained with regularity in patients with heart disease and may be diminished by certain extracardiac influences. A more sensitive method for the assessment of cardiocirculatory function has been maximal treadmill exercise with determination of the cardiac output achieved at the pulmonary arterial oxygen saturation of 30 percent.[61] At this level of oxygen extraction in the pulmonary artery, patients with diminished cardiac reserve exhibit cardiac output of less than 4.0 L/min/M^2, whereas the normal response is characterized by a cardiac index above 7.0 L/min/M^2. Further, another important difference between normal subjects and patients with impaired cardiac function in response to exhausting exercise is the level to which the mixed systemic venous oxygen saturation falls.[61] Patients with heart disease extract greater quantities of oxygen from systemic arterial blood and achieve pulmonary arterial oxygen saturations that usually are less than 15 percent, whereas in normal subjects this level is greater than 20 percent.

Although intense levels of treadmill exercise allow detection of mild degrees of cardiac impairment, these exercise studies, which employ various measurements of total body oxygen utilization relative to cardiac output, do not differentiate between abnormalities of ventricular loading and contractility. It also has become apparent that cardiocirculatory responses are substantially influenced not only by the intensity of exercise, but also by position and type of exercise performed.[62] The cardiocirculatory responses—and the differences in these responses—in normal subjects and patients with impaired cardiac function are substantially in-

fluenced by the choice of supine versus upright exercise and bicycle versus treadmill exercise.

Ventricular Function Curves

As discussed in chapter 9, the characterization of ventricular function within the concept of the Frank-Starling principle, which relates stroke work to ventricular end-diastolic volume (see Figure 1 in chapters 9 and 20), has provided a useful means for the qualitative evaluation of directional differences in ventricular contractility between patients and in individual patients in response to interventions.[44-47,59,60] The ventricular function curve consists of a principal ascending limb on which increases in end-diastolic volume produce elevations of stroke work (Figure 10). This ascending limb is terminated at a level of end-diastolic volume that produces no further increase in stroke work. In experimental animals, the peak of the ventricular function curve is followed by a short descending limb on which further increases in end-diastolic volume cause reductions in stroke work.

In normal subjects, the apex of the ventricular function curve is traditionally considered to be at a LVEDP of about 12 mm Hg, whereas in patients with depressed ventricular contractility this level is considerably elevated (Figure 10). When contractility becomes depressed—as in congestive heart failure—the entire ventricular function curve shifts downward and to the right with an ascending limb that is prolonged and less steep, an apex that is shifted to the right and a descending limb that has a depressed slope (Figure 10). Current evidence suggests that the failing human ventricle does not usually operate on the descending limb of the ventricular function curve for prolonged periods of time. In patients with heart failure, the descending limb of the depressed ventricular function curve has been demonstrated by increasing preload transiently. However, it usually has not been possible to show that these ventricles chronically perform on the descending limb, since decreases in preload have not augmented cardiac output or stroke work.[65] However, chronic operation of the diseased ventricle on a descending limb has been shown in a few patients,[66] and this is thought to represent slippage be-

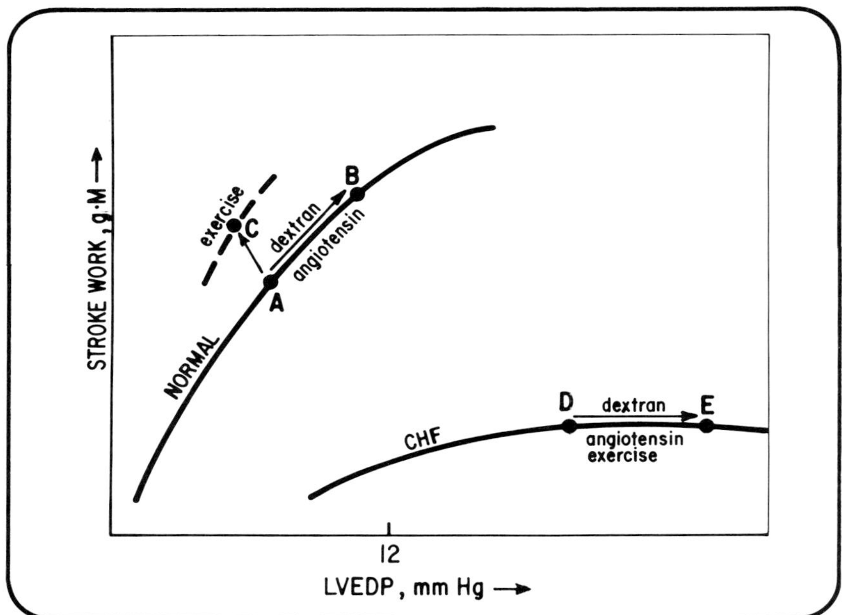

FIGURE 10. Representative left ventricular function curves, relating left ventricular stroke work to left ventricular end-diastolic pressure (LVEDP), in normal subjects and in patients with congestive heart failure (CHF) due to depressed contractility. Comparative responses to increments in preload (dextran infusion) and afterload (angiotension infusion) and to supine leg exercise are shown. In normal subjects, with the resting left ventricle operating at **point A,** elevations of left ventricular loading with dextran or angiotensin produce a large increase in stroke work concomitant with a relatively small rise in LVEDP **(point B),** thereby defining a steep ascending limb of the ventricular function curve characterized by normal contractility. In contrast, elevations of left ventricular loading with dextran or angiotensin produce little rise or no change in stroke work concomitant with a large increase in LVEDP **(point D** to **point E),** thereby defining a flat and depressed ventricular function curve due to marked decrease in contractility. In normal subjects, exercise results in a substantial increase in contractility **(point A** to **point C),** indicated by a rise in stroke work and a decline in LVEDP, with the left ventricle operating on an enhanced, steeper function curve **(broken lines).** In contrast, exercise in CHF due to depressed contractility does not result in an increase in contractile state **(point D** to **point E),** indicated by the further elevation of LVEDP without a rise in stroke work.

tween myofibrils and cardiac fibers rather than overstretch at the sarcomere level.[67] It is pointed out that alterations in preload are indicated by changes of position on the same curve and that alterations of contractility are documented by shifts of the entire ventricular function curve.

In clinical practice, a segment of the ascending limb is obtained by determining two points on the ventricular function curve at different end-diastolic volumes (Figure 10). Thus it is necessary to obtain cardiac output and LVEDP measurements in the control state and during a maneuver that alters end-diastolic volume. Since it is difficult to measure end-diastolic volume, LVEDP is utilized as an estimation of end-diastolic fiber length. One of several systolic performance characteristics of the ventricle is em-

ployed on the ordinate: stroke volume, cardiac output or, traditionally, stroke work. Stroke work is the product of stroke volume and integrated left ventricular systolic pressure, and thus stroke work includes both the flow and pressure work of the ventricle.

Within the structure of the Frank-Starling concept, only the preload and contractility determinants of ventricular performance are considered. Further, in the traditional determination of a single ventricular function curve, only preload is altered; contractile state, afterload and heart rate should remain constant. In studies of the effects of an intervention on contractility in an individual patient, the control function curve is obtained, the event undergoing investigation is carried out, and preload and contractility—but not afterload or heart rate—are allowed to vary; the ventricular function curve is then redetermined in the same manner as was the control curve, by alterations of preload alone.

When alterations of afterload or heart rate are used to change preload, or when afterload and heart rate are not controlled during a maneuver that changes preload in the determination of a ventricular function curve, or when the intervention being evaluated in an individual patient alters afterload or heart rate, there are certain limitations in the interpretation of alterations of stroke work and stroke output in the assessment of cardiac contractility within the Frank-Starling concept. Thus, the performance characteristics of the heart might be influenced by the changes in afterload and heart rate themselves besides the alteration of preload, while the function curve is obtained, and in addition to alterations of preload and contractility, during the intervention under investigation. The problem presented by inconstant afterload is that stroke volume and cardiac output vary inversely with impedance to ejection; thus reductions in impedance and afterload allow stroke output to rise, which might be incorrectly deduced to represent an increase in contractility. In the presence of changing afterload, stroke work is a better performance variable than is stroke output for use in the Frank-Starling analysis, since stroke volume is altered inversely whereas ventricular pressure is altered in the same direction in response to afterload, resulting in opposing influences on stroke work and relatively less dependence of stroke work on afterload. In contrast to the substantial effects of acute changes in afterload on variables of cardiac performance, the principal response of the ventricle to chronically increased afterload appears to be the development of ventricular hypertrophy. Thus, variations in afterload per se among different ventricles do not cause large changes in the shape and position of ventricular function curves in interpatient studies.

In describing the slope of the ascending limb of ventricular function curves and the ability of the ventricle to augment the position of the entire curve, three general approaches have been employed clinically: alterations in (1) preload; (2) afterload; and (3) exercise.

Preload Alterations: The inflation of a balloon-tip catheter in the inferior vena cava, which partially obstructs venous return to the heart, provides a means of decreasing LVEDP, thereby lowering the point on the function curve at which the ventricle operates and allowing determination of the slope of the ascending limb.[68] In normal subjects, small decreases in filling pressure of the left ventricle result in marked diminution of stroke volume. In contrast, in patients with disease of the myocardium and depressed contractility, large decrements of LVEDP result in little or no decline in cardiac performance, indicating a flattened and depressed ventricular function curve and reduced myocardial contractility.

The integrity of the ventricular function curve obtained by direct alteration of preload can also be assessed by leg raising, which produces an elevation in LVEDP. In addition, the ascending limb can be obtained by increasing LVEDP with infusion of low molecular weight dextran[69] (Figure 10) or injection of angiographic dye.[70] In this latter maneuver, determination of the second point of the function curve should be delayed for several minutes after injection of the contrast dye to allow dissipation of alterations in contractility and compliance produced by the contrast substance itself.[71–73] It has also been demonstrated that meaningful ventricular function curves can be obtained by changes in preload, stroke volume and myocardial oxygen requirements induced by atrial pacing in studies of cardiac performance in coronary heart disease.[74–76]

Afterload Alterations: Another intervention allowing definition of a segment of the ventricular function curve—and thereby qualitative assessment of myocardial contractile state—is the infusion of the arteriolar constrictor substance angiotensin or methoxamine.[65] By increasing afterload with these agents, increased resistance to left ventricular ejection causes a small rise in LVEDP, and thus ventricular preload is indirectly augmented (Figure 10). Despite the increased afterload, the resultant increase in preload causes relatively large elevation of stroke volume in normal patients, resulting in a steep ascending limb of the function curve. In contrast, in patients with heart failure and depressed contractility, marked elevations of LVEDP cause little change in stroke volume, resulting in a flattened and depressed ventricular function curve.

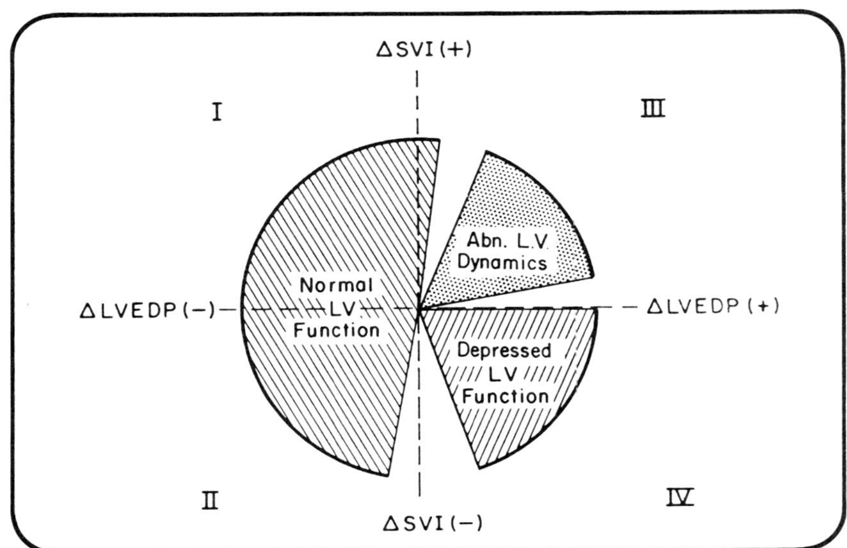

FIGURE 11. Left ventricular function response to supine muscular exercise relating patterns of changes in stroke volume index (SVI) to left ventricular end-diastolic pressure (LVEDP). Normal left ventricular (LV) function (quadrants I and II, **hatched area**) includes a variable change in SVI, usually an increase, with a decrease or no change in LVEDP. Mild to moderate decrease in left ventricular performance (quadrant III, **stippled area**) is associated with an increase in SVI and an increase in LVEDP. Severely depressed LV function (quadrant IV, **hatched area**) is characterized by no change or a decrease in SVI with an increase in LVEDP. (Reproduced by permission from Ross et al.[77])

Exercise: Although the exercise techniques described previously, in which cardiac output is related to total body oxygen consumption, suggest the degree to which the pump function of the heart is capable of satisfying the increased metabolic demands of physical stress, they are not helpful in differentiating abnormalities of loading from inotropic factors that may limit the cardiac output response. A useful method for the qualitative differential evaluation of these factors is the study of left ventricular performance by determination of the effects of supine leg exercise on cardiac output, stroke volume or stroke work and LVEDP.[77] The integrity of cardiac performance in response to the stress of muscular exercise can be analyzed by alteration of the position of the ventricular function curve (Figure 10). Thus, augmentation of sympathetic activity occurring with exercise normally increases myocardial contractility and thereby changes the shape and position of the entire curve, so that its ascending slope is steeper and elevated compared with the control curve. In contrast, patients with depressed ventricular contractility exhibit a depressed and flat curve with little change or decline in cardiac performance despite development of high levels of LVEDP. Thus, a characteristic of the ventricle with diminished contractility is impairment of its ability to augment contractile state in response to positive inotropic stimulation.

A simplified and useful means of assessment of these leg exercise data is the comparison of the changes of stroke volume and end-diastolic pressure with the resting levels of these variables[6,77,78] (Figure 11). In normal subjects during exercise, the LVEDP does not exceed 12 mm Hg and usually decreases or increases by no more than 2 mm Hg accompanied by an increase in stroke volume. In contrast, patients with abnormal myocardial contractility exhibit a decrease in stroke volume despite excessive increments in LVEDP, which reaches total levels of more than 12 mm Hg (see Figure 7 in chapter 9). An intermediate response consisting of a rise in stroke volume accompanied by an excessive elevation of LVEDP is considered to be due to abnormal ventricular compliance or to a lesser impairment of contractility with increased use of ventricular preload as a compensatory mechanism to achieve an increase in cardiac output in response to exercise.

Left ventricular function also has been evaluated by forearm isometric exercise accomplished by sustained handgrip. Both central hemodynamic and myocardial mechanical responses have been evaluated.[79-82] The isometric maneuver imposes an afterload burden on the left ventricle accompanied by sympathetic stimulation to the myocardium. Normal subjects respond to this increased afterload principally by enhancement of the contractile state. In contrast, patients with diminished myocardial contractility demonstrate reduced ability to augment the depressed inotropic state and, instead, use the Frank-Starling preload mechanism for compensation.

Left Ventricular Volume, Ejection Fraction, Work, Power and Mass

Angiographic techniques allow determination of chamber dimensions, volume, wall thickness and mass of the left ventricle that, when combined with measurements of intraventricular pressure and cardiac output, provide detailed assessment of the function of the heart as a pump.[83-88] By analysis of these complex variables and their interrelationships, it is possible qualitatively to evaluate contractile state separately from abnormalities of ventricular loading.

Ejection Fraction: The relation of stroke volume to left ventricular end-diastolic volume provides important information concerning ventricular contractility. Employing angiographic methods, the normal left ventricular end-diastolic volume index is 70 ± 20 SD cc/M^2, and the normal systolic ejection fraction is 0.56 to 0.78.[89] Although the systolic ejection fraction is dependent on acute variations of systemic arterial resistance, the ventricle utilizes the development of hypertrophy rather than an increase of end-diastolic volume in its adjustment to chronic elevation of resistance to ejection. Thus, the ejection fraction is little influenced by chronic alterations of afterload per se.[85] A reduced ejection fraction suggests rel-

atively more ventricular dilation than can be accounted for by excessive preload alone and thereby indicates the presence of reduced myocardial contractility.

Ventricular Work and Power: The instantaneous relation of left ventricular pressure and volume throughout the cardiac cycle constitutes the pressure-volume curve or loop of the ventricle[90-93] (Figure 12). Analysis of the shape and position of these pressure-volume curves affords qualitative evaluation concerning depressed myocardial contractility and loading abnormalities due to valvular heart disease. Integration of the pressure-volume loop during contraction—including the diastolic portion above the base line—represents systolic work (stroke work). The diastolic area below the curve is diastolic work and constitutes the energy expended in distending the ventricle during the resting stage of the cardiac cycle. When contractility is reduced, increased diastolic work is necessary to distend the ventricle. Net work is the difference between systolic and diastolic work, and net work decreases with reduced left ventricular contractility.

The rate at which ventricular systolic work is performed is ventricular power, calculated as the product of instantaneous intraventricular pressure and the rate of ventricular ejection, which in turn is determined from the rate of change of ventricular volume during systole.[85,94] The left ventricular power curve can be constructed during the cardiac cycle and peak systolic power determined; this is normally about 600 g/M/sec and is substantially reduced with depressed myocardial contractile state.

Ventricular Mass: Knowledge of left ventricular wall thickness, chamber dimensions and volume provides the calculation of left ventricular mass, which is normally 92 ± 16 SD g/M^2 by this method.[95,96] In chronic systolic pressure overloading of the left ventricle, hypertrophy often occurs with little or no increase in chamber volume; conversely, in chronic systolic volume overloading of the left ventricle, ventricular dilation occurs to a proportionally greater degree than does hypertrophy. However, in both chronic systolic pressure and volume overloading, the extent of left ventricular mass correlates with stroke work.[83,85]

Ventricular Stress Relations: Reductions in the ratio of ejection fraction to ventricular end-diastolic volume and of ventricular power relative to end-diastolic volume indicate depressed left ventricular contractility.[83,85] Ventricular stroke work and power are maintained at a normal level at the expense of ventricular dilation by the Frank-Starling mechanism and at the expense of diminished cardiac reserve in terms of the capacity for further ventricular dilation. Since left ventricular mass correlates with diastolic volume in chronic systolic volume overloading when contractile state is maintained at a normal level, the relation of ventricular mass to diastolic work is inappropriately large with diminished myocardial contractility and increased preloading. Also, inappropriately increased ventricular dilation and elevated end-diastolic volume per unit of stroke work (the Frank-Starling principle) indicate depressed ventricular contractility.

Since there is a positive correlation between left ventricular mass and stroke work in patients with chronic valvular heart disease—resulting in pressure or volume overloading of the ventricle—excessive development of ventricular hypertrophy or mass relative to stroke work indicates an associated decrease in myocardial contractility in these conditions as well as in primary cardiomyopathies. Patients with depressed left ventricular contractility and loading abnormalities have low values of stroke work per unit mass, diminished values of peak power per unit mass and reduced ejection fraction related to end-diastolic volume.[83,85,97] Thus, assessment of cardiac performance in these terms of the heart as a pump provides qualitative evaluation of contractility by relating stroke volume, rate of ejection, stroke work and stroke power to left ventricular end-diastolic volume and left ventricular mass. Inappropriate dilation—chronically increased afterload or hypertrophic cardiomyopathy—indicates diminished contractility.

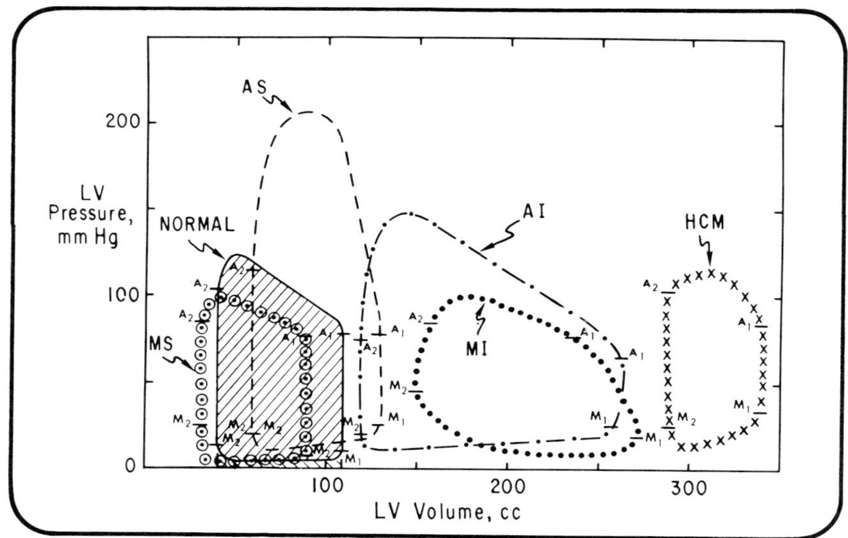

FIGURE 12. Representative comparison of pressure-volume (work) curves of the left ventricle (LV) in mitral stenosis (MS), normal subject, aortic stenosis (AS), aortic regurgitation (AI), mitral regurgitation (MI) and hypertrophic cardiomyopathy (HCM). Systolic pressure-volume work is determined from the systolic pressure-volume relations, and work expended in distending the diastolic left ventricle is obtained from pressure-volume relations during diastole. Systolic work in the normal subject, is shown by the area containing the **right upward diagonal lines;** diastolic work, by the **right downward diagonal lines;** and net work, by systolic work minus the diastolic work. The height of each pressure-volume loop is determined by systolic pressure and the width by stroke volume of the LV. The smallest curves occur in MS, due to diminished preload, and in HCM, due to depressed contractility with cardiac output supported in part by end-diastolic dilation. Wide loops, due to volume overloading, are observed in MI and in AI, and the tall curve of pressure overloading is seen in AS. A_1 = aortic valve opening; A_2 = aortic valve closure; M_1 = mitral valve closure; and M_2 = mitral valve opening. (Reproduced by permission from Mason et al.[45])

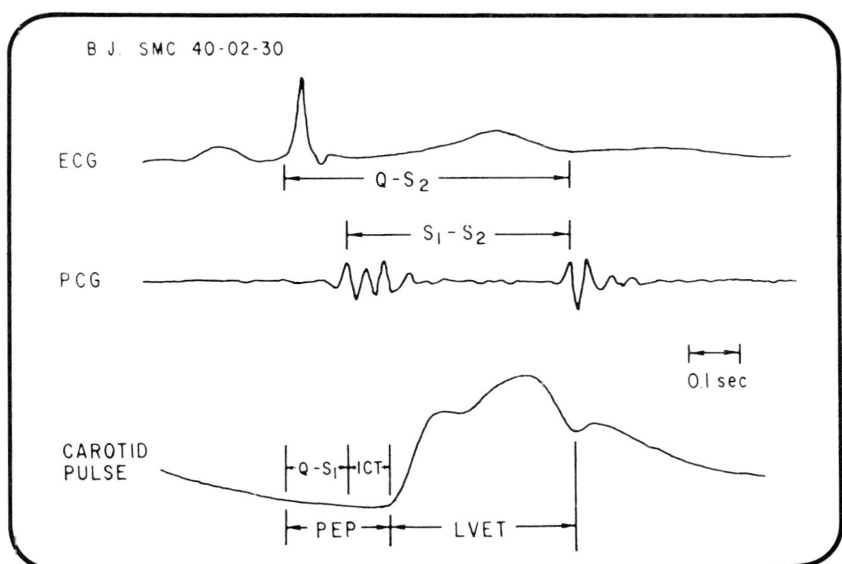

FIGURE 13. Recording of electrocardiogram (ECG), phonocardiogram (PCG) and indirect carotid arterial pulse demonstrating the systolic time intervals, Q–S$_2$, S$_1$–S$_2$ and Q–S$_1$; isovolumic contraction time (ICT); pre-ejection period (PEP); and left ventricular ejection time (LVET). (Reproduced by permission from Mason et al.[45])

Systolic Time Intervals

Attention has been focused recently on the development of noninvasive techniques for the evaluation of cardiac function that can be applied with ease at the bedside. The simultaneous recording of the electrocardiogram, phonocardiogram and carotid arterial pulsations allows indirect determination of total electromechanical systole (Q–S$_2$ interval—beginning of QRS complex to the first high-frequency vibration of the second heart sound), left ventricular ejection time (LVET—onset of upstroke to incisural notch on the carotid tracing; normal, 415 ± 10 SD msec) and the pre-ejection period (PEP—electromechanical systole minus ejection time; normal, 132 ± 12 SD msec)[98–101] (Figure 13).

In patients with primary and secondary abnormalities of myocardial contractility—often before the onset of overt congestive heart failure —the pre-ejection period usually lengthens while the ejection time shortens. Thus, the ratio of the pre-ejection period to ejection time (PEP/LVET; normal, 0.35 ± 0.04 SD) provides a useful index of cardiac function permitting relative separation of patients with diminished contractility from normal subjects. In patients with heart disease, the PEP/LVET ratio appears to be sensitive to diminished contractile state in the cardiomyopathies, systemic arterial hypertension and chronic coronary artery disease. In valvular heart disease, however, the index is somewhat less accurate due to concomitant chronic pressure and volume overload. Acute myocardial infarction usually results in normal or variable PEP whereas the LVET is abbreviated.[102–104] In serial studies in an individual patient, PEP is altered by acute changes of preload or afterload alone, in addition to changes in contractility.[105] Digitalis tends to shorten both PEP and LVET.[106] Leg exercise in patients with angina pectoris due to coronary artery disease leads to an increase of LVET, whereas this interval is unchanged with exercise in normal subjects; PEP normally shortens with exercise and remains unchanged in patients with angina.[107]

Left intraventricular conduction defects produce lengthening of PEP without alterations of LVET. In the presence of left ventricular conduction disturbances, determination of the isovolumic contraction time as the measure of pre-ejection duration appears to offer potential advantages over PEP, since the isovolumic con-

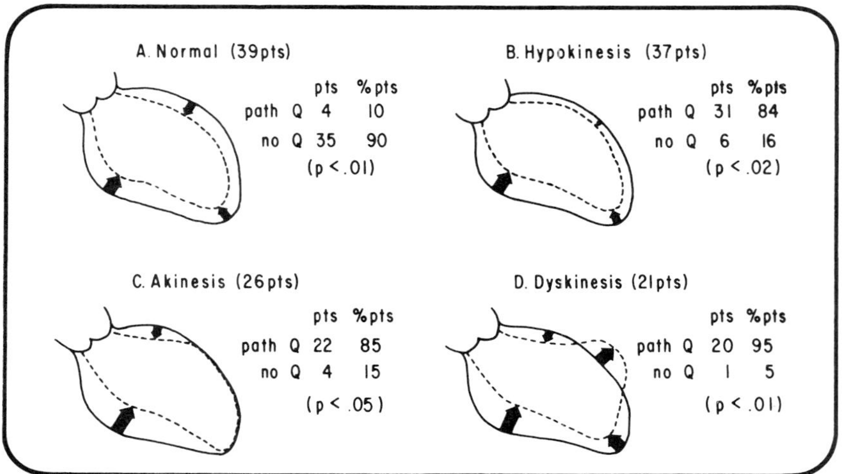

FIGURE 14. Nature of dyssynergy related to the presence (path Q = pathologic Q waves) or absence (no Q) of ECG-documented myocardial infarction. Normal contraction pattern (**A**) was associated with no Q; in hypokinesis (**B**), akinesis (**C**) and dyskinesis (**D**), path Q was more common. (Reproduced by permission from Miller et al.[181])

traction time is not influenced by variations of QRS depolarization time among different ventricles[108] (Figure 13).

Ventricular Dyssynergy

The normal pattern of left ventricular excitation and contraction takes place in a coordinated manner with integrated inward movement of the ventricular wall during ejection. However, disturbances of electrical conduction within the ventricle, as in left bundle branch block, result in disorderly distribution of contraction, which in itself compromises ventricular function and cardiac output even when each zone of myocardium has normal contractile properties.[109]

Abnormal sequence of wall motion is also produced by localized disturbances in muscle function even in the presence of normal spread of electrical activation.[109-112] Segmental abnormalities of the pattern of ventricular contraction are observed most commonly in coronary artery disease—and sometimes in cardiomyopathies, which contribute to cardiac dysfunction on a mechanical basis. Thus, in coronary artery disease, cardiac performance may be impaired by dyssynergy due to a combination of delayed regional electrical conduction and abnormal lo-

cal wall movement, as well as by segmental depression of contractility.

Regional disturbances in ventricular wall motion in patients with coronary artery disease can be appreciated readily by left ventricular cineangiography[112] (Figure 14). Four different types of localized disorders of systolic wall motion have been described: (1) hypokinesis, or diminished regional inward motion; (2) akinesis, or absent movement of part of the wall; (3) dyskinesis, or paradoxical outward local wall motion during contraction, as seen with ventricular aneurysms; and (4) asynchrony, or disturbed sequence of the temporal phases of contraction with alternating zones of contraction and expansion (See Figure 6 in chapter 11). Dyssynergy is a general term referring to any or a combination of these subtypes of abnormal segmental wall motion during contraction.

In addition to local depression of cardiac contractility in regional disease of the ventricular myocardium, dyssynergy itself modifies the cardiac pumping action due to unfavorable geometric effects on the mechanical mechanism of ejection. In addition, these regional abnormalities place a mechanical burden on the normal areas of the left ventricle that provides the stimulus for hypertrophy in coronary artery disease.[87] Inherent in the stimulus for hypertrophy is the need for the residual nonischemic heart muscle to shorten to a greater extent; thus, in this hyperdynamic segment, a portion of ventricular wall shortening is expended in stretching the poorly contractile muscle rather than in ejecting stroke volume.

Ventricular Muscle Function

More recently it has become possible clinically to examine ventricular performance and contractility in terms of muscle mechanics that describe the force, velocity and length properties of the ventricular myocardium. In the numeric assessment of contractile state, the mechanical events occurring during both the isovolumic and ejection phases of systole have been characterized.[44–48,113–116] Thus, measures of inotropic state have been developed along two general lines: (1) isovolumic indexes utilizing dp/dt—rate of ventricular pressure rise; and (2) ejection indexes employing V_{CF}—rate of circumferential fiber shortening.

Currently, there is considerable discussion concerning the advantages and limitations of derived mechanical variables in the examination of contractile state. It has been difficult to evaluate the validity and sensitivity of various indexes of contractility in the intact heart since there is no standard measure with which they can be compared; thus, considerable discussion has consisted of circular reasoning. Nevertheless, certain isovolumic and ejection mechanical indexes provide qualitative and quantitative estimation of contractility alterations in response to interventions in individual patients and of resting contractile state among different patients.

Isovolumic Mechanical Indexes (dp/dt)

The high sensitivity of the rate of ventricular pressure rise (dp/dt) to inotropic state has stimulated intense interest in isovolumic indexes employing dp/dt for the clinical assessment of contractility[114] (Figure 15).

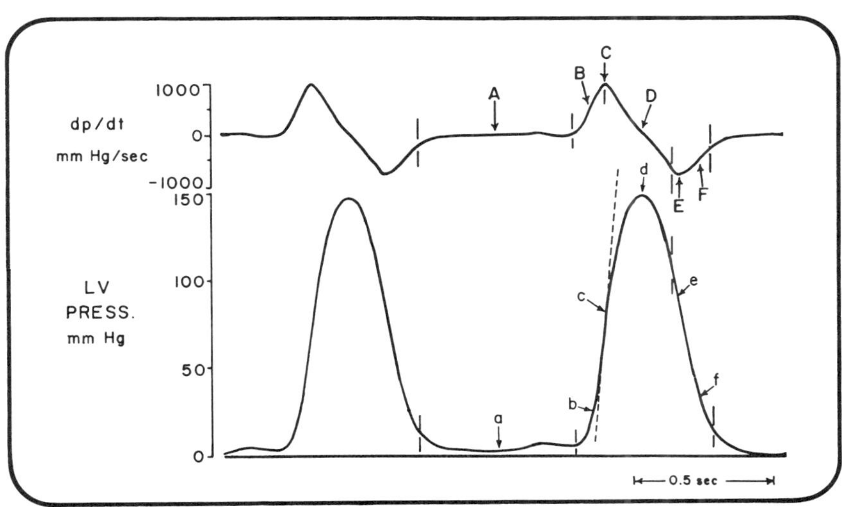

FIGURE 15. Simultaneous high-fidelity recordings of left ventricular (LV) pressure and its first derivative (dp/dt) in a patient with an aortic valve prosthesis. The various portions of the first derivative and corresponding segments of the pressure recording from which they were continuously computed are labeled. During ventricular filling when rate of change of ventricular pressure is minimal, dp/dt is flat at a level near zero **(segment A)**. With the onset of isovolumic contraction, dp/dt rises slowly and then rapidly **(segment B)** to reach the peak dp/dt **(point C)**—the maximal rate of pressure rise—indicated by the slope of the **diagonal broken line.** Peak dp/dt usually occurs at the instant of opening of the semilunar valves—at peak isovolumic ventricular pressure. During the early and middle phases of ventricular ejection, dp/dt descends to the baseline; during late ejection, as intraventricular pressure decreases, dp/dt becomes negative **(segment D)**. The rate of decrease of ventricular pressure is maximal at **point E** during isovolumic relaxation **(segment F)**. Left ventricular pressure was recorded by direct needle puncture. (Reproduced by permission from Mason.[114])

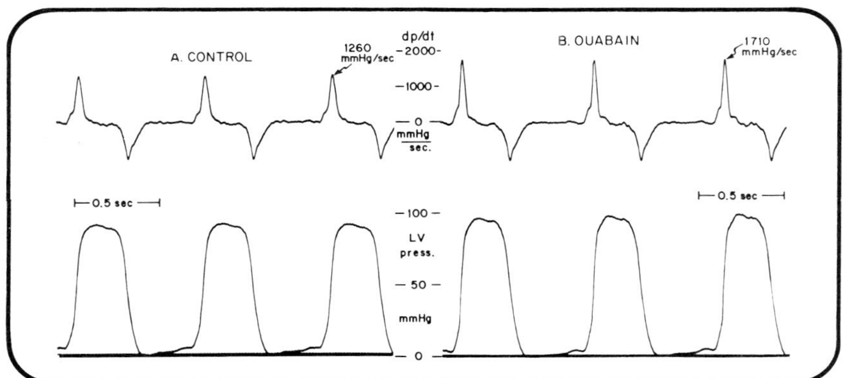

FIGURE 16. Simultaneous high-fidelity recordings of left ventricular (LV) pressure and of its rate of pressure change (dp/dt) during the control period **(A)** and after digitalis **(B)** in a patient with a small atrial septal defect. Left ventricular pressure was recorded with the Telco intracardiac micro-manometer. (Reproduced by permission from Mason.[114])

Peak dp/dt: Peak dp/dt itself is a valid and sensitive measure for the study of ventricular inotropic state in serial studies in an individual patient when loading conditions are constant.[114] With stable ventricular loading, peak dp/dt correlates directly with the contractile state of the ventricle in the study of interventions in an individual patient[117] (Figure 16). However, peak dp/dt is a complex function also directly dependent on preload (LVEDP) and afterload (arterial diastolic pressure in the case of peak dp/dt). An increase in LVEDP causes an elevation of instantaneous dp/dt throughout the course of isovolumic contraction, including peak dp/dt. Since changes in loading conditions of the ventricle ordinarily occur in response to most physiologic and pharmacologic interventions in individual patients and in the resting state among different patients, usually it is not possible to evaluate precisely ventricular contractile state clinically by the determination of peak dp/dt alone.

Time-to-Peak dp/dt: The recognition that dp/dt is influenced by preload and afterload variations has led to the development of contractility indexes in which dp/dt is modified by certain hemodynamic and mechanical variables that tend to cancel the changes in dp/dt caused by inconstant loading.[114] By correlating these loading-related correction factors with dp/dt, it is possible to employ dp/dt in the assessment of contractility despite concurrent alterations in loading. One approach that is useful in serial studies in an individual patient is the examination of the time interval from the onset of ventricular contraction to maximal dp/dt (time-to-peak dp/dt) in relation to peak dp/dt itself[118] (Figure 17). Alterations in contractility produce opposite changes in time-to-peak dp/dt and peak dp/dt, whereas variations in loading result in directionally similar changes in these two variables. Although directionally opposite changes in time-to-peak dp/dt and peak dp/dt indicate a qualitative alteration of contractility, large concomitant changes in LVEDP or arterial diastolic pressure might obscure alterations in inotropic state analyzed in this manner.

In the presence of changes in LVEDP not associated with variations of arterial diastolic pressure, alterations in contractility can be studied using the ratios: peak dp/dt to integrated systolic isovolumic tension,[119] peak dp/dt to peak isovolumic pressure (PIP),[120] peak dp/dt to maximal isovolumic ventricular tension,[121] peak dp/dt to LVEDP[122] and (peak dp/dt)/PIP related to left ventricular end-diastolic circumferential fiber length.[123] As with peak dp/dt, these ratios are dependent on arterial diastolic pressure.

Relation of dp/dt to Common Peak Isovolumic Pressure: When LVEDP is nearly constant and arterial diastolic pressure varies, the relation of dp/dt to common peak developed isovolumic pressure (CPIP) correlates directly with contractile state independent of afterload varia-

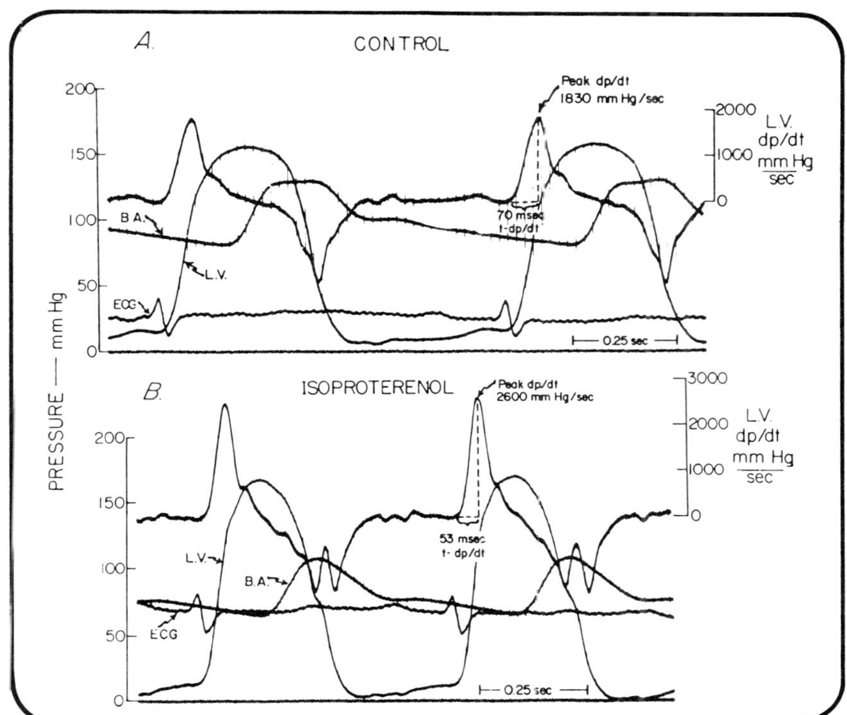

FIGURE 17. Simultaneous high-fidelity recordings of left ventricular (LV) pressure, its first derivative (dp/dt) and brachial arterial pressure (BA) during the control period **(A)** and after contractility was increased with isoproterenol **(B)** in a patient with an aortic valve prosthesis. The interval from the onset to peak dp/dt (t-dp/dt) is indicated. Left ventricular pressure was recorded by direct needle puncture. (Reproduced by permission from Mason.[114])

tions[116] (Figure 18). The relation between dp/dt and simultaneously developed pressure during the course of isovolumic contraction can also be applied in the assessment of resting contractile state among different patients.[56] Thus dp/dt determined at the developed isovolumic ventricular pressure of 50 mm Hg common to each ventricle corrects for differences in arterial diastolic pressure. Since the preload of the different ventricles varies widely, dp/dt at common developed isovolumic pressure of 50 mm Hg is modified by relating it to left ventricular end-diastolic volume index $(LVEDV/M^2)^{45}$ (Figure 19). This ratio $(dp/dt_{CPIP})/(LVEDV/M^2)$ is analogous to contractile element velocity (V_{CE}) corrected for its preload dependence at an isopressure point on the pressure-velocity curve to be described.

Ventricular Pressure-Velocity Curves: In the myocardium, the mechanical properties of contraction can be considered conceptually by muscle models containing a contractile element (CE) with distensible series elastic (SE) and parallel elastic (PE) springs. The finding that isovolumic V_{CE} can be determined from high-fidelity ventricular pressure and its dp/dt alone[124] has provided a new practical approach to the quantification of left ventricular contractile state relatively free of loading variations both in serial comparisons in individual patients[115] and in comparisons among different patients.[56] In the intact heart during isovolumic contraction, V_{CE} can be considered essentially equivalent to the rate of SE elongation (V_{SE}). In the calculation of isovolumic ventricular V_{SE}—and thereby V_{CE}—knowledge of tension or stress is not necessary; only the value of isovolumic pressure is required since pressure is the single independent variable and chamber radius and wall thickness cancel in the equation for isovolumic V_{SE}.[115]

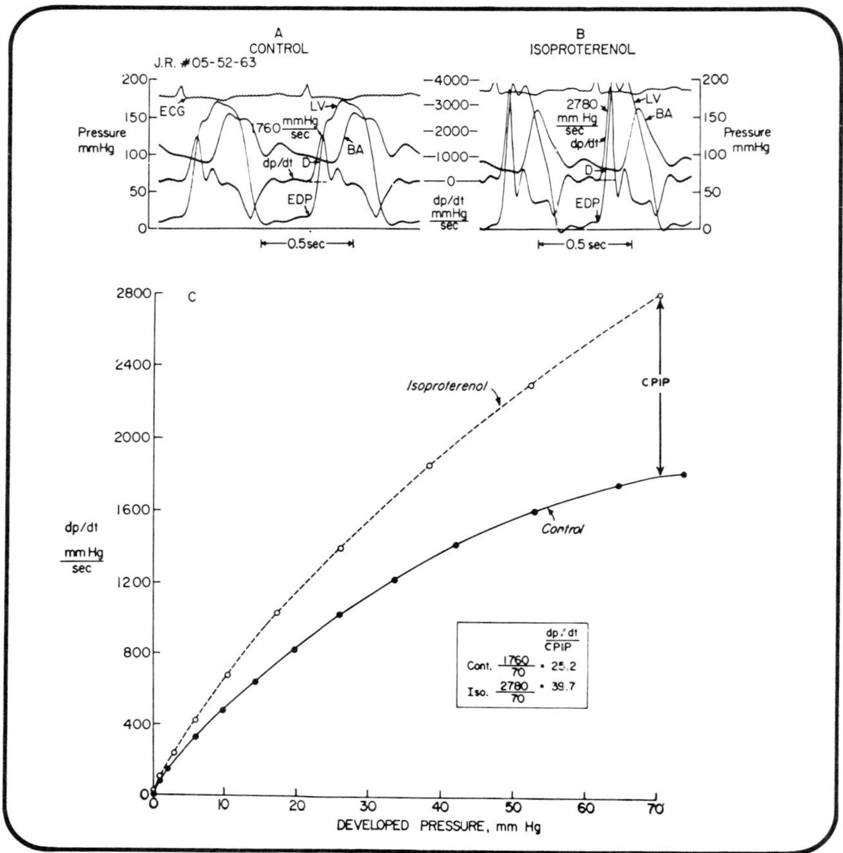

FIGURE 18. A and **B,** simultaneous high-fidelity recordings of left ventricular (LV) pressure, its first derivative (dp/dt), brachial arterial pressure (BA) and electrocardiogram during the control period (**A**) and during administration of isoproterenol (**B**). EDP = LV end-diastolic pressure; D = peak isovolumic LV pressure. The numerical values of dp/dt indicated are at the highest developed isovolumic pressure common to both beats (CPIP). **C,** relation between LV dp/dt and developed isovolumic pressure at 5 msec intervals throughout isovolumic systole of the contractions shown in the **top panel** in the control period (cont) and during isoproterenol administration (iso). The **arrows** indicating CPIP of both curves are the points at which the ratios (dp/dt)/CPIP shown in the insert were calculated. (Reproduced by permission from Mason et al.[116])

Therefore, isovolumic V_{CE} in ejecting beats can be determined entirely from isovolumic ventricular pressure (IP) and corresponding dp/dt by use of the equation for isovolumic V_{SE}: (dp/dt)/(K × IP)[115] with K at body temperature the SE stiffness component of 32/muscle length (ML).[125] Thus, from single beats, segments of isovolumic pressure-V_{CE} curves can be constructed (Figure 20) that are related to force-velocity properties of the ventricle. Extrapolation of the pressure-velocity descending limb to zero pressure allows estimation of the independent inotropic index, maximal V_{CE} (Vmax). Importantly, ventricular pressure-velocity and tension-velocity curves of a given contraction extrapolate to identical values of Vmax.[126,127]

The pressure-velocity method of assessing ventricular contractile state can be applied in evaluation of resting contractility in different patients, as well as in studies of interventions in individual patients, since V_{CE} is expressed in terms of muscle units (ML/sec) and extrapolated V_{CE} (Vmax) is free of differences of ventricular geometry and wall thickness and relatively in-

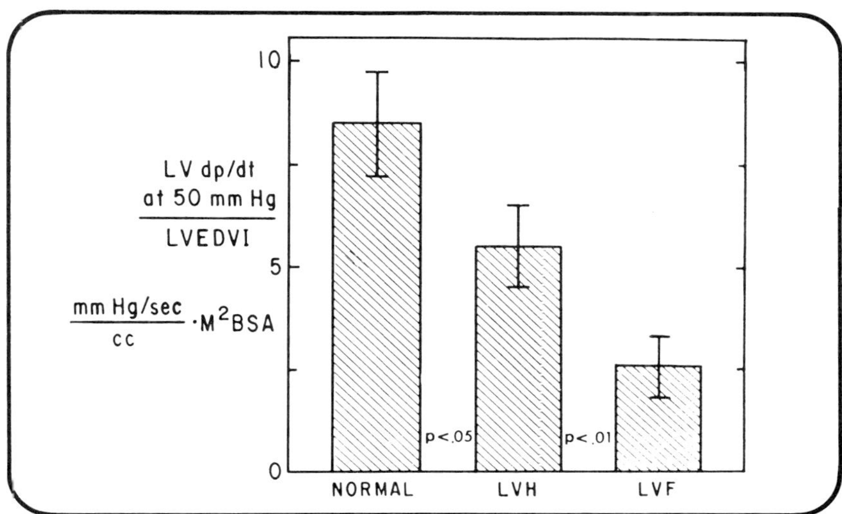

FIGURE 19. Comparative average values of the ratio of left ventricular (LV) dp/dt at the common isovolumic pressure of 50 mm Hg related to left ventricular end-diastolic volume index (LVEDVI) in normal subjects, in patients with compensated left ventricular hypertrophy (LVH) secondary to valvular aortic stenosis and in patients with left ventricular hypertrophy and decompensated congestive heart failure (LVF) due to valvular aortic stenosis. (Reproduced by permission from Mason et al.[56])

sensitive to loading.[115,127] Utilizing total pressure-velocity analysis for determination of Vmax in patients with primary and secondary ventricular hypertrophy, a spectrum of decreasing inotropic state has been shown between those without failure and those with failure[56] (Figure 21).

The isovolumic total pressure-velocity method for the evaluation of contractile state is based on the two-component Hill model in which CE and SE are connected in series. It has been suggested that the PE component should also be considered during isovolumic contraction by subtracting LVEDP from total isovolumic pressure to obtain developed isovolumic pressure for use in the V_{CE} equation and on the abscissa of the pressure-velocity curve[128] (Figure 22). With the isovolumic developed pressure-velocity curve obtained by utilization of the three-component model, V_{CE} is infinitely high at very small developed isovolumic pressures, and therefore, the first point on the descending pressure-velocity limb is usually arbitrarily taken at 10 mm Hg. Employing developed pressure-derived Vmax, it has been shown clinically that contractility is more depressed in primary hypertrophy of idiopathic cardiomyopathies than

in secondary hypertrophy of aortic stenosis,[129] and that contractility is lower in chronic volume overloading of mitral or aortic regurgitation compared with long-standing pressure overloading of aortic stenosis.[130] It is also possible to estimate right ventricular contractility by application of this developed pressure-V_{CE} approach, since this method allows description of a descending limb at relatively low isovolumic pressures.[131] In contrast, the onset of the total pressure-V_{CE} descending curve is delayed until development of full active state of the ventricle (Figure 22).

In decreasing order, the degree of sensitivity to contractility and preload of the principal contractility indexes employing isovolumic dp/dt is: (1) peak dp/dt; (2) (dp/dt)/CPIP; (3) total and then (4) developed pressure-V_{CE} methods. At the top of this spectrum, peak dp/dt is very sensitive to inotropism but is somewhat responsive to loading; at the other end, developed pressure V_{CE} is not altered by large changes in end-diastolic volume but is relatively insensitive to contractility. Contractility indexes designed to eliminate loading influences become inherently less sensitive to contractility.

Although physiologic changes in preload,

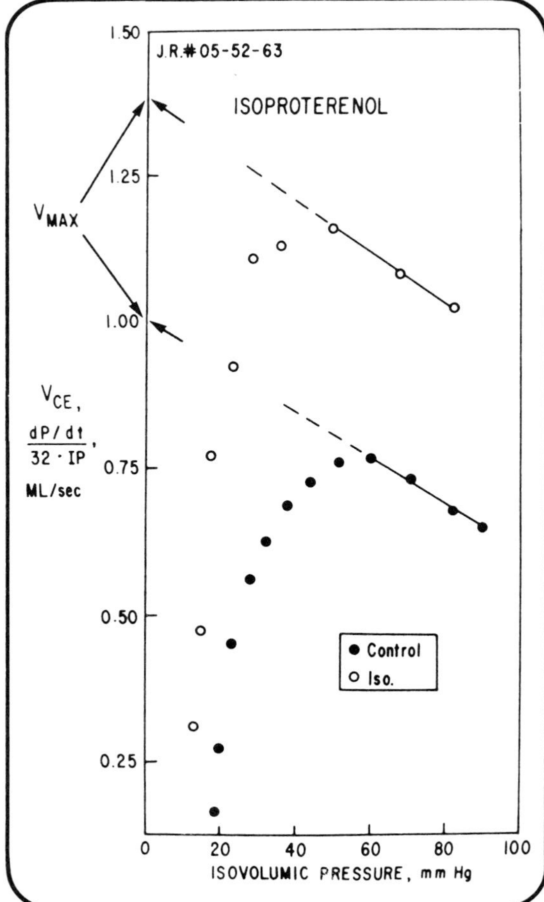

FIGURE 20. Total pressure-velocity relation during isovolumic contraction before and after isoproterenol (iso) infusion in a patient with an aortic valve prosthesis. High-fidelity left ventricular pressure was recorded by direct needle puncture. The **diagonal broken lines** indicate extrapolation of the isovolumic segment to Vmax (unloaded V_{CE}). V_{CE} is expressed in terms of muscle lengths (ML) per second (sec). IP = total LV isovolumic pressure. (Reproduced by permission from Mason et al.[115])

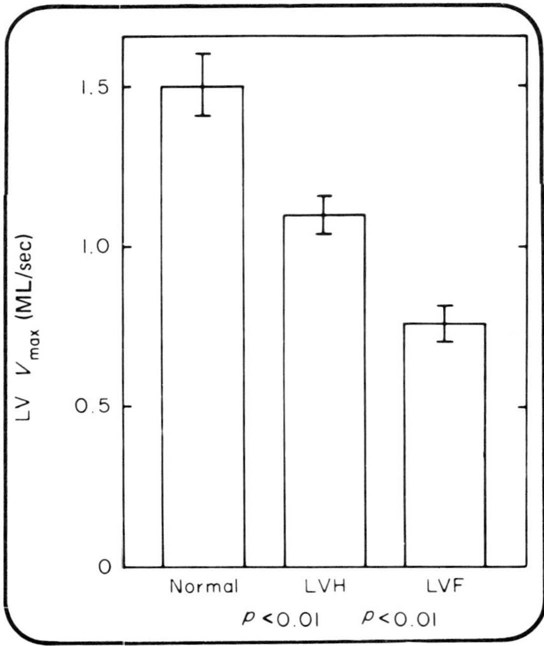

FIGURE 21. Comparative average values of left ventricular (LV) Vmax in normal subjects, in patients with compensated left ventricular hypertrophy (LVH) due to aortic stenosis and in patients with left ventricular hypertrophy and decompensated congestive heart failure (LVF) due to aortic stenosis. (Reproduced by permission from Mason et al.[56])

compliance variations, dyssynergy, nonisovolumic systole (mitral regurgitation) and segmental necrosis may considerably affect loaded V_{CE} prior to aortic valve opening, the accompanying alterations of the slope of the total and developed pressure-V_{CE} curves are such that extrapolated Vmax is minimally influenced or undisturbed.[132–135] Thus, as a contractility index, Vmax has been useful in these settings, including coronary heart disease. It now appears that these previously held problems largely represent "biologic noise" concerning the clinical application of Vmax from isovolumic pressure-velocity curves as an index estimating contractile state. Conversely, the use of peak measured V_{CE} (Vpm) in these situations is limited since loaded V_{CE} is substantially affected. Furthermore, it is important to note that in these particular conditions, marked disparity between ventricular hemodynamic performance and contractility assessed as Vmax appropriately may occur.[136,137]

Ejection Mechanical Indexes

The systolic ejection techniques applied to analysis of ventricular force-velocity properties and contractile state examine fiber-shortening rate (circumferential fiber-shortening velocity) to determine V_{CE} according to the principles of isotonic mechanics elucidated in isolated muscle.[47]

Epicardial Motion: One approach to the analysis of V_{CF} in serial studies in an individual patient is the cinegraphic determination of the rate of change of epicardial dimensions by measurement of the velocity of movement, frame by frame, of roentgenopaque markers previously sutured to the surface of the ventricle at therapeutic operation.[138,139] Other techniques for the study of external border motion are the measurement of epicardial segmental velocity as determined by movement of branch points of coronary arteries during angiography[140] and noninvasively by radarkymography.[141,142]

V_{CF} at Peak Tension: A more promising approach to the evaluation of V_{CE} and contractility during ejection is the study of endocardial wall motion. Angiographic study of instantaneous tension-velocity-length relations during ejection[143] provides determination of V_{CF} at peak midwall tension at which V_{SE} is zero; thereby V_{CF} at peak midwall tension equals V_{CE} at peak tension. Thus, a single V_{CE}-tension relation is established that identifies a point on the force-velocity curve of the ventricle, similar to the manner in which a point is determined on the isotonic force-velocity curve of papillary muscle by determination of peak fiber-shortening rate at peak tension from a single isotonic contraction.[47] The electromagnetic velocity catheter in the ascending aorta has also been used recently in determining instantaneous V_{CF} related to corresponding tension in the ejecting ventricle.[144–146] Ventricular V_{CE} at peak midwall tension correlates well with cardiac function, and V_{CE} values of less than 1.30 circumferences per second indicate depressed contractility. Although it is loading-dependent and not Vmax, V_{CE} at peak tension is applicable in nonisovolumic contractions and does obviate the need for the SE constant.

Mean V_{CF}: It has been shown that mean V_{CF}, determined angiographically as the relation of extent of internal wall shortening (end-diastolic volume minus end-systolic volume, corrected for end-diastolic volume) to duration of ejection, provides a good correlation with the more difficult calculation of V_{CE} at peak tension.[147–149] Furthermore, V_{CF} determined by echocardiographic measurements of left ventricular endocardial dimensions (described in chapter 15) relates closely to mean V_{CF} calculated by angiographic means.[150]

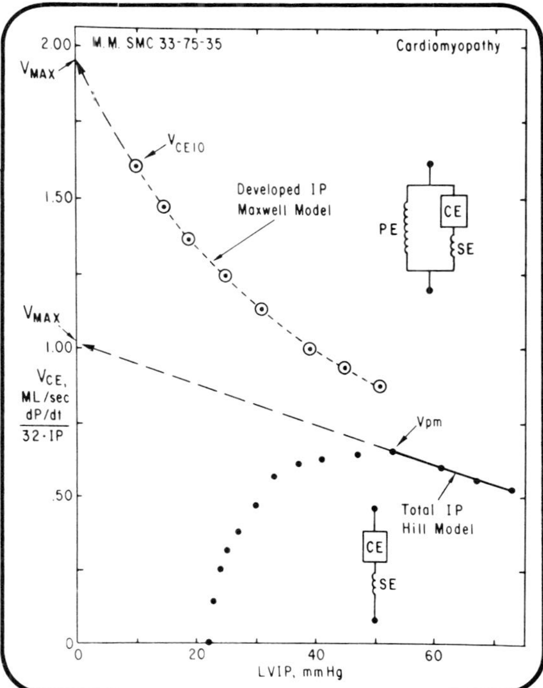

FIGURE 22. Left ventricular (LV) pressure-velocity relation during isovolumic contraction (LVIP) obtained by the use of total instantaneous isovolumic pressure (IP) in the calculation of instantaneous V_{CE} (two-component Hill model) and on the abscissa for LVIP (**closed dots** and **solid lines**) compared with the isovolumic pressure-velocity relation obtained by the use of developed instantaneous isovolumic pressure in the V_{CE} equation (three-component Maxwell model) and on the abscissa for LVIP (**open circles** and **short broken lines**). The extrapolations to Vmax are shown by the **long broken lines** and **arrows**. The appropriate muscle models are shown. The 2 pressure-velocity curves were obtained from the same LV beat in a patient with a cardiomyopathy. Vpm = peak measured V_{CE} using total IP; V_{CE10} = V_{CE} at 10 mm Hg developed IP. (Reproduced by permission from Mason et al.[47])

Nuclear Cardiology

In addition to the radionuclidic techniques for measuring cardiac output and evaluating intracardiac shunts described previously, a variety of new techniques have been developed that employ radioactive isotopes in the clinical evaluation of other aspects of cardiac function and structure. Three major areas of application of these techniques are: (1) noninvasive determination of ejection fraction and abnormalities of regional wall motion; (2) evaluation of regional myocardial perfusion, either in conjunction with left heart catheterization, using intracoronary injection of ^{133}Xe or ^{99m}Tc-labeled albumin particles, or noninvasively, using peripheral venous injection of potassium 43 ([43]K) or rubidium 81 ([81]Rb); and (3) identification of acute myocardial infarction with radiopharmaceuticals that accumulate in the infarcted myocardium, such as ^{99m}Tc pyrophosphate and related agents.

Ejection Fraction and Regional Contraction: Utilizing the Anger scintillation camera, the technique of radioisotopic angiocardiography was developed in 1969.[151,152] In 1971 a noninvasive radionuclidic method was described using gated cardiac blood pool imaging with the scintillation camera for estimating ejection fraction and segmental contraction.[153,154] More recently, ejection fraction has been measured by using scintillations obtained with the camera within an area of interest encompassing the left ventricular chamber.[155–157] Measurement of ejection fraction is also possible using a single precordial probe with a strip-chart recorder.[158] Unlike the gated blood pool imaging method, these area-counts methods fail to provide information regarding regional contraction patterns. Both the imaging and area-counts techniques offer the advantage of noninvasiveness, as each requires simply a venous injection.

In our laboratories we recently have developed an improved method of gated blood pool imaging for measuring ejection fraction and assessing regional contraction patterns in patients.[159] The validity of this imaging technique has been established by correlation with selective left ventricular cineangiography in a large group of patients, and its practicality and usefulness in directing clinical decisions have been demonstrated by our experience in several patients.

The essential components of the method are as follows. With the patient in a supine position beneath the detector of a scintillation camera equipped with a high-resolution collimator and rotated 30 degrees to the right anterior oblique position, a bolus injection of 15 to 20 mCi of ^{99m}Tc-tagged autologous red blood cells[160] is made through a short plastic catheter in an antecubital vein. The scintigraphic data obtained during the initial minute after injection are collected without gating on videotape for subsequent validation of the location of the aortic and mitral annuli. After the first minute, an R wave-triggered gating device activates the oscilloscope of the scintillation camera for a 60 msec period representing end-systole and subsequent end-diastole. The phonocardiogram is used for the precise timing of the end-systolic gating interval, which consists of the 60 msec period immediately preceding the first high-frequency component of the second heart sound. End-diastole is chosen as the 60 msec interval immediately after the R wave and is obtained by setting the delay control of the gating apparatus at zero. Thus, the end-diastolic interval always occurs immediately after the QRS complex and is independent of R-R interval. Polaroid film is used to record 500,000 count gated images of end-systole and end-diastole from 500 to 1,000 cardiac cycles, requiring approximately 10 minutes per picture. After the initial end-systolic and end-diastolic imaging, gated images can be obtained in the modified left anterior oblique position for observation of septal and posterior wall motion, or repeated right anterior oblique gated images can be obtained after the administration of sublingual nitroglycerin to assess viability of abnormally contracting segments.[161] These additional procedures do not require repeated injection of the radiopharmaceutical.

The gated images are interpreted by outlining the borders of the left ventricle on the gated images with a paraffin pencil. In most patients, all margins of the left ventricle—including the aortic and mitral valve planes—are determined by inspection of the end-systolic and end-diastolic gated images. In some patients, it is necessary to use the initial transit image of the left ventricle to determine these planes. Transparent 35 mm photographs of the outlined end-systolic and end-diastolic images and of calibration images are projected to life-size, and the superimposed outlines of the left ventricle in systole and diastole are traced onto paper. From this tracing, regional contraction patterns are observed, and the end-systolic and end-diastolic volumes are determined by the area-length method. Ejection fraction is calculated by dividing stroke volume by the end-diastolic volume.

In the large group of patients in whom the

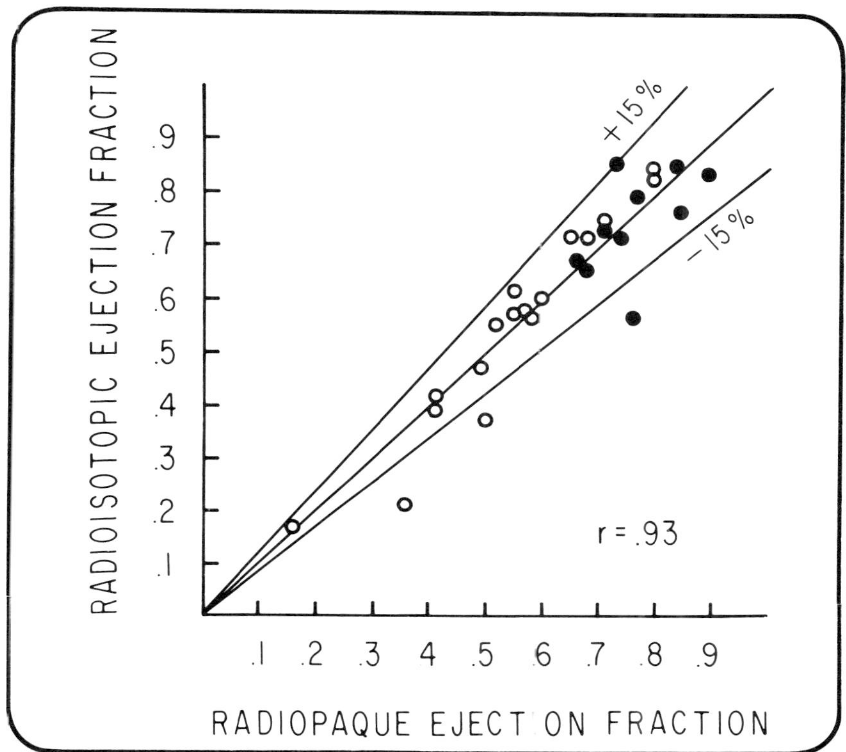

FIGURE 23. Comparison of left ventricular ejection fraction measurements obtained by radioisotopic (intravenous ^{99m}Tc-tagged autologous red blood cells) and radiopaque (biplane left ventriculography) methods in 27 patients. **Closed circles** = normal contraction pattern; **open circles** = abnormal contraction patterns in patients with chronic coronary heart disease. The **center line** is the line of identity; the **outer lines** represent 15 percent distribution limits.

scintigraphic method was compared with left ventricular cineangiography, excellent correlations of ejection fraction and abnormal contraction patterns were demonstrated[159] (Figure 23). An example of the use of this technique in evaluating the viability of dyssynergic segments is illustrated in scintigraphic images obtained before and after sublingual nitroglycerin in a patient with preinfarction angina pectoris (Figure 24). The radionuclidic technique has also been utilized in the assessment of pump performance after surgical coronary revascularization.[159] In the patient shown in Figure 24, gated scintigraphy performed two weeks after aortocoronary bypass objectively documented surgical efficacy without cardiac catheterization (Figure 25). With respect to abnormalities in the region of the septum, a striking example of the diagnostic capabilities of this procedure is shown by the right anterior oblique and modified left anterior oblique images obtained in a patient with idiopathic hypertropic subaortic stenosis (Figures 26 and 27).

Both the gated blood pool imaging and the area-counts methods have been shown to correlate well for ejection fraction with left ventricular cineangiography;[153,155–159,162] however, there are certain advantages and limitations of each technique. The principal advantage of the imaging techniques is that in addition to ejection fraction, regional contraction patterns of the left ventricle can be observed. The importance of this ability to identify ventricular dyssynergy was clearly demonstrated in our study in which a significant number of patients with normal ejection fraction mani-

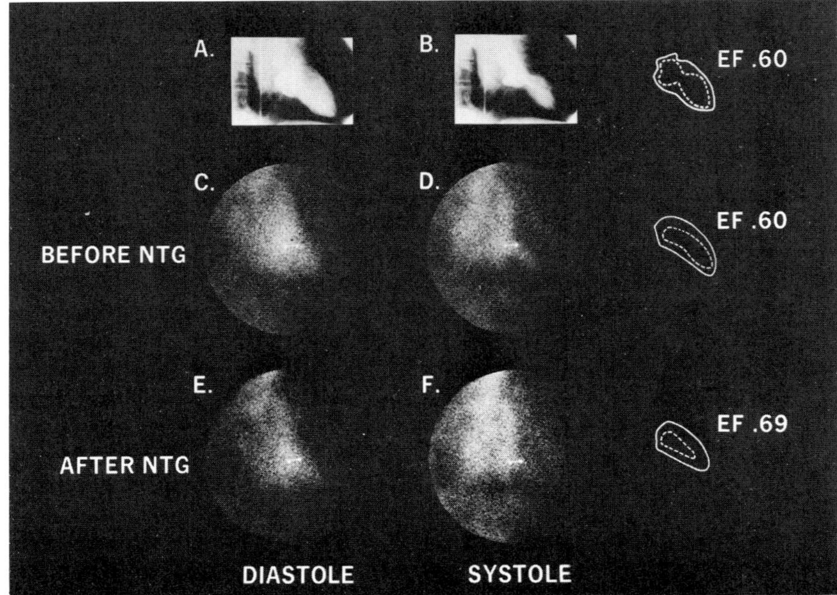

FIGURE 24. Left ventricular scintigraphic images (right anterior oblique, RAO) obtained with intravenous 99mTc-tagged autologus red blood cells before (**C** and **D**) and after (**E** and **F**) sublingual nitroglycerin (NTG) in a patient with the preinfarction angina syndrome. Left ventricular radiopaque RAO cineangiograms before NTG are shown in diastole (**A**) and systole (**B**). The superimposed end-diastolic (**solid lines**) and end-systolic (**broken lines**) silhouettes and ejection fractions (EF) are given on the **right**. The scintigraphic images show that the systolic movement of the hypokinetic left ventricular apex (**D**) was improved after NTG (**F**), indicating ischemic involvement rather than infarction of this area.

fested regional contraction abnormalities (Figure 23). Furthermore, the gated blood pool technique allows assessment of dynamic interventions such as the administration of nitroglycerin without requiring a second injection or a time delay for physical or biologic decay of the radiopharmaceutical (Figure 24). Conversely, the chief advantage of most of the area-counts methods is that the outlines of the left ventricle are determined during the initial transit of the radioactive bolus—at a time when the adjacent cardiac structures do not contain radioactivity —making precise definition of the aortic and mitral valve planes easier than in the gated blood pool studies. These two techniques can easily be combined, using a single injection. The first-pass area-counts method provides determination of ejection fraction, and subsequent gated end-systolic and end-diastolic images allow evaluation of regional wall motion and response of abnormal wall motion to nitroglycerin or other interventions.

Regional Myocardial Perfusion: Radionuclidic techniques for assessing regional myocardial perfusion have also found widespread clinical application. These techniques can conveniently be divided into invasive methods requiring intracoronary injection and noninvasive methods requiring peripheral venous injection.

The invasive methods are performed in conjunction with cardiac catheterization. One technique uses regional ^{133}Xe washout curves obtained with a scintillation camera and analyzed by computer.[163] Since the washout curves are obtained immediately after injection of the radioactive gas, the scintillation camera must be located in the catheterization laboratory. Also, in order to use the technique to determine regional perfusion rather than overall myocardial perfusion, a computer is required to generate washout curves from multiple areas of interest. When these facilities are present, this technique can be used to obtain semi-quantitative information regarding regional myocardial blood flow.

After intracoronary injection, the distribution of radioactive human serum albumin particles

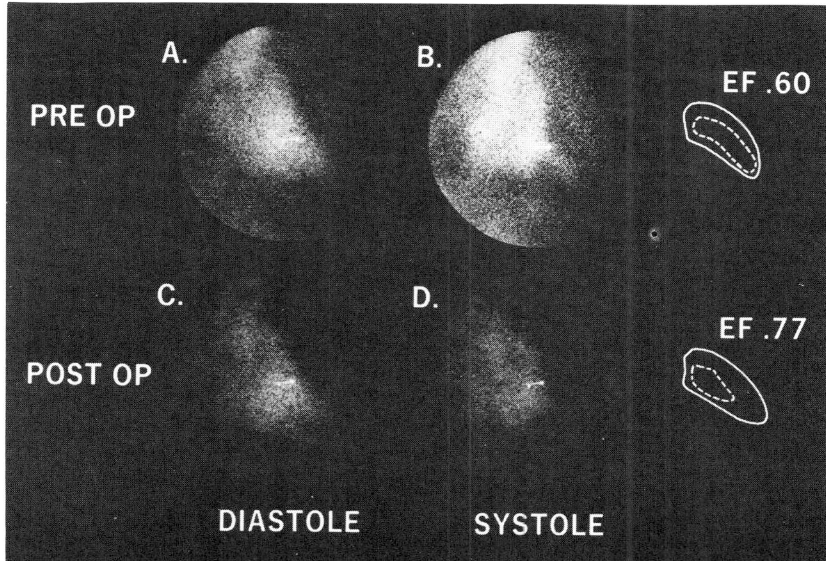

FIGURE 25. Scintigraphic right anterior oblique images obtained with intravenous ^{99m}Tc-tagged autologous red blood cells before (**A** and **B**) and after (**C** and **D**) coronary artery bypass surgery in the patient shown in Figure 24. Marked improvement in systolic apical motion of the left ventricle is evident postoperatively (**D**). The superimposed end-diastolic and end-systolic images and ejection fractions (EF) are shown on the **right.**

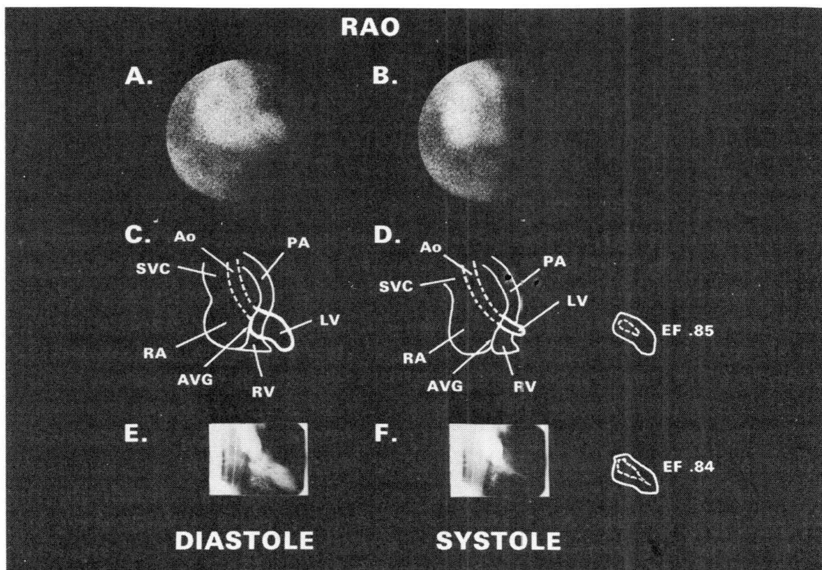

FIGURE 26. Scintigraphic right anterior oblique (RAO) cardiac images obtained with intravenous ^{99m}Tc-tagged autologous red blood cells at end-diastole (**A**) and at end-systole (**B**) in a patient with idiopathic hypertrophic subaortic stenosis (IHSS). Diagrams derived from the radionuclidic images are given in **C** and **D**. Left ventricular radiopaque RAO cineangiograms are shown in **E** and **F**. Systolic obliteration of the apical portion of the left ventricular cavity is evident (**B, D** and **F**). The superimposed end-diastolic and end-systolic images and ejection fractions (EF), are shown on the **right.** Ao = ascending aorta; AVG = atrioventricular groove; LV = left ventricle; PA = pulmonary artery; RA = right atrium; RV = right ventricle; SVC = superior vena cava.

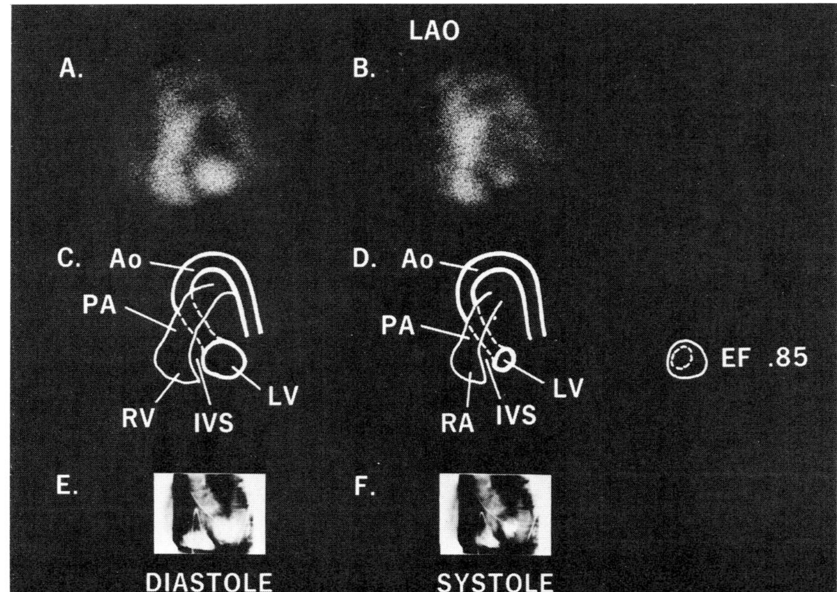

FIGURE 27. Scintigraphic cardiac images obtained with intravenous 99mTc-tagged autologous red blood cells in the modified left anterior oblique view (LAO) at end-diastole (**A**) and at end-systole (**B**) in the patient with IHSS shown in Figure 26. Diagrams drawn from the radionuclidic images are given in **C** and **D**. Bi-ventricular radiopaque LAO cineangiograms (simultaneous RV and LV injections) are illustrated in **E** and **F**. Asymmetric thickening of the interventricular septum (IVS) is clearly documented in the systolic and diastolic scintigraphic and angiographic pictures. Ao = ascending aorta; LV = left ventricle; PA = pulmonary artery; RA = right ventricle.

can be used for evaluation of regional myocardial perfusion at rest.[164,165] Recently, a method with improved sensitivity for detection of ischemia has been described that uses particles labeled with two different radionuclides, one injected before and the other after injection of contrast medium into a coronary artery.[166,167] This constitutes a rest and stress examination since the injection of contrast material normally is associated with reactive hyperemia. In coronary arteries with significant stenosis, reactive hyperemia does not occur; the lack of normal reactive hyperemia is reflected in the pattern of the image obtained from the radionuclide injected after the contrast medium compared with the image from the radionuclide injected at rest. An advantage of these particle techniques over the ^{133}Xe gas washout technique is that images can be obtained in the nuclear medicine laboratory after cardiac catheterization has been completed.

The noninvasive methods for assessing regional myocardial perfusion with radionuclides involve the peripheral venous injection of ^{43}K or its analogue ^{81}Rb or more recently ^{201}Tl (thallium 201), taking advantage of the fact that these elements are avidly extracted by the myocardium. Although radionuclidic imaging of the myocardium at rest with these and other related agents can be employed to detect infarction, the use of resting images alone does not allow detection of coronary disease before infarction has occurred. Recently, a technique for evaluating myocardial ischemia has been described that combines treadmill stress testing, with scintigraphy utilizing either ^{43}K or ^{81}Rb and the rectilinear scanner.[168-170] Radioactive cesium (^{137}Cs), although adequate for myocardial imaging at rest, is not suitable for combined rest and exercise studies, since it is not extracted as efficiently on the first transit as is ^{43}K or ^{81}Rb (22 percent for ^{137}Cs versus 71 percent for ^{43}K and 65 percent for ^{81}Rb).[171] Of these four agents, only ^{43}K, ^{81}Rb and ^{201}Tl are extracted efficiently enough to be distributed during the time of exercise-induced ischemia.

The sensitivity of combined rest and exercise myocardial perfusion imaging using the scintillation camera and intravenously administered [81]Rb has recently been compared in our laboratories with that of exercise electrocardiography in the detection of myocardial ischemia in a large group of patients with arteriographically documented coronary artery disease.[172] For each rest or exercise study, 4 mCi of [81]Rb was injected into a peripheral vein after a 12 hour fast. For the exercise portion of the study, maximal cardiac stress was achieved by either graded treadmill exertion or transvenous cardiac pacing, both performed in the nuclear medicine laboratories and carried to the point of angina pectoris, maximal heart rate or severe fatigue, at which time the [81]Rb was injected. Exercise was continued an additional 30 seconds after injection. Beginning 2 minutes after injection, multiple myocardial images were obtained using the scintillation camera equipped with a pinhole collimator and a specially constructed lead shield. Images were taken in the anterior, left anterior oblique and left lateral positions (Figure 28).

These images were evaluated for evidence of regional myocardial ischemia, which was manifested by an area of decreased accumulation of radioactivity after exercise when compared with results during rest (Figure 29, A and B). During the stress tests, four-lead electrocardiographic tracings were continuously monitored and evaluated for evidence of myocardial ischemia, using the criterion of horizontal ST depression of 1 mm or more in any lead. All patients had selective coronary arteriography performed during clinically indicated cardiac catheterization.

In a large group of patients with more than 75 percent stenosis of at least one of the three major coronary vessels, rest and exercise [81]Rb imaging detected myocardial ischemia (Figure 29, A and B) in 88 percent of patients, whereas simultaneous exercise electrocardiographic monitoring was positive in only 58 percent of patients.[172] Of special interest, some patients in our group with arteriographically proved coronary obstruction exhibited positive [81]Rb exercise scans but had neither angina nor positive results on exercise treadmill testing. In some additional patients without obstruction of a major coronary vessel

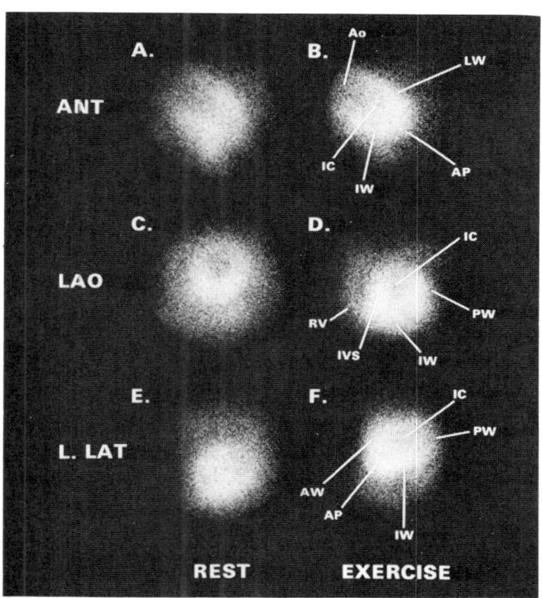

FIGURE 28. Scintigraphic myocardial images obtained with intravenous [81]Rb at rest (**A, C** and **E**) and after treadmill exercise (**B, D** and **F**) in a patient with normal coronary arteriograms. The central area of decreased radioactivity seen most prominently in the LAO view represents the left ventricular chamber (IC). In the anterior view (ANT), decrease in activity is seen in the upper left of the image representing the aortic outflow tract (Ao). Homogeneous distribution of radioactivity throughout the left ventricular (LV) myocardium at rest and after exercise characterizes this normal study. AP = left ventricular apex; AW = anterior left ventricular wall; IVS = interventricular septum; IW = inferior left ventricular wall; L. LAT = left lateral view; LW = lateral left ventricular wall; PW = posterior left ventricular wall; RV = right ventricular wall.

on arteriography, the exercise [81]Rb image was without perfusion abnormalities, although the exercise electrocardiogram was positive. These latter patients with positive results on exercise electrocardiography had normal coronary vessels on selective arteriography. Therefore, rest and exercise [81]Rb myocardial imaging appears to offer enhanced sensitivity and specificity compared with exercise electrocardiography in the noninvasive identification of stenosis of the coronary arteries.

In our laboratories, [81]Rb imaging at rest and during exercise has successfully been extended to the evaluation of therapeutic modalities in patients with coronary artery disease.[173,174] We have employed radionuclidic determinations of

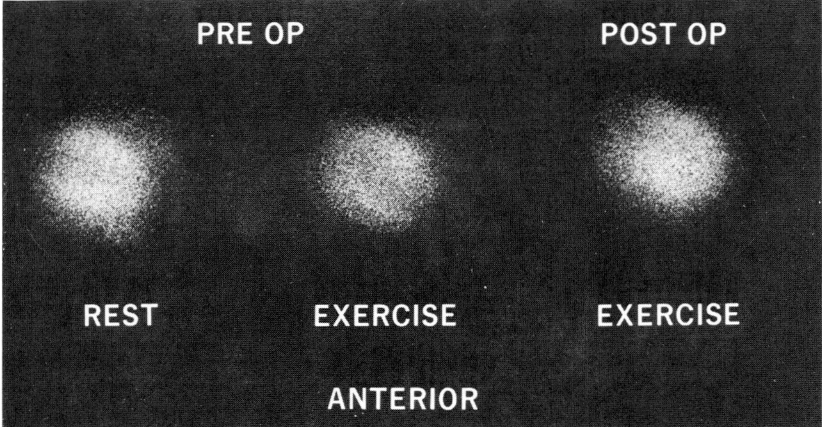

FIGURE 29. Anterior scintigraphic images obtained with intravenous [81]Rb preoperatively at rest (**left**) and after treadmill exercise (**middle**) and postoperatively after treadmill exercise (**right**) in a patient with chronic angina pectoris without myocardial infarction. The preoperative resting scintigram is normal. However, the preoperative exercise scintigram demonstrates an apical filling defect, corresponding to 90 percent proximal stenosis of the left anterior descending coronary artery by selective coronary arteriography. Coronary arteriography also revealed 90 percent stenosis of the left circumflex coronary artery and 75 percent stenosis of the right coronary artery. The postoperative exercise scintigram is normal, objectively documenting the efficacy of surgical myocardial revascularization by coronary artery saphenous vein bypass grafts in this patient.

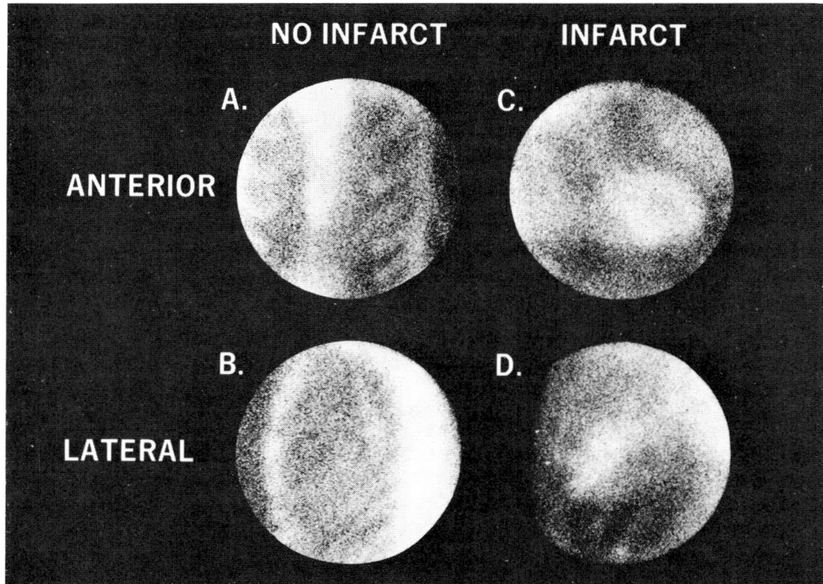

FIGURE 30. Precordial scintigraphic images obtained 2 hours after intravenous injection of ^{99m}Tc pyrophosphate in 2 patients with chest pain. Anterior (**A** and **C**) and left lateral (**B** and **D**) views are shown. The patient in the left column (**A** and **B**) had no clinical evidence of acute myocardial infarction, and the scintigrams demonstrated no abnormal concentration of radioactivity in the heart. In contrast, the patient in the right column (**C** and **D**) had acute subendocardial myocardial infarction 4 days prior to this study, and the radionuclidic images revealed intense abnormal increased concentration of radioactivity throughout the anterior left ventricular wall (**C** and **D**).

myocardial perfusion patterns in the objective assessment of the efficacy of pharmacologic treatment[173] and aortocoronary bypass surgery[174] (Figure 29). Our findings and those of others demonstrate that [81]Rb imaging at rest and with exercise is a valuable addition to the noninvasive evaluation of myocardial perfusion and enhances the sensitivity and specificity of stress electrocardiography. The major limitations of the widespread application of this technique at present are the expense of the radioisotope and its physical characteristics necessitating the use of special lead shielding. A radiopharmaceutical currently undergoing clinical trial for this application is ^{201}Tl, which allows high-resolution camera imaging without special shielding.[175,176]

Acute Myocardial Infarction: An exciting new development in the field of nuclear cardiology has been the application of hot-spot imaging techniques for the diagnosis of acute myocardial infarction. Employing the knowledge that calcium accumulates in irreversibly damaged myocardium, myocardial infarction imaging has been carried out in experimental animals by using ^{99m}Tc pyrophosphate.[177] After initial success in detecting experimental infarctions, this technique has now been extended successfully to patients with acute myocardial infarction.[178]

In clinical practice, the technique can easily be performed without special patient preparation. Intravenous injection of 15 mCi of ^{99m}Tc pyrophosphate (or polyphosphate or diphosphonate) is performed at the bedside. Multiple views of the heart are obtained with the scintillation camera 1 to 2 hours after injection. The procedure takes approximately 20 minutes, and risks are negligible. The radiation dose is approximately equivalent to a chest roentgenogram. Interpretation of the images is also simple, since in the absence of acute myocardial infarction there is no detectable uptake of the radiopharmaceutical in the heart (Figure 30, A and B). In the presence of myocardial infarction, the radiopharmaceutical accumulates in the heart and is visible as a hot spot (Figure 30, C and D). Uptake is first noted approximately 12 hours after the acute episode, reaches a maximum at 24 to 48 hours and then begins to decrease gradually (Figure 31, A, B and C). Imag-

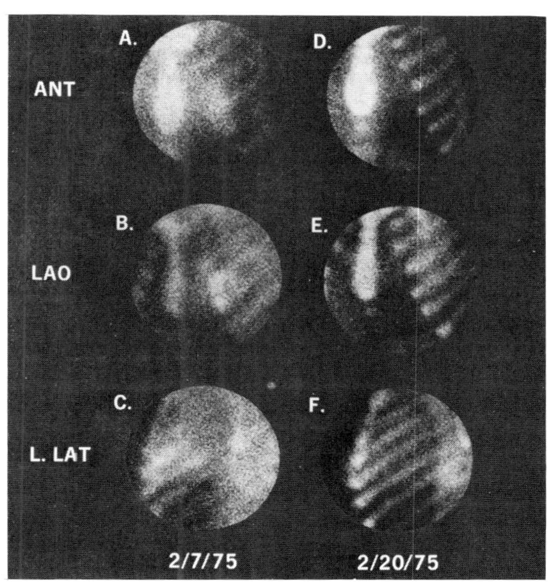

FIGURE 31. Precordial scintigraphic images obtained with ^{99m}Tc pyrophosphate in a 31 year old man 5 days (**A, B** and **C**) and 18 days (**D, E** and **F**) after acute transmural anterior myocardial infarction. Abnormal accumulation of radioactivity is seen in the anterior left ventricular wall (**A, B** and **C**) at the t me of the first study. In contrast, at the time of the second study prior to hospital discharge, complete clearing of the previously abnormal myocardial pattern of radioactive uptake was noted (**D, E** and **F**). ANT = anterior view; LAO = left anterior oblique view; L. LAT = left lateral view.

ing performed before 24 hours or after 6 days may provide false-negative results (Figure 31, D, E and F). The pattern of acute myocardial infarction may be either a localized or diffuse increase in myocardial uptake of the ^{99m}Tc pyrophosphate.

The exact mechanism of myocardial accumulation is unknown, but it is believed to be related to the deposition of calcium in and around the mitochondria in regions of irreversible ischemia.[179] The principal clinical application of this technique is the detection of acute infarctions that are difficult to diagnose by standard electrocardiographic and enzymatic methods, such as in patients with left bundle branch block, subendocardial myocardial infarction (Figure 30, C and D), true posterior myocardial infarction, intraoperative infarction and new infarction adjacent to regions of old myocardial necrosis; the technique also can be used to evaluate the course of acute infarction.

Summary

The rapid advancement in knowledge of the dynamics of the normal and diseased heart has resulted from the development of practical techniques for cardiac catheterization. The ability to obtain pressure pulses, angiographic visualization and other essential information from within the cardiac chambers has been responsible for the elucidation of a variety of physiologic and pathologic states and has strongly stimulated the expansion of medical and surgical means for the treatment of heart diseases. To provide perspective and understanding of the many procedures that now constitute the specialized science of cardiac catheterization and related methodology in the precise evaluation of cardiac disorders, the present status and recent advances in several techniques and the determination of hemodynamic variables related to the assessment of cardiac performance have been considered in the foregoing discussion—analysis of intracardiac pressure pulses, cardiac output, intravascular shunts, pulmonary vascular resistance, and valvular stenosis and regurgitation; intracardiac phonocardiography and electrocardiography and nuclear cardiology; and evaluation of systolic time intervals, ventricular segmental contraction abnormalities and ventricular function.

In regard to the assessment of ventricular function, the determinant of myocardial contractility can be evaluated clinically by indexes of pump performance (hemodynamic measures of pressure and flow) and muscle mechanical properties (isovolumic indexes utilizing dp/dt and ejection indexes employing V_{CF}). Characterization of cardiac pump hemodynamics describes contractile state in qualitative terms, whereas determination of muscular properties provides a quantitative approach that appears to be more sensitive and specific. Contractility indexes designed to eliminate the influence of loading changes become inherently less sensitive to contractility. Since there are specific advantages and limitations with each of the hemodynamic methods and mechanical indexes, the properly selected approach according to the conditions of study allows assessment of right and left ventricular contractility in serial studies in individual patients and in comparisons among numbers of patients.

Acknowledgment: This work was supported in part by Research Program Project Grant HL-14780 from the National Heart and Lung Institute, National Institutes of Health.

The authors gratefully acknowledge the technical assistance of Robert Kleckner, Arthur Lewis and Leslie Silvernail.

References

1. **Rockoff SD, Mason DT:** The spectrum of congenital heart disease associated with cyanosis in adults; angiographic findings. Amer J Roentgen 91:326, 1964
2. **Mason DT, Braunwald E:** Hemodynamic techniques in the investigation of cardiovascular function in man. In, Clinical Cardiopulmonary Physiology, third edition (Gordon B, ed). New York, Grune & Stratton, 1969, p 153
3. **Abrams HL, Adams DF:** The coronary arteriogram: structural and functional aspects. New Eng J Med 281:1276, 1336, 1969
4. **Ross J Jr:** Considerations regarding the technique for transseptal left heart catheterization. Circulation 34:391, 1966
5. **Brockenbrough EC, Morrow AG, Talbert J, et al:** Percutaneous puncture of the left ventricle. Brit Heart J 23:643, 1961
6. **Mason DT, Ross J Jr, Gault JH, et al:** Combined prosthetic replacement of the mitral and aortic valves: pre- and post-operative hemodynamic studies including left ventricular responses to muscular exercise. Circulation 35 suppl I:15, 1967
7. **Cohn LH, Mason DT:** Determinants of the height of the left atrial contraction wave in mitral stenosis. Amer J Cardiol 18:724, 1966
8. **Tatooles CJ, Gault JH, Mason DT, et al:** Reflux of oxygenated blood into the pulmonary artery in severe mitral regurgitation. Amer Heart J 75:102, 1968
9. **Roberts WG, Mason DT, Wright LD:** The nondistensible right atrium of carcinoid heart disease. Amer J Clin Path 44:627, 1965
10. **Braunwald E, Awe WC:** The syndrome of severe mitral regurgitation with normal left atrial pressure. Circulation 27:29, 1963
11. **Morrow AB, Braunwald E, Haller JA, et al:** Left atrial pressure pulse in mitral valve disease: a correlation of pressures obtained by transbronchial puncture with the valvular lesion. Circulation 16:399, 1957
12. **Mason DT, Cohen LS, Braunwald E:** Diagnostic value of the configuration of the transaortic pressure gra-

dient for the differentiation between idiopathic hypertrophic subaortic stenosis and the discrete forms of left ventricular outflow obstruction. Ann Intern Med 68:1159, 1968

13. **Gabe IT, Mason DT, Gault JH, et al:** Effect of respiration on venous return and stroke volume in cardiac tamponade. Brit Heart J 32:592, 1970

14. **Mason DT, Braunwald E, Ross J Jr, et al:** Diagnostic value of the first and second derivatives of the arterial pressure pulse in aortic valve disease and in hypertrophic subaortic stenosis. Circulation 30:90, 1964

15. **Ross J Jr, Braunwald E, Gault JH, et al:** The mechanism of the intraventricular pressure gradient in idiopathic hypertrophic subaortic stenosis. Circulation 34:558, 1966

16. **Visscher MB, Johnson JA:** The Fick principle: analysis of potentia errors in its conventional application. J Appl Physiol 5:635, 1953

17. **Hamilton WF:** The physiology of the cardiac output. Circulation 8:527, 1953

18. **Glick G, Schreiner BF Jr, Luria MN, et al:** Determination of cardiac output by means of radioisotopic dilution technic. Progr Cardiovasc Dis 4:586, 1962

19. **Kloster RE, Bristow JD, Starr A, et al:** Serial cardiac output and blood volume studies following cardiac valve replacement. Circulation 33:528, 1966

20. **Berman DS, Salel AF, DeNardo GL, et al:** Non-invasive radioisotopic determination of cardiac output utilizing a single probe and a computer model. J Nucl Med 15:478, 1974

21. **Barnett GO, Greenfield JC Jr, Fox SM:** The technique of estimating the instantaneous aortic blood velocity in man from the pressure gradient. Amer Heart J 62:359, 1961

22. **Gault JH, Ross J Jr, Mason DT:** Patterns of brachial arterial blood flow in conscious human subjects with and without cardiac dysfunction. Circulation 34:833, 1966

23. **Mason DT, Gabe IT, Mills CJ, et al:** Applications of the catheter-tip electromagnetic flowmeter in the study of the central circulation in man. Amer J Med 49:465, 1970

24. **Wood EH:** Diagnostic applications of indicator-dilution techniques in congenital heart disease. Circ Res 10:531, 1962

25. **Zelis R, Mason DT, Fisher RD, et al:** Anomalous pulmonary venous drainage from the entire left lung without cardiac malformations. Arch Intern Med 124:91, 1969

26. **Frommer DL, Plaff WW, Braunwald E:** The use of ascorbate dilution curves in cardiovascular diagnosis. Circulation 24:1227, 1961

27. **Mason DT, Braunwald E:** Diagnosis of congenital heart disease. In, Nuclear Medicine (Bland WH, ed). New York, McGraw-Hill, 1965, p 411

28. **Alazraki NP, Ashburn WL, Hagan A, et al:** Detection of left-to-right cardiac shunts with the scintillation camera pulmonary dilution curve. J Nucl Med 13:142, 1972

29. **Weber PM, Dos Remedios LV, Jasko IA:** Quantitative radioisotopic angiocardiography. J Nucl Med 13:815, 1972

30. **Maltz DL, Treves S:** Quantitative radionuclide angiocardiography. Determination of Qp:Qs in children. Circulation 47:1049, 1973

31. **Wesselhoeft H, Hurley PJ, Wagner HN Jr, et al:** Nuclear angiocardiography in the diagnosis of congenital heart diseases in infants. Circulation 45:77, 1972

32. **Bosnjakovic VB, Bennett LR, Greenfield LD, et al:** Dual-isotope method for diagnosis of intracardiac shunts. J Nucl Med 14:514, 1973

33. **Strauss WH, Hurley PJ, Rhodes BA, et al:** Quantification of right-to-left transpulmonary shunts in man. J Lab Clin Med 74:597, 1969

34. **Frommer PL, Ross J Jr, Mason DT, et al:** Clinical applications of an improved, rapidly responding fiberoptic catheter. Amer J Cardiol 15:672, 1965

35. **Rockoff SD, Braunwald E, Ross J Jr, et al:** Simultaneous recording of oscillographic and radiologic events on cine film: applications of the cinetrace during cardiac catheterization. Amer J Cardiol 16:708, 1965

36. **Braunwald E, Goldblatt A, Long RTL, et al:** The krypton-85 inhalation test for the detection of left-to-right shunts. Brit Heart J 24:47, 1962

37. **Hugenholtz PG, Schwark T, Monroe RG, et al:** The clinical usefulness of hydrogen gas as an indicator of left-to-right shunts. Circulation 28:542, 1963

38. **Gorlin R, Gorlin SG:** Hydraulic formula for calculation of the area of the stenotic mitral valve, and other cardiac valves, and central circulatory shunts. Amer Heart J 41:1, 1951

39. **DeMaria A, Chung G, Zelis R, et al:** Comparison of in vitro aortic orifice size with calculated valve area in aortic stenosis. Circulation 46 suppl II:145, 1972

40. **Cohn LH, Mason DT, Ross J Jr, et al:** The preoperative assessment of aortic regurgitation in patients with mitral valve disease. Amer J Cardiol 19:177, 1967

41. **Dodge HT, Sandler H, Baxley WA, et al:** Usefulness and limitations of radiographic methods for determining left ventricular volume. Amer J Cardiol 18:10, 1966

42. **Cohen LS, Mason DT, Gault JH, et al:** The diagnosis of congenital cardiac defects using a fiberoptic catheter-pressure-cinefilm system. Amer J Cardiol 25:238, 1970

43. **Narula OS:** Advances in clinical electrophysiology: contributions of His bundle recordings. In, Cardiac Pacing (Samet P, ed). New York, Grune & Stratton, 1973, p 331

44. **Mason DT, Spann JF Jr, Zelis R, et al:** Alterations of hemodynamics and myocardial mechanics in patients with congestive heart failure: pathophysiologic mechanisms and assessment of cardiac function and ventricular contractility. Progr Cardiovasc Dis 12:507, 1970

45. **Mason DT, Zelis R, Amsterdam EA, et al:** Clinical determination of left ventricular contractility by hemodynamics and myocardial mechanics. In, Progress in Cardiology (Yu P, Goodwin J, ed). Philadelphia, Lea & Febiger, 1972, p 121

46. **Mason DT:** Regulation of cardiac performance in clinical heart disease: interactions between contractile state, mechanical abnormalities and ventricular compensatory mechanisms. Amer J Cardiol 32:437, 1973

47. **Mason DT, Zelis R, Amsterdam EA, et al:** Mechanisms

of cardiac contraction: structural, biochemical and functional relations in the normal and diseased heart. In, Pathologic Physiology, fifth edition (Sodeman WA Jr, Sodeman WA, ed). Philadelphia, WB Saunders, 1974, p 206

48. **Mason DT, Zelis R:** Clinical quantification of cardiac contractility by mechanical properties of isovolumic systole. In, Proceedings of Symposium on Left Ventricular Performance in Man (Besse P, Bricaud H, ed). Paris, Expansion Scientifique Francaise, 1975, p 9

49. **Gaasch WH, Battle WE, Oboler AA, et al:** Left ventricular stress and compliance in man. Circulation 45:746, 1972

50. **Fester A, Samet P:** Passive elasticity of the human left ventricle. Circulation 50:609, 1974

51. **Gaasch WH, Cole JS, Quinones MA, et al:** Dynamic determinants of left ventricular diastolic pressure-volume relations in man. Circulation 51:317, 1975

52. **Miller RR, DeMaria AN, Amsterdam EA, et al:** Improvement of reduced left ventricular diastolic compliance in ischemic heart disease following successful coronary artery bypass. Amer J Cardiol 35:11, 1975

53. **Forrester JS, McHugh TJ, Diamond G, et al:** Rapid assessment of cardiopulmonary hemodynamics in acutely ill patients utilizing a single right heart catheter. Amer J Cardiol 26:633, 1970

54. **Swan HJC, Ganz W, Forrester J, et al:** Catheterization of the heart in man with use of a flow-directed balloon-tipped catheter. New Eng J Med 283:447, 1970

55. **Cohn JN, Tristani FE, Khatri IM:** Studies in clinical shock and hypotension. VI. Relationship between left and right ventricular function. J Clin Invest 48:2008, 1969

56. **Mason DT, Spann JF Jr, Zelis R, et al:** Comparison of the contractile state of the normal, hypertrophied, and failing heart in man. In, Cardiac Hypertrophy (Alpert NR, ed). New York, Academic Press, 1971, p 433

57. **Levine HJ, Neill WA, Wagman RJ, et al:** The effect of exercise on mean left ventricular ejection rate in man. J Clin Invest 41:1050, 1962

58. **Ross J Jr, Linhart JW, Braunwald E:** Effects of changing heart rate in man by electrical stimulation of the right atrium. Circulation 32:549, 1965

59. **Ferrer ME, Harvey RM, Cathcart RT, et al:** Hemodynamic studies in rheumatic heart disease. Circulation 6:688, 1952

60. **Chapman CB, Mitchell JH, Sproule BJ, et al:** The maximal oxygen intake test in patients with predominant mitral stenosis: a pre-operative and post-operative study. Circulation 22:4, 1960

61. **Epstein SE, Beiser GD, Stampfer M, et al:** Characterization of the circulatory response to maximal upright exercise in normal subjects and patients with heart disease. Circulation 35:1049, 1967

62. **Epstein SE, Beiser GD, Stampfer M, et al:** Exercise in patients with heart disease: effects of body position and type and intensity of exercise. Amer J Cardiol 23:572, 1969

63. **Braunwald E, Chidsey CA, Pool PE, et al:** Congestive heart failure: biochemical and physiological considerations. Ann Intern Med 64:904, 1966

64. **Braunwald E, Ross J Jr, Gault JH, et al:** Assessment of cardiac function. Ann Intern Med 70:369, 1969

65. **Ross J Jr, Braunwald E:** The study of left ventricular function in man by increasing resistance to ventricular ejection with angiotensin. Circulation 29:739, 1964

66. **Potanin C, Sinclair-Smith B:** Patterns of cardiac output response to acute reduction of ventricular preload and afterload pressures. Amer J Cardiol 25:662, 1970

67. **Ross J Jr, Sonnenblick EH, Taylor RR, et al:** Diastolic geometry and sarcomere lengths in the chronically dilated canine left ventricle. Circ Res 28:49, 1971

68. **Ross J Jr, Braunwald E:** Studies on Starling's law of the heart. IX. Effects of impeding venous return on performance of normal and failing human left ventricle. Circulation 30:719, 1964

69. **Russell RO Jr, Rackley CE, Pombo J, et al:** Effects of increasing left ventricular filling pressure in patients with acute myocardial infarction. J Clin Invest 49:1539, 1970

70. **Brundage BH, Cheitlin MD:** Left ventricular angiography as a function test. Chest 64:70, 1973

71. **Mason DT, Spann JF Jr, Beiser GD, et al:** Effects of angiographic dye on isometric contraction and force-velocity characteristics of cat papillary muscle. Clin Res 16:239, 1968

72. **Zelis R, Mason DT, Spann J, et al:** The effects of angiographic dye on cardiac contractility and the peripheral circulation in man. Amer J Cardiol 25:137, 1970

73. **Mullins CB, Leshin SJ, Mierzwiak DS, et al:** Changes in left ventricular function produced by the injection of contrast media. Amer Heart J 83:373, 1972

74. **Linhart JW:** Pacing-induced changes in stroke volume in the evaluation of myocardial function. Circulation 43:253, 1971

75. **Parker JO, Khaja F, Case RB:** Analysis of left ventricular function by atrial pacing. Circulation 43:241, 1971

76. **Linhart JW:** Atrial pacing in coronary artery disease. Amer J Med 53:64, 1972

77. **Ross J Jr, Gault JH, Mason DT, et al:** Left ventricular performance during muscular exercise in patients with and without cardiac dysfunction. Circulation 34:597, 1966

78. **Ross J Jr, Morrow AG, Mason DT, et al:** Left ventricular function following replacement of the aortic valve: hemodynamic responses to muscular exercise. Circulation 33:507, 1966

79. **Kivowitz C, Parmley WW, Donoso R, et al:** Effects of isometric exercise on cardiac performance. Circulation 44:994, 1971

80. **Krayenbuehl HP, Rutishauser W, Schoenbeck M, et al:** Evaluation of left ventricular function from isovolumic pressure measurements during isometric exercise. Amer J Cardiol 29:323, 1972

81. **Siegel W, Gilbert CA, Nutter DO, et al:** Use of isometric handgrip for the indirect assessment of left ventricular function in patients with coronary atherosclerotic heart disease. Amer J Cardiol 30:48, 1972

82. **Stefadouros MA, Grossman W, Shahawy ME, et al:** The effect of isometric exercise on the left ventricular volume in normal man. Circulation 49:1185, 1974

83. **Dodge HT, Baxley WA:** Hemodynamic aspects of heart failure. Amer J Cardiol 22:24, 1968

84. **Hood WP Jr, Rackley CE, Rolett EL:** Wall stress in the normal and hypertrophied human left ventricle. Amer J Cardiol 22:550, 1968

85. **Dodge HT, Baxley WA:** Left ventricular volume and mass and their significance in heart disease. Amer J Cardiol 23:528, 1969

86. **Hood WP Jr, Thomson WJ, Rackley CE, et al:** Comparison of calculations of left ventricular wall stress in man from thin-walled and thick-walled ellipsoidal models. Circ Res 24:575, 1969

87. **Rackley CE, Dear HD, Baxley WA, et al:** Left ventricular chamber volume, mass, and function in severe coronary artery disease. Circulation 41:605, 1970

88. **Gentzler RD, Briselli MF, Gault JH:** Angiographic estimation of right ventricular volume in man. Circulation 50:324, 1974

89. **Kennedy JW, Baxley WA, Figley MM, et al:** Quantitative angiocardiography. The normal left ventricle in man. Circulation 34:272, 1966

90. **Dodge HT, Sandler H, Hay RE:** Left ventricular pressure-volume loops in man with valvular heart disease. Circulation 24:920, 1961

91. **Bunnell IL, Grant C, Greene DG:** Left ventricular function derived from the pressure-volume diagram. Amer J Med 39:881, 1965

92. **Dodge HT, Sandler H, Baxley WA, et al:** Usefulness and limitations of radiographic methods for determining left ventricular volume. Amer J Cardiol 18:10, 1966

93. **Rackley CE, Behar WS, Whalen RE, et al:** Biplane cineangiographic determinations of left ventricular function: pressure-volume relationships. Amer Heart J 74:766, 1967

94. **Chapman CB, Baker O, Mitchell JH:** Left ventricular function at rest and during exercise. J Clin Invest 38:1202, 1959

95. **Kennedy JW, Reichenbach DD, Baxley WA, et al:** Left ventricular mass. A comparison of angiocardiographic measurements with autopsy weight. Amer J Cardiol 19:221, 1967

96. **Rackley CE, Dodge HT, Coble YD, et al:** A method for determining left ventricular mass in man. Circulation 29:666, 1964

97. **Russell RO Jr, Porter CM, Frimer M, et al:** Left ventricular power in man. Amer Heart J 81:799, 1971

98. **Weissler AM, Harris WS, Schoenfeld CD:** Systolic time intervals in heart failure in man. Circulation 37:149, 1968

99. **Weissler AM, Harris WS, Schoenfeld CD:** Bedside technics for the evaluation of ventricular function in man. Amer J Cardiol 23:577, 1969

100. **Garrard CL Jr, Weissler AM, Dodge HT:** The relationship of alterations in systolic time intervals to ejection fraction in patients with cardiac disease. Circulation 42:455, 1970

101. **Weissler AM, Garrard CL Jr:** Systolic time intervals in cardiac disease. Mod Conc Cardiovasc Dis 40:1, 1971

102. **Bennett ED, Smithen CS, Sowton GE:** Systolic time intervals in acute myocardial infarction. Amer J Cardiol 26:625, 1970

103. **Diamant B, Killip T:** Indirect assessment of left ventricular performance in acute myocardial infarction. Circulation 42:579, 1970

104. **Inoue K, Young GM, Grierson AL, et al:** Isometric contraction period of left ventricle in acute myocardial infarction. Circulation 42:79, 1970

105. **Talley RC, Meyer JF, McNay JL:** Evaluation of the pre-ejection period as an estimate of myocardial contractility in dogs. Amer J Cardiol 27:384, 1971

106. **Weissler AM, Schoenfeld CD:** Effect of digitalis on systolic time intervals in heart failure. Amer J Med Sci 259:4, 1970

107. **Pouget JM, Harris WS, Mayran BR, et al:** Abnormal responses of the systolic time intervals to exercise in patients with angina pectoris. Circulation 43:289, 1971

108. **Metzger CC, Chough CB, Kroetz FW, et al:** True isovolumic contraction time: its correlation with two external indices of ventricular performance. Amer J Cardiol 25:434, 1970

109. **Gorlin R, Sonnenblick EH:** Regulation of performance of the heart. Amer J Cardiol 22:16, 1968

110. **Herman MV, Heinle RA, Klein MD, et al:** Localized disorders in myocardial contraction. New Eng J Med 277:222, 1967

111. **Klein MD, Herman MV, Gorlin R:** Hemodynamic study of left ventricular aneurysm. Circulation 35:614, 1967

112. **Herman MV, Gorlin R:** Implications of left ventricular asynergy. Amer J Cardiol 23:538, 1969

113. **Levine HJ, Britman NA:** Force-velocity relations in the intact dog heart. J Clin Invest 43:1383, 1964

114. **Mason DT:** Usefulness and limitations of the rate of rise of intraventricular pressure (dp/dt) in the evaluation of myocardial contractility in man. Amer J Cardiol 23:516, 1969

115. **Mason DT, Spann JF, Zelis R:** Quantification of the contractile state of the intact human heart. Amer J Cardiol 26:248, 1970

116. **Mason DT, Braunwald E, Covell JW, et al:** Assessment of cardiac contractility: the relation between the rate of pressure rise and ventricular pressure during isovolumic systole. Circulation 44:47, 1971

117. **Mason DT, Braunwald E:** Studies on digitalis. IX. Effects of ouabain on the nonfailing human heart. J Clin Invest 42:1105, 1963

118. **Mason DT, Sonnenblick EH, Ross J Jr, et al:** Time to peak dp/dt: a useful measurement for evaluating the contractile state of the human heart. Circulation 32 suppl II:145, 1965

119. **Seigel JH, Sonnenblick EH, Judge RD, et al:** The quantification of myocardial contractility in dog and man. Cardiologia (Basel) 45:189, 1964

120. **Veragut UP, Krayenbuhl HP:** Estimation and quantification of myocardial contractility in the closed chest dog. Cardiologia (Basel) 47:96, 1965

121. **Frank MJ, Levinson GE:** Measurement of myocardial contractility in man. Clin Res 12:182, 1964

122. **Reeves TJ, Hefner LL, Jones WB, et al:** The hemodynamic determinants of the rate of change in pressure of the left ventricle during isometric contraction. Amer Heart J 64:525, 1962

123. **Frank MJ, Levinson GE:** An index of the contractile

state of the myocardium in man. J Clin Invest 47:1615, 1968

124. **Mason DT, Spann JF, Zelis R:** The maximum intrinsic velocity of the myocardium in man: estimation from the rate of pressure rise and intraventricular pressure throughout isovolumic left ventricular systole. Circulation 38 suppl VI:134, 1968

125. **Yeatman LA, Parmley WW, Sonnenblick EH:** Effects of temperature on series elasticity and contractile element motion in heart muscle. Amer J Physiol 217:1030, 1969

126. **Mirsky I, Ellison RC, Hugenholtz PG:** Assessment of myocardial contractility in man from ventricular pressure recordings. Clin Res 17:255, 1969

127. **Wolk MJ, Keefe JF, Bing OHL, et al:** Estimation of Vmax in auxotonic systoles from the rate of relative increase of isovolumic pressure: (dp/dt)kP. J Clin Invest 50:1276, 1971

128. **Urschel CW, Henderson AH, Sonnenblick EH:** Model dependency of ventricular force-velocity relations: importance of developed pressure. Fed Proc 29:719 1970

129. **Mason DT, Spann JF, Zelis R, et al:** Comparison of inotropic state and compensatory mechanisms between patients with primary and secondary ventricular hypertrophy. Circulation 42 suppl III:85, 1970

130. **Mason DT, Salel A, Amsterdam EA, et al:** The evaluation of pump and muscle function in patients with left ventricular pressure and volume overloads. Circulation 43 and 44 suppl II:126, 1971

131. **Salel AF, Kamiyama T, Peng CL, et al:** Quantification of right ventricular contractility by developed isovolumic pressure-velocity index. Clin Res 21:447, 1973

132. **Capone RJ, Mason DT, Amsterdam EA, et al:** The effect of mitral regurgitation and ventricular aneurysm on Vmax calculated from pressure-velocity data during isovolumic systole. Circulation 44 suppl II:96, 1971

133. **Zelis R, Amsterdam EA, Mason DT:** Isometric Vmax as an index of contractility independent of series elastic and fiber shortening. Implications concerning pressure-velocity data in myocardial fibrosis, valvular regurgitation, ventricular aneurysm and ventricular septal defect. Circulation 43 and 44 suppl II:89, 1971

134. **DeMaria A, Kamiyama T, Peng CL, et al:** Alterations of ventricular function and myocardial contractility indices induced by ventricular asynchrony. Clin Res 21:414, 1973

135. **Zelis R, Salel AF, Capone RJ, et al:** Evaluation of muscle function in the human myocardium by contractility measurements: coronary artery disease. In, Proceedings of International Symposium on Chronic Diseases of the Heart, Frieberg, Germany (Roskam H, Reindell H, ed). Stuttgart, FK Schattauer Verlag, 1973, p 379

136. **Salel A, Mason DT, Amsterdam EA, et al:** Abnormalities of muscle mechanics in coronary artery disease before the development of congestive heart failure. Clin Res 20 suppl III:395, 1972

137. **Parmley WW, Tomoda H, Diamond G, et al:** Dissociation between indices of pump performance and contractility in patients with coronary artery disease and acute myocardial infarction. Chest 67:141, 1975

138. **Glick G, Sonnenblick EH, Braunwald E:** Myocardial force-velocity relations studied in intact unanesthetized man. J Clin Invest 44:978, 1965

139. **Sonnenblick EH, Williams JF Jr, Glick G, et al:** Studies on digitalis. XV. Effects of cardiac glycosides on myocardial force-velocity relations in the non-failing human heart. Circulation 34:532, 1966

140. **Kong Y, Morris JJ Jr, McIntosh HD:** Assessment of regional myocardial performance from biplane coronary cineangiograms. Amer J Cardiol 27:529, 1971

141. **DeMaria A, Bonanno JA, Amsterdam EA, et al:** Radarkymography. In, Noninvasive Cardiology (Weissler AM, ed). New York, Grune & Stratton, 1974, p 275

142. **Levitsky S, Schuette WH, Kempner KM, et al:** Experimental and early clinical evaluation of heart tracking (radarkymography) as a noninvasive method for measuring myocardial contractility. Amer J Cardiol 32:156, 1973

143. **Gault JH, Ross J Jr, Braunwald E:** Contractile state of the left ventricle in man. Circ Res 22:451, 1968

144. **Gabe IT, Gault JH, Ross J Jr, et al:** Measurement of instantaneous blood flow velocity and pressure in conscious man with a catheter-tip velocity probe. Circulation 40:603, 1969

145. **Peterson KL, Uther JB, Shabetai R, et al:** Assessment of left ventricular performance in man. Circulation 47:924, 1973

146. **Hammermeister KE, Brooks RC, Warbasse JR:** The rate of change of left ventricular volume in man. Circulation 49:729, 1974

147. **Karliner JS, Gault JH, Eckberg D, et al:** Mean velocity of fiber shortening. Circulation 44:323, 1971

148. **Hernandez-Lattuf PR, Quinones MA, Gaasch WH:** Usefulness and limitations of circumferential fiber shortening velocity in evaluating segmental disorders of left ventricular contraction. Brit Heart J 36:1167, 1974

149. **Peterson KL, Skloven D, Ludbrood P, et al:** Comparison of isovolumic and ejection phase indices of myocardial performance in man. Circulation 49:1088, 1974

150. **Cooper RH, O'Rourke RA, Karliner JS, et al:** Comparison of ultrasound and cineangiographic measurements of the mean rate of circumferential fiber shortening in man. Circulation 46:914, 1972

151. **Mason DT, Ashburn WL, Harbert JC, et al:** Rapid sequential visualization of the heart and great vessels in man using the wide field Anger scintillation camera. Radioisotope-angiography following the intravenous injection of technetium-99m. Circulation 39:19, 1969

152. **Mullins CB, Mason DT, Ashburn WL, et al:** Determination of left ventricular volume by radioisotope-angiography. Amer J Cardiol 24:72, 1969

153. **Strauss HW, Zaret BL, Hurley PJ, et al:** A scintiphotographic method for measuring left ventricular ejection fraction in man without cardiac catheterization. Amer J Cardiol 28:575, 1971

154. **Zaret BL, Strauss HW, Hurley PJ, et al:** A noninvasive scintiphotographic method for detecting regional ventricular dysfunction in man. New Eng J Med 284:1165, 1971

155. **Van Dyke D, Anger HO, Sullivan RW, et al:** Cardiac evaluation from radioisotope dynamics. J Nucl Med 13:585, 1972

156. **Weber PM, dos Remedios LV, Jasko IA:** Quantitative radioisotopic angiocardiography. J Nucl Med 13:815, 1972

157. **Secker-Walker RH, Resnick L, Kunz H, et al:** Measurement of left ventricular ejection fraction. J Nucl Med 14:798, 1973

158. **Steele PP, Van Dyke D, Trow RS, et al:** Simple and safe bedside method for serial measurement of left ventricular ejection fraction, cardiac output, and pulmonary blood volume. Brit Heart J 36:122, 1974

159. **Berman DS, DeNardo GL, Salel AF, et al:** High resolution scintigraphy of cardiac systole and diastole. J Nucl Med 15:478, 1974

160. **Eckelman W, Richards P, Hauser W, et al:** Technetium-labeled red blood cells. J Nucl Med 12:22, 1971

161. **Salel AF, Berman DS, DeNardo GL, et al:** Noninvasive radioisotopic evaluation of regional dyskinesis and pump performance in coronary disease: use of nitroglycerin in detection of reversible segmental ischemia. Circulation 50 suppl III:26, 1974

162. **Ashburn WL, Kostuk WJ, Karliner JS, et al:** Left ventricular volume and ejection fraction determination by radionuclide angiography. Semin Nucl Med 3:165, 1973

163. **Cannon PJ, Dell RB, Dwyer EM:** Measurement of regional myocardial perfusion in man with ^{133}xenon and a scintillation camera. J Clin Invest 51:964, 1972

164. **Ashburn WL, Braunwald E, Simon AL, et al:** Myocardial perfusion imaging with radioactive-labeled particles injected directly into the coronary circulation of patients with coronary artery disease. Circulation 44:851, 1971

165. **Jansen C, Judkins MP, Grames GM, et al:** Myocardial perfusion color scintigraphy with MAA. Radiology 109:369, 1973

166. **Gould KL, Hamilton GW, Lipscomb K, et al:** Method for assessing stress-induced regional malperfusion during coronary arteriography. Amer J Cardiol 34:557, 1974

167. **Gould KL, Lipscomb K, Hamilton GW:** Physiologic basis for assessing critical coronary stenosis. Amer J Cardiol 33:87, 1974

168. **Zaret BL, Strauss HW, Martin ND, et al:** Noninvasive regional myocardial perfusion with radioactive potassium: study of patients at rest, with exercise, and during angina pectoris. New Eng J Med 288:809, 1973

169. **Strauss HW, Zaret BL, Martin ND, et al:** Noninvasive evaluation of regional myocardial perfusion with potassium-43: technique in patients with exercise-induced transient myocardial ischemia. Radiology 108:85, 1973

170. **Martin ND, Zaret BL, McGowan RL, et al:** Rubidium-81: a new myocardial scanning agent: noninvasive regional myocardial perfusion scans at rest and exercise and comparison with potassium-43. Radiology 111:651, 1974

171. **Love WD, Ishihara Y, Lyon LD, et al:** Differences in the relationship between coronary blood flow and myocardial clearance of isotopes of potassium, rubidium, and cesium. Amer Heart J 76:353, 1968

172. **Berman DS, Salel AF, DeNardo GL, et al:** Rubidium-81 imaging at rest and after exercise: screening test for myocardial ischemia. Circulation 50 suppl III:26, 1974

173. **Salel AF, Berman DS, DeNardo GL, et al:** Clinical effects of tolamolol on myocardial ischemia assessed by rest and exercise rubidium-81 imaging. In, Clinical Experience with Tolamolol, a Cardioselective Beta-Blocking Agent (Lown B, Mason D, Nager F, et al, ed). Amsterdam, Excerpta Medica, 1975, p 38

174. **Salel AF, Berman DS, DeNardo GL, et al:** Effects of saphenous vein bypass surgery on myocardial perfusion in coronary artery disease: evaluation by rest and exercise rubidium-81 scintigraphy. Clin Res 13:84A, 1975

175. **Lebowitz E, Greene MW, Fairchild R, et al:** Thallium-201 for medical use. I. J Nucl Med 16:151, 1975

176. **Bradley-Moore PR, Lebowitz E, Greene MW, et al:** Thallium-201 for medical use. II. Biologic behavior. J Nucl Med 16:156, 1975

177. **Bonte FJ, Parkey RW, Graham KD, et al:** A new method for radionuclide imaging of myocardial infarcts. Radiology 110:473, 1974

178. **Parkey RW, Bonte FJ, Meyer SL, et al:** A new method for radionuclide imaging of acute myocardial infarction in humans. Circulation 50:540, 1974

179. **Bonte FJ, Parkey RW, Graham KD, et al:** Distributions of several agents useful in imaging myocardial infarcts. J Nucl Med 16:132, 1975

180. **Bonanno JA, Amsterdam EA, Mason DT:** Pericarditis. In, Infectious Diseases (Hoeprich P, ed). New York, Harper and Row, 1972, p 1073

181. **Miller RR, Amsterdam EA, Bogren HG, et al:** Electrocardiographic and cineangiographic correlations in assessment of the location, nature and extent of abnormal left ventricular segmental contraction in coronary artery disease. Circulation 49:447, 1974

Catheterization Evaluation of Cardiac Function in Acute and Chronic Coronary Artery Disease

Charles E. Rackley, MD, FACC
Richard O. Russell, Jr, MD, FACC
Roger E. Moraski, MD
John A. Mantle, MD
Bolling J. Feild, MD
McKamy Smith, MD, PhD, FACC

In coronary artery disease impaired ventricular performance often produces symptoms of heart failure during acute episodes of ischemic pain or on a chronic basis. In recent years investigators have utilized newly developed instrumentation and cardiac catheterization techniques to measure ventricular performance in patients with acute myocardial infarction as well as in those with chronic stages of coronary artery disease. This information has proved valuable in the management of patients during acute disturbances and also in the selection and evaluation of medical and surgical interventions in patients with chronic coronary artery disease. This chapter describes the catheterization methods and results of measurement of left ventricular function in patients with acute myocardial infarction and those with chronic, stable coronary artery disease. Observations made during acute myocardial infarction and subsequent follow-up study are presented, since a number of measurements have been obtained in these areas.

Techniques in Acute Myocardial Infarction

Patients with acute myocardial infarction admitted to coronary care units with specialized facilities can now have measurement of intracardiac pressures and cardiac output and constant monitoring of these parameters.[1] After local anesthesia is induced in the antecubital area, a venous cutdown can be performed and a Swan-Ganz catheter advanced to the pulmonary artery under fluoroscopic visualization or pressure monitoring. A cutdown or percutaneous puncture of the brachial artery allows insertion of a catheter for the recording of arterial pressure. Other available techniques include puncture of the femoral artery with retrograde passage of the catheter into the left ventricle.[2] These techniques can provide measurements of pulmonary arterial systolic, diastolic and wedge pressure as well as right atrial pressure. Systemic arterial pressures and, in the case of retrograde entry into the left ventricle, left ventricular diastolic pressures can also be recorded. Cardiac output can be measured using the green dye or thermodilution technique. In the green dye method, the indicator is injected into the pulmonary artery, and the sample is collected from a peripheral artery. With the thermodilution technique, a cold solution is injected into the right atrium, and the temperature is sampled and recorded from a thermistor located near the tip of the pulmonary artery catheter. These measurements of pressure and cardiac output can be repeated as frequently as necessary during the first 48 to 72 hours or longer in coronary care units that have the facilities for hemodynamic pressure monitoring. Left ventricular performance can be further evaluated by relating the left ventricular filling pressure to the cardiac output or other parameters before and after expansion of the blood volume.[3] Dextran or other volume expanders can be infused rapidly into the pulmonary artery to permit monitoring of left ventricular filling pressure as pulmonary arterial end-diastolic pressure. Determinations of cardiac output are repeated (1) after the pulmonary arterial end-diastolic pressure has risen more than 4 mm Hg; (2) after each 200 ml infusion; or (3) when the pulmonary arterial end-diastolic pressure rises to 20 mm Hg. The left ventricular filling pressure can be related to the cardiac index, stroke index, stroke work index or stroke power index to construct the respective ventricular function curves.

Techniques in Chronic Coronary Heart Disease

In patients with stable coronary artery disease, cardiac catheterization is performed with techniques similar to those employed in the acute studies. In addition to the measurement of intracardiac pressures and cardiac output, coronary angiography is performed using Sones' or Judkins' technique.[7,8] Both cineangiograms and large cut films are used for filming the opacified coronary arteries. Ventriculograms can be obtained after the injection of contrast material into the left ventricle with either single or biplane cineangiography or biplane angiocardiography. The methods for calculation of left ventricular volume include biplane angiocardiography, biplane cineangiocardiography and single plane cineangiocardiography.[9-11] These quantitative angiographic techniques provide measurements of end-diastolic and end-systolic volumes, left ventricular stroke volume and ejection fraction—the ratio of left ventricular stroke volume to end-diastolic volume. In addition to measurement of chamber dimensions on the angiocardiograms, the free or lateral left ventricular wall thickness can be determined. The left ventricular wall thickness is added to chamber dimensions to estimate left ventricular mass.[12]

The method of Feild and associates[13] can be utilized to superimpose the diastolic and systolic angiocardiograms in the anteroposterior and lateral positions to estimate the percentage of the abnormally contracting segment. In Figure 1, lateral and anteroposterior (AP) views in a patient with chronic coronary artery disease are superimposed. The black dot represents the central x-ray beam and the edges of the cut films are aligned. There is movement from the diastolic silhouette both along the walls of the left ventricle as well as at the aortic valve. However, areas on the lateral view and two areas on the AP view exhibit either no movement—designated akinesis—or paradoxical movement—expansion of systolic silhouette beyond the diastolic margin. The circumference is measured on the superimposed films, and the length of the akinetic or dyskinetic portion of the diastolic circumference is related to the total end-diastolic circumference to obtain the percentage of the abnormally contracting segment. Abnormally contracting segments obtained for the lateral and the AP projections are averaged to yield a single measurement of the abnormally contracting segment.

The method of Smith et al[14] can then be utilized to calculate left ventricular compliance, which can be assessed by 4 formulas:

(1) $\Delta V / \Delta P$

(2) $\dfrac{\Delta V / ESV}{\Delta P}$

(3) $\dfrac{dV}{dP_{ed}}$

(4) $\dfrac{dV}{dP_{ed}} \times \dfrac{1}{EDV/BSA}$

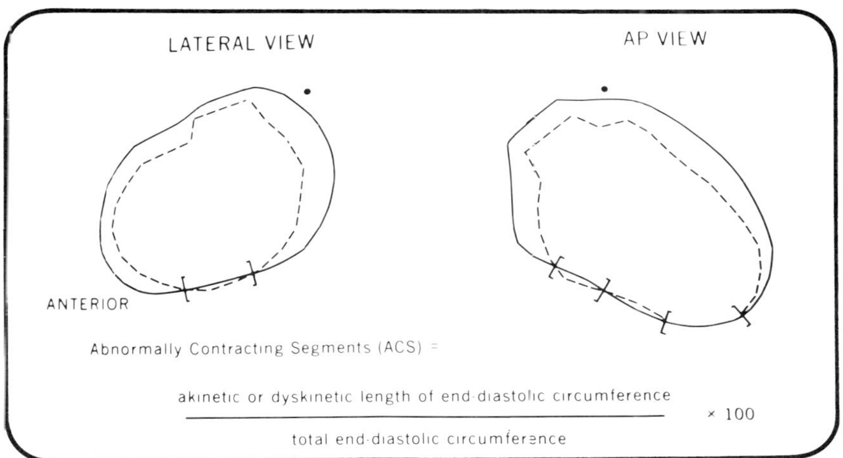

FIGURE 1. The anteroposterior (AP) and lateral biplane angiocardiograms are superimposed to demonstrate the method for calculating the abnormally contracting segment. The calculation for each projection is averaged to yield an estimate of the abnormally contracting segment. (Reproduced by permission from Feild et al.[13])

where ΔV = the left ventricular diastolic volume change or the angiographic stroke volume calculated as the end-diastolic volume (EDV) minus the end-systolic volume (ESV) in milliliters; ΔP = the left ventricular pressure change calculated at the end-diastolic pressure minus the lowest early diastolic pressure; $\Delta V/ESV$ = the diastolic volume change divided by the end-systolic volume to calculate diastolic fractional volume change; dV/dP_{ed} = the reciprocal of the slope of the diastolic pressure volume curve at end-diastole calculated according to the method of Gaasch et al,[15] which assumes a linear log pressure versus volume relationship and a constant positive pressure intercept at zero volume for all subjects; BSA = body surface area in meters squared.

Left Ventricular Function in Acute Myocardial Infarction

Figure 2 illustrates simultaneous left ventricular and pulmonary arterial pressure recordings in a patient with acute myocardial infarction.[1]

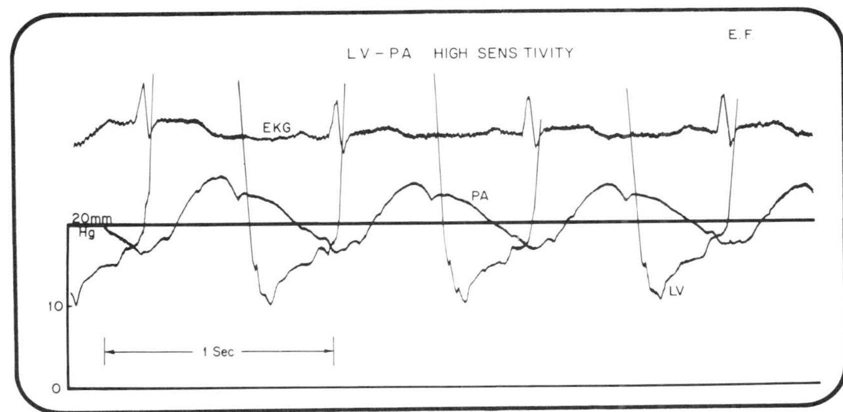

FIGURE 2. Simultaneous left ventricular (LV) and pulmonary artery (PA) pressure recordings in a patient with acute myocardial infarction demonstrate the similarity between left ventricular and pulmonary artery end-diastolic pressures (Reproduced by permission from Rackley et al.[1])

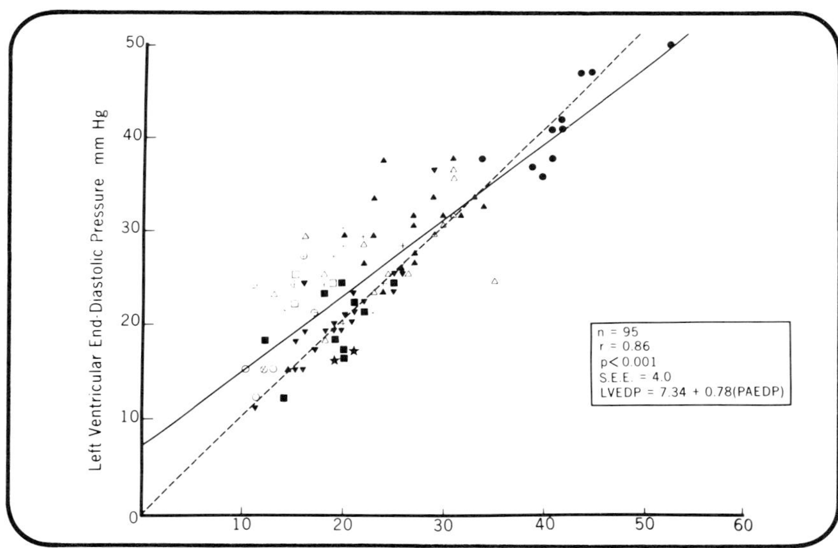

FIGURE 3. The statistical relationship for 95 individual comparisons of left ventricular (LVEDP) and pulmonary artery end-diastolic pressure in 12 patients with acute myocardial infarction is shown. (Reproduced by permission from Russell et al.[16])

The pulmonary arterial end-diastolic and the left ventricular end-diastolic pressures equilibrate. This observation suggests that the pulmonary arterial end-diastolic pressure can be used to estimate left ventricular end-diastolic pressure. The pulmonary capillary or wedge pressure and the mean left atrial pressure are considered the left ventricular filling pressure and, in the absence of mitral valve obstruction or pulmonary vascular disease, usually equate to the left ventricular end-diastolic or pulmonary arterial end-diastolic pressure.

As shown in Figure 3, simultaneous pulmonary arterial and left ventricular pressures were recorded in 12 patients with acute myocardial infarction.[16] The end-diastolic pressures in the pulmonary artery and left ventricle were analyzed statistically, and a linear relationship was demonstrated at normal and moderately and severely elevated pressures. These observations suggest that in acute circulatory disturbances in the absence of severe pulmonary vascular disease or mitral valve disease, pulmonary arterial end-diastolic pressure can be substituted for left ventricular end-diastolic pressure. This relationship has additional clinical application since the pulmonary arterial end-diastolic pressure

can be monitored over prolonged periods of time without the risks of an indwelling catheter in the left ventricle with the potential for systemic emboli.

Although the central venous pressure has been monitored to estimate the adequacy of blood volume in acute circulatory disorders, this measurement must be interpreted with caution in patients with acute myocardial infarction.[17-20] In Figure 4, the mean right atrial pressure or central venous pressure is compared with the left ventricular filling pressure measured as pulmonary arterial or left ventricular end-diastolic pressure in patients with acute myocardial infarction.[1] A wide range of values for left ventricular filling pressure may be encountered for similar right atrial or central venous pressures. Studies by Rapaport and Scheinman[17] and Hamosh and Cohn[18] have shown that the central venous pressure does not bear a consistent relationship to the left ventricular filling pressure in patients with acute myocardial infarction. The central venous pressure reflects the characteristics of diastolic filling in the right ventricle, and in myocardial infarction it is generally increased as a result of right ventricular overload secondary to left ventricular failure.

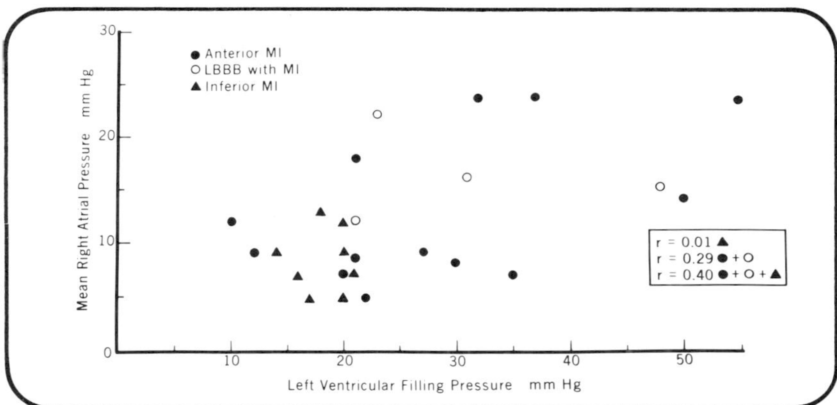

FIGURE 4. The lack of correlation between mean right atrial pressure (central venous pressure) and left ventricular filling pressure measured as pulmonary artery or left ventricular end-diastolic pressure is shown in patients presenting with acute myocardial infarction (MI). LBBB = left bundle branch block. (Reproduced by permission from Rackley et al.[1])

Occasionally patients may have abnormal elevations of right atrial pressure in acute myocardial infarction when the process involves significant portions of the ventricular septum and right ventricular wall.

The measurement of left ventricular filling pressure and cardiac output provides two traditional parameters for the assessment of left ventricular performance. In patients with clinically uncomplicated acute myocardial infarction—without evidence of left ventricular failure or shock—several studies have revealed a high incidence of abnormal elevations in left ventricular filling pressure and reductions in cardiac index. Hunt and co-workers[21] initially reported that patients with uncomplicated infarction frequently had abnormal elevations of left ventricular filling pressure. In a series of 21 patients with clinically uncomplicated infarction, 14 had pulmonary arterial end-diastolic pressures ranging from 13 to 28 mm Hg.[22] In 8 of these 14 patients, the cardiac index was less than 2.5 L/min/M². Rotman and co-workers have reported abnormal elevations of the pulmonary arterial end-diastolic pressure in 47 percent of patients without pulmonary rales or a ventricular gallop. Heart failure consisting of basilar lung rales and a left ventricular gallop is associated with higher elevations in left ventricular filling pressure and a greater reduction in cardiac index than occur in the absence of these clinical findings.[24] A higher left ventricular filling pressure and heart rate and a lower stroke index and stroke work index have been observed in patients with anterior myocardial infarctions when compared with patients with inferior infarctions.[16]

In patients who have cardiogenic shock with acute myocardial infarction, measurements of left ventricular filling pressure and cardiac output have also been recorded.[25-29] A frequently employed definition of cardiogenic shock requires a systolic blood pressure of less than 90 mm Hg or a decline of more than 80 mm Hg from a previously documented hypertensive level of systolic pressure. In addition, the patient must exhibit clinical evidence of impaired organ perfusion—notably cold, clammy, cyanotic skin, altered mentation and reduced urine output. Finally, hypotension secondary to significant arrhythmias or analgesics must be excluded. In Figure 5, the initial measurements of cardiac index and pulmonary arterial or left ventricular end-diastolic pressure are presented for 43 patients with cardiogenic shock complicating a documented acute myocardial infarction.[29] There is a wide scatter of values for both left ventricular filling pressure and cardiac index. Analysis of the left ventricular filling pressure and cardiac index reveals 4 subsets of cardiogenic shock in terms of prognosis. In patients with a left ventricular filling pressure of more

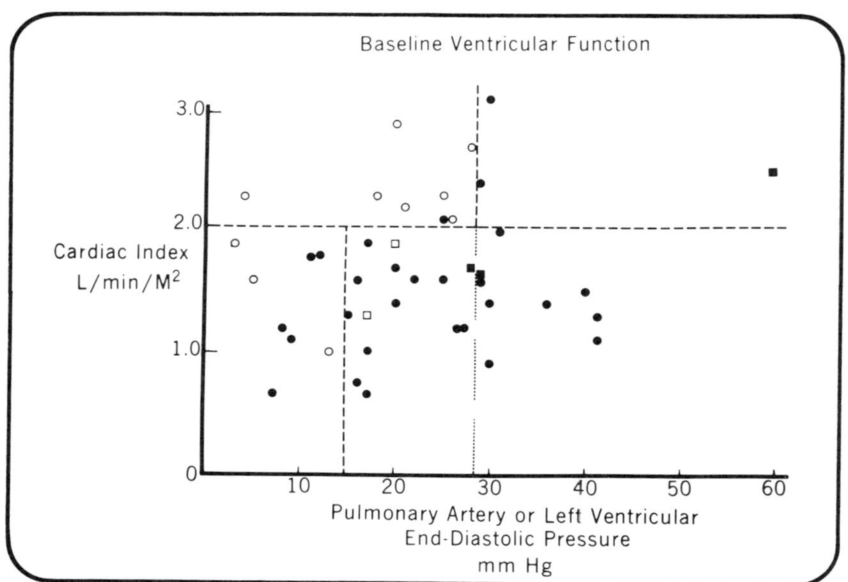

FIGURE 5. The initial pulmonary arterial or left ventricular end-diastolic pressure and cardiac index are shown for 43 patients who presented with cardiogenic shock complicating acute myocardial infarction. The **open symbols** represent survivors, and the **solid symbols** represent nonsurvivors. (Reproduced by permission from Rackley et al.[29])

than 29 mm Hg, the hospital mortality was 100 percent. Among patients who demonstrated a left ventricular filling pressure of more than 15 mm Hg and a cardiac index of less than 2.0 L/min/M², mortality was 92 percent. A third group of patients had a normal or near normal left ventricular filling pressure of less than 15 mm Hg and a cardiac index of less than 2.0 L/min/M². These patients are often considered hypovolemic, and in a significant number the circulatory dynamics responded dramatically to the expansion of blood volume. Mortality was 63 percent in this third category. Finally, in a fourth group with a left ventricular filling pressure of less than 29 mm Hg and a cardiac index of more than 2.0 L/min/M², the mortality was a surprisingly low 13 percent. Although patients in this latter category may have alterations in peripheral vascular tone and a lesser extent of myocardial damage than that in the other three categories, the clinical presentation of cardiogenic shock is indistinguishable. Therefore, in patients presenting with cardiogenic shock complicating acute myocardial infarction, the initial measurement of left ventricular filling pressure and cardiac index can be useful in determining the immediate prognosis.

In addition to the initial measurements of left ventricular filling pressure and cardiac index, studies involving a mild form of stress to the left ventricle have utilized the rapid expansion of blood volume with an agent such as low molecular weight dextran. Figure 6 shows the initial pulmonary arterial end-diastolic pressure and cardiac index and the alterations produced by the infusion of 500 ml of low molecular weight dextran into the pulmonary artery.[1] The elevation in the left ventricular filling pressure is associated with a significant increase in cardiac index. These changes persist for approximately 6 hours before the pulmonary arterial end-diastolic pressure and the cardiac index return to their respective control values. Such studies suggest that the expansion of blood volume in patients with acute myocardial infarction can provide a mild stress that increases the preload of the resting myocardial fiber. Dependent on the mechanical status of the noninfarcted myocardium, this increase in preload can produce an increase in cardiac output and systolic performance.

Since the rapid infusion of low molecular weight dextran and the expansion of the blood volume can produce changes in the left ventricular filling pressure and cardiac output in patients with acute myocardial infarction, these measurements can be analyzed further to assess left ventricular performance. Figure 7 shows the initial measurements of pulmonary arterial diastolic pressure and cardiac index and the serial changes associated with the rapid infusion of 3 200 ml increments of low molecular weight dextran into the pulmonary artery.[1] Minimal change in heart rate was associated with the infusion. The line connecting the changes in filling pressure and cardiac index describes a ventricular function curve. The ventricular function curve is depressed or flat on the first day after acute infarction in this patient and reveals that expansion of the blood volume produced an elevation in filling pressure relatively greater than the increase in cardiac index. Additional systolic parameters analyzed include the stroke index, the stroke work index and the stroke power index, and respective function curves can be constructed. The initial increase in these parameters was produced by the dextran infusion, but a subsequent decrease in all parameters described a descending limb to the left ventricular function curve.

Figure 8 shows repeated measurements made on day 3 in the patient with acute infarction whose hemodynamics are reported in Figure 7.[1] Analysis of the initial resting filling pressure and cardiac index reveals a slight fall in resting pulmonary artery end-diastolic pressure associated with a minimal increase in cardiac index. The repeated infusion of the same amounts of low molecular weight dextran resulted in a higher cardiac output on day 3 than on day 1. This produced a steeper slope to the ventricular function curve. Furthermore, the function curves describing stroke index, stroke work index and stroke power index had no descending limb and exhibited a steeper slope to the curve than those on day 1. These observations suggest that spontaneous improvement in left ventricular performance occurred during the initial 3 day period after acute myocardial infarction in this patient.

In Figure 9, the ventricular function curves in a group of patients with acute myocardial infarction are shown, and the stroke index is related to the left ventricular or pulmonary arterial end-diastolic pressure.[3] Analysis of the slopes in

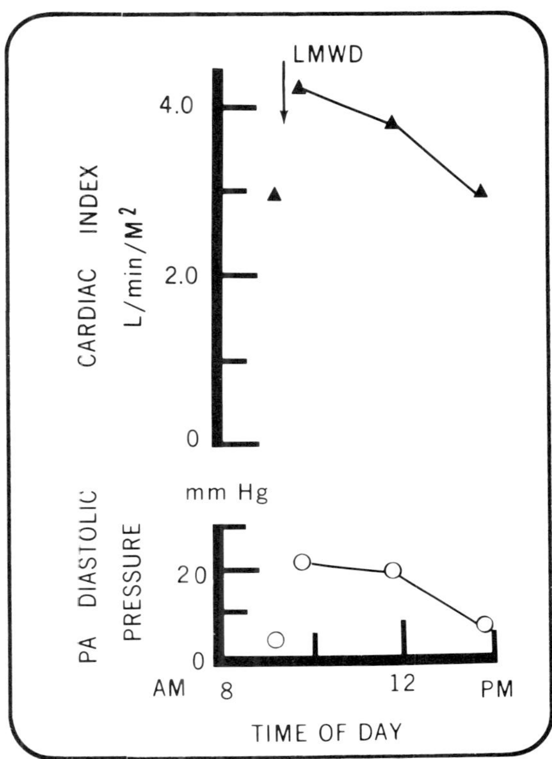

FIGURE 6. The alterations in pulmonary arterial end-diastolic pressure and cardiac index produced by the rapid infusion of 500 ml of low molecular weight dextran (LMWD) are shown. (Reproduced by permission from Rackley et al.[1])

these 19 patients with either 1 or 2 determinations of ventricular function curves indicates that the majority of the function curves exhibited a plateau between 20 and 24 mm Hg. At a left ventricular filling pressure above 24 mm Hg, patients exhibited not only depressed or descending limbs to the ventricular function curves, but also had clinically evident dyspnea and rales indicating pulmonary edema. The peak of these left ventricular function curves would suggest that the optimal left ventricular or pulmonary arterial end-diastolic pressure in patients with acute myocardial infarction is in the range of 20 to 24 mm Hg.

In relating the hemodynamic findings to the clinical assessment of the patient, a number of studies have analyzed the examination of the lungs, auscultation of the heart and interpreta-

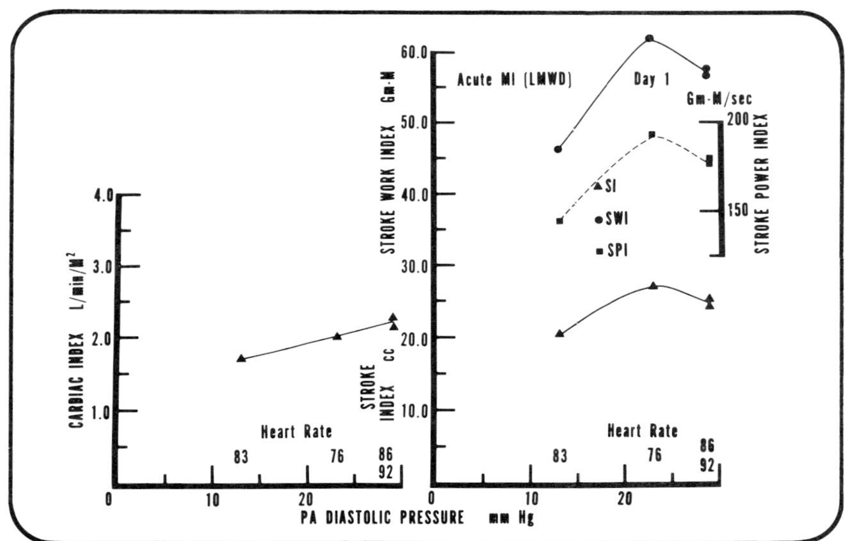

FIGURE 7. The serial changes in pulmonary arterial end-diastolic pressure and cardiac index associated with the rapid infusion of 3 200 ml increments of low molecular weight dextran are connected on the **left** to describe a ventricular function curve. On the **right,** ventricular function curves for stroke index (SI), stroke work index (SWI) and stroke power index (SPI) describe descending limbs. These measurements were obtained on the first day after acute infarction. (Reproduced by permission from Rackley et al.[1])

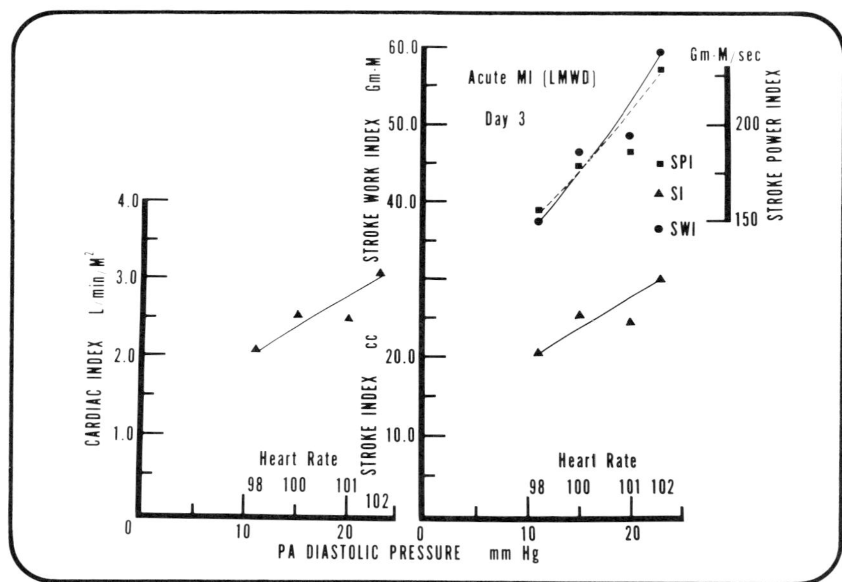

FIGURE 8. Repeated left ventricular function curves in the patient shown in Figure 7 obtained on day 3 after acute infarction reveal an upward shift on the **left** and absence of the descending limbs on the **right.** (Reproduced by permission from Rackley et al.[1])

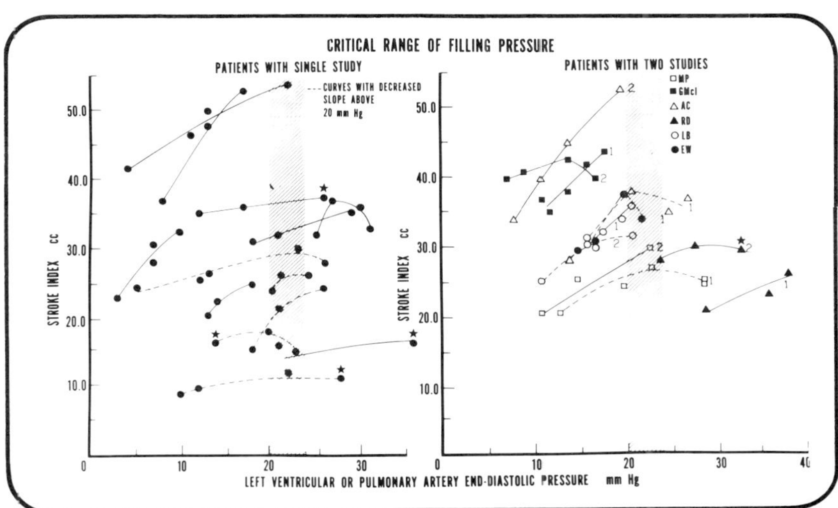

FIGURE 9. Analysis of the slopes of the ventricular function curves in 19 patients with single curves **(left)** or with two studies **(right)** indicate that the plateau or peak of the function curves developed with a left ventricular filling pressure of 20 to 24 mm Hg. (Reproduced by permission from Russell et al.[3])

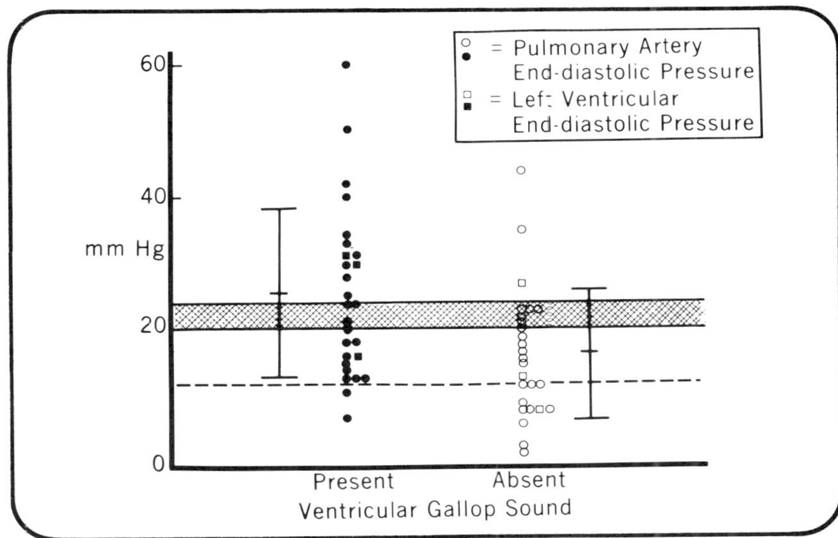

FIGURE 10. The initial pulmonary arterial or left ventricular end-diastolic pressure was measured in 53 patients and separated according to the presence or absence of a ventricular gallop sound. Of the 27 patients with a ventricular gallop sound, 25 were found to have abnormally elevated left ventricular filling pressures above 12 mm Hg **(dashed line).** (Reproduced by permission from Riley et al.[30])

tion of the chest x-ray film for comparison with hemodynamic measurements. In our experience, the single most sensitive finding on clinical or radiographic examination that relates to hemodynamic measurements is the presence of the left ventricular, or S_3, gallop. In Figure 10, the initial measurements of left ventricular filling pressure either as pulmonary arterial end-diastolic pressure or left ventricular end-diastolic pressure are shown for 53 patients.[30] In 26 patients a ventricular gallop was not audible, and approximately one-third of these patients

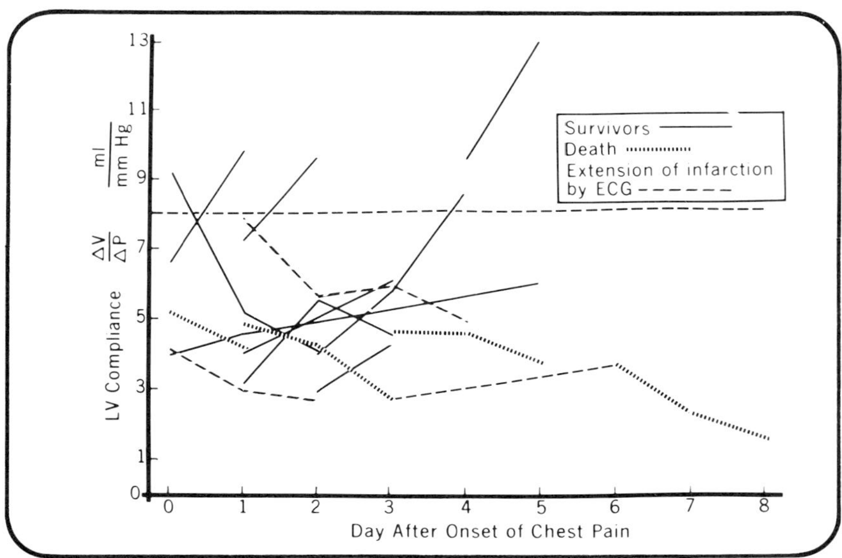

FIGURE 11. Left ventricular filling pressure measured as pulmonary arterial end-diastolic pressure is related to the left ventricular diastolic dimension obtained from echocardiography to estimate left ventricular compliance. A de-crease in compliance in the days after acute infarction was associated with extension of the infarction or death. (Reproduced by permission from Smith et al.[6])

had a normal left ventricular filling pressure of 12 mm Hg or less. Another one-third of this group revealed mild elevations of left ventricular filling pressure from 13 to 20 mm Hg, and the remaining patients presented with values above 20 mm Hg. Therefore, in the absence of a left ventricular gallop, the left ventricular filling pressure could be normal or mildly or severely elevated. In contrast, 25 of 27 patients with an audible ventricular gallop exhibited an abnormally elevated left ventricular filling pressure of more than 12 mm Hg, ranging from 13 to 60 mm Hg. As shown in Figure 9, the optimal range of left ventricular filling pressure in patients with acute myocardial infarction appeared to range between 20 and 24 mm Hg. Therefore, in patients with ventricular gallop, measurement of left ventricular filling pressure would identify those who might have improved cardiac performance with cautious expansion of blood volume that raised the filling pressure to 20 to 24 mm Hg. In those patients with a left ventricular filling pressure of more than 24 mm Hg, phlebotomy or diuresis is required to reduce the filling pressure to the optimal range. Finally, the left ventricular filling pressure could

be monitored and maintained within this optimal range during the initial period of management in patients with acute infarction to insure optimal loading or preload of the left ventricle. This form of monitoring and volume expansion or reduction then provides a precise clinical tool for augmenting impaired left ventricular performance with acute myocardial infarction.

Although abnormal elevations in left ventricular filling pressure have traditionally been interpreted as evidence of failing or impaired ventricular performance, the abnormalities in elastic properties or compliance of the ventricle must also be considered. Figure 11 shows the results of measuring left ventricular filling pressure through a Swan-Ganz catheter and relating it to the left ventricular diastolic diameter determined by echocardiography to obtain a measure of left ventricular compliance expressed as the change in volume related to the change in pressure.[6] These measurements were obtained in 14 patients with acute myocardial infarction over an 8 day period. The large changes in the pulmonary arterial end-diastolic pressure during the period of observation were associated with minimal or no alterations in the echocardiographic left ventricular end-diastolic dimension and thereby implied acute changes in ventricular compliance. Patients surviving the acute myocardial infarction demonstrated an increase in left ventricular compliance during the early days of convalescence. Those patients who exhibited an extension of the infarction on the electrocardiogram or those who did not survive generally exhibited a fall or reduction in left ventricular compliance.

Left Ventricular Function in Chronic Coronary Heart Disease

In patients with a history of myocardial infarction, several investigators have reported correlations between the electrocardiogram, coronary arteriogram and ventriculogram. The electrocardiographic location of QRS abnormalities consistent with a previous infarction correlate with the anatomic site of the coronary artery disease.[13,31,32] In addition, the areas of abnormal wall motion can be estimated from the electrocardiographic changes. Rarely, patients with a history of infarction reveal no coronary anatomic lesions. However, abnormally contracting segments in the left ventricle have been described in patients without a history of myocardial infarction.[33]

In patients with severe coronary artery disease as demonstrated by coronary arteriography, changes may occur in ventricular dimensions and wall thickness. These measurements are expressed as end-diastolic volume, ejection fraction and left ventricular mass. Figure 12 shows that in 23 patients with severe coronary artery disease demonstrated by angiography, a relationship exists between the end-diastolic volume and the left ventricular mass.[34] An abnormal increase in the left ventricular end-diastolic volume would be dilatation and an increase in left ventricular mass would be hypertrophy. As dilatation develops after acute infarction and myocardial scarring, there is an associated increase in left ventricular mass. In Figure 13, the relationship between left ventricular mass and end-diastolic volume is illustrated for patients with a range of ejection fraction values. Patients with an ejection fraction of more than 0.50 similarly exhibited normal values for end-diastolic volume and left ventricular

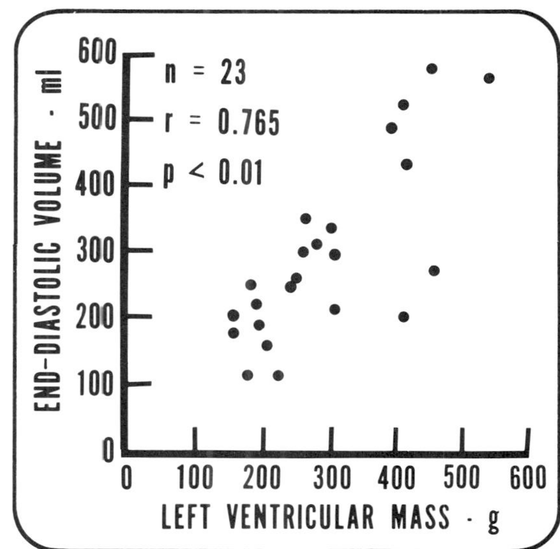

FIGURE 12. In 23 patients with severe coronary artery disease on angiography, a relationship is shown between left ventricular end-diastolic volume and left ventricular mass. (Reproduced by permission from Rackley et al.[34])

mass. In patients with mild to moderate reductions in ejection fraction—ranging from 0.30 to 0.49—early dilatation in terms of increased end-diastolic volume was associated with abnormally increased left ventricular mass. Finally, in patients with severe reductions in ejection fraction—less than 0.30—there was more marked left ventricular dilatation and hypertrophy. These observations suggest that in the chronic stage of severe coronary artery disease, depression of the mechanical performance as expressed by the ejection fraction is associated with an increase in end-diastolic volume, or dilatation, and an increase in left ventricular mass, or hypertrophy. Thus, dilatation and hypertrophy represent 2 major compensatory mechanisms for depressed ventricular performance in chronic coronary artery disease.

In Figure 14, the size of the abnormally contracting segment is related to the ejection fraction in patients with previous acute myocardial infarction. A curvilinear relationship exists between the ejection fraction and abnormally contracting segment, and as the size of the abnormally contracting segment or scar increases after acute myocardial infarction, there is an as-

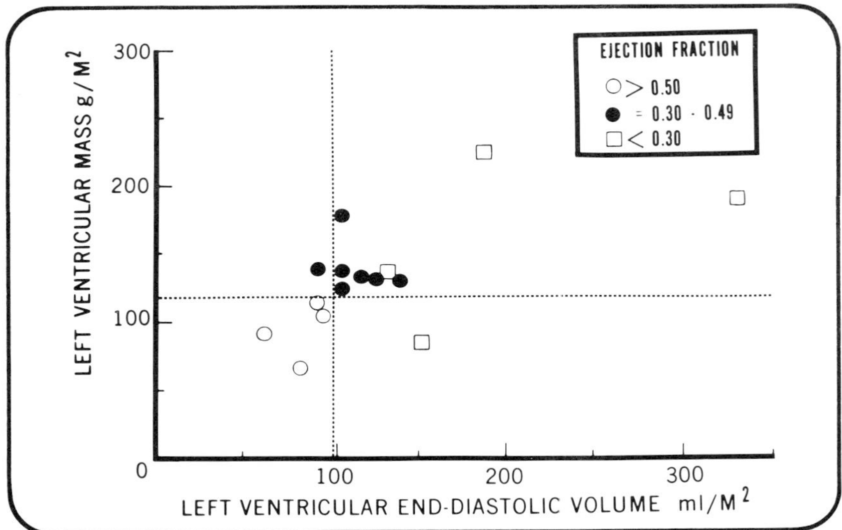

FIGURE 13. In patients studied within a year after myocardial infarction, a reduction in the ejection fraction (EF) below 0.50 was associated with abnormal increases in left ventricular mass and left ventricular end-diastolic volume. The **dotted lines** indicate the limits of normal for left ventricular mass and volume.

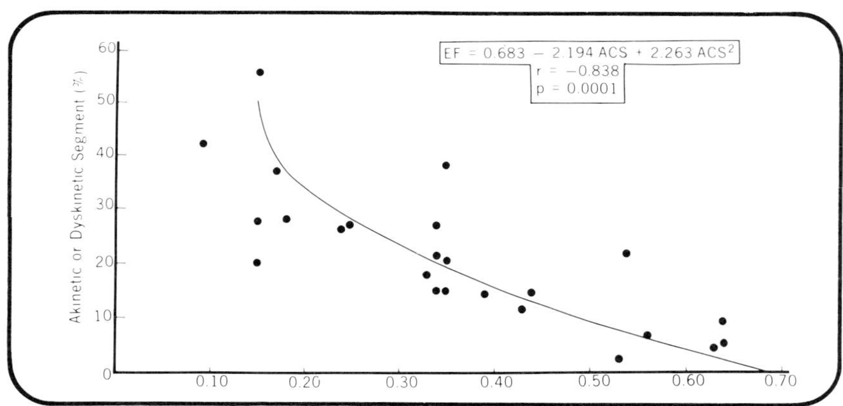

FIGURE 14. The size of the akinetic or dyskinetic segment is significantly related to the ejection fraction in patients with previous acute myocardial infarction.

sociated reduction in ejection fraction. The size of the abnormally contracting segment or residual scar after myocardial infarction can also be related to the compliance of the left ventricle expressed as the change in volume per end-systolic volume related to the change in end-diastolic pressure. As illustrated in Figure 15, a curvilinear relationship is found between the size of the abnormally contracting segment and left ventricular specific compliance.[14] Generally, normal values of left ventricular specific compliance were encountered in patients in whom the size of the abnormally contracting segment was less than 8 percent.

In these patients—studied 2 to 12 months after acute myocardial infarction—a relationship between size of the residual scar or abnormally contracting segment and left ventricular compliance, end-diastolic pressure, end-diastolic volume and the clinical manifestations of heart failure has been shown. When the size of the abnormally contracting segment exceeds 8 per-

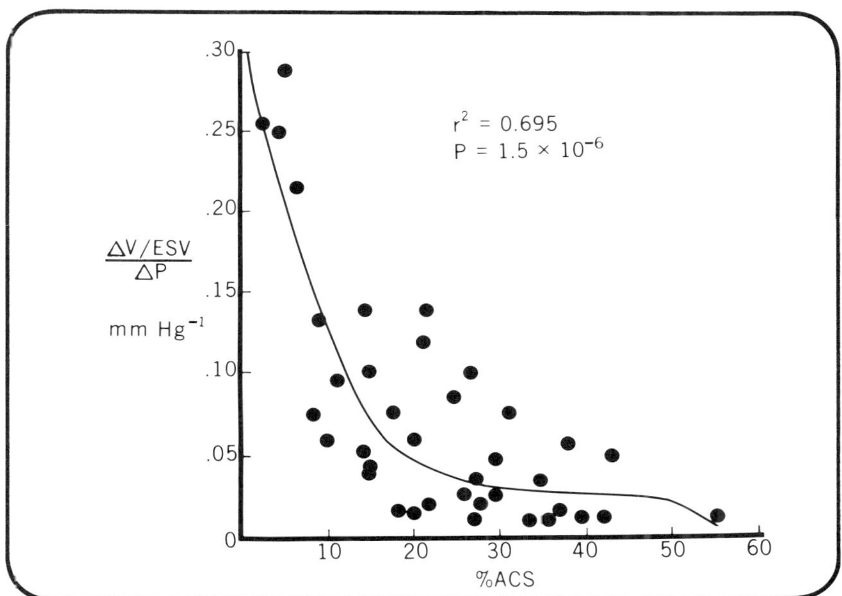

FIGURE 15. A significant curvilinear relationship exists between the size of the abnormally contracting segment (ACS) and left ventricular specific compliance $\frac{\Delta V/ESV}{\Delta P}$ in patients studied in the months after acute myocardial infarction. (Reproduced by permission from Smith et al.[14])

cent, there is an abnormal reduction in left ventricular compliance. An abnormally contracting segment larger than 15 percent is associated with an abnormal elevation in the left ventricular end-diastolic pressure. When the abnormally contracting segment is larger than 17 percent, an abnormal increase in the left ventricular end-diastolic volume, or left ventricular dilatation, is observed. Patients generally complain of dyspnea or orthopnea or have an audible ventricular gallop when the size of the myocardial scar exceeds 23 percent. Therefore, the size of the residual left ventricular scar after myocardial infarction appears related to left ventricular compliance, dilatation, hypertrophy and the clinical manifestation of heart failure.

In Figure 16, the contributions of akinesis and hypokinesis to overall ventricular performance are illustrated in 2 patients, and the lateral and AP biplane angiocardiograms are superimposed.[13] In the patient whose angiocardiograms are shown in the upper portion of the illustration, the abnormally contracting segment was 19.8 percent, compared with that in the patient represented in the lower portion of the figure, in whom it was 21.7 percent. Although these seg-

ment scars are similar in size, there is a significant difference in the ejection fractions in the two patients. The patient represented in the upper portion exhibited an extremely depressed ejection fraction of 0.15, whereas the patient represented in the lower portion of the illustration had an ejection fraction of 0.54. It is obvious that hypokinesis of the contracting myocardium contributes significantly to the overall reduction in ejection fraction. Therefore, although the residual scar or abnormally contracting segment is important, the area of hypokinesis also contributes to the determination of overall mechanical performance.

Figure 17 shows results obtained in 3 patients studied after acute myocardial infarction, in whom ventricular function curves were determined and left ventricular end-diastolic pressure was compared with the cardiac index during the rapid infusion of dextran. In the patient with a normal angiographic ejection fraction of 0.63, the ventricular function curve exhibits an ascending or normal slope. In the patient with a moderately depressed ejection fraction of 0.39, the slope of the ventricular function curve is depressed. In the patient with an extremely re-

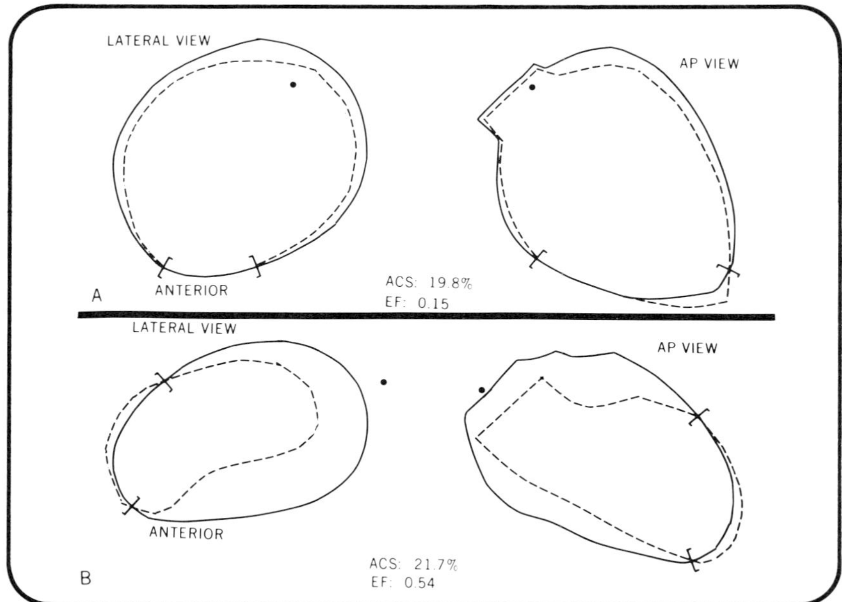

FIGURE 16. The contributions of akinesis and hypokinesis to overall ventricular performance are illustrated in 2 patients with superimposed anteroposterior (AP) and lateral biplane angiocardiograms. The abnormally contracting segments (ACS) are similar but the ejection fractions (EF) differ due to the areas of hypokinesis. (Reproduced by permission from Feild et al.[13])

duced ejection fraction of 0.18, there is a flat ventricular function curve indicating that volume expansion is associated primarily with an increase in filling pressure and minimal change in cardiac index. In addition to the analysis of the ejection fraction and left ventricular function curve, the relations between left ventricular A-wave amplitude and left ventricular dimensions, compliance, systolic performance and the abnormally contracting segments have been examined in patients after myocardial infarction.[35] The highest correlations were found between A-wave height and the left ventricular end-diastolic pressure, compliance, ejection fraction and abnormally contracting segment. In patients studied during dextran infusion, values for the diastolic pressure-volume slope and A-wave amplitude increased with the infusion. These observations indicate that increased left ventricular A-wave amplitudes in patients after myocardial infarction signified a decrease in both left ventricular diastolic compliance and systolic function.

As shown in Figure 18, the changes in ejection fraction and the increase in end-diastolic volume after myocardial infarction do not result in cardiac enlargement on standard chest x-ray films until moderately severe alterations in ventricular function have occurred.[36] Significant depression of the ejection fraction can develop before the cardiothoracic ratio exceeds 0.50, the limits of normal. In the 42 patients studied angiographically 2 to 12 months after the acute infarction, the ejection fraction was usually less than 0.30 for patients who exhibited symptoms of left ventricular failure; however, since cardiomegaly was not consistently present until the end-diastolic volume exceeded 150 ml/M^2, both normal heart size and cardiomegaly were at times associated with congestive heart failure.

Value of Hemodynamic Studies in Acute Coronary Disease

Methods for assessing the hemodynamic status of patients presenting with acute myocardial infarction have improved considerably over the past few years. Significant developments have been the introduction of the Swan-Ganz balloon-tipped catheter and the incorporation of a thermistor into the catheter. Computer programs are now available for measuring, analyzing and displaying pressures, cardiac outputs and the changes brought about by pharmacologic interventions and for serial monitoring of these parameters. The necessary instrumentation is current y being developed for the bedside analysis of these measurements.

Hemodynamic studies in patients with acute myocardial infarction have revealed a high incidence of abnormalities in patients without clinical findings. The hemodynamic parameters have proved useful in determining the prognosis of the patient. Approximately two-thirds of patients without clinical evidence of impaired left ventricular performance have been shown to have abnormal elevations in the left ventricular filling pressure. About half the patients may have moderate reductions in resting cardiac output. Serial measurements of the left ventricular filling pressure and the cardiac index have demonstrated spontaneous improvement over the initial 48 to 72 hours after the acute episode. The left ventricular filling pressure can fall and the cardiac index can increase in certain pa-

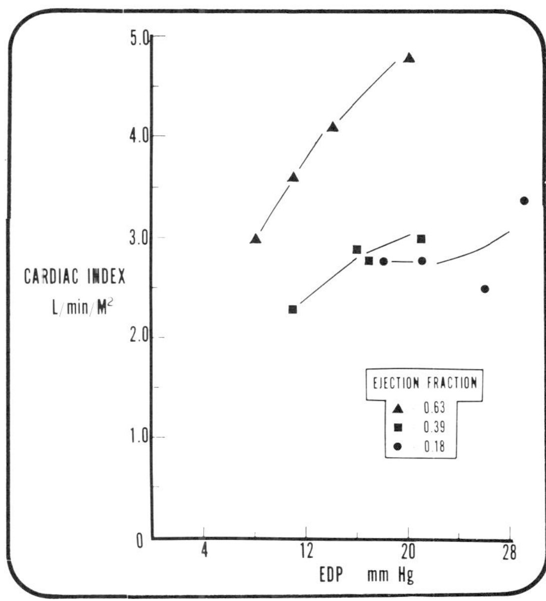

FIGURE 17. Left ventricular function curves in 3 patients studied within a year after myocardial infarction were compared with the ejection fraction. The slopes of the function curves correlated with the values for ejection fraction and ind cate that these are sensitive methods for assessing left ventricular performance. EDP = end-diastolic pressure.

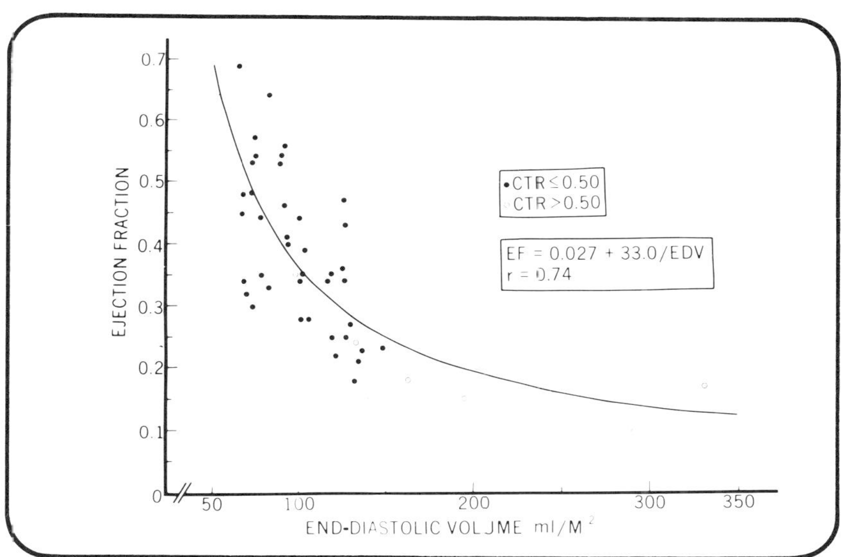

FIGURE 18. In patients studied after acute myocardial infarction, significant depression of the ejection fraction (EF) as well as a moderate increase in the end-diastolic volume (EDV) can occur before the radiographic manifestations of cardiomegaly become apparent by a cardiothoracic ratio (CTR) of more than 0.50.

tients during the initial period after myocardial infarction. Furthermore, ventricular function curves have demonstrated an increase in the slope of the curve during the second and third days after the infarction. Patients with normal or near normal cardiac performance may exhibit a depressed ventricular function curve during the first 12 to 24 hours after the infarction, but a higher mortality has been observed in patients in whom the left ventricular function curve remains depressed. In patients presenting with a pulmonary arterial end-diastolic pressure of more than 20 mm Hg, a 66 percent mortality has been observed during the acute hospital phase. In patients presenting with cardiogenic shock as a complication of acute myocardial infarction, the initial hemodynamic measurements have proved useful in determining the prognosis. Although the overall mortality in cardiogenic shock remains above 75 percent, it is possible to identify subgroups in terms of mortality. Therefore, two groups of patients in cardiogenic shock with high mortality rates of 100 and 92 percent can be identified. A third subset of patients may exhibit a relative hypovolemic state with normal or near normal left ventricular filling pressures and a mortality of 63 percent. These patients often respond impressively to volume expansion. Finally, a group with clinical features indistinguishable from cardiogenic shock may exhibit an extremely low mortality of 13 percent. These patients probably have smaller areas of infarction and destruction of left ventricular muscle and disturbances in peripheral vasomotor control may contribute to the shock state. Therefore, measurements of left ventricular filling pressure and cardiac output in patients with acute myocardial infarction can provide very useful prognostic information.

Efforts to correlate the clinical findings on both physical examination and chest x-ray films with hemodynamic findings have been made by several groups. In patients with acute myocardial infarction, pulmonary rales may be caused by chronic bronchitis with smoking, depressed respiration due to analgesics, elevated diaphragm and reduced diaphragmatic excursion due to the recumbent position or, finally, left ventricular failure. The comparison of the presence of pulmonary rales with hemodynamic abnormalities has not yielded significant correlation. Similarly, the comparison of the chest x-ray film and various venous patterns with left ventricular filling pressure has shown directional changes but not a highly significant correlation. Ventricular gallop in patients with acute myocardial infarction on admission has been shown to have a high correlation with abnormal elevations of the left ventricular filling pressure. In contrast, atrial gallop has not been found to have a significant relationship with left ventricular hemodynamics, and this sound is quite frequently observed in patients with ischemic heart disease. Therefore, with the exception of the ventricular gallop, clinical correlations have not been impressive in predicting abnormalities in hemodynamic measurements. There is a high incidence of abnormal values for left ventricular filling pressure and cardiac index without the physical findings of left ventricular failure.

Value of Hemodynamic Studies in Chronic Coronary Disease

Studies during the chronic stage of disease in patients surviving acute myocardial infarction have revealed anatomic, hemodynamic and wall motion abnormalities and relationships among these observations. The majority of patients surviving acute myocardial infarction exhibit significant anatomic lesions in the coronary arteries, which are associated with measurable areas of abnormal wall motion on the ventriculogram. The size of the abnormally contracting segment or scar after the myocardial infarction is related to the development of abnormal compliance values, abnormal elevations in left ventricular end-diastolic pressure, increases in left ventricular end-diastolic volume, increases in left ventricular mass and the clinical symptoms of heart failure. Investigations have shown that a reduction in overall left ventricular mechanical performance as measured by the ejection fraction is related to the development of dilatation and hypertrophy. Furthermore, in the chronic studies, the mechanical expression of the ejection fraction has been shown to relate to the slope of the ventricular function curve determined at that time. These two independent expressions of left ventricular performance therefore bear a significant relationship in chronic coronary artery disease.

Subsequent myocardial infarctions and possibly the subclinical scarring process in the myocardium caused by chronic coronary artery disease can continue to contribute to a progressive increase in the size of the abnormally contracting segment or segments in the left ventricle. As shown in previous studies, the size of the scar contributes to mechanical abnormalities of left ventricular function. Although the area of the abnormally contracting segment on the ventriculogram usually relates to the previous site of coronary arterial narrowing or occlusion in patients with acute infarction, these scars have been observed in patients without previous clinically documented myocardial infarction. The area of normally contracting segment or the viable myocardium may also contribute to overall depression of ventricular function, and the wall motion during the cardiac cycle is reduced. In this manner, hypokinetic areas of myocardium can also contribute to overall depression of ejection fraction and ventricular performance.

In chronic coronary artery disease, as in acute myocardial infarction, there may be significant depression of left ventricular performance before symptoms of heart failure develop or cardiomegaly is evident on x-ray films. The initial alteration in left ventricular mechanical performance would be an increase in end-systolic volume, which occurs with acute infarction and may lead to alterations in compliance and elevation of left ventricular end-diastolic pressure. During the chronic stages of convalescence, dilatation may develop with a lowering of end-diastolic pressure. In the early phase after infarction, the ejection fraction may be maintained even though both the end-diastolic and end-systolic volumes are increased. However, as the size of the abnormally contracting segment or residual scar increases, there are serial and progressive abnormalities in compliance, dilatation and hypertrophy. Eventually, left ventricular failure can develop, and these symptoms are manifested clinically when the ejection fraction is less than 0.30. This degree of depressed ventricular function is also associated with a left ventricular gallop as well as dyspnea and orthopnea. As shown in previous studies, cardiomegaly may not become apparent on standard x-ray films until the ejection fraction has been depressed near the range of 0.30 and end-diastolic volume has exceeded the normal limits. In chronic coronary artery disease, clinical assessment by physical examination and radiologic evaluation may not reveal the early depression of left ventricular performance.

Summary

Acute myocardial infarction in patients with coronary artery disease significantly influences the hemodynamic performance of the left ventricle. These abnormalities may not be detectable by bedside evaluation of the patient. Serial changes in ventricular performance occur during the early recovery phase from myocardial infarction. Initial hemodynamic measurements of left ventricular filling pressure and cardiac output can be useful in determining the immediate prognosis, particularly in patients with cardiogenic shock. Chronic studies performed in these patients as examples of long-standing coronary artery disease have revealed that the size of the residual scar after the infarction influences various mechanical parameters of ventricular performance, such as compliance, dilatation, hypertrophy and ejection fraction, as well as the clinical manifestations of heart failure. Contributions of abnormal wall motion and myocardial scar in the left ventricle secondary to myocardial infarction as well as chronic coronary artery disease may initially produce minimal abnormalities in ventricular performance. Subsequent infarctions as well as the progressive course of coronary disease may be additive; as additional myocardium is affected, the compensatory mechanisms of dilatation, hypertrophy and other mechanisms for the support of ventricular performance fail. Thus, the catheterization evaluation of cardiac function in acute and chronic coronary artery disease can provide important clinical information for the management of the patient.

Acknowledgment: This work was supported in part by the Myocardial Infarction Research Unit Program, Contract Number HL 43-67-1441, the Cardiovascular Research and Training Center, Program Project Grant Number HL 11-310 (Division of Heart and Vascular Diseases, National Heart and Lung Institute) and the Clinical Research Unit Grant Number RR-32 (General Clinical Research Centers Program, Division of Research Resources, National Institutes of Health).

References

1. **Rackley CE, Russell RO Jr:** Coronary Care: Invasive Techniques for Hemodynamic Measurements. American Heart Association. In press
2. **Cohn JN, Khatri IM, Hamosh P:** Bedside catheterization of the left ventricle. Amer J Cardiol 25:66, 1970
3. **Russell RO Jr, Rackley CE, Pombo J, et al:** Effects of increasing left ventricular filling pressure in patients with acute myocardial infarction. J Clin Invest 49:1539, 1970
4. **Ratshin RA, Rackley CE, Russell RO Jr:** Serial evaluation of left ventricular volumes and posterior wall movement in the acute phase of myocardial infarction using diagnostic ultrasound. Amer J Cardiol 29:286, 1972
5. **Pombo JF, Russell RO Jr, Rackley CE, et al:** Comparison of stroke volume and cardiac output determination by ultrasound and dye dilution in acute myocardial infarction. Amer J Cardiol 27:630, 1971
6. **Smith M, Ratshin RA, Harrell FE Jr, et al:** Early sequential changes in left ventricular dimensions and filling pressure in postmyocardial infarction patients. Amer J Cardiol 33:363, 1974
7. **Sones FM Jr, Shirey EK:** Cine coronary arteriography. Mod Conc Cardiovasc Dis 31:735, 1962
8. **Judkins MP:** Percutaneous transfemoral selective coronary arteriography. Radiol Clin N Amer 6:467, 1968
9. **Dodge HT, Sandler H, Ballew DW, et al:** The use of biplane angiocardiography for the measurement of left ventricular volume in man. Amer Heart J 60:762, 1960
10. **Rackley CE, Behar VS, Whalen RE, et al:** Biplane cineangeographic determinations of left ventricular function: pressure-volume relationships. Amer Heart J 74:766, 1967
11. **Greene DG, Carlisle R, Grant C, et al:** Estimation of left ventricular volume by one-plane cineangiography. Circulation 35:61, 1967
12. **Rackley CE, Dodge HT, Coble YD Jr, et al:** A method for determining left ventricular mass in man. Circulation 29:666, 1964
13. **Feild BJ, Russell RO Jr, Dowling JT, et al:** Regional left ventricular performance in the year following myocardial infarction. Circulation 46:679, 1972
14. **Smith M, Russell RO Jr, Feild BJ, et al:** Left ventricular specific compliance and abnormally contracting segments following myocardial infarction. Chest 65:368, 1974
15. **Gaasch WH, Battle WE, Oboler AA, et al:** Left ventricular stress and compliance in man: with special reference to normalized ventricular function curves. Circulation 45:746, 1972
16. **Russell RO Jr, Hunt D, Rackley CE:** Left ventricular hemodynamics in anterior and inferior myocardial infarction. Amer J Cardiol 32:8, 1973
17. **Rapaport E, Scheinman M:** Rationale and limitations of hemodynamic measurements in patients with acute myocardial infarction. Mod Conc Cardiovasc Dis 38:55, 1969
18. **Hamosh P, Cohn JN:** Left ventricular function in acute myocardial infarction. J Clin Invest 50:523, 1971
19. **Rackley CE, Russell RO Jr:** Left ventricular function in acute myocardial infarction and its clinical significance. Circulation 45:231, 1972
20. **Rackley CE, Russell RO Jr:** Right ventricular function in acute myocardial infarction. Amer J Cardiol 33:927, 1974
21. **Hunt D, Potanin C, Pombo J, et al:** Left ventricular function in clinically uncomplicated myocardial infarction. Clin Res 18:313, 1970
22. **Rackley CE, Russell RO Jr, Mantle JA:** Hemodynamic measurements in clinically uncomplicated myocardial infarction. In, Hemodynamic Monitoring in a Coronary Intensive Care Unit (Russell RO Jr, Rackley CE, ed). Mount Kisco, New York, Futura, 1974, p 191
23. **Rotman M, Chen JTT, Seningen RP, et al:** Pulmonary arterial diastolic pressure in acute myocardial infarction. Amer J Cardiol 33:357, 1974
24. **Rackley CE, Russell RO Jr, Mantle JA:** Hemodynamic measurements of heart failure in patients with myocardial infarction. In Ref 22, p 203
25. **Gunnar RM, Cruz A, Boswell J, et al:** Myocardial infarction with shock. Hemodynamic studies and results of therapy. Circulation 33:753, 1966
26. **Cohn JN, Luria MH, Daddario RC, et al:** Studies in clinical shock and hypotension. V. Hemodynamic effects of dextran. Circulation 35:316, 1967
27. **Scheidt S, Ascheim R, Killip T:** Shock after acute myocardial infarction. Amer J Cardiol 26:556, 1971
28. **Ratshin RA, Rackley CE, Russell RO Jr:** Hemodynamic evaluation of left ventricular function in shock complicating myocardial infarction. Circulation 45:127, 1972
29. **Rackley CE, Russell RO Jr, Ratshin RA, et al:** Cardiogenic shock in patients with myocardial infarction. In Ref 22, p 223
30. **Riley CP, Russell RO Jr, Rackley CE:** Left ventricular gallop sound and acute myocardial infarction. Amer Heart J 86:598, 1973
31. **Williams RA, Cohn PF, Vokonas PS, et al:** Electrocardiographic, arteriographic and ventriculographic correlations in transmural myocardial infarction. Amer J Cardiol 31:595, 1973
32. **Miller RR, Amsterdam EA, Bogren HG, et al:** Electrocardiographic and cineangiographic correlations in assessment of the location, nature and extent of abnormal left ventricular segmental contraction in coronary artery disease. Circulation 49:447, 1974
33. **Moraski RE, Russell RO Jr, Feild BJ, et al:** Localized left ventricular contraction abnormalities in patients with nonocclusive coronary artery disease and no myocardial infarction. Clin Res 22:9a, 1974
34. **Rackley CE, Dear HD, Baxley WA, et al:** Left ventricular chamber volume, mass and function in severe coronary artery disease. Circulation 41:605, 1970
35. **Smith M, Russell RO Jr, Moraski RE, et al:** Left ventricular A-wave amplitude in patients after myocardial infarction. Amer J Cardiol 33:370, 1974
36. **Feild BJ, Russell RO Jr, Moraski RE, et al:** Left ventricular size and function and heart size in the year following myocardial infarction. Circulation (in press)

PART III: TREATMENT

Chapter 18

Management of Chronic Refractory Congestive Heart Failure

Dean T. Mason, MD, FACC
Richard R. Miller, MD, FACC
David O. Williams, MD
Anthony N. DeMaria, MD, FACC
Leigh D. Segel, PhD
Ezra A. Amsterdam, MD, FACC

In some patients with severe, chronic cardiac dysfunction, proper application of the standard therapeutic measures of rest, diet, digitalis and diuretics does not ameliorate the congestive heart failure state. Unresponsiveness in these patients is termed refractory or intractable chronic heart failure. The clinician's approach to this problem consists of two general considerations—evaluation of the diagnosis and assessment of the adequacy of treatment. Successful management of long-standing abnormal cardiac performance that is unresponsive to the usual medical means requires thorough knowledge of the specific cardiac diseases, clear understanding of the altered physiologic mechanisms involved, appreciation of the extracardiac factors that may perpetuate heart failure and complete information concerning available therapy.

Pathophysiology of Chronic Heart Failure

In general, chronic congestive heart failure is the result of severe primary depression of myocardial contractility or extreme ventricular hemodynamic overloading combined with a secondary diminution of contractile state.[1] Cardiac decompensation occurs when primary or secondary impairment of contractility becomes marked. As delineated in chapter 9 on the regulation of cardiac performance in heart disease, the function of the heart is controlled by the four principal determinants that govern stroke volume and cardiac output: (1) preload—ventricular filling pressure; (2) afterload—ventricular tension during ejection; (3) contractility—contractile force independent of loading; and (4) heart rate. The general terms "cardiac performance" and "ventricular function" refer to the combined effects of these factors and not necessarily to the specific determinant of contractility.

The abnormal mechanism operative in each type of heart disease can be analyzed as an isolated or a combined disorder of the four major determinants of cardiac performance. Moreover, appreciation of the determinants of cardiac function provides the physiologic basis for an improved understanding of the manner in which various types of heart disease lead to disturbed pump performance and for an organized approach to the dimensions and integration of therapy in the management of congestive heart failure.[3]

The final clinical expression of deteriorating cardiac performance—decompensated congestive heart failure (functional class IV, New York Heart Association classification)—is the heart's inability to maintain a normal cardiac output in the basal state.[1] Compensated congestive left heart failure occurs when left ventricular function is depressed but the resting cardiac output is preserved, with marked (class III) or moderate (class II) elevations of pulmonary venous pressure. Mild degrees of cardiac dysfunction are observed when normal cardiac output is delivered at rest and during exercise without circulatory congestion (class I).

When chronic hemodynamic overloading or a primary contractility defect is imposed on the heart, there are three principal inherent compensatory mechanisms for the fundamental goal of maintaining a normal cardiac output at rest:[1,4] (1) ventricular dilation—Frank-Starling principle, by which increased ventricular preload improves depressed pump output; (2) ventricular hypertrophy—increased number of contractile units provided by elevated protein synthesis; and (3) increased activity of the sympathetic nervous system—enhanced heart rate, contractility, venous return and partitioning of regional blood flow. Deleterious symptoms necessarily accompany the operation of the compensatory mechanisms in their primary role of sustaining basal stroke volume, and these symptoms—dyspnea due to left ventricular dilation, angina pectoris due to cardiac hypertrophy and tachycardia due to adrenergic activity—may limit the extent to which these adaptive systems can be employed.

In compensated left heart failure (New York Heart Assocation classes II and III), the compensatory reserve mechanisms achieve normal basal cardiac output from the dysfunctioning heart at the expense of increased ventricular end-diastolic and pulmonary venous pressures.[1] Decompensated congestive heart failure (class IV) evolves with chronic low cardiac output causing resting fatigue and oliguria, when the pump function of the heart becomes too impaired to eject a normal basal stroke output despite maximal use of the compensatory mecha-

nisms, resulting in persistent congestive symptoms at rest. Thus, in the decompensated failing heart, marked depression of cardiac performance exceeds the capacity of preload, hypertrophy and adrenergic protection to support resting cardiac output even at the lower limit of normal. It is reemphasized, as discussed in chapter 9, that the conventional symptomatic classification of congestive heart failure is based principally on symptoms consequent to secondary factors (compensatory mechanisms) in the heart failure state, rather than on the critical hemodynamic variable (cardiac output) and the fundamental cause (depressed contractility) of decompensated heart failure.

Determination of Specific Heart Disease

Specific heart diseases result in chronic refractory heart failure through three different primary mechanisms of cardiac dysfunction: (1) contractility defect, as in idiopathic or ischemic myocardial diseases; (2) diastolic mechanical inhibition of ventricular filling, as in mitral stenosis or pericardial tamponade; and (3) systolic hemodynamic overload either by excessive pressure loading, as in aortic stenosis or systemic hypertension, or by excessive volume loading, as in mitral regurgitation. In general, heart failure indicates severe primary diminution of cardiac contractility or substantial secondary reduction of contractility in combination with primary hemodynamic overloading.[5]

Surgical Intervention and Special Medical Therapy

At the onset of the discussion of the evaluation and management of chronic refractory heart failure, it is important to emphasize that cardiac dysfunction should not be allowed to become refractory to medical therapy in congenital heart disease or acquired valvular disorders. Indeed, definitive evaluation by cardiac catheterization and appropriate surgical intervention are generally carried out electively before symptoms develop in congenital heart disease and when cardiac symptoms occur with ordinary activity (more than stable class II symptoms) in chronic rheumatic valvular heart disease. In severe valvular malfunction, valve replacement should not be delayed until the development of refractory congestive heart failure, since the secondary abnormalities in ventricular contractility remain after surgical correction of the ventricular mechanical burden in patients with chronic cardiac symptoms occurring with mild activity (class III) or at rest (class IV) prior to heart surgery.[6,7]

In patients with chronic refractory heart failure, even when idiopathic cardiomyopathy is suspected, it is our policy to carry out detailed right and left heart catheterization to establish positively the type of heart disease involved and to quantify the extent of cardiac and myocardial dysfunction. In patients with unsuspected congenital or acquired heart disease, corrective or palliative surgery may be possible. Numerous such conditions may be present, including: patent ductus arteriosus, atrial and ventricular septal defects, pulmonary stenosis,[8] mitral and aortic valvular diseases, cor triatriatum,[9] coarctation of the aorta, idiopathic hypertrophic subaortic stenosis,[10,11] carcinoid heart disease,[12] traumatic valvular disease, atrial myxoma,[13] peripheral arteriovenous fistula, rupture of mitral chordae terdineae,[14] papillary muscle insufficiency,[15] ventricular aneurysm,[16] constrictive pericarditis[17] and pericardial tamponade.[18]

Some of the more common entities overlooked in adult patients with refractory heart failure and to which special medical and surgical therapeutic measures can be applied are: masked hyperthyroidism, recurrent pulmonary emboli, constrictive pericarditis,[17] atrial septal defect, left-to-right shunting patent ductus arteriosus with pulmonary hypertension,[19] mitral stenosis, idiopathic hypertrophic subaortic stenosis[11] (Figure 1), ventricular aneurysm,[16] papillary muscle insufficiency[15] and myxedema with pericardial effusion.

Identification of patients with cardiomyopathies due to the toxic effect of specific substances, as in chronic alcoholism[20,21] (Figure 2) or hemachromatosis, and recognition of myocardial involvement in systemic diseases, such as sarcoidosis or nutritional, metabolic, hematologic, neoplastic and collagen vascular diseases, may allow the application of special medical therapy that may be useful in arresting or attenuating cardiac muscle damage. Thia-

mine deficiency is a specific cause of the rare entity of beriberi heart disease[22] and has been postulated to contribute to alcoholic cardiomyopathy associated with nutritional inadequacies. Acute rheumatic carditis and the viral, diphtherial, idiopathic and related forms of myocarditis are especially refractory to therapy during their active inflammatory stages.[23]

Mitral replacement has been helpful in some patients with cardiomyopathies and marked secondary mitral regurgitation (Figure 3), despite the increased operative risk, prolonged convalescence and incomplete benefit. In chronic coronary artery disease, elective saphenous vein bypass by itself has not consistently produced improvement in chronic ventricular dysfunction,[16,24] except in occasional patients with frequent angina in whom satisfactory anastomosis substantially improves blood flow to the ischemic regions of the ventricle. Patients with refractory heart failure due to chronic coronary artery disease, however, usually do not have prominent anginal symptoms since they have little potentially normally functioning myocardium that is ischemic.[16,25] Rather, heart failure in these patients is more often due to muscle necrosis and fibrosis with generalized abnormalities of wall motion.

Identification of Extracardiac Factors Exacerbating Heart Failure

In heart failure unresponsive to standard medical therapy, in addition to the systematic evaluation of the nature and degree of heart disease, careful consideration of the possibility of noncardiac conditions simulating or perpetuating cardiac dysfunction is essential. The common abnormalities that mimic heart disease include: pulmonary embolism, other bronchopulmonary disorders, thyrotoxicosis, pheochromocytoma, adrenal tumors and insufficiency, metastatic carcinoma, various forms of anemia and hepatic and renal diseases.

Further, several conditions may contribute to the persistence of the heart failure state in any type of heart disease: hyperthyroidism, hypothyroidism, anemias, atrial fibrillation[26,27] and other tachyarrhythmias[28] (Figure 4), heart block, pulmonary embolism, bacterial endocarditis, pulmonary and urinary tract infections, hepatic and

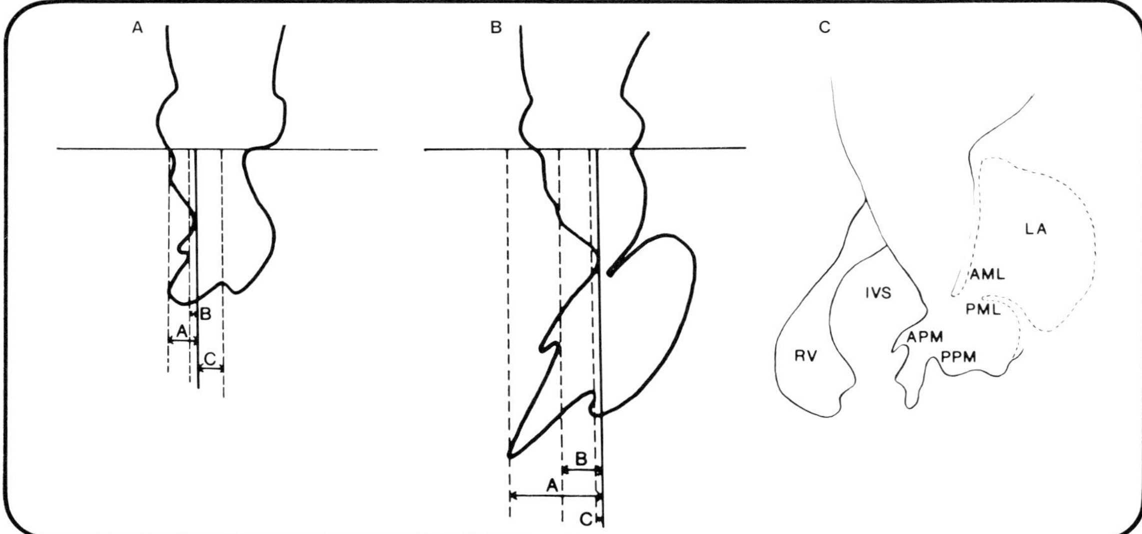

FIGURE 1. A, left anterior oblique diagram of the left ventricular cavity and ascending aorta from a cineangiographic frame obtained in mid-ejection from a patient with asymmetric hypertrophy of the interventricular septum without aortic outflow obstruction (ASH). The nearly **horizontal solid line** is drawn at the level of the aortic valve annulus, with the ascending aorta above and the left ventricle below. The nearly **vertical solid line** perpendicular to the aortic annulus and extending inferiorly through the left ventricular cavity just touching the posterior aspect of the interventricular septum serves as a line of reference for the parallel broken lines. The **left** side of the figure is anterior and the **right** side posterior. The **left broken line** perpendicular to the aortic annulus traverses the inner border of the left ventricular apex; distance A is shown between this broken line and the septal reference line. The **middle broken line** perpendicular to the aortic annulus is through the tip of the anterior papillary muscle; distance B is between this broken line and the septal line. The **right broken line** perpendicular to the aortic annulus is through the tip of the posterior papillary muscle; distance C is between this broken line and the septal line. **B,** left anterior oblique diagram of the left ventricular cavity and ascending aorta from a cineangiographic frame taken in mid-ejection from a patient with idiopathic hypertrophic subaortic stenosis (IHSS). The solid line through the aortic annulus and the solid septal reference line are drawn as in **A.** The broken lines are also drawn through the same left ventricular structures as described in **A.** Distance A is between the left ventricular apex line and the septal line; distance B is between the anterior papillary muscle line and the septal line; distance C is between the posterior papillary muscle line and the septal line. The **left** side of the diagram

is anterior and the **top** is superior in orientation. In IHSS (in contrast to ASH), the left ventricular apex and anterior papillary muscle are markedly anterior to the septal line of reference, and the posterior papillary muscle is also anterior to this line. The apex of the left ventricle is directed toward the mitral valve **(B)** in IHSS, whereas the left ventricular apex is directed toward the aortic valve **(A)** in ASH, idiopathic left ventricular hypertrophy, secondary left ventricular hypertrophy in chronic systolic hemodynamic overload (as in aortic valvular stenosis) and the normal left ventricle. **C,** left anterior oblique diagram of the left and right ventricular inner walls, demonstrating the configuration of the interventricular septum (IVS), from a cineangiographic frame taken in mid-ejection at the time of simultaneous contrast dye opacification of the left and right ventricles (biventricular cineangiogram) in a patient with IHSS. AML = anterior mitral leaflet; APM = anterior papillary muscle; LA = left atrium; PML = posterior mitral leaflet; PPM = posterior papillary muscle. The interventricular septum in IHSS is more markedly hypertrophied in its superior midsegment than in its inferior portion. In addition, the anterior papillary muscle is pulled beneath the superior midseptal bulge during mid-ejection, thereby producing tension and traction on the chordae tendineae attached to the anterior mitral leaflet which results in abnormal systolic forward motion of the anterior mitral leaflet. Consequently, the anterior mitral leaflet encroaches on the hypertrophied septal bulge, causing the dynamic subaortic stenosis characteristic of IHSS. This anterior-superior systolic malposition of the anterior papillary muscle is accentuated by positive inotropic agents such as isoproterenol. (Reproduced by permission from Mason et al.[1])

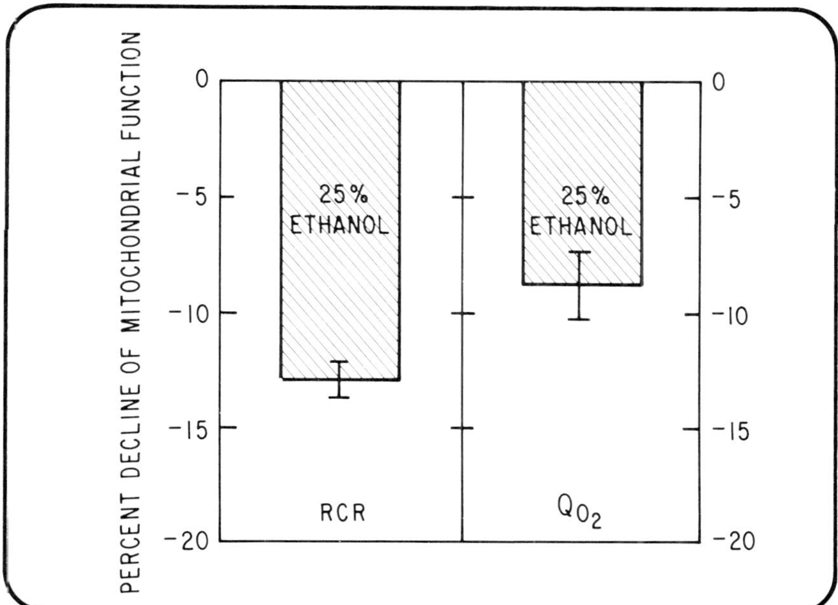

FIGURE 2. Effects of chronic alcohol ingestion on cardiac mitochondrial function in rats that received 32 percent of their daily caloric intake as 25 percent ethanol for 6 months. Results are expressed as percent decrease in function compared with values in matched control animals. RCR = respiratory control ratio (ratio of oxygen consumption rate with ADP added to that after ADP phosphorylation); QO_2 = respiratory quotient (natoms of oxygen consumed with ADP phosophorylation/sec/mg mitochondrial protein).

renal diseases, hypertension, ingestion of large quantities of alcohol[29,30] (Figure 5), obesity,[31] excessive physical activity, increased salt and water intake, electrolyte disturbances, abnormalities of acid-base balance and excessive use of opiates. In addition, complications of cardiovascular drug therapy may perpetuate or worsen pump function, such as cardiac depression due to large doses of antiarrhythmic agents,[32] relatively low blood volume because of too vigorous diuretic therapy and rhythm and conduction disturbances induced by digitalis toxicity.[33,34]

Myocardial Oxygen Consumption and Ischemic Heart Disease

An important consideration in the management of cardiac dysfunction—particularly in coronary heart disease—is the effect of therapy on myocardial energetics. The three principal determinants of myocardial oxygen consumption are:[35] (1) left ventricular wall tension—a product of systolic pressure and volume of the ventricle; (2) left ventricular contractility; and (3) heart rate.

Although a rise in myocardial oxygen demand attends increased inotropism as such,[36] the indirect effects of positive contractile agents in reducing ventricular size and tension when administered in the heart failure state may lead to overall reduction of myocardial oxygen consumption[37] (see Figure 5, chapter 9). Thus, in chronic congestive heart failure due to coronary disease, digitalis is usually of substantial hemodynamic benefit and does not result in increased ischemia, since the glycoside tends to lower myocardial oxygen requirements by diminishing the size and tension of the dilated heart. Although there has been concern that the positive inotropic properties of digitalis increase the size of the myocardial infarct,[38] this is not the case with acute coronary obstruction occurring in chronic ischemic heart disease in a patient taking digitalis. Thus, the indirect effect of digitalis—lowering the myocardial oxygen de-

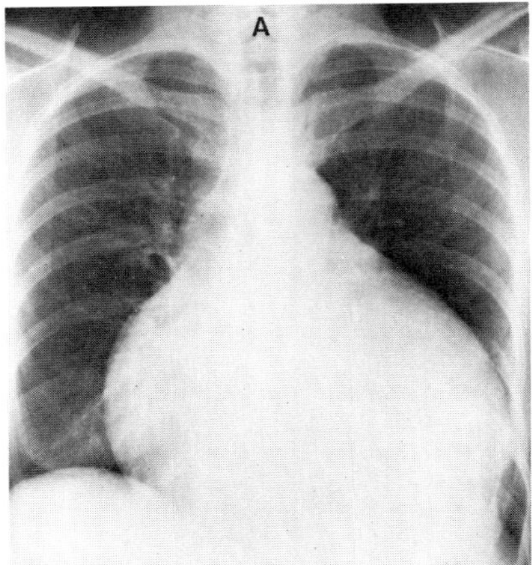

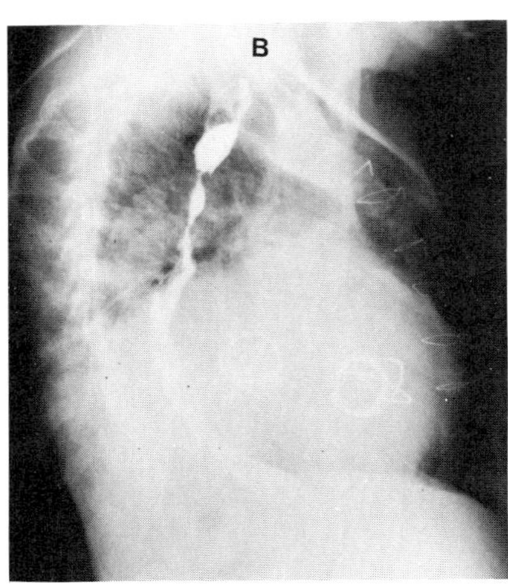

FIGURE 3. Chest roentgenograms in an adult patient with idiopathic cardiomyopathy, severely depressed cardiac function and refractory biventricular congestive heart failure. Cardiac catheterization revealed left ventricular end-diastolic pressure of 25 mm Hg, left atrial mean pressure of 30 mm Hg with peak V waves of 40 mm Hg, pulmonary artery systolic pressure of 60 mm Hg, right atrial mean pressure of 16 mm Hg and cardiac index of 2.15 L/min/M²; ventriculography demonstrated marked mitral and tricuspid valvular regurgitation. Operative intervention with combined mitral and tricuspid valvular prostheses resulted in substantial clinical improvement; functional capacity increased from complete incapacity to symptoms of heart failure on mild to moderate physical exertion. At operation, the atrioventricular valve leaflets per se were normal, but severe regurgitation was evident due to dilation of the atrioventricular annuli and malfunction of the papillary muscle/chordae tendineae apparatus because of marked ventricular enlargement. As anticipated, postoperative convalescence was difficult and prolonged due to severe depression of ventricular contractility. **A,** preoperative frontal view demonstrating marked generalized cardiomegaly; **B,** postoperative lateral view showing the mitral and tricuspid prosthetic heart valves.

mands of the dilated ventricle in chronic coronary disease with congestive heart failure—reduces the area of acute ischemia and necrosis.[39]

In heart failure resulting from acute myocardial infarction (see chapter 22 on myocardial infarction shock), the abnormal mechanisms and therapeutic considerations necessarily differ from those in congestive heart failure associated with chronic coronary heart disease.[40–44] Often relatively little left ventricular enlargement accompanies acute heart failure due to infarction. An increase in contractility induced by a positive inotropic agent in peri-infarct ischemic regions might aggravate the extent of ischemia and necrosis, particularly in the non-dilated heart.

Improved understanding of the factors governing myocardial oxygen consumption has recently led to experimental evaluation—with some extension to clinical trials—of a number of treatment modalities designed to reduce the extent of acute myocardial infarction.[45,46] Minimizing the area of infarction and ischemia improves left ventricular function and diminishes the incidence of tachyarrhythmias. Therapeutic approaches to the limitation of infarct size include: (1) reduction of myocardial oxygen needs by propranolol,[47–49] nitroglycerin,[50–56] long-acting nitrates,[56–58] nitroprusside,[59–62] phentolamine[62,63] and trimethaphan (Arfonad®);[64] (2) improvement of myocardial oxygen delivery by phenylephrine,[52,53,65] norepinephrine,[40,41] external counterpulsation,[66] internal balloon counterpulsation,[67–70] inspiration of oxygen-enriched air,[71] thrombolytic agents[72] and coronary artery bypass reperfusion;[16,73,74] (3) decrease in myocardial edema and inflammation by hydrocortisone,[75] hyaluronidase,[76] hypertonic mannitol[77–30] and cobra venom;[81] and (4) augmentation of myocardial anaerobic metabolism by glucose-insulin-potassium[82–85] and hypertonic glucose.[86,87]

The clinical value of many of these manipulations in acute myocardial infarction remains to be firmly established. In addition, as discussed in chapter 22, their use in patients must be individualized, and application depends upon the hemodynamic setting associated with the acute coronary episode. Propranolol is effective in protecting the ischemic myocardium in preinfarction angina[88] but should not be employed in heart failure due to acute infarction because of its depression of pump function.[48] Nitroprusside is useful in reducing myocardial oxygen requirements in preinfarction angina and in also improving pump performance in heart failure with acute infarction,[59-61] whereas the drug may not be applicable in hypotension associated with myocardial infarction shock. In the latter situation, norepinephrine may be necessary to maintain coronary perfusion pressure;[40,42] however, this agent should not be employed in the absence of refractory hypotension. Nitrates are beneficial in decreasing cardiac oxygen needs in the intermediate coronary syndrome and in also reducing pulmonary congestion in myocardial infarction with normal cardiac output;[55] however, because of their potential cardiac output-lowering effect, they are hazardous in low output heart failure and cardiogenic shock due to myocardial infarction.[55]

In myocardial infarction with congestive heart failure, certain combinations of therapy, such as nitroprusside and dopamine with counterpulsation, may be employed to optimize pump function by achieving the most favorable alterations of contractility and peripheral vascular resistance, while attempting to protect the ischemic myocardium. Further, in therapeutic trials designed to limit the size of the acute infarct, phenylephrine has been added to nitroglycerin to counteract the hypotension and reflex tachycardia resulting from the nitrate.[53] Concerning the effects of inotropic stimuli on the function of the ischemic heart, a difference in response has been observed in experimental animals with global ischemia produced by partial obstruction of the left main coronary artery compared with animals with segmental ventricular ischemia caused by occlusion of the left circumflex coronary artery.[89,90] Isoproterenol depressed left ventricular function in global ischemia because of the inotropism-induced increase in myocardial oxygen demand without a concomitant increase in coronary blood flow,[89] whereas the catecholamine improved cardiac performance in segmental ischemia.[90] In con-

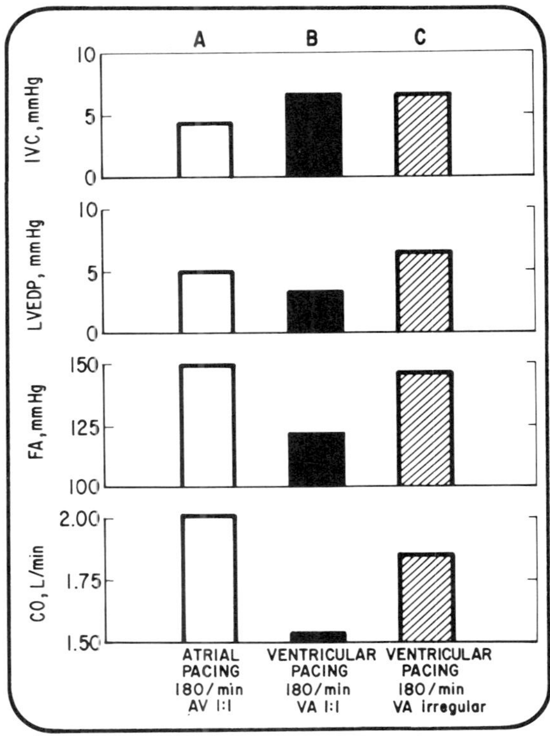

FIGURE 4. Deleterious hemodynamic consequences of ventricular tachycardia with (**B**) and without (**C**) retrograde 1:1 ventriculoatrial (VA) conduction. Control hemodynamics are shown during atrial pacing (**A**) with 1:1 atrioventricular (AV) conduction. Atrial or ventricular pacing rates were constant at 180/min in this representative canine preparation. Cardiac function was more disturbed in ventricular tachycardia with retrograde VA 1:1 conduction (**B**) since not only was ventricular preload reduced by loss of synchronous atria contraction in late ventricular diastole, but also the large regularly occurring cannon atrial contractions appeared to cause transient retrograde flow in the vena cavae and pulmonary veins, further lowering left ventricular end-diastolic pressure (LVEDP) and cardiac output (CO). In ventricular tachycardia with irregular VA conduction (**C**), cardiac function was disturbed to a lesser degree than in **B** but remained below normal (**A**) due to ventricular dyssynergy of contraction combined with the loss of regular atrial contribution to ventricular filling. FA = femoral artery systolic pressure; IVC = mean inferior vena cavae pressure.

trast, propranolol or nitroglycerin enhanced cardiac function in global ischemia due to a reduction of myocardial oxygen requirements.[90] Finally, it should be pointed out that the positive inotropic action of cardiotonic agents may be attenuated in the ischemic ventricle[91-94] and

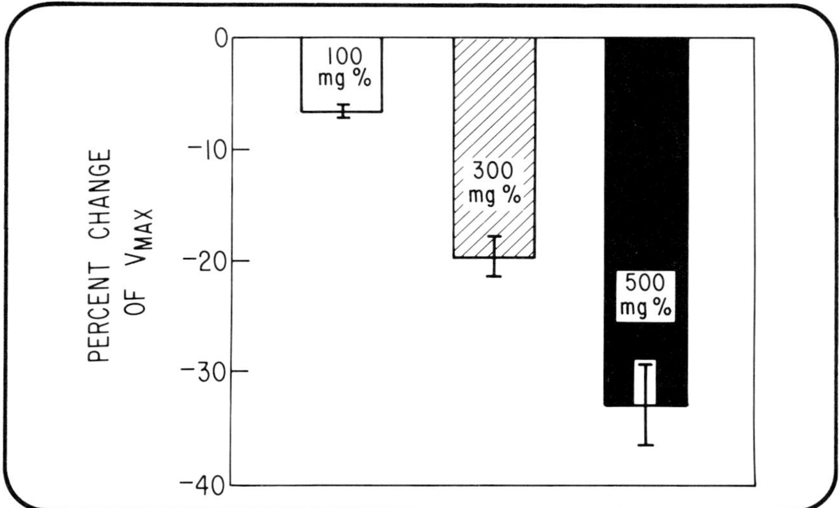

FIGURE 5. Effect of alcohol on myocardial contractility in heart failure. Negative inotropic action of acute ethanol on right ventricular papillary muscles of cats in which chronic right ventricular hypertrophy and failure were induced by constriction of the main pulmonary artery. Peak velocity of contractile element shortening (Vmax) represents the index of contractile state. The concentration of ethanol in the myograph bath was 100, 300 and 500 mg/100 ml (%). **Vertical lines** with cross bars indicate ± 1 standard error of the mean (SEM).

that myocardial depression by negative inotropic agents may be enhanced in coronary heart disease.[95]

Therapeutic Approach to Chronic Heart Failure due to Cardiomyopathy

In many instances of chronic refractory heart failure, careful reevaluation of the history and results of physical examination, laboratory tests and cardiac catheterization does not reveal previously unrecognized diseases or conditions in which special medical or surgical therapy can be applied. Thus, chronic refractory heart failure in such patients is caused by myocardial heart disease—the specific, idiopathic and ischemic cardiomyopathies—with severe reduction in contractility without chronic hemodynamic overload. Ventricular dysfunction may be largely irreversible in these situations. The remainder of this discussion of the management of refractory heart failure deals with the difficult and relatively incomplete therapeutic modalities that can be employed in chronic pump dysfunction due entirely to markedly depressed inotropic state. The special problems of acute intractable congestive heart failure induced by myocardial infarction are considered in chapter 22 on cardiogenic shock.

Medical therapy is somewhat limited and nonspecific in chronic congestive heart failure due to primary ventricular muscle dysfunction. Nevertheless, salutary effects can be achieved in most instances. The physiologic approach to treatment is based on improving the four dimensions of cardiac function. The four principal determinants of cardiac performance—preload, contractility, afterload and heart rate—are therapeutically adjusted to provide optimal circumstances for the depressed contractile force of the failing pump to deliver a normal cardiac output.

Treatment is best initiated in the hospital, with decreased physical activity and the use of bed rest. Management usually centers on improving two principal aspects of the congestive failure state—impaired contractility and body salt and water retention. In addition, certain electrical measures may sometimes be applied to optimize heart rate and improve ventricular filling. Further, reduction of the impedance to left ventricular ejection by the use of peripheral vasodilator agents constitutes a new therapeutic approach to increasing low stroke output.

Positive Inotropic Agents

Since the basic abnormality of the failing myocardium leading to refractory circulatory congestion is marked disturbance of contractile state, the first principle of management is consideration of positive inotropic agents for enhancing cardiac performance. Improvement of depressed contractility elevates the entire ventricular function curve toward normal, as a result of an increase in the lowered cardiac output and a decrease in the excessive left ventricular end-diastolic pressure (see Figure 1, chapters 9 and 20).

Digitalis: Rational treatment generally begins with the digitalis glycosides (see chapter 20). Since the beneficial effects of these agents stem from their direct stimulatory action on the force of contraction of the myocardium, these drugs produce some improvement in the depressed contractile state and in the lowered cardiac output.[96,97] Furthermore, the glycosides exert an overall indirect effect of vasodilation in congestive heart failure; increased peripheral vascular resistance is reduced by the elevation of diminished cardiac output, allowing withdrawal of sympathetically mediated vasoconstriction, which overrides the mild direct vasoconstrictor action of digitalis.[98] Although the favorable hemodynamic effects of the glycosides reduce severe heart failure, these drugs alone often are not sufficient to reverse the refractory congestive failure state. Indeed, this refractory condition usually develops in cardiac patients who are already receiving digitalis in doses approaching the level of toxicity.

Isoproterenol: The powerful sympathomimetic isoproterenol is sometimes useful in refractory heart failure.[40] Stimulation of contractility and heart rate by the agent is produced by its direct action on beta adrenergic receptors in the heart. The maximal inotropic effect of isoproterenol usually exceeds that of digitalis prior to the onset of toxicity.[99] Furthermore, the elevation of cardiac output at comparable levels of enhanced contractility is greater with isoproterenol than with digitalis, since the cathecholamine produces direct vasodilation by its stimulation of beta receptors in the peripheral arteriolar beds.[99] The influence of isoproterenol on blood pressure varies. When the depressed contractile state of the diseased ventricle can be improved, the drug produces a small rise in cardiac output relative to the greater decline in peripheral vascular resistance. Thus, there may be a tendency for blood pressure to decrease.

Since isoproterenol reduces systemic resistance to left ventricular ejection, it may be of special benefit when mitral regurgitation complicates severe cardiomyopathies. Isoproterenol has been more useful in chronic refractory heart failure due to causes other than coronary artery disease. The agent is given by slow intravenous drip for several hours at an initial rate of 1 to 3 μg/min. Isoproterenol must be administered cautiously because of the rapid heart rate, ventricular tachyarrhythmias and hypotension it may provoke. In our experience, it has been valuable during the recovery period in patients with the low cardiac output syndrome after cardiac surgery.[40] In addition, in patients with aortic stenosis who have delayed corrective surgery too long, isoproterenol has been useful in causing sufficient reduction of considerably elevated blood urea nitrogen levels due to markedly lowered cardiac output to allow safer cardiac catheterization and valve replacement. Isoproterenol may also provide temporary improvement of impaired organ perfusion in chronic cardiomyopathies.

Dopamine: The biologic precursor of norepinephrine, dopamine, possesses certain advantages over isoproterenol.[100–103] The beta receptor-stimulating property of dopamine exerts a positive inotropic effect, and there is mild reduction of total peripheral vascular resistance. The action of dopamine is somewhat similar to that of epinephrine, with elevation of cardiac output and a directional change of arteriolar resistance intermediate between that of the vasodilation of isoproterenol and the vasoconstriction induced by norepinephrine. In addition, dopamine possesses the beneficial effect of direct, non-beta receptor-mediated renal vasodilation.[104] Dopamine is administered slowly by intravenous drip at an initial rate of 2 to 5 μg/kg/min. Epinephrine can be given in the same manner at an initial rate of 1 to 2 μg/min.[43] In order to obtain the desired effects on cardiac output and blood pressure, the simultaneous use of dopamine and isoproterenol—or phentolamine and dopamine or norepinephrine/ may be more effective than is any single agent.[103,105]

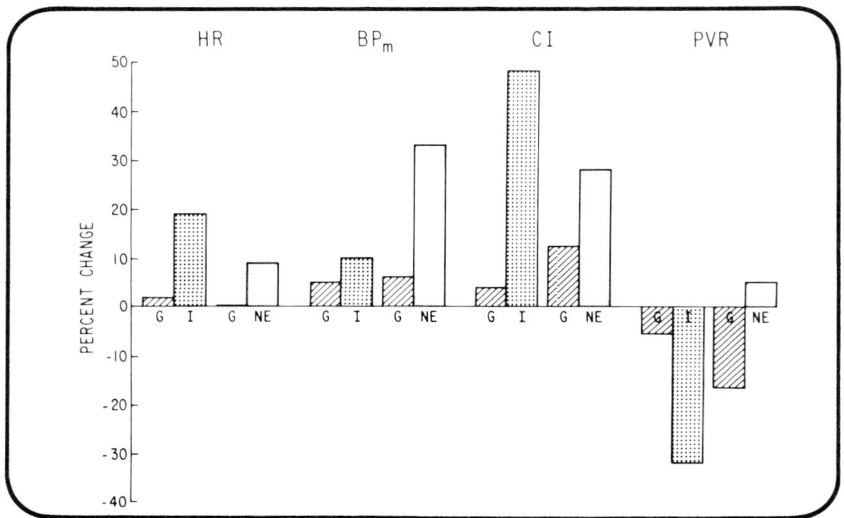

FIGURE 6. Comparative effects of glucagon (G) and sympathomimetic amines (I = isoproterenol; NE = norepinephrine) in patients with chronic congestive heart failure. BP_M = mean systemic intraarterial blood pressure (mm Hg); CI = cardiac output (L/min/M²); HR = heart rate (beats/min); PVR = total peripheral vascular resistance (dynes sec cm⁻⁵). (Reproduced by permission from Amsterdam et al.[112])

Glucagon: Extensive investigations of this direct adenylate cyclase-stimulating agent have established that it possesses a positive inotropic effect independent of beta adrenergic receptor activation[106-110] and mildly dilates peripheral resistance vessels.[111] Its positive contractile effect is considerably greater in experimental animals than in man. In our experience, glucagon has not been useful in patients with chronic refractory congestive heart failure.[112] Although we administered this hyperglycemic agent to fully tolerated levels, we observed only small and inconsistent improvement of abnormal hemodynamics. Furthermore, the beneficial hemodynamic effects of dopamine or isoproterenol were greater than those of glucagon (Figure 6). It has been reported that glucagon is of some value in acute heart failure[113] and that the agent enhances other positive inotropic drugs.

Other Agents: Aminophylline also exerts a positive inotropic action,[114] apparently by its influence on the intracellular beta-sympathomimetic pathway.[115] Thus the agent inhibits the enzyme phosphodiesterase that deactivates cyclic adenosine monophosphate (cAMP), tending to prolong the action of cAMP within the myocardial cell. Aminophylline has been shown experimentally to augment the positive inotropic effects of sympathomimetic agents.[115] The recently synthesized sympathomimetic agent, dobutamine, possesses the advantage of relatively selective myocardial beta receptor stimulation that produces substantial positive inotropic effect with little influence on peripheral vascular resistance and heart rate.[116,117]

A unique approach in the therapy of ventricular dysfunction has been provided by a new class of positive inotropic compounds, termed ionophores, that alter the permeability of cardiac cell membranes.[118,119] These agents augment cardiac contractility through enhanced calcium delivery to the contractile proteins, by increasing transport of calcium ions into the cell and by releasing calcium from sarcoplasmic reticulum.[118,119] The ionophores are microbial metabolites that concentrate in the lipid of cell membranes where they form ionophore-cation complexes, thereby serving as mobile cation carriers across the membrane surface. In experimental studies, the intravenous administration of the calcium ionophore RO 2-2985 (X537A), an antibiotic produced from a Streptomyces strain, has been shown to result in a sustained, marked increase in myocardial contractility and cardiac output, accompanied by a rise in systemic arterial pressure with little or no change in systemic vascular resistance and heart rate.[118,119] Considerable attention presently is being focused on the therapeutic potential of calcium ionophores in the therapy of heart failure and cardiogenic shock.

Experimental studies have indicated that synthetic dextrothyroxine increases cardiac contractility without the excessive increase of body and myocardial metabolic rate induced by the natural thyroid hormone levothyroxine.[120] Thyroid hormone acts directly on adenylate cyclase[121] to elevate the level of the intracellular regulatory substance cAMP, which appears in turn to increase contractile state by stimulation of intracellular calcium release from sarcoplasmic reticulum.[122] Levodopa, the levorotatory isomer of the dopamine precursor dihydroxyphenylalanine (dopa), which has been used extensively in the treatment of Parkinson's disease, also possesses cardiovascular actions by causing increased generation of dopamine through tissue decarboxylation of dopa.[123–125] Therefore, the effects of levodopa on the myocardium are those of beta adrenergic stimulation by dopamine and by increased release of norepinephrine.[123] Since there are no positive inotropic agents suitable for oral administration, other than the digitalis glycosides, that are sufficiently effective in enhancing contractile state for periods of several hours, oral dextrothyroxine or oral levodopa might be considered for possible benefit in improving contractility in the treatment of nonischemic congestive heart failure. Levodopa has shown a natriuretic effect in clinical heart failure, apparently because of the peripheral circulatory action of dopamine causing renal vasodilation.[123]

Corticosteroids have been reported to help promote diuresis in some patients with refractory cardiac edema.[126] However, steroids do not directly enhance contractility and therefore, are not used to increase pump function in refractory heart failure. Although it has been suggested that steroids might have a favorable anti-immune action in chronic heart failure due to primary myocardial diseases, these agents are not of special benefit in these conditions—with the rare exception of an occasional case of active, rapidly progressive myocarditis.

Although morphine sulfate has been utilized effectively for more than a century in the rapid relief of acute pulmonary edema due to left heart failure and in the amelioration of chest pain in acute myocardial infarction, the precise manner by which the agent influences cardiocirculatory dynamics has not been elucidated until recently. Experimental and clinical data available at this time indicate that the cardiovascular effects of morphine sulfate are largely produced indirectly by central nervous system inhibition of sympathetic activity.[127,128] This process of central sympatholysis results in dilation of both arterioles and veins in the peripheral vascular beds. However, total peripheral vascular reflex activity and venomotor responses remain intact. Blood pressure is usually well maintained in the supine position, and the agent can safely be administered with appropriate caution when its beneficial actions are required in myocardial infarction and in acute pulmonary edema. In regard to the analgesic action of morphine in myocardial infarction, the indirect peripheral vasodilator actions of the agent may aid in the relief of ischemic pain by reducing myocardial oxygen requirements through a decrease in ventricular size and tension. The salutary effects of morphine in alleviating the severe dyspnea associated with acute pulmonary edema of congestive left heart failure appear to be the result of the narcotic's actions on the central nervous system, reducing both anxiety and sympathetic activity and thereby decreasing respiratory center discharge and promoting peripheral pooling of blood due to venodilation.

Electrical Measures

Application of electrical methods to improve cardiac pump function in the management of refractory heart failure includes cardioversion of tachyarrhythmias and pacemaker catheters in sinus bradycardia and complete heart block.

Cardioversion: Restoration of atrial transport after direct current electroconversion of atrial fibrillation may substantially improve ventricular preload and raise lowered cardiac output in heart failure due to hypertrophic cardiomyopathies, coronary artery disease and systolic ven-

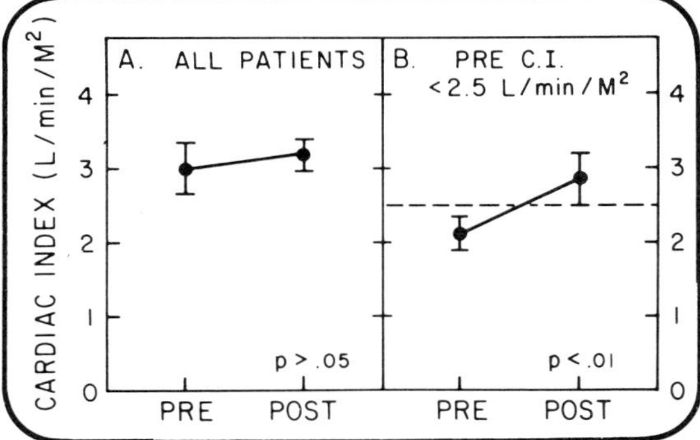

FIGURE 7. Response of cardiac index (CI) to elective direct current electric cardioversion from atrial fibrillation (pre) to normal sinus rhythm (post) in patients with chronic coronary heart disease or cardiomyopathies without valvular dysfunction. Cardiac output was measured echographically. **A** illustrates the mean pre- and postconversion levels of cardiac index for all of the patients studied, whereas **B** depicts those for the subgroup of patients with precardioversion depression of cardiac index to less than 2.5 L/min/M². Horizontal broken line in **B** indicates the lower limit of normal of cardiac index. (Reproduced by permission from DeMaria et al.[27])

tricular pressure overloading prior to the advanced stage of decompensation in which marked ventricular dilation occurs[26,27] (Figure 7). Although it is difficult to maintain normal sinus rhythm when the pressure or volume of the left atrium is increased,[26] elective electroconversion of atrial fibrillation should be attempted in these types of heart disease. Occasionally, even short periods of sinus rhythm are associated with reduction in heart failure, which affords improved management of congestive failure even upon return of atrial fibrillation. As discussed in chapter 23 on antiarrhythmic therapy, in patients receiving therapeutic doses of digitalis, elective defibrillation can safely be carried out without induction of digitalis toxicity by using initially small, incrementally increased levels of countershock.[129]

Cardiac Pacemakers: Increasing the frequency of contraction by electrical pacing catheters may improve cardiac performance in some patients with ventricular dysfunction. Thus, raising heart rate to normal levels in those with relatively slow rates—and sometimes to the upper limits of normal in patients with normal resting rates—may enhance cardiac output, by the increased frequency of stroke volume delivered from the heart and the inherent increase in inotropism associated with a rise in heart rate.

Electroaugmentation of Contraction: Electroaugmentation of contractile force by postextrasystolic inotropic potentiation induced by the technique of paired electrical stimulation has been evaluated in clinical heart failure.[130] However, the increased contractility is usually not translated into elevation of cardiac output, apparently because of interference with diastolic ventricular filling by the weak contraction induced by the second electrical stimulus.

Another electrical technique potentially applicable in refractory heart failure is rapid atrial pacing in an attempt to inhibit release of antidiuretic hormone.[131] However, this approach has not produced diuresis in patients.[132]

Afterload Reduction

The salutary effects of producing alterations in cardiac loading with peripheral vasodilator drugs have been recognized recently in the therapy of chronic—as well as acute—cardiac failure in certain clinical conditions. Thus, in congestive heart failure due to acute myocardial infarction, reducing ventricular afterload with intravenous nitroprusside or phentolamine has been shown to elevate low cardiac output, decrease high left ventricular filling pressure and diminish myocardial oxygen demands.[59,60,133,134]

The concept of decreasing the impedance to left ventricular ejection has also been extended recently to chronic congestive heart failure,[61,62,135] as discussed in chapter 21 on ventricular unloading by systemic vasodilator therapy. Intravenous nitroprusside can raise reduced cardiac output and lower markedly elevated ventricular filling pressures in chronic heart failure due to coronary artery disease, cardiomyopathies and essential hypertension.[61,62,135,136] Stroke volume may be especially enhanced by this agent when these conditions are associated with mitral regurgitation.[137]

To achieve the increase in stroke volume with nitroprusside or other peripheral vasodilator drugs, it may be necessary for the depressed ventricle to operate near the beginning of the apex of its function curve by maintenance of a relatively high preload with volume expansion at a left ventricular end-diastolic pressure of approximately 15 mm Hg.[61] In addition, as delineated in chapter 21, the benefits of hemodynamic unloading of the dysfunctioning ventricle may be extended to oral therapy and thereby maintained on a chronic basis by use of sublingual or oral long-acting nitrates.[57,58] Further, in hypertensive heart disease, chronic antihypertensive therapy reduces the increased afterload on the left ventricle and improves pump performance through long-term control of elevated systemic blood pressure.[138]

Diuretic Management

With reduced renal blood flow, which may occur in heart disease even prior to a decline in resting cardiac output due to the cardiac compensatory mechanism of increased adrenergic activity with redistribution of total blood flow within the body,[1] the kidneys retain sodium and water with consequent increased intra- and extravascular volume. As discussed in chapter 13 on renal function in heart failure, congestion in this condition results initially from elevated venous pressure, and with subsequent reduction of renal blood flow, retention of salt and water by the kidneys largely underlies the remainder of pulmonary and systemic fluid accumulation. In heart failure, blood flow to the kidneys is diminished to a greater extent than is the glomerular filtration rate, thereby elevating the filtration fraction with an increase in the reabsorption of sodium in the proximal convoluted tubules.[126] In addition, the increased reabsorption of sodium in congestive heart failure may result, in part, from insufficiency of an undefined hormonal substance that usually causes proximal renal tubular sodium rejection.[139] Furthermore, with more advanced heart failure, the renin-angiotension-aldosterone system is activated[140] and inappropriately increased secretion of antidiuretic hormone may also occur,[141] leading to enhanced sodium and water reabsorption in the distal tubules and collecting ducts.

Although it may be difficult to correct the basic defect in refractory heart failure by improving depressed contractile state, usually it is possible to alter excessive body salt and fluid accumulation by rational selection of diuretic agents. In refractory congestive heart failure, it is often necessary to restrict daily intake of salt to less than 1 gm and of water to less than 1 L. The development of the potent oral diuretic drugs—chlorothiazide, ethacrynic acid, furosemide and spironolactone—in the past decade has greatly enhanced the ease and success of relieving relatively intractable circulatory congestion.

Thiazides: Modern diuretic therapy begins with oral thiazides.[142] These agents interfere with dilution of urine (inhibiting free water formation) in the ascending loop of Henle and distal tubule by preventing reabsorption of sodium, chloride and potassium with resultant excretion of these ions with water.

Aldosterone Antagonists: If the thiazides prove inadequate, an oral aldosterone antagonist should be added.[126] Either spironolactone or triamterene is the agent employed. The more potent aldosterone antagonist amiloride is not yet available for general use. The aldosterone antagonists inhibit exchange of potassium for sodium in the distal tubules, resulting in excretion of sodium while potassium is retained.[126] Aldosterone antagonism is competitive with spironolactone and noncompetitive with triamterene and amiloride.[126] The aldosterone inhibitors are less powerful than are the thiazides, ethacrynic acid and furosemide, but they promote considerable natriuresis when administered daily for several weeks. An aldosterone antagonist combined with a thiazide makes potassium supplementation hazardous.

Loop Diuretics: If the combination of chlorothiazide with spironolactone or triamterene is unsuccessful, one of the most potent oral diuretics, ethacrynic acid[143] or furosemide,[144] is substituted for the thiazide. These newer agents—ethacrynic acid and furosemide—block sodium transport from the ascending loop of Henle, thereby interfering with urine-concentrating ability by rendering the renal medullary interstitium less hypertonic for water reabsorption in the collecting ducts. These loop diuretics also possess the thiazide action of inhibiting dilution of urine in the ascending loop of Henle and distal tubules. In some refractory conditions, initiation of diuresis appears to be aided by beginning ethacrynic acid or furosemide therapy by the intravenous route.

Organomercurials: Although the organomercurials remain useful and powerful diuretics that inhibit isosmotic reabsorption of salt and water in the proximal and distal tubules,[126] they must be given intramuscularly to be effective. For potent diuresis in resistant congestion, there is no longer need for the complex combined regimens of acidifying chlorides, carbonic anhydrase inhibitors (to prevent proximal tubular urine acidification, thereby inhibiting exchange of hydrogen for sodium and reducing sodium reabsorption), mercurials and aminophylline (to increase renal blood flow).

Mannitol and Steroids: In the rare instance when marked edema is refractory to the regimen of loop diuretics and aldosterone antagonists, volume expanders such as the osmotic diuretic mannitol or albumin together with the low sodium-retaining corticosteroids may be added[126] to enhance renal blood flow and glomerular filtration in order to provide a more favorable setting for the beneficial actions of ethacrynic acid or furosemide and the aldosterone antagonists. Renal and peritoneal dialysis have been employed in the therapy of chronic refractory congestive heart failure, but these measures are impractical.

Mechanical Assist Devices and Cardiac Homotransplantation

When chronic end-stage congestive heart failure that is truly refractory to the judicious use of all medical measures develops in patients with ischemic or primary cardiomyopathies in whom a palliative operation is not applicable, it is not imprudent to consider the possibility of cardiac homotransplantation—after careful selection and at medical centers highly experienced with this procedure.[145–147] However, cardiac homotransplantation is quite restricted in availability and also limited in success. Mechanical cardiac assist devices[41,70,148–150] have not been useful in the management of chronic heart failure, although such devices have provided at least temporary benefit in the treatment of severe cardiac dysfunction due to acute myocardial infarction (see chapter 22). The major inroads in the management of absolutely intractable myocardial failure incompatible with life in chronic coronary heart disease and the cardiomyopathies must await the development of a successful permanently implantable artificial heart.

Summary

Management of chronic refractory congestive heart failure is based on firm knowledge of the pathophysiologic mechanisms involved, identification of the specific type of cardiac disease responsible, and correction of extracardiac factors that may contribute to the unresponsive condition. In general, cardiac catheterization is performed to determine the cause of heart disease and to delineate the degree of abnormal ventricular performance. Therapy of severe myocardial dysfunction requires the skillful correction of disorders of the four principal cardiac pump determinants: (1) preload; (2) afterload; (3) contractility; and (4) heart rate. Thus, medical treatment of chronic severe congestive heart failure, in which no special operative intervention is applicable, usually consists of therapeutic combinations from among digitalis and dopamine to increase depressed inotropic state; diuretics and nitrates to relieve circulatory congestion; maintenance of ventricular filling pressure at the upper limit of normal, with volume expansion if necessary, to provide optimal preload; reduction of increased ventricular afterload by systemic vasodilation with nitroprusside; and establishment of normal ventricular rate and cardiac rhythm by antiarrhythmic agents, direct current cardioversion, and pacemakers. Special consideration is required of the effects of therapy on myocardial oxygen consumption in coronary heart disease.

Acknowledgment: This work was supported in part by Research Program Project Grant HL 14780 from the National Heart and Lung Institute, National Institutes of Health, and Research Grant AA-00270 from the National Institute on Alcohol Abuse and Alcoholism, National Institute of Mental Health.

The authors gratefully acknowledge the technical assistance of Robert Kleckner, Arthur Lewis and Leslie Silvernail.

References

1. **Mason DT, Spann JF, Zelis R, et al:** Alterations of hemodynamics and myocardial mechanics in patients with congestive heart failure: pathophysiologic mechanisms and assessment of cardiac function and ventricular contractility. Progr Cardiovasc Dis 12:507, 1970

2. **Mason DT, Zelis R, Amsterdam EA, et al:** Clinical determinations of left ventricular contractility by hemodynamics and myocardial mechanics. In, Progress in Cardiology (Yu P, Goodwin J, ed). Philadelphia, Lea & Febiger, 1972, p 121

3. **King JF, Salel AF, Amsterdam EA, et al:** Recent advances in therapy for refractory congestive heart failure. Geriatrics 28:94, 1973

4. **Mason DT, Zelis R, Amsterdam EA, et al:** Mechanisms of cardiac contraction: structural, biochemical and functional relations in the normal and diseased heart. In, Pathologic Physiology, fifth edition (Sodeman WA Jr, Sodeman WA, ed). Philadelphia, WB Saunders, 1974, p 206

5. **Mason DT, Spann JF, Zelis R, et al:** Comparison of the contractile state of the normal, hypertrophied, and failing heart in man. In, Cardiac Hypertrophy (Alpert NR, ed). New York, Academic Press, 1971, p 433

6. **Mason DT, Ross J, Gault JH, et al:** Combined prosthetic replacement of the mitral and aortic valves: pre- and post-operative hemodynamic studies including left ventricular responses to muscular exercise. Circulation 35 suppl I:15, 1967

7. **Mason DT, Fisher RD, Ross J, et al:** Left ventricular performance following isolated and combined replacement of the aortic and mitral valves. In, Prosthetic Heart Valves (Brewer L, ed). Springfield, Illinois, Charles C Thomas, 1969, p 352

8. **Roberts WC, Mason DT, Morrow AG, et al:** Calcific pulmonic stenosis. Circulation 37:973, 1968

9. **Maguire LB, Nolan TB, Reeve R, et al:** Cor triatriatum as a problem of adult heart disease. Circulation 31:263, 1965

10. **Mason DT, Braunwald E, Ross J:** Effects of changes in body position on the severity of obstruction to left ventricular outflow in idiopathic hypertrophic subaortic stenosis. Circulation 33:374, 1966

11. **Mason DT, King JF, Reis RL, et al:** Idiopathic hypertrophic subaortic stenosis: recent progress in elucidation of the mechanism of obstruction. In, New Horizons in Cardiovascular Practice (Russek HI, ed). Baltimore, University Park Press, 1975, p 403

12. **Roberts WC, Mason DT, Wright LD:** The nondistensible right atrium of carcinoid heart disease. Amer J Clin Path 44:627, 1965

13. **Yarnell PR, Spann JF, Dougherty M, et al:** Episodic central nervous system ischemia of undetermined cause: relation to occult left atrial myxoma. Stroke 2:35, 1971

14. **Cohen LS, Mason DT, Braunwald E:** The significance of an atrial gallop sound in mitral regurgitation: a clue to the diagnosis of ruptured chordae tendineae. Circulation 35:122, 1967

15. **Vismara LA, Miller RR, DeMaria A, et al:** Mitral regurgitation in patients with coronary artery disease: relation to extent of myocardial dysfunction. Amer J Cardiol 33:175, 1974

16. **Amsterdam E, Hughes JL, Iben A, et al:** Surgery for acute myocardial infarction. In, Shock in Myocardial Infarction (Gunnar RM, Loeb HS, Rahimtoola SH, ed). New York, Grune & Stratton, 1974, p 257

17. **Bonanno JA, Amsterdam EA, Mason DT:** Pericarditis. In, Infectious Diseases (Hoeprich PD, ed). New York, Harper & Row, 1972, p 1073

18. **Gabe IT, Mason DT, Gault JH, et al:** Effects of respiration on venous return and stroke volume in cardiac tamponade. Brit Heart J 32:592, 1970

19. **Tikoff G, Echegaray HM, Schmidt AM, et al:** Patent ductus arteriosus complicated by heart failure. Amer J Med 46:43, 1969

20. **Burch GE, DePasquale HP:** Alcoholic cardiomyopathy. Amer J Cardiol 23:723, 1969

21. **Segel LD, Rendig SW, Choquet Y, et al:** Effects of chronic ethanol consumption on the metabolism, ultrastructure and mechanical function of the rat heart. Cardiovasc Res 9:649, 1975

22. **Blankenhorn MA:** The diagnosis of beriberi heart disease. Ann Intern Med 23:398, 1945

23. **Bonanno JA, Zelis R, Mason DT:** Myocarditis. In, Ref 17, p 1061

24. **Mason DT, Amsterdam EA, Miller RR, et al:** Consideration of the therapeutic roles of pharmacologic agents, collateral circulation and saphenous vein bypass in coronary artery disease. Amer J Cardiol 28:608, 1971

25. **Roberts WC, Buja LM, Bukley BH, et al:** Congestive heart failure and angina pectoris: opposite ends of the spectrum of symptomatic ischemic heart disease. Amer J Cardiol 34:870, 1974

26. **Fisher RD, Mason DT, Morrow AG:** Restoration of sinus rhythm after mitral valve replacement: correlations with left atrial pressure and size. Circulation 37 suppl II:173, 1968

27. **DeMaria AN, Lies JE, King JF, et al:** Echographic assessment of atrial transport, mitral movement and ventricular performance following electroversion of supraventricular arrhythmias. Circulation 51:273, 1975

28. **DeMaria A, Tabaie H, Kamiyama T, et al:** The deleterious hemodynamic consequences of retrograde ventriculoatrial conduction in ventricular tachycardia. Circulation 46 suppl II:118, 1972

29. **Mason DT, Spann JF, Beiser GD:** Effects of ethanol on the contractile state of the myocardium. Clin Res 15:451, 1967

30. **Mason DT, Spann JF, Zelis R, et al:** Alcohol and the heart. Heart Bulletin 20:1, 1971

31. **Alexander JK, Peterson KL:** Cardiovascular effects of weight reduction. Circulation 45:310, 1972

32. **Mason DT, Spann JF, Zelis R, et al:** The clinical pharmacology and therapeutic applications of the antiarrhythmic drugs. Clin Pharmacol Ther 11:460, 1970

33. **Mason DT, Zelis R, Lee G, et al:** Current concepts and treatment of digitalis toxicity. Amer J Cardiol 27:546, 1971

34. **Massumi RA, Amsterdam EA, Zelis R, et al:** The digi-

talis glycosides: contractile and electrophysiologic actions, clinical indications, precautions and toxicity. Semin Drug Ther 2:221, 1972

35. **Braunwald E:** Control of myocardial oxygen consumption: physiologic and clinical considerations. Amer J Cardiol 27:416, 1971

36. **Coleman HN:** Role of acetylstrophanthidin in augmenting myocardial oxygen consumption: relation of increased oxygen consumption to changes in velocity of contraction. Circ Res 21:487, 1967

37. **Covell JW, Braunwald E, Ross J, et al:** Studies on digitalis. XVI. Effects on myocardial oxygen consumption. J Clin Invest 45:1535, 1966

38. **Maroko PR, Braunwald E:** Modification of myocardial infarction size after coronary occlusion. Ann Intern Med 79:720, 1973

39. **Watanabe T, Covell JW, Maroko PR, et al:** Effects of increased arterial pressure and positive inotropic agents on the severity of myocardial ischemia in the acutely depressed heart. Amer J Cardiol 30:371, 1972

40. **Mason DT, Spann JF, Zelis R:** Pathogenesis and treatment of the low cardiac output syndrome. In, Pre- and Postoperative Management of the Cardiopulmonary Patient (Oaks WW, ed). Philadelphia, FA Davis, 1970, p 328

41. **Amsterdam EA, Massumi RA, Zelis R, et al:** Evaluation and management of cardiogenic shock. I. Approach to the patient. Heart and Lung 1:402, 1972

42. **Amsterdam EA, Massumi RA, Zelis R, et al:** Evaluation and management of cardiogenic shock. II. Drug therapy. Heart and Lung 1:663, 1972

43. **Amsterdam EA, Massumi RA, Zelis R, et al:** Evaluation and management of cardiogenic shock. III. The roles of cardiac surgery and mechanical assist. Heart and Lung 2:122, 1973

44. **Mason DT, Amsterdam EA, Miller RR, et al:** Recent advances in pathophysiology and therapy of myocardial infarction shock. In, Cardiovascular Disease: New Concepts in Diagnosis and Therapy (Russek H, ed). Baltimore, University Park Press, 1974, p 143

45. **Braunwald E, Maroko PR:** The reduction of infarct size—an idea whose time (for testing) has come. Circulation 50:206, 1974

46. **Braunwald E, Maroko PR, Libby P:** Reduction of infarct size following coronary occlusion. Circ Res 35 suppl III:192, 1974

47. **Maroko PR, Kjekshus JK, Sobel BE, et al:** Factors influencing infarct size following experimental coronary artery occlusion. Circulation 43 suppl III:67, 1971

48. **Amsterdam EA, Williams DO, Caudill C, et al:** Hemodynamic effects of propranolol in acute myocardial infarction: beneficial and deleterious actions. Clin Res 22:257A, 1974

49. **Mueller HS, Ayres SM, Religa A, et al:** Propranolol in the treatment of acute myocardial infarction. Circulation 49:1078, 1974

50. **Mason DT, Spann JF, Zelis R, et al:** Physiologic approach to the treatment of angina pectoris. New Eng J Med 281:1225, 1969

51. **Mason DT, Zelis R, Amsterdam EA:** Actions of the nitrites on the peripheral circulation and myocardial oxygen consumption: significance in the relief of an-

gina pectoris. Chest 59:296, 1971

52. **Smith ER, Redwood DR, McCarron WE, et al:** Coronary artery occlusion in the conscious dog. Effects of alterations in arterial pressure produced by nitroglycerin, hemorrhage, and alpha-adrenergic agonists on the degree of myocardial ischemia. Circulation 47:51, 1973

53. **Hirshfeld JW, Boxer JS, Goldstein RE, et al:** Reduction in severity and extent of myocardial infarction when nitroglycerin and methoxamine are administered during coronary occlusion. Circulation 49:291, 1974

54. **Epstein SE, Kent KM, Goldstein RE, et al:** Reduction of ischemic injury by nitroglycerin during acute myocardial infarction. New Eng J Med 292:29, 1975

55. **Williams DO, Amsterdam EA, Mason DT:** Hemodynamic effects of nitroglycerin in acute myocardial infarction: decrease in ventricular preload at the expense of cardiac output. Circulation 51:421, 1975

56. **Capone R, Mason DT, Amsterdam EA, et al:** A comparison of the action of short and long-action nitrites on the peripheral circulation. Clin Res 20:204, 1972

57. **Franciosa JA, Mikulic E, Cohn JN, et al:** Hemodynamic effects of orally administered isosorbide dinitrate in patients with congestive heart failure. Circulation 50:1020, 1974

58. **Willis WH, Russell RO, Mantle JA, et al:** Hemodynamic response to sublingual isosorbide dinitrate in unstable angina pectoris. Amer J Cardiol 33:179, 1974

59. **Franciosa JA, Guiha NH, Limas CJ, et al:** Improved left ventricular function during nitroprusside infusion in acute myocardial infarction. Lancet 1:650, 1972

60. **Chatterjee K, Parmely WW, Ganz W, et al:** Hemodynamic and metabolic responses to vasodilator therapy in acute myocardial infarction. Circulation 48:1183, 1973

61. **Miller RR, Vismara LA, Zelis R, et al:** Clinical use of sodium nitroprusside in chronic ischemic heart disease. Circulation 51:328, 1975

62. **Williams DO, Hilliard GK, Cantor SA, et al:** Comparative mechanisms of ventricular unloading by systemic vasodilator agents in therapy of cardiac failure: nitroprusside versus phentolamine. Amer J Cardiol 35:177, 1975

63. **Kelly DT, Delgado CE, Taylor DR, et al:** Use of phentolamine in acute myocardial infarction associated with hypertension and left ventricular failure. Circulation 47:729, 1973

64. **Shell WE, Sobel BE:** Protection of jeopardized ischemc myocardium by reduction of ventricular afterload. New Eng J Med 291:481, 1974

65. **Redwood DR, Smith ER, Epstein SE:** Coronary artery occlusion in the conscious dog. Effects of alterations in heart rate and arterial pressure on the degree of myocardial ischemia. Circulation 46:323, 1972

66. **Soroff HS, Cloutier CT, Birtwell WC, et al:** External counterpulsation. JAMA 229:1441, 1974

67. **Maroko PR, Bernstein EF, Libby P, et al:** The effects of intra-aortic balloon counterpulsation on the severity of myocardial ischemic injury following acute coronary occlusion. Counterpulsation and myocardial injury. Circulation 45:1150, 1972

68. **DeLaria GA, Johnsen KH, Sobel BE, et al:** Delayed evolution of myocardial ischemic injury after intra-aortic balloon counterpulsation. Circulation 50 suppl II:242, 1974

69. **O'Rourke MF, Chang VP, Windsor HM, et al:** Acute severe cardiac failure complicating myocardial infarction. Brit Heart J 37:169, 1975

70. **Willerson JT, Curry GC, Watson JT, et al:** Intraaortic balloon counterpulsation in patients in cardiogenic shock, medically refractory left ventricular failure and/or recurrent ventricular tachycardia. Amer J Med 58:183, 1975

71. **Maroko PR, Hale SL, Braunwald E:** The influence of oxygen inhalation on the severity of myocardial ischemic injury following experimental coronary occlusion. Circulation 48 suppl IV:128, 1973

72. **Poliwoda H:** The thrombolytic therapy of acute myocardial infarction. Angiology 17:528, 1966

73. **Maroko PR, Libby P, Ginks WR, et al:** Coronary artery reperfusion. I. Early effects on local myocardial function and the extent of myocardial necrosis. J Clin Invest 51:2710, 1972

74. **Ginks WR, Sybers HD, Maroko PR:** Coronary artery reperfusion. II. Reduction of myocardial infarct size at one week after coronary occlusion. J Clin Invest 51:2717, 1972

75. **Libby P, Maroko PR, Sobel BE, et al:** Reduction of experimental myocardial infarct size by corticosteroid administration. J Clin Invest 52:599, 1973

76. **Maroko PR, Davidson DM, Libby P, et al:** Effects of hyaluronidase administration on myocardial ischemic injury in acute infarction. Ann Intern Med 82:516, 1975

77. **Amsterdam EA, Foley D, Massumi RA, et al:** Influence of increased glucose availability and mannitol on performance of hypoxic myocardium. J Clin Invest 51:4a, 1972

78. **Atkins JM, Wildenthal K, Horwitz LD:** Cardiovascular responses to hyperosmotic mannitol in anesthetized and conscious dogs. Amer J Physiol 225:132, 1973

79. **Willerson JT, Weisfeldt ML, Sanders CA, et al:** Influence of hyperosmolar agents on hypoxic cat papillary muscle function. Cardiovasc Res 8:8, 1974

80. **Hutton I, Marynick SP, Fixler DE, et al:** Changes in regional coronary blood flow with hypertonic mannitol in conscious dogs. Cardiovasc Res 9:47, 1975

81. **Maroko PR, Capenter CB:** Reduction in infarct size following acute coronary occlusion by the administration of cobra venom factor. Clin Res 21:950, 1973

82. **Amsterdam EA, Foley D, Massumi R, et al:** Effects of glucose loading and insulin on myocardial function during experimental hypoxia. Fifth International Congress on Pharmacology, San Francisco, 1972, p 6

83. **Maroko PR, Libby P, Sobel BE, et al:** The effect of glucose-insulin-potassium infusion on myocardial infarction following experimental coronary artery occlusion. Circulation 45:1160, 1972

84. **Sybers HD, Maroko PR, Ashraf M, et al:** The effect of glucose-insulin-potassium on cardiac ultrastructure following acute experimental coronary occlusion. Amer J Pathol 70:401, 1973

85. **Stanley AW, Moraski RE, Russell RO, et al:** Alteration of myocardial fuel and oxygen extraction by glucose-insulin-potassium. Clin Res 22:13A, 1974

86. **Amsterdam EA, Foley D, Massumi RA, et al:** Enhancement of myocardial function during hypoxia by increased glucose availability. Amer J Cardiol 29:251, 1972

87. **Amsterdam EA, Zelis R, Miller RR, et al:** Pathophysiology of angina pectoris. In, Atherosclerosis and Coronary Heart Disease (Likoff W, Segal W, Insull W, et al, ed). New York, Grune & Stratton, 1972, p 178

88. **Amsterdam EA, DeMaria AN, Miller RR, et al:** Intermediate coronary syndrome: clinical and angiographic considerations and results of medical versus surgical therapy. Clin Res 23:76A, 1975

89. **Vatner SF, McRitchie RJ, Maroko PR, et al:** Effects of catecholamines, exercise, and nitroglycerin on the normal and ischemic myocardium in conscious dogs. J Clin Invest 54:563, 1974

90. **Braunwald E, Maroko PR, Davidson S, et al:** Effects of inotropic stimuli on the function of the ischemic myocardium. Thirteenth Annual Meeting of Association of University Cardiologists, Arizona, 1974, p 5

91. **Amsterdam EA, Choquet Y, Lenz J, et al:** Attenuation of positive inotropic action of digitalis by hypoxia and comparison with isoproterenol. Circulation 46:124, 1972

92. **Maroko PR, Libby P, Braunwald E:** Effect of pharmacologic agents on the function of the ischemic heart. Amer J Cardiol 32:930, 1973

93. **Serur JR, Urschel CW:** Attenuation of inotropic interventions by myocardial ischemia. Cardiovasc Res 7:458, 1973

94. **Davidson S, Maroko PR, Braunwald E:** Effects of isoproterenol on contractile function of the ischemic and anoxic heart. Amer J Physiol 227:439, 1974

95. **Amsterdam EA, Zelis R, Kohfeld DB, et al:** Effect of morphine on myocardial contractility: negative inotropic action during hypoxia and reversal by isoproterenol. Circulation 44 suppl II:135, 1971

96. **Mason DT, Spann JF, Zelis R:** New developments in the understanding of the actions of digitalis glycosides. Progr Cardiovasc Dis 11:443, 1969

97. **Mason DT:** Digitalis pharmacology and therapeutics: recent advances. Ann Intern Med 80:520, 1974

98. **Mason DT, Braunwald E:** Studies on digitalis. X. Effects of ouabain on forearm vascular resistance and venous tone in normal subjects and in patients with heart failure. J Clin Invest 43:532, 1964

99. **Beiser GD, Epstein SE, Goldstein RE, et al:** Comparison of the peak inotropic effects of a catecholamine and a digitalis glycoside in the intact canine heart. Circulation 42:805, 1970

100. **Amsterdam EA, Bonanno J, Mansour E, et al:** Effects of dopamine on hemodynamics and myocardial metabolism in patients with coronary artery disease. Clin Res 20:202, 1972

101. **Rosenblum R, Tai AR, Lawson D:** Dopamine in man: cardiorenal hemodynamics in normotensive patients with heart disease. J Pharmacol Exp Ther 183:256, 1972

102. **Holzer J, Karliner JS, O'Rourke RA, et al:** Effectiveness of dopamine in patients with cardiogenic shock.

Amer J Cardiol 32:79, 1973

103. **Goldberg LI:** Dopamine—clinical uses of an endogenous catecholamine. New Eng J Med 291:707, 1974

104. **McNay JL, McDonald RH, Goldberg LI:** Director renal vasodilation produced by dopamine in the dog. Circ Res 16:510, 1965

105. **Rabinowitz B, Parmley WW, Bonnoris G, et al:** Interaction of phentolamine and noradrenaline on myocardial contractility and adenyl cyclase activity. Cardiovasc Res 8:243, 1974

106. **Glick G, Parmley WW, Wechsler AS, et al:** Glucagon—its enhancement of cardiac performance in the cat and dog and persistence of its inotropic action despite beta adrenergic blockade with propranolol. Circ Res 22:789, 1968

107. **Manchester JH, Parmley WW, Matloff JM, et al:** Effects of glucagon on myocardial oxygen consumption and coronary blood flow in man and in dog. Circulation 41:579, 1970

108. **Nord HJ, Fontanes AL, Williams JF:** Treatment of congestive heart failure with glucagon. Ann Intern Med 72:649, 1970

109. **Epstein SE, Levey GS, Skelton CL:** Adenyl cyclase and cyclic AMP. Circulation 43:437, 1971

110. **Hopkins BE, Taylor RR:** Digitalis-induced increase in aortic regurgitation and the contrasting effects of glucagon in the sedated dog. J Clin Invest 53:1716, 1974

111. **Zelis R, Amsterdam EA, Spann JF, et al:** The peripheral vasodilator action of glucagon: an indirect non-adrenergic mechanism. Fed Proc 29:388, 1970

112. **Amsterdam EA, Mansour E, Hughes JL, et al:** Present status of glucagon and bretylium tosylate. In, Changing Concepts in Cardiovascular Disease (Russek H, ed). Baltimore, Williams & Wilkins, 1972, p 215

113. **Parmley WW, Glick G, Sonnenblick EH:** Cardiovascular effects of glucagon in man. New Eng J Med 279:12, 1968

114. **Amsterdam EA, Zelis R, Spann JF, et al:** Aminophylline: effects in isolated cardiac muscle and intact human heart. Circulation 42 suppl III:129, 1970

115. **Marcus ML, Skelton CL, Prindle KH, et al:** Potentiation of the inotropic effects of glucagon by theophylline. J Pharmacol Exp Ther 179:331, 1971

116. **Bodem R, Skelton CL, Sonnenblick EH:** Inotropic and chronotropic effects of dobutamine on isolated cardiac muscle. Europ J Cardiol 2:2:181, 1974

117. **Vatner SF, McRitchie RJ, Braunwald E:** Effects of dobutamine on left ventricular performance, coronary dynamics, and distribution of cardiac output in conscious dogs. J Clin Invest 53:1265, 1974

118. **DeGuzman NT, Pressman BC:** The inotropic effects of the calcium ionophore X-537A in the anesthetized dog. Circulation 49:1072, 1974

119. **Schwartz A, Lewis RM, Hanley HG, et al:** Hemodynamic and biochemical effects of a new positive inotropic agent: antibiotic ionophore RO 2-2985. Circ Res 34:102, 1974

120. **Gunning JF, Harrison CE, Coleman HN:** Myocardial contractility and energetics following treatment with d-thyroxine. Amer J Physiol 226:1166, 1974

121. **Levey GS, Epstein SE:** Myocardial adenyl cyclase: activation by thyroid hormones and evidence for two adenyl cyclase systems. J Clin Invest 48:1663, 1969

122. **Katz AM, Tada M, Repke DE, et al:** Adenylate cyclase: its probable localization in sarcoplasmic reticulum as well as sarcolemma of the canine heart. J Molec Cell Cardiol 6:73, 1974

123. **Finlay GD, Whitsett TL, Cucinell EA, et al:** Augmentation of sodium and potassium excretion, glomerular filtration rate and renal plasma flow by levodopa. New Eng J Med 284:865, 1971

124. **Goldberg LI, Whitsett TL:** Cardiovascular effects of levodopa. Clin Pharmacol Ther 12:376, 1971

125. **Watanabe AM, Parks LC, Kopin IJ:** Modification of the cardiovascular effects of L-dopa by decarboxylase inhibitors. J Clin Invest 50:1322, 1971

126. **Laragh JH:** Diuretics in the management of congestive heart failure. Hosp Pract 5:43, 1970

127. **Vismara LA, Mason DT, Amsterdam EA:** Cardiocirculatory effects of morphine sulfate: mechanisms of action and therapeutic application. Heart and Lung 3:495, 1974

128. **Zelis R, Mansour EJ, Capone RJ, et al:** The cardiovascular effects of morphine. J Clin Invest 54:1247, 1974

129. **Hughes JL, Mansour E, Salel AF, et al:** Elective conversion of atrial fibrillation: relation of energy level, digitalis, and lidocaine to post-shock rhythm. Amer J Cardiol 26:639, 1970

130. **Braunwald E, Ross J, Frommer PL:** Clinical observations on paired electrical stimulation of the heart: effects on ventricular performance and heart rate. Amer J Med 37:700, 1964

131. **Wood P:** Polyuria in paroxysmal tachycardia and paroxysmal atrial flutter and fibrillation. Brit Heart J 25:273, 1963

132. **Mason DT, Bartter FC:** Autonomic regulation of blood volume. Anesthesiology 29:681, 1968

133. **Majid PA, Sharma B, Taylow SH:** Phentolamine for vasodilator treatment of severe heart failure. Lancet 2:719, 1971

134. **Walinshy P, Chatterjee K, Forrester J, et al:** Enhanced left ventricular performance with phentolamine in acute myocardial infarction. Amer J Cardiol 33:37, 1974

135. **Guiha NH, Cohn JN, Mikulic E, et al:** Treatment of refractory heart failure with infusion of nitroprusside. New Eng J Med 291:587, 1974

136. **Schlant RC, Tsagaris TS, Robertson RJ:** Studies on the acute cardiovascular effects of intravenous sodium nitroprusside. Amer J Cardiol 9:51, 1962

137. **Chatterjee K, Parmley WW, Swan HJC, et al:** Beneficial effects of vasodilator agents in severe mitral regurgitation due to dysfunction of subvalvular apparatus. Circulation 48:684, 1973

138. **Cohn JN:** Blood pressure and cardiac performance. Amer J Med 55:351, 1973

139. **Martinez-Maldonado M, Kurtzman NA, Rector FC, et al:** Evidence for a hormonal inhibitor of proximal tubular readsorption. J Clin Invest 46:1091, 1967

140. **Carpenter CE, Davis JO, Wallace CR, et al:** Acute effects of cardiac glycosides on aldosterone secretion in dogs with hyperaldosteronism secondary to chronic right heart failure. Circ Res 10:178, 1962

141. **Bartter FC, Schwartz WB:** The syndrome of inappro-

priate secretion of antidiuretic hormone. Amer J Med 42:790, 1967

142. **Laragh JH, Heinemann HO, Demartini FE:** Effect of chlorothiazide on electrolyte transport in man. Its use in the treatment of edema of congestive heart failure, nephrosis, and cirrhosis. JAMA 166:145, 1958

143. **Cannon PJ, Heinemann HO, Stason WB, et al:** Ethacrynic acic. Effectiveness and mode of diuretic action in man. Circulation 31:5, 1965

144. **Stason WB, Cannon PJ, Heinemann HO, et al:** Furosemide, a clinical evaluation of its diuretic action. Circulation 34:910, 1966

145. **Clark DA, Stinson EB, Griepp RB, et al:** Cardiac transplantation in man. VI. Prognosis of patients selected for cardiac transplantation. Ann Intern Med 75:15, 1971

146. **Griepp, RB, Stinson EB, Doug E, et al:** Acute rejection of the allografted human heart: diagnosis and treatment. Ann Thorac Surg 12:113, 1971

147. **Grahan AF, Schroeder JS, Griepp RB, et al:** Does cardiac transplantation significantly prolong life and improve its quality? Circulation 53 suppl III:116, 1973

148. **Kantrowitz A, Krahauer JS, Butner AM:** Phase-shift balloon pumping in cardiogenic shock. Prog Cardiovasc Dis 12:293, 1969

149. **Soroff HS, Cloutier CT, Birtwell WC, et al:** Clinical evaluation of external counterpulsation in cardiogenic shock. Circulation 45 suppl II:75, 1972

150. **Mueller H, Giannelli S, Ayres SM:** Mechanical cardiac assistance in shock following acute myocardial infarction. In, Ref 16, p 229

Chapter 19

New Developments and Therapeutic Applications of Cardiac Stimulating Agents

John F. Williams, Jr, MD, FACC

It is evident from this monograph that our knowledge of the biochemistry and physiology of heart failure has advanced considerably in recent years. Unfortunately, the development of pharmacologic agents with clinically useful positive inotropic cardiac effects has not kept pace. Digitalis glycosides, catecholamines and glucagon remain the only drugs with more than limited therapeutic usefulness, and only the glycosides can be used for more than brief periods. Nevertheless, continued interest in the pharmacodynamics of these agents and further studies of their effects in various cardiac disorders have provided new information that has significantly improved techniques for using them in patients with heart failure.

Digitalis Glycosides

The development of methods for accurately measuring the concentration of digitalis glycosides and their metabolites in various tissues and fluids has permitted a major expansion in the understanding of glycoside metabolism, actions and uses. Since available evidence indicates that the only differences in cardiac effects among glycosides are those attributable to differences in rates of absorption, metabolism and excretion, this discussion will be limited to the most commonly used glycosides, digitoxin and digoxin.

Absorption, Metabolism, Excretion: Both digoxin[1] and digitoxin[2] apparently are absorbed from the gastrointestinal tract by a passive, nonsaturable transport process. Digoxin is absorbed primarily in the proximal small intestine, whereas digitoxin is absorbed equally well from the proximal and distal small bowel.[2] Digoxin is not bound significantly to serum proteins, does not undergo extensive enterohepatic recycling or metabolism by the liver and is excreted primarily unchanged by the kidneys.[3] A maximum of 80 to 90 percent of a given dose of digoxin can be absorbed,[3] but preparations of different manufacturers vary greatly in the extent to which they are absorbed.[5] Digitoxin is completely absorbed, tightly bound to serum proteins, has a significant enterohepatic circulation and undergoes metabolic degradation primarily by the liver.[3] Of the absorbed digitoxin, approximately 8 percent is converted to digoxin and 30 percent is excreted unchanged; the remainder is degraded to metabolites of lesser biological activity that are excreted by the kidneys.[4] The extensive enterohepatic circulation and serum protein binding of digitoxin are thought to contribute to its longer duration of action; its serum half-life is approximately three times that of digoxin.[3] Interruption of this recirculation by the use of cholestyramine can reduce both serum levels and inotropic effects in man,[6] an observation with obvious therapeutic implications.

Renal dysfunction has a more significant effect on digoxin kinetics than on digitoxin kinetics,[4] and chronic liver disease has an insignificant effect on digoxin metabolism.[7] Sur-

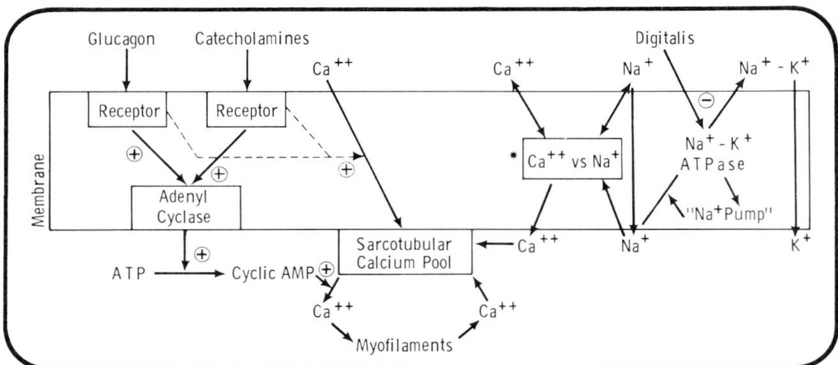

FIGURE 1. Proposed mechanisms by which glucagon catecholamines and digitalis glycosides produce their positive inotropic cardiac effects. AMP = adenosine monophosphate; ATP = adenosine triphosphate; Ca^{++} = calcium; K^+ = potassium; Na^+ = sodium; Na^+-K^+ ATPase = sodium-potassium-activated adenosine triphosphatase; *indicates sites for which Ca^{++} and Na^+ are in competition; + and − indicate positive and negative modifications, respectively, of the particular process.

prisingly, the effect of hepatic dysfunction on digitoxin metabolism has not been clearly defined.

Mechanisms of Action: The myocardial binding site of the glycosides has not been determined conclusively, but it may be the transverse tubular system of the sarcoplasmic reticulum.[8] It is clear that the glycosides do not exert their positive inotropic effects by releasing myocardial catecholamines or stimulating beta adrenergic receptors.[9] Schwartz and co-workers[10] have presented evidence that the inotropic effect is related to the inhibition of sodium- and potassium-activated adenosine triphosphatase (Na^+,K^+–ATPase) (Figure 1). Inhibition of this enzyme reduces Na^+ pumping and results in an increase in intracellular Na^+. Intracellular Na^+ and Ca^{++} compete for binding sites; thus, the increment in Na^+ results in an increase in intracellular Ca^{++}. Langer[11] recently discussed the role of ionic factors in the intrinsic control of myocardial contraction and the importance of intracellular Ca^{++} in coupling excitation to contraction. The observation that a significant correlation exists between the inhibition of this enzyme and the increase in cardiac contractile force following glycoside administration[12] supports this proposed mechanism of action.

Clinical Use: Recent studies have altered understanding of the loading dose of digoxin and digitoxin. Jelliffe et al.[4,13] have reported that patients given effective maintenance doses of these agents had, after equilibrium had been attained, total body stores that were significantly smaller than the commonly used loading doses. This finding indicates that much of the loading dose must be excreted. Thus, a loading dose smaller than that ordinarily administered should be as effective and less hazardous to the patient. In fact, loading doses are not always necessary. In one study, patients who received maintenance doses of digoxin for 6 to 7 days, without a previous loading dose, had serum levels and calculated total body stores equal to those of patients who received a loading dose followed by a comparable maintenance dose.[14] Therefore, the decision to employ a loading dose should be based primarily on how quickly one wishes to obtain a therapeutic effect. In view of the data just cited, doses currently recommended for the inotropic effect of digoxin and digitoxin are presented in Table I. These are average doses that may be affected by many factors, particularly the ability of the kidneys to excrete the glycosides. On the basis of kinetic studies, Jelliffe and co-workers have constructed graphs that relate maintenance doses of digoxin[13] and digitoxin[4] to creatinine clearance. With these graphs, appropriate adjustments in glycoside dosage can be made for patients with renal dysfunction.

Understanding of the indications for the administration of the glycosides has advanced little in recent years. It is still not known whether the administration of digitalis to patients with heart disease will retard development of the clinical manifestations of heart failure, although results of animal studies[15] suggest that it may. The routine use of glycosides in the treatment of various forms of shock thought to be associated with acute pump failure also cannot be condemned or supported on the basis of existing evidence. However, recent studies suggest caution in the use of glycosides in patients with coronary atherosclerosis unless heart failure exists. The glycosides increase myocardial oxygen requirements by their positive inotropic action in both the failing and nonfailing heart. In the former condition, a reduction in ventricular volume and wall tension may also occur, whereas little change may occur in the nonfailing heart. Since ventricular wall tension is a major determinant of myocardial oxygen consumption, the glycosides may not affect the oxygen requirement in the failing heart but increase it in the nonfailing heart.[16] The potential significance of this observation is emphasized by the report[17] that an increase in both the magnitude and extent of ischemia occurred after administration of ouabain to animals with acute coronary artery occlusion.

Toxicity: Since the subject of glycoside toxicity recently has been reviewed,[18] this discussion will be limited to a recent advance in means of diagnosis—the measurement of serum concentrations of the glycosides. Smith and Haber[19] and Doherty[20] have discussed the different methods available for measuring the minute quantities of circulating glycosides and their clinical application. The radioimmunoassay technique, which is sensitive and specific and can be performed relatively rapidly, is currently the most widely used method. Although determination of serum levels is helpful in determining whether a given arrhythmia is digitalis-induced, no sharp separation exists between toxic and nontoxic levels. Smith[21] observed serum levels of 26 ng/ml or more in all six patients with evidence of digitoxin toxicity, whereas similar values were found in 17 percent of patients without toxicity. Ninety percent of patients who were receiving digoxin and had no evidence of toxicity had serum levels of 2.0 ng/ml or less, whereas 87 percent of patients with definite evidence of toxicity had values ex-

TABLE I

***Average* Recommended Oral Doses of Glycosides**

	Loading	Maintenance	No Loading
Digoxin	1.0-1.5 mg in 24 hours	0.25-0.5 mg	0.25-0.5 mg (6 to 8 days)
Digitoxin	1.0-1.5 mg in 24-72 hours	0.1-0.15 mg	0.1-0.15 mg (25 to 30 days)

( ) = number of days required for body stores to attain kinetic equilibrium.

ceeding 2.0 ng/ml.[22] Unfortunately, the serum values in patients without toxicity and in those with equivocal evidence of toxicity demonstrated considerably more overlap, and the latter patients pose the more difficult problem.

It should not be surprising that one cannot use the serum levels of glycosides to separate clearly patients with toxic and nontoxic conditions. Although a linear relation normally exists between serum levels and myocardial content of the glycoside after equilibration,[23] alterations in this ratio can occur.[19] More importantly, there is significant individual variation in "sensitivity" of the myocardium to the action of the glycosides. The failure to observe a significant correlation between serum levels of digoxin and the ventricular rate in a large series of patients with atrial fibrillation further emphasizes this clinically well known fact.[24]

The development of digitalis antibodies, which are necessary in the radioimmunoassay of the glycosides, has opened another potentially fruitful area of research. Reversal of digoxin-induced arrhythmias by administration of specific antibodies has now been demonstrated in the dog.[25]

Catecholamines

Norepinephrine, epinephrine and isoproterenol are widely used cardiac stimulating agents, whereas dopamine, the immediate precursor of norepinephrine, is currently undergoing clinical trials.

Mechanism of Action: Our understanding of the mechanism of action of the catecholamines results largely from the pioneering work of Ahlquist,[26] who devised a functional definition of adrenergic receptors, and of Sutherland et al.,[27] who found that cyclic adenosine monophosphate (cyclic AMP) serves as the intracellular mediator of hormone action. The role of cyclic AMP and Ca^{++} in cellular responses[28] and, specifically, their role in mediating the cardiac effects of the catecholamines[29] have been reviewed recently. Our present concept of this latter role is illustrated in Figure 1 and can be summarized as follows: In the heart, catecholamines combine with a beta adrenergic receptor that activates adenyl cyclase and increases the conversion of adenosine triphosphate (ATP) to cyclic AMP. Cyclic AMP enhances the mobilization of Ca^{++} from sarcotubular stores, thereby augmenting myocardial contraction. In addition, there is evidence that the interaction of the catecholamines with their receptor may increase the permeability of the cell membrane to Ca^{++}.[28] A critical step in this concept, the demonstration that cyclic AMP augments myocardial contractility, was not previously possible since cyclic AMP does not readily cross cell membranes. However, by administering cyclic AMP with dimethylsulfoxide, Kjekshus et al.[30] were recently able to obtain an intracellular effect of cyclic AMP in the perfused guinea pig heart, as evidenced by an increase in phosphorylase activation. No increase in myocardial contractility was observed. These investigators postulate that catecholamines activate adenyl cyclase, which results in conversion of membrane-bound ATP to cyclic AMP with release of Ca^{++} from a Ca^{++}-membrane-ATP complex. The augmentation of myocardial contractility results from an increase in intracellular Ca^{++} but one that is not produced by cyclic AMP.

Clinical Uses: Catecholamines obviously have a limited role in the treatment of patients with chronic heart failure. Their major use is in the treatment of conditions thought to be produced by or associated with acute pump failure, such as low cardiac output state after cardiac surgery and shock associated with sepsis or acute myocardial infarction. Although isoproterenol is probably the most commonly used cardiac stimulating agent in the treatment of post-surgical low output states and septic shock, there is considerable disagreement as to which sympathomimetic agent should be employed

initially in the treatment of shock after myocardial infarction. This controversy involves primarily the use of norepinephrine or isoproterenol and has arisen principally from theoretical considerations based on the opposite effects these agents have on peripheral resistance vessels. Recently Maroko et al.[17] observed that isoproterenol increased the magnitude and extent of ischemia in animals with acute coronary arterial occlusion, whereas the pure alpha stimulator methoxamine reduced ischemia by increasing arterial pressure. This observation does not indicate that methoxamine is the drug of choice in the treatment of shock after myocardial infarction, but it further emphasizes the urgency of maintaining coronary perfusion pressure in this condition, particularly when administering agents that augment myocardial oxygen consumption. For similar reasons, caution has been suggested when using isoproterenol in the treatment of hypotension associated with massive pulmonary embolism. Increments in pulmonary arterial obstruction in the dog resulted in a corresponding decline in right ventricular function that was much more pronounced in animals with a restricted blood supply to the right ventricle. In contrast, if the coronary vessels supplying the right ventricle were hyperperfused, right ventricular dysfunction was reversed.[31] Results of clinical studies in patients with shock after myocardial infarction are not conclusive, but the trend appears to be toward use of agents with combined alpha and beta adrenergic stimulating actions.[32,33]

The role of dopamine in the treatment of pump failure in man is only now being defined. Dopamine does have theoretical advantages over other catecholamines in that, in addition to its stimulating actions on alpha and beta adrenergic receptors, it also produces nonadrenergically mediated vasodilatation in mesenteric[34] and renal vascular[35] beds. Loeb et al.[36] demonstrated hemodynamic improvement during infusion of dopamine in patients with cardiogenic shock due to various causes or shock due to infection. Their study also compared the effect of dopamine on hemodynamics and urinary flow rates with the effects of isoproterenol or norepinephrine in the same patients. An obvious superiority of dopamine over the other agents was not apparent. However, in general, dopamine produced a comparable or greater increase in urinary flow, whereas its effect on cardiac output was intermediate; the greatest increase occurred with isoproterenol. The results were similar in patients with cardiogenic shock or sepsis. In patients with cardiogenic shock, too few measurements of left ventricular end-diastolic pressure were made for a meaningful interpretation. In patients with septic shock, the highest level of left ventricular end-diastolic pressure occurred with norepinephrine, the lowest with isproterenol and intermediate levels with dopamine.

Glucagon

Since Farah and Tuttle[37] first described the positive inotropic cardiac effects of glucagon, there has been considerable interest in the possible role of this agent in the treatment of heart disease in man.

Mechanism of Action: The effect of glucagon on adenyl cyclase, cyclic AMP and intracellular calcium in the heart is similar to that of catecholamines,[29] but these hormones have a different receptor[38] (Figure 1). Glucagon stimulates catecholamine release. What role, if any, this action plays in the inotropic response in man has not been determined, although it is clearly not the sole factor responsible for the effect of glucagon in animals.[38]

Clinical Use: The early clinical studies with glucagon were encouraging because improvement in cardiac performance was observed without significant adverse effects.[39,40] However, subsequent studies indicated that the clinical role of glucagon as a cardiac stimulating agent will be limited. Glucagon is relatively ineffective in patients with chronic congestive heart failure.[41] It has been shown experimentally that under such conditions glucagon does not activate adenyl cyclase or produce a positive inotropic effect.[42] Current evidence suggests that increasing duration and severity of the heart disease may adversely effect the response to glucagon.[41,43] Catecholamines activate adenyl cyclase and increase contractility in chronically failing hearts unresponsive to glucagon.[42] Furthermore, compared with glucagon, isoproterenol produces greater increments in cardiac output and greater reductions in left ventricular end-diastolic pressure in patients with heart disease. However, glucagon may have a role in the treatment of acute heart failure. A positive inotropic effect and improvement in pump function have been demonstrated in patients with low cardiac output after cardiac surgery[44] and in those with heart failure after acute myocardial infarction.[45] In addition, the administration of glucagon under these conditions may permit the use of smaller amounts of more potent inotropic agents, thereby reducing the frequency of adverse effects from the latter. The persistence of cardiac effects after beta adrenergic blockade suggests that glucagon might be of benefit in patients with cardiotoxicity due to propranolol.

Although cardiac arrhythmias have not been reported after administration of glucagon in human, no systematic studies of the electrophysiologic effects of glucagon in patients with heart disease have been reported. Therefore we recently undertook such a study in patients with impaired impulse formation or conduction.[46] Single intravenous injections of 5 mg of glucagon in patients with complete heart block have produced no significant effects on ventricular or nodal automaticity or on the threshold for ventricular stimulation. Glucagon also did not affect atrioventricular conduction in patients with first or second degree heart block or atrial fibrillation. These findings suggest that glucagon also may be of value in some patients with congestive heart failure and digitalis-induced arrhythmias.

None of the presently available cardiac stimulating agents approach the ideal for the treatment of patients with myocardial dysfunction, and greater emphasis is needed on the development of such drugs. In the meantime, studies to further refine and define the use of currently available agents must continue.

Summary

Digitalis glycosides, catecholamines and glucagon remain the only cardiac stimulating drugs with significant therapeutic use. Considerable information is now available concerning the metabolism of absorption and excretion of the glycosides and the mechanism by which these drugs produce their cardiac effects. Such information has resulted in major modification in the use of loading doses. The role of serum assays in the diagnosis of digitalis toxicity has been more clearly defined, and recent studies have demonstrated conditions in which the use of the glycosides may be hazardous.

The pathways by which the catecholamines produce their positive inotropic effects have been further delineated. Controversy continues as to which sympathomimetic agent is the drug of choice in patients with shock associated with acute pump failure. Dopamine has actions that theoretically make it superior to other catecholamines, and initial clinical studies with this agent are encouraging.

Results of both experimental and clinical studies indicate that the major role of glucagon is as an adjunct to other agents in the treatment of acute pump failure. In addition, theoretical considerations suggest that glucagon may be beneficial in some patients with congestive heart failure and digitalis toxicity or in patients with cardiotoxicity caused by beta receptor blocking agents.

References

1. **Caldwell JH, Martin JF, Dutta S, et al:** Intestinal absorption of digoxin-^{3}H in the rat. Amer J Physiol 217:1747, 1969
2. **Greenberger NJ, MacDermott RP, Martin JF, et al:** Intestinal absorption of six tritium-labeled digitalis glycosides in rats and guinea pigs. J Pharmacol Exp Ther 167:265, 1969
3. **Doherty JE, Hall WH, Murphy ML, et al:** New information regarding digitalis metabolism. Chest 59:433, 1971
4. **Jelliffe RW, Buell J, Kalaba R, et al:** An improved method of digitoxin therapy. Ann Intern Med 72:453, 1970
5. **Lindenbaum J, Mellow MH, Blackstone MO, et al:** Variation in biologic availability of digoxin from four preparations. New Eng J Med 285:1344, 1971
6. **Caldwell JH, Bush CA, Greenberger NJ:** Interruption of the enterohepatic circulation of digitoxin by cholestyramine. II. Effect on metabolic disposition of tritium-labeled digitoxin and cardiac systolic intervals in man. J Clin Invest 50:2638, 1971
7. **Marcus FI, Kapadia GG:** The metabolism of tritiated digoxin in cirrhotic patients. Gastroenterology 47:517, 1964
8. **Sonnenblick EH, Spotnitz HM, Spiro D:** Role of the sarcomere in ventricular function and the mechanism of heart failure. Circ Res 15 suppl II:70, 1964
9. **Koch-Weser J:** Beta-receptor blockade and myocardial effect of cardiac glycosides. Circ Res 28:109, 1971
10. **Schwartz A, Allen JC, Harigaya S:** Possible involvement of cardiac Na$^+$, K$^+$-adenosine triphosphatase in the mechanism of action of cardiac glycosides. J Pharmacol Exp Ther 168:31, 1969
11. **Langer GA:** The intrinsic control of myocardial contraction-ionic factors. New Eng J Med 285:1065, 1971
12. **Akera T, Larsen FS, Brody TM:** Correlation of cardiac sodium and potassium-activated adenosine triphosphatase activity with ouabain-induced inotropic stimulation. J Pharmacol Exp Ther 173:145, 1970
13. **Jelliffe RW:** An improved method of digoxin therapy. Ann Intern Med 69:703, 1968
14. **Marcus FI, Burkhalter L, Cuccia C, et al:** Administration of tritiated digoxin with and without a loading dose. A metabolic study. Circulation 34:865, 1966
15. **Williams JF Jr, Braunwald E:** Studies on digitalis. XI. Effects of digitoxin on the development of cardiac hypertrophy in the rat subjected to aortic constriction. Amer J Cardiol 16:534, 1965
16. **Covell JW, Braunwald E, Ross J Jr, et al:** Studies on digitalis. XVI. Effects on myocardial oxygen consumption. J Clin Invest 45:1535, 1966
17. **Maroko PR, Kjekshus JK, Sobel BE, et al:** Factors influencing infarct size following experimental coronary artery occlusion. Circulation 43:67, 1971
18. **Mason DT, Zelis R, Lee G, et al:** Current concepts and treatment of digitalis toxicity. Amer J Cardiol 27:546, 1971
19. **Smith TW, Haber E:** Current techniques for serum or plasma digitalis assay and their potential clinical application. Amer J Med Sci 259:301, 1970
20. **Doherty JE:** Digitalis serum levels: clinical use. Ann Intern Med 74:787, 1971
21. **Smith TW:** Radioimmunossay for serum digitoxin concentration: methodology and clinical experience. J Pharmacol Exp Ther 175:352, 1970
22. **Smith TW, Haber E:** Digoxin intoxication: the relationship of clinical presentation to serum digoxin concentration. J Clin Invest 49:2377, 1970
23. **Doherty JE, Perkins WH, Flanigan WJ:** The distribution and concentration of tritiated digoxin in human tissues. Ann Intern Med 66:116, 1967
24. **Chamberlain MJ, White RJ, Howard MR, et al:** Plasma digoxin concentrations in patients with atrial fibrillation. Brit Med J 3:429, 1970
25. **Schmidt DH, Butler VP:** Reversal of digoxin toxicity with specific antibodies. J Clin Invest 50:1738, 1971
26. **Ahlquist RP:** Study of adrenotropic receptors. Amer J Physiol 153:586, 1948
27. **Sutherland EW, Robison GA:** The role of cyclic-3,5'-AMP in responses to catecholamines and other hormones. Pharmacol Rev 18:145, 1966

28. **Rasmussen H:** Cell communication, calcium ion, and cyclic adenosine monophosphate. Science 170:404, 1970

29. **Epstein SE, Skelton CL, Levey GS, et al:** Adenyl cyclase and myocarcial contractility. Ann Intern Med 72:561, 1970

30. **Kjekshus JK, Henry PD, Sobel BE:** Activation of phosphorylase by cyclic AMP without augmentation of contractility in the perfused guinea pig heart. Circ Res 29:468, 1971

31. **Brooks H, Kirk ES, Vokonas PS, et al:** Performance of the right ventricle under stress: relation to right coronary flow. J Clin Invest 50:2176, 1971

32. **Shubin H, Weil MH:** Practical considerations in the management of shock complicating acute myocardial infarction. Amer J Cardiol 26:603, 1970

33. **Kuhn LA:** Shock in myocardial infarction—medical treatment. Amer J Cardiol 26:578, 1970

34. **Eble JN:** A proposed mechanism for the depressor effect of dopamine in the anesthetized dog. J Pharmacol Exp Ther 145:64, 1964

35. **McNay JL, Goldberg LI:** Comparison of the effects of dopamine, isoproterenol, norepinephrine and bradykinin on canine renal and femoral blood flow. J Pharmacol Exp Ther 151:23, 1966

36. **Loeb HS, Winslow EBJ, Rahimtoola SH, et al:** Acute hemodynamic effects of dopamine in patients with shock. Circulation 44:163, 1971

37. **Farah A, Tuttle R:** Studies on the pharmacology of glucagon. J Pharmacol Exp Ther 129:49, 1960

38. **Glick G. Parmley WW, Wechsler AS:** Glucagon: its enhancement of cardiac performance in the cat and dog and persistence of its inotropic action despite beta receptor blockade with propranolol. Circ Res 22:789, 1968

39. **Parmley WW, Glick G, Sonnenblick EH:** Cardiovascular effects of glucagon in man. New Eng J Med 279: 12, 1968

40. **Williams JF Jr, Childress RH, Chip JN, et al:** Hemodynamic effects of glucagon in patients with heart disease. Circulation 39:38, 1969

41. **Nord HJ, Fontanes AL, Williams JF Jr:** Treatment of congestive heart failure with glucagon. Ann Intern Med 72:649, 1970

42. **Gold HK, Prindle KH, Levey GS, et al:** Effects of experimental heart failure on the capacity of glucagon to augment myocardial contractility and activate adenyl cylcase. J Clin Invest 49:999, 1970

43. **Armstrong PW, Gold HK, Daggett WM, et al:** Hemodynamic evaluation of glucagon in symptomatic heart disease. Circulation 44:67, 1971

44. **Parmley WW, Matloff JM, Sonnenblick EH:** Hemodynamic effects of glucagon in patients following prosthetic valve replacement. Circulation 39 suppl I:163, 1969

45. **Diamond G, Forrester J, Danzig R, et al:** Acute myocardial infarction in man. Comparative hemodynamic effects of norepinephrine and glucagon. Amer J Carciol 27:612, 1971

46. **Nishimura A, Fortner RB, Williams JF Jr:** Effect of glucagon on automaticity, threshold for stimulation and junctional conduction in patients with impaired impulse formation or conduction. Amer Heart J 84:359, 1972

Chapter 20

Digitalis Glycosides
Clinical Pharmacology and Therapeutics

Dean T. Mason, MD, FACC
Ezra A. Amsterdam, MD, FACC
Garrett Lee, MD

For nearly two centuries, the digitalis glycosides have been employed widely in clinical medicine as the principal drug in the treatment of congestive heart failure. Although certain aspects of these agents continue to excite controversy, many important advances in the past few years have considerably improved our understanding of their physiologic and subcellular mechanisms of action, their pharmacodynamics and their application in patients. This chapter focuses attention on those recent findings that are of particular significance to the clinician in affording a more rational use of these agents.

Cardiotonic Action

It is now well founded that the beneficial effects of digitalis in patients with congestive heart failure result from its direct stimulation of depressed contractile state.[1-4] Digitalis augments the low cardiac output and reduces the elevated ventricular end-diastolic pressure of the dysfunctioning heart, as depicted by the series of ventricular function curves in Figure 1 relating a performance characteristic of the heart—in this example, stroke work—to ventricular filling pressure. The steepest curve (on the left) represents normal cardiac performance. With decline of contractility—the fundamental disturbance of the failing myocardium[5,6]—ven-

tricular function becomes depressed as shown by the lowest curve (on the right). At normal end-diastolic pressure, the failing heart is unable to deliver adequate cardiac output. Therefore, the ventricle must dilate to operate at an abnormally high filling pressure (point A) to pump a normal cardiac output, the level of which is indicated by the horizontal broken line. With the administration of digitalis, the positive inotropic action of the drug raises ventricular function toward normal, shown by the intermediate ventricular function curve in Figure 1. Thus, the glycoside improves the fundamental physiologic defect causing ventricular failure—depressed contractility[5,6]—and this increase in contractile state allows less Frank-Starling preload compensation, so that a normal cardiac output can be delivered at a substantially lower ventricular filling pressure (point B).

Although there is now general agreement that digitalis stimulates the force of contraction of the failing myocardium, there has been considerable confusion concerning its effects on the nonfailing heart. This problem has been resolved by the demonstration that the glycoside directly elevates the contractile state of the normal ventricle,[7-10] although the increased contractile state is not translated into an increase in cardiac output. In Figure 2, high-fidelity recordings of left ventricular pressure and its simulta-

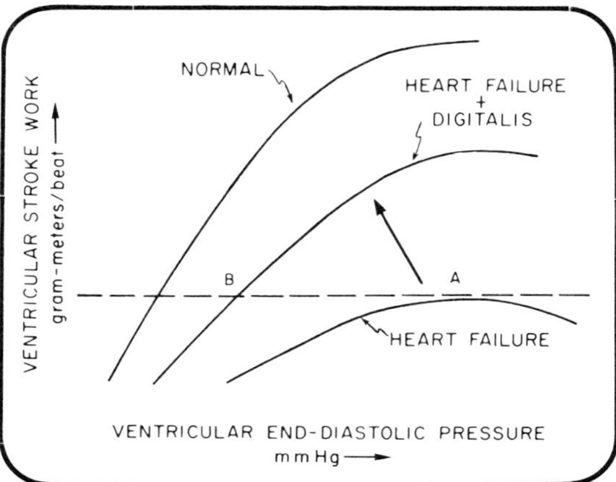

FIGURE 1. Effects of digitalis on ventricular function. In the heart failure state, the work capacity of the myocardium at any given end-diastolic volume or pressure is diminished. Digitalis results in a shift of this abnormal ventricular function curve upwards and to the left (**arrow**), indicating that the drug increases the force of systolic ejection and thus cardiac contractility. Therefore, as a result of the more forceful contraction and augmented work capacity provided by digitalis, the residual systolic blood volume is reduced and end-diastolic pressure is correspondingly diminished; the same stroke work can be delivered from a markedly lowered filling pressure—point B in contrast to point A.

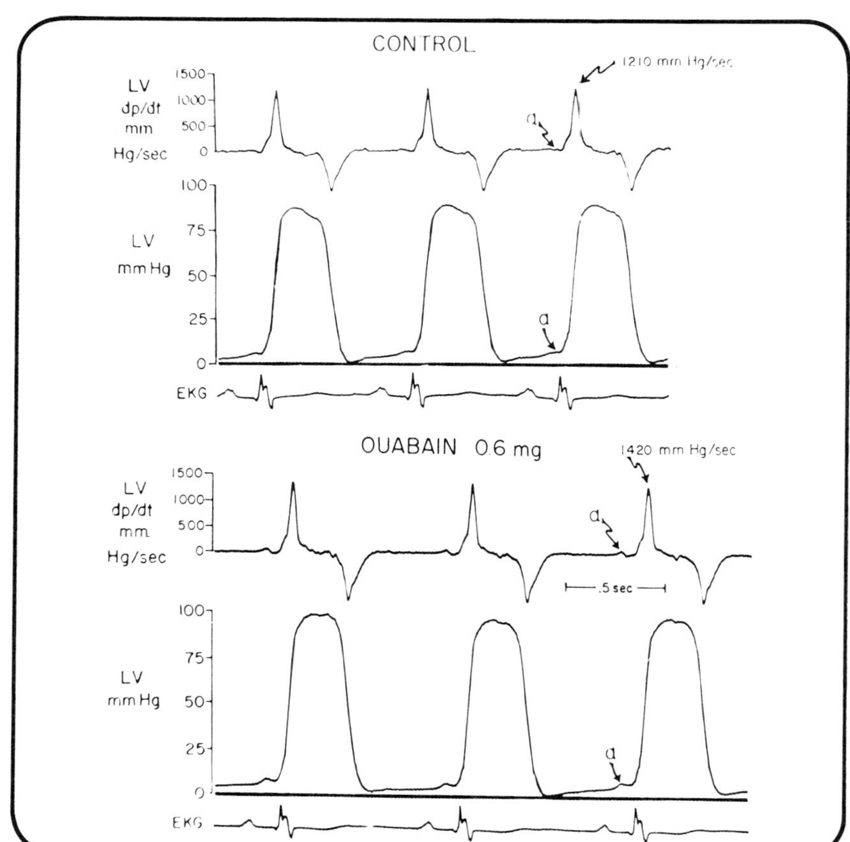

FIGURE 2. Simultaneous high-fidelity recordings of left ventricular (LV) pressure and its rate of pressure change (dp/dt) during the control period (**top**) and 30 minutes after the administration of 0.6 mg of ouabain (**bottom**) in a patient with normal left heart function; a = accentuation of LV late-diastolic pressure by left atrial contraction. After ouabain, the a deflection was increased thereby suggesting that ouabain also improved the strength of left atrial contraction. (Reprinted by permission from Mason et al.[8])

neous rate of pressure change (dp/dt) are shown before and after administration of ouabain in a patient with normal cardiac performance. Ouabain increased left ventricular peak dp/dt, signifying that digitalis augments contractility of normal heart muscle since the loading variables influencing peak dp/dt of end-diastolic pressure and arterial diastolic pressure remained constant.[10]

In addition to stimulation of ventricular contractility, digitalis also directly increases the force of contraction of the atrial myocardium.[11] Augmentation of left atrial contractility by ouabain is shown in Figure 3 in a patient with pure mitral stenosis in normal sinus rhythm. Left atrial pressure and its dp/dt are illustrated before (top) and after administration of the drug (bottom). After ouabain, the height, amplitude and rate of rise of the atrial contraction wave (a) and corresponding dp/dt (arrow) are augmented, indicating that the agent stimulates the inotropic state of the atrium.

From these observations concerning the direct stimulating action of digitalis on normal and diseased ventricular and atrial myocardium, it is apparent that the glycosides exert the same fundamental contractile action on both normal and failing hearts. Therefore, the notion held previously that the drug has a harmful inotropic effect on the nonfailing ventricle can no longer be maintained.

Vasoconstrictor Action

The observation that the digitalis-induced increase in contractility in the normal heart does not result in a rise in cardiac output suggests possible extracardiac vascular effects of the glycosides.[12] As shown in Figure 4, intravenous ouabain in a normal subject caused a rise in mean blood pressure, a decrease in forearm blood flow measured plethysmographically, an elevation of forearm vascular resistance and an increase in forearm venous tone, whereas total peripheral vascular resistance rose and cardiac output fell slightly. Thus, digitalis exerts a moderate direct constrictor action on peripheral arterial and venous smooth muscle.[13]

After consideration of the direct cardiac and peripheral vascular actions of digitalis, it is possible to synthesize the overall effects of

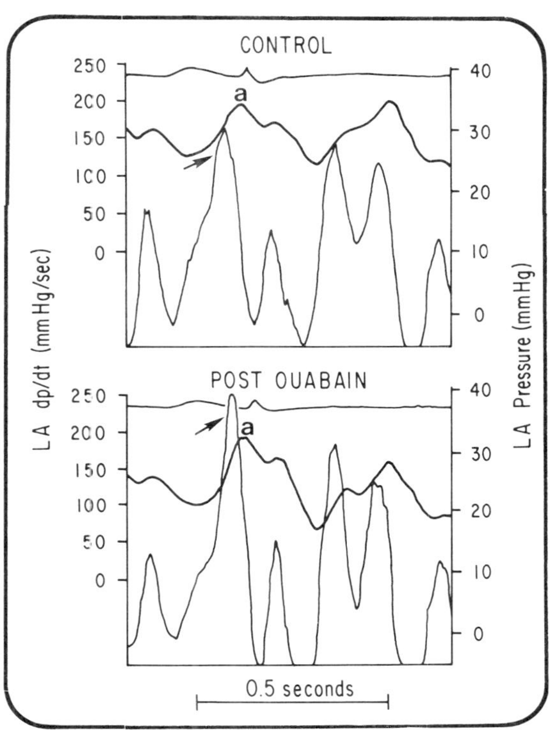

FIGURE 3. Simultaneous high-fidelity recordings of left atrial (LA) pressure and its pressure change (dp/dt) during the control period (**top**) and after intravenous administration of digitalis (**bottom**) in a patient with mitral stenosis and normal sinus rhythm. In both panels, phasic LA pressure is the top tracing and LA dp/dt the bottom recording.

the agent on the pump function of the normal heart.[3,4,12] The normal cardiocirculation is illustrated in Figure 5. The positive inotropic action of digitalis is not observed as an increase in cardiac output, since the elevated contractile force is opposed by increased impedance to ventricular ejection resulting from the digitalis-induced peripheral arteriolar constriction.[13] Thus, the increase in ventricular afterload may mask or override the cardiotonic effect of the glycoside in the normal heart, resulting in no change or even a slight decline in cardiac output.

Cardiocirculatory Effects

In Heart Failure: In contrast to its effects in the normal heart, digitalis results in an overall reduction of peripheral vasoconstriction in

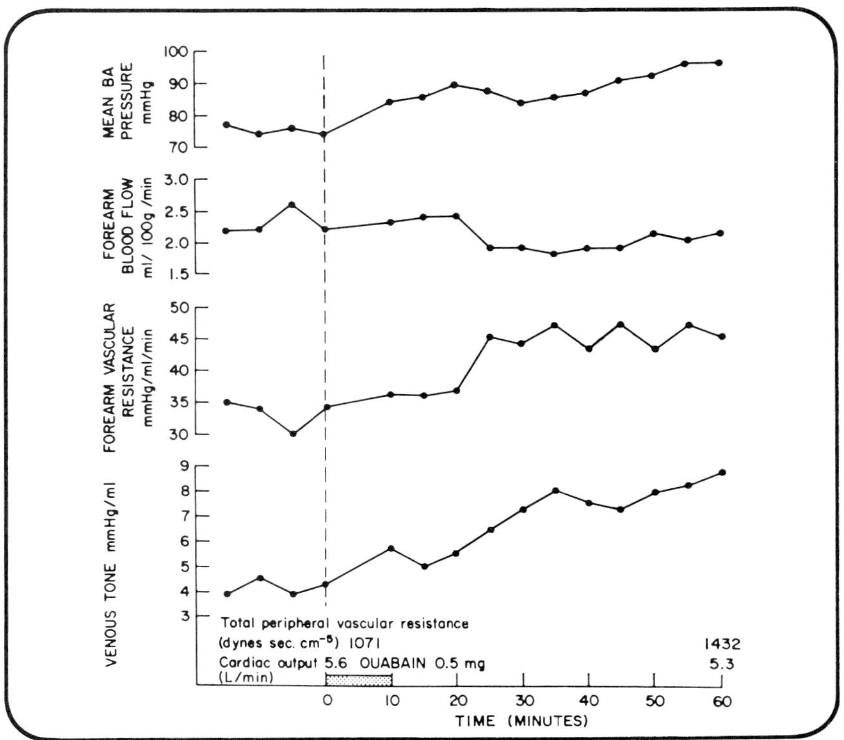

FIGURE 4. Serial determinations of brachial arterial pressure (BA), forearm blood flow, forearm vascular resistance and venous tone, cardiac output and systemic vascular resistance before and after ouabain in a normal subject. (Reprinted by permission from Mason et al.[13])

congestive heart failure.[13] As shown in Figure 6, intravenous ouabain in a patient with congestive heart failure caused a slight decline in mean blood pressure, a rise in the low forearm blood flow, a decrease in the high forearm vascular resistance and reduction of both elevated forearm venous tone and elevated central venous pressure, whereas the high total peripheral vascular resistance fell and the low cardiac output increased. Thus, digitalis results in peripheral arteriolar and venous dilation in congestive heart failure.

Figure 7 represents the cardiovascular system in congestive heart failure. The elevations in systemic vascular resistance and venous tone represent characteristic compensatory mechanisms in the heart failure state that are largely produced by increased activity of the sympathetic nervous system.[5] With the administration of digitalis, its direct positive inotropic action results in augmentation of the low cardiac output with decline in cardiac enlargement. The large rise in cardiac output allows reflex withdrawal of increased sympathetic activity in the peripheral vascular beds, leading to systemic arterial and venous dilation.[3,4,13] This indirect vasodilation is greater in magnitude than is the glycoside stimulation of vascular smooth muscle and thereby overrides the lesser direct vasoconstrictor action of digitalis.

These observations indicate that digitalis possesses both direct and indirect cardiac and peripheral vascular effects, and the overall alterations of hemodynamics depend on the integration of these effects and the cardiac functional status of the patient prior to administration of the agent (Figure 8). Direct vasoconstriction occurs in consort with the increase in contractility in the normal heart, resulting in no change in cardiac output. In contrast, the digitalis-induced increase in contractility effects improvement in cardiac output in the failing heart so that indirect dilation predominates in the peripheral vascular beds.

The glycosides are of limited value in heart failure principally due to mechanical disturbances, such as constrictive pericarditis, pure valvular aortic stenosis and isolated mitral stenosis in normal sinus rhythm.[11,14] The glycosides are of most clinical benefit in improving cardiac function when heart failure results from chronic primary and secondary depression of ventricular contractility, such as in nonobstructive cardiomyopathies, coronary artery disease, systemic hypertension, acquired valvular regurgitation and types of congenital heart disease with chronic ventricular volume overload.[4]

In Compensated Heart Disease: In patients with heart disease without failure, the cardiac reserve mechanisms of ventricular dilation, hypertrophy and adrenergic stimulation maintain cardiac output at a normal level.[5,6] Further, recently it has been shown experimentally and clinically that contractile state is diminished in chronic hemodynamic overload and in cardiomyopathies even before the onset of overt congestive heart failure.[15] Thus, as shown in Figure 3 in chapter 9 on the regulation of cardiac performance, the diseased but compensated heart is characterized by the moderately depressed ventricular function curve 3, intermediate to the severely flattened performance curve 4 of the failing heart and the steep curve 1 of the normal heart. Digitalis in patients with ventricular dysfunction without failure does not elevate the cardiac output above normal (horizontal broken line); instead, the upward shifted ventricular function curve 2 provided by the positive inotropic effect of digitalis allows normal cardiac output to be maintained at a substantially lower ventricular filling pressure (point B in contrast to point C). Thus, the drug allows less encroachment on cardiac compensatory mechanisms, reduces ventricular dilation and improves effort dyspnea even in the absence of overt pulmonary congestion. In compensated heart disease, the direct constrictor and indirect relaxing actions of the glycoside are equally balanced and thus no alteration in peripheral vascular resistance occurs.[4]

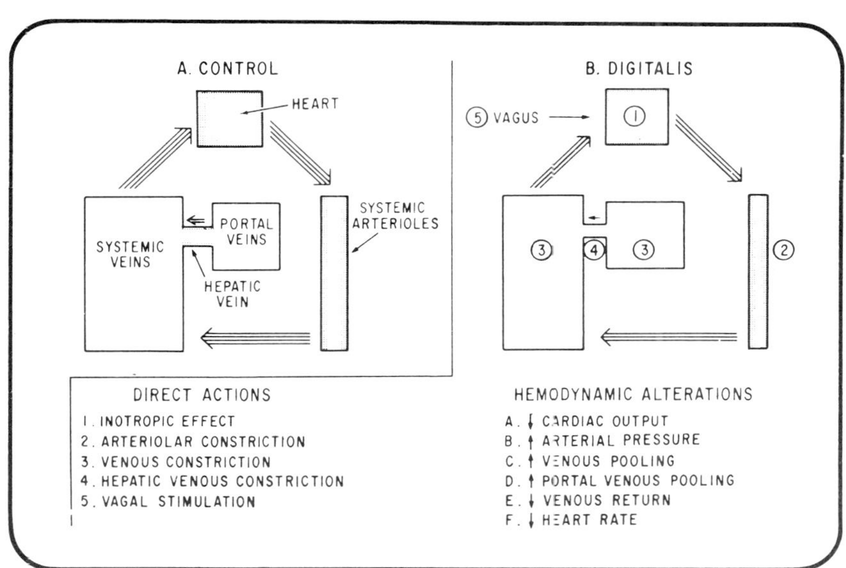

FIGURE 5. Diagrammatic representation of the hemodynamic effects of digitalis in a normal subject. The cardiocirculation is shown in the control state in **A** and after digitalis in **B**. On the **bottom left** are shown the direct actions of the glycoside on the heart, peripheral vessels and the vagus; on the **bottom right** are the hemodynamic alterations resulting from the direct actions of the agent. The **circled numbers** in **B** refer to direct actions of digitalis. The width of the **arrows** indicates the relative quantity of blood flow. (Reprinted by permission from Mason et al.[5])

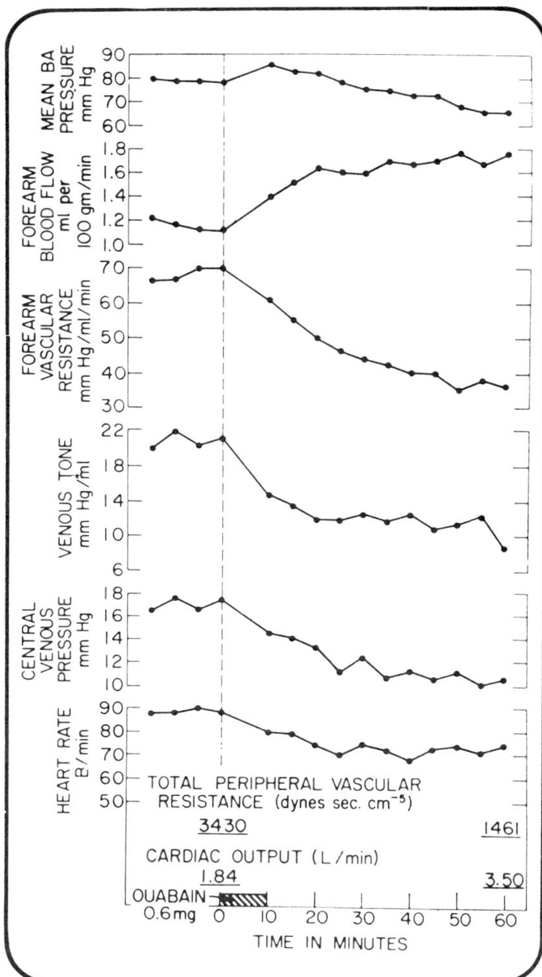

FIGURE 6. Serial measurements of cardiocirculatory dynamics before and after ouabain in a patient with rheumatic mitral regurgitation and chronic congestive heart failure. (Reprinted by permission from Mason et al.[13])

Myocardial Oxygen Consumption

It is now acknowledged that the oxygen consumption of the heart is largely regulated by the interplay among three major hemodynamic-related determinants[16] shown in Figure 9. Most important is intramyocardial tension, which is governed by ventricular systolic pressure and the radius of the ventricle. The other two major variables controlling cardiac oxygen requirements are the heart rate and contractile state.

The positive inotropic effect of digitalis is known to elevate myocardial oxygen consumption.[17,18] In the normally functioning heart, the predominant effect of digitalis on myocardial energetics is an increase in cardiac oxygen demands (see Figure 5 in chapter 9). Conversely, digitalis reduces overall myocardial oxygen consumption and increases cardiac efficiency in the failing heart[17] (see Figure 5 in chapter 9). Thus, in the enlarged dysfunctioning heart, ventricular tension is diminished by the reduction in heart size resulting from the inotropic action of the glycoside. In terms of cardiac oxygen needs, this indirect decline in wall tension is greater than is the direct increase in contractility produced by digitalis. Thus, in chronic ischemic heart disease with ventricular dysfunction, digitalis may exert an antianginal effect. It is pointed out that this improvement in myocardial energetics in heart failure brought about by digitalis is not a fundamental property of the agent; rather, in this condition, it overrides the energy-wasting effect normally associated with the direct positive inotropic action of the glycoside.

Studies in experimental animals have shown that raising myocardial oxygen requirements in the normal ventricle by stimulating contractility with digitalis increases the extent of ventricular ischemia and necrosis after subsequent coronary occlusion.[19] In contrast, in the presence of ventricular dysfunction and cardiomegaly, treatment with the glycoside prior to coronary obstruction reduces the area of myocardial ischemia and infarction.[20]

Acute Myocardial Infarction

There has been considerable debate concerning the role of digitalis therapy in acute myocardial infarction. In cardiogenic shock when the ventricle is largely destroyed, it is of little value —as is the case with other cardiotonic agents. Conversely, in acute congestive heart failure without shock in the immediate period after infarction, studies in our coronary care unit have shown that intravenous ouabain or digoxin produced substantial improvement in ventricular function in the majority of patients (Figure 10), although the results were somewhat inconsistent.[21] Elevated left ventricular end-diastolic

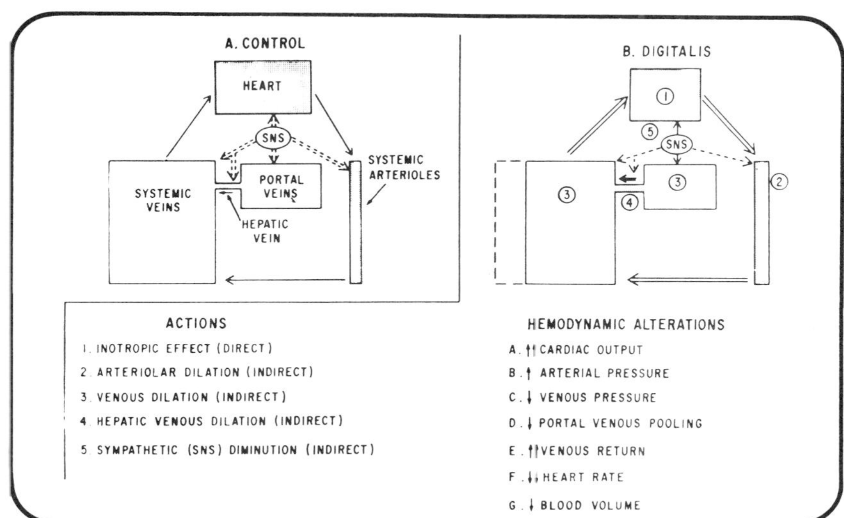

FIGURE 7. Diagrammatic representation of the hemodynamic effects of digitalis in a patient with congestive heart failure. The **broken arrows** represent activity of the sympathetic nervous system (SNS). The **circled numbers** in **B** refer to the direct and indirect actions of digitalis. The **broken line** indicating expansion of the systemic venous reservoir in **B** represents an initial increase in blood volume in this compartment; later the size of this compartment is reduced after diuresis with decline in total blood volume. The width of the **arrows** indicates the degree of blood flow. (Reprinted by permission from Mason et al.[5])

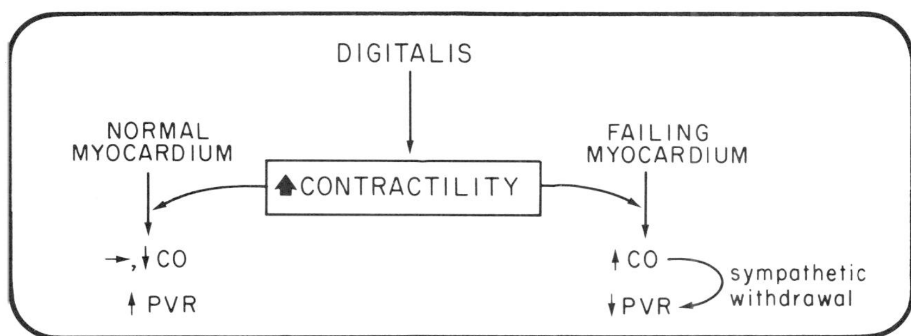

FIGURE 8. Diagrammatic representation of the different hemodynamic translation of the positive cardiac inotropic action of digitalis in the normal heart (**left**) compared with that in the failing heart (**right**). CO = cardiac output; PVR = peripheral vascular resistance.

pressure was reduced while low cardiac output rose or normal cardiac output was maintained in most patients.

In the management of congestive heart failure due to acute myocardial-infarction, it is our current practice to use intravenous furosemide to relieve pulmonary congestion when the left ventricular filling pressure—measured by Swan-Ganz catheterization of the pulmonary artery—is greater than 18 to 20 mm Hg (Figure 11). Mild to moderate elevations of left ventricular filling pressure (12 to 18 mm Hg) usually do not require therapy and return to normal levels in about 5 days with improvement of diminished compliance after infarction. In patients with filling pressures exceeding 18 to 20 mm Hg in whom sufficient reduction of this variable is not achieved with furosemide, intravenous digoxin is given in approximately two-thirds of its standard parenteral digitalizing dose.

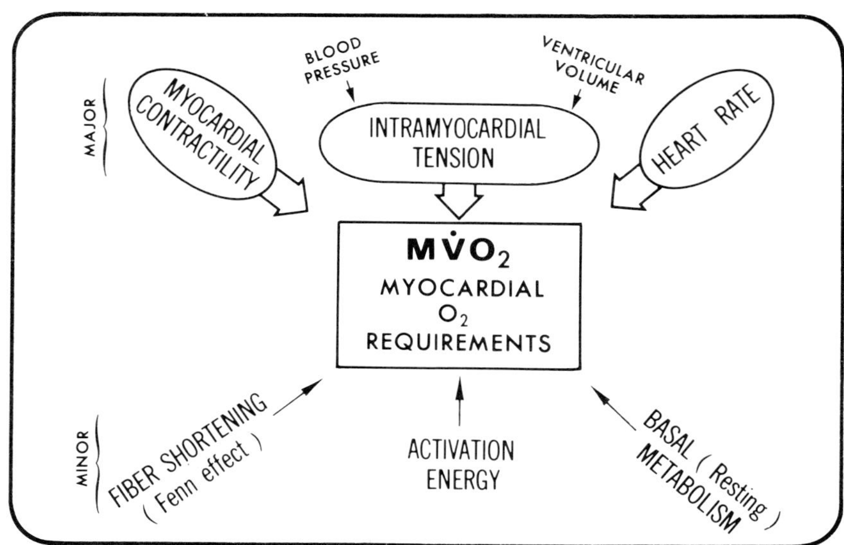

FIGURE 9. Diagram showing the three major and three minor determinants of myocardial oxygen consumption ($M\dot{V}O_2$). (Reprinted by permission from Mason.[112])

To evaluate some of the factors contributing to the inconsistent cardiotonic response to digitalis in acute myocardial infarction, the inotropic effect of ouabain was evaluated in our laboratories in a preparation of isolated right ventricular papillary muscle from cats in which the myocardium was made hypoxic.[22] It was found that the increase in peak tension caused by ouabain during normal oxygenation was markedly attenuated during hypoxia (Figure 12), whereas isoproterenol retained its full positive inotropic action at the level of hypoxia. Therefore, the ability to respond to digitalis-inotropic stimulation is impaired in the hypoxic myocardium. This inherent impaired response to inotropic stimulation by digitalis in hypoxic heart muscle is additive to reduced contractile response resulting from decreased binding of the agent to ischemic myocardium induced by coronary occlusion.[23] Nevertheless, at least some enhancement of depressed contractility is achieved in acutely ischemic myocardium surrounding the necrotic area, as shown in our laboratories after experimental coronary occlusion in the intact canine heart.[24] That dyssynergy of the infarcted ventricular segment might be worsened by glycoside-inotropic stimulation remains speculative clinically. Among all the factors responsible for the reduced hemodynamic response to digitalis in the infarcted heart, the most important appears to be that the normal portion of the ventricle is already operating at a near-peak level of increased contractile state due to cardiac sympathetic stimulation and elevated blood-borne levels of endogenous catecholamines, coupled with the fact that the necrotic muscle zone is incapable of physiologically meaningful responses to cardiovascular drugs.

Pharmacodynamics

Pharmacodynamic studies using tritiated digoxin have shown that oral digoxin is absorbed considerably better than was previously appreciated.[25,26] Since 80 percent of an oral dose is absorbed, the total oral digitalizing dose should now be only 2 mg. In contrast to digitoxin, digoxin is poorly bound to serum proteins; therefore, after absorption, digoxin is rapidly bound to the myocardium and other tissues, resulting in a ratio of myocardial to serum levels of approximately 30:1.[27]

Digitalis slowly accumulates within the body after institution of a daily maintenance regimen without an initial loading dose. The body re-

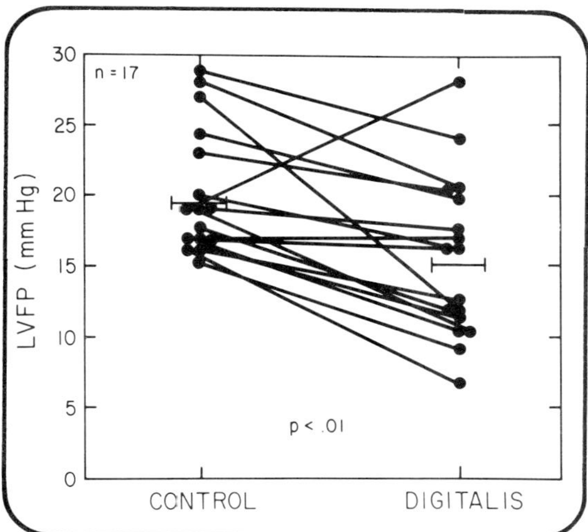

FIGURE 10. Effects of intravenous digitalis on left ventricular end-diastolic pressure (LVFP) in patients with acute myocardial infarction in whom the pre-glycoside LVFP was above normal (greater than 12 mm Hg). All patients had congestive heart failure without cardiogenic shock.

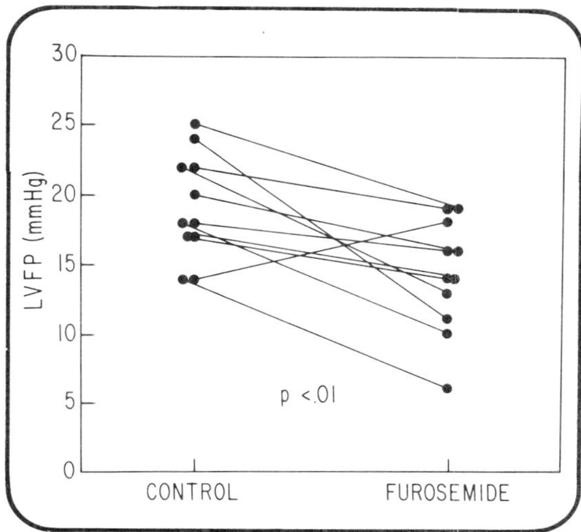

FIGURE 11. Effects of intravenous furosemide on left ventricular end-diastolic pressure (LVFP) in patients with acute myocardial infarction in whom the pre-diuretic LVFP was above normal (greater than 12 mm Hg). All patients had congestive heart failure without cardiogenic shock.

tains a certain constant percentage of the quantity of systemic glycoside daily—30 percent in the case of digoxin. In normal subjects taking 0.5 mg of oral tritiated digoxin daily, the plateau concentration of radioactive digoxin in the blood is the same after 6 days whether or not an initial loading dose is given.[28] Consequently, only maintenance doses of digoxin are required to achieve therapeutic concentrations over a period of a few days.

Whereas digitoxin is metabolized in the liver and excreted in the bile,[26,29] digoxin—which is water-soluble—is removed from the body in the unaltered state by the kidneys.[26,30] Thus, patients with renal failure are highly susceptible to the development of digoxin toxicity.[26,31–33] Urinary digoxin clearance correlates closely with glomerular filtration rate as estimated by creatinine clearance, and digoxin clearance may be depressed even before elevation of blood urea nitrogen levels.[34] Digoxin dosage should be determined on the basis of lean body weight; obese patients should not be administered large doses based on total body weight.[35] In contrast, digitoxin is lipid-soluble, and its dosage is related to total body weight in obesity. Elderly patients generally have an increased

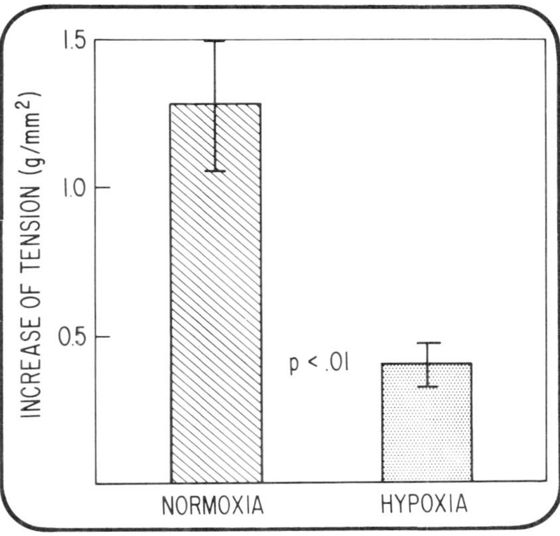

FIGURE 12. Comparison of the positive inotropic properties of digitalis in isolated ventricular myocardium during normal oxygenation (**left**) and hypoxic conditions (**right**). The contractile action of digitalis was markedly attenuated during a level of tissue hypoxia at which isoproterenol retained its full positive inotropic action.

susceptibility to digoxin toxicity because of their relative impairment of renal excretion and smaller body size.[36]

Dose-Contractile Response: The traditional concept of the relation between the dose and the positive contractile action of digitalis has been that (1) little contractile benefit is achieved until a certain digitalizing dose is reached, and (2) the positive contractile action of the glycosides then diminishes as higher doses are administered and toxicity is approached. However, recent evidence indicates a linear relation between therapeutic dose and contractile response.[37–40] This linear dose-response relation has been demonstrated in our laboratories in isolated ventricular papillary muscles from cats for digoxin, ouabain and acetylstrophanthidin.[39,40] Thus, small or large quantities of the glycosides have the same qualitative contractile action, the extent of which is proportional to the dose employed. Therefore, a patient need not receive a maximally tolerated dose of digitalis to achieve some salutary effect. Even small amounts of the glycoside provide some therapeutic action—a point to be kept in mind when the agent is used in patients who may be prone to toxicity.

Temporal Course of Contractile Action: The time to maximal inotropic effect in patients differs widely among the various glycosides, even after intravenous administration. To investigate the time course of contractile action of the glycosides, we determined the temporal inotropic responses of papillary muscles to doses producing a 50 percent increase in peak tension of acetylstrophanthidin, ouabain and digoxin in oxygenated Krebs solution for periods of two hours.[40] It was found that the contractile force responses to equivalent doses of the three agents increased similarly to a plateau after 1.5 hours.[40] Therefore, it appears that the differences in onset and peak action among these glycosides administered parenterally is largely the result of their different serum protein binding or metabolism and not due to differential effects of the preparations on heart muscle.

Relation to Potassium: The serum potassium concentration is known to importantly influence the actions of digitalis. Both the toxic and contractile actions of digitalis are increased in

the presence of hypokalemia.[41–44] Consistent with this observation is the finding that both the toxic and contractile effects of digitalis are reduced when the glycoside is administered during hyperkalemia.[41,44–46] The relationship between potassium and the contractile action of digitalis was recently examined in isolated, supported cat papillary muscles in our laboratories.[39] The linear dose-contractile response curve for acetylstrophanthidin added to a muscle bath with an extracellular potassium concentration of 3.5 mM was markedly depressed when the drug was added to an extracellular bath of 7.0 mM potassium concentration, demonstrating attenuation of inotropic stimulation by digitalis after pretreatment with potassium. In contrast, increasing the extracellular potassium concentration in the muscle bath from 3.5 to 7.0 mM after pretreatment with digitalis did not alter the force of cardiac muscle contraction.[39]

From these[39,41–46] and related[47,48] observations, potassium and digitalis appear to compete for myocardial binding sites. However, potassium is relatively loosely bound to the myocardium, and it delays subsequent digitalis binding. In contrast, digitalis is firmly bound to myocardial receptors, and thus potassium has little effect on glycoside already attached to the heart when potassium is administered. Translated into the clinical setting, alterations in serum potassium levels effected before treatment with digitalis have marked influences on the toxic and contractile actions of the glycoside. However, potassium has relatively little influence on the toxic and contractile effects of digitalis when it is given after the glycoside has been taken up by the heart.

Electrophysiologic Effects: The influences of digitalis on the electrophysiologic properties of heart muscle are complex.[41,49] The effects vary considerably with dose, type of cardiac tissue involved and autonomic activity. The middle panel of Figure 13 is a diagrammatic representation of the transmembrane electrical potential recorded from a microelectrode implanted in a single automatic cardiac cell in the atrial, junctional or ventricular myocardium. The associated transcellular membrane movements of sodium and potassium cations during the cardiac cycle are shown on the bottom, and the

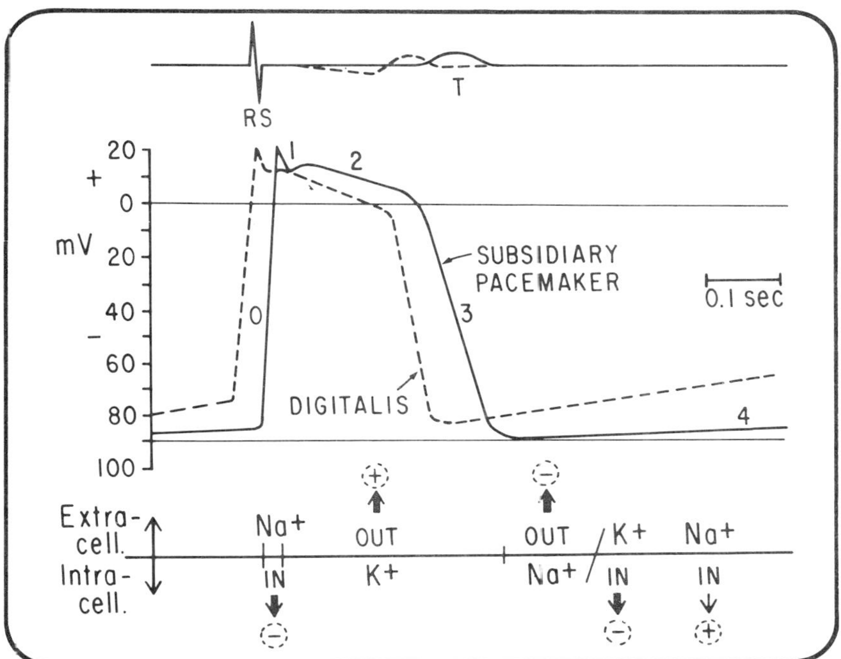

FIGURE 13. Diagrammatic representation of the transmembrane electrical potential (**middle**), unipolar electrocardiogram (**top**) and transmembrane cation movement (**bottom**) of a spontaneously depolarizing conductive fiber in the atrial, junctional or ventricular myocardium (**solid line**) and after administration of digitalis (**broken line**). The ST segment depression and QT interval shortening effected by digitalis are shown by the **broken line** in the **top** panel. **Top:** RS wave occurs at the time of depolarization and the T wave during the final phase of repolarization. **Middle:** 0 = depolarization; 1, 2 and 3 = phases of repolarization; 4 = resting period exhibiting diastolic depolarization; mV = millivolts. **Bottom:** The **horizontal line** represents the sarcolemma cell membrane; the **arrows** indicate transmembrane flux of Na^+ and K^+ during depolarization, repolarization and the resting period. At the onset of the resting period is shown the active exit ($\uparrow$) of Na^+ extracellularly (extracell) accompanied by active entrance ($\downarrow$) of K^+ intracellularly (intracell). During the remainder of the resting period, diastolic depolarization takes place with passive Na^+ movement into the cell. The size of each arrow is directly related to large or small movement of cations. The effects of digitalis on these cation fluxes are shown by the sign within the **broken circles.** Transmembrane influx of Ca^{++} is thought to take place during phase 2. (Reprinted by permission from Mason et al.[41])

standard surface electrocardiogram is on the top. The effects of digitalis on these variables are demonstrated by the broken lines.

In diastole during intracellular negativity, excitability is raised by reduction in resting potential. Also in diastole, digitalis stimulates automaticity by increasing the phase 4 slope of diastolic depolarization,[50] thereby enhancing subsidiary ectopic pacemakers (Figure 13). Concerning the process of depolarization, the phase 0 rate of rise of the action potential determining conduction velocity is diminished by digitalis (Figure 13), particularly in the atrioventricular (A-V) node,[51] leading to various degrees of heart block. Since the speed of the phase 0 depolarization spike is directly related to the level of resting membrane potential, digitalis depresses membrane responsiveness. The reduction of conduction velocity in the A-V node by digitalis is of major therapeutic significance in slowing rapid ventricular rate in atrial fibrillation, thereby furthering decremental conduction and increasing the functional refractory period of the A-V node.

Phases 1, 2 and 3 of the repolarization process are altered by digitalis. The duration of the

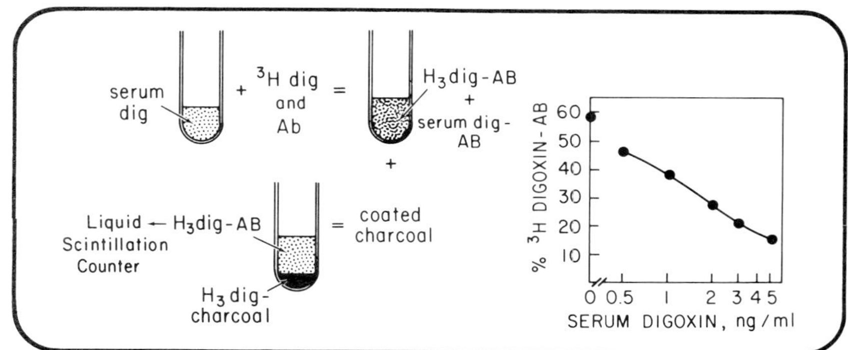

FIGURE 14. Diagrammatic representation of the radioimmunoassay method for the quantification of serum digoxin concentrations. On **left,** known amounts of tritiated digoxin and digoxin antibodies are added to the serum containing the nonradioactive glycoside. Since the digitalis antibodies bind to both radioactive and nonradioactive digoxin, the extent of radioactive digoxin-to-antibody binding (determined by scintillation counting) is inversely proportional to the concentration of nonradioactive digoxin in the serum, as obtained from a standardized curve (**right,** reprinted by permission from Smith et al.[53])

action potential in cardiac tissues is shortened by the glycoside (Figure 13), leading to decreased refractoriness in myocardial conductive fibers,[51] which, in the ventricles, is observed by narrowing of the QT interval on the surface electrocardiogram. Also, digitalis changes the slope of phases 1 and 2 of the action potential plateau, which is manifested as an ST segment shift on the electrocardiogram. The actions of digitalis on conduction velocity and refractory period underlie the drug's provocation of reentrant tachyarrhythmias.[52]

Radioimmunoassay: One of the most important advances in clinical digitalis pharmacology has been the recent development of the radioimmunoassay technique for the accurate quantification of glycoside concentrations. Since the original development of the immunologic method for digoxin by Butler, Smith and Haber[53,54] and for digitoxin by Oliver et al,[55] radioimmunoassay has become available for routine clinical use in many medical centers. Recently, a radioimmunoassay for ouabain also has been developed.[56]

The digoxin assay is based on competition between serum nonradioactive digoxin and a constant amount of tritiated digoxin for a constant number of digoxin antibody-binding sites (Figure 14, left). Since nonradioactive digoxin interferes with tritiated digoxin binding, radioactive digoxin-bound antibody is reduced with higher concentrations of serum digoxin, as determined in a liquid scintillation counter. The precise concentration of serum digoxin is then determined from a standard curve (Figure 14, right).

Digitalis Toxicity

It is now recognized that digitalis intoxication is among the most common adverse drug reactions and may provoke arrhythmias and conduction disturbances in as many as one-fourth of patients receiving this drug for treatment of congestive heart failure.[57-61] Although the most common and earliest side effects are related to the gastrointestinal tract—due to action of the glycosides on the central nervous system rather than local gastric irritation—disorders of cardiac rhythm are the most important toxic manifestations, and they are the first adverse features of the agents in one-third of patients. It has been estimated that arrhythmias and conduction disturbances are provoked in up to four-fifths of patients in whom toxic effects are observed. Both retrospective and prospective clinical studies of digitalis overdosage have demonstrated considerable variability of cardiac and extracardiac manifestations without predictability concerning the rhythm disorder produced, even with administration of the identical glycoside preparation in the same patient.[57-63] All the digitalis preparations are equally capable of producing digitalis toxicity, and no special advantage is achieved by the use of certain glycosides regarding earlier onset of extracardiac reactions relative to rhythm disturbances or reduced incidence of serious arrhythmias.

Considerable variability has recently been found in the biologic availability of oral digoxin tablets produced by different manufacturers.[64] Digoxin serum concentrations varied widely after ingestion of different brands with the same digoxin content, which indicated nonequivalent absorption due to variations in product formulation leading to unequal disintegration and dissolution rates. Lanoxin® is now recognized to be the brand of digoxin providing uniform and optimal potency.

Patients receiving daily maintenance doses of 0.25 to 0.50 mg oral digoxin without toxicity usually have therapeutic concentrations between 1 and 2 ng/ml of serum, whereas approximately 90 percent of patients with electrical toxicity have serum levels above 2 ng/ml.[31,32,65] Although the range of overlap between nontoxicity and toxicity is 1.5 to 3.0 ng/ml, in the presence of levels above 2 ng/ml, it is generally prudent to discontinue digoxin until the serum level falls below this concentration. Diminished renal function appears to largely account for elevated concentrations of digoxin in patients intoxicated with this glycoside.[31] However, no significant difference in renal function has been observed in patients with toxicity from digitoxin, which is excreted in the bile.[66]

Patients with atrial fibrillation who require more than 0.50 mg of digoxin daily for rate control appear relatively less susceptible to toxicity, and they may have levels above 2 ng/ml.[31] Other conditions in which digitalis dosage may be increased include hyperthyroidism,[67] impaired intestinal absorption in malabsorption syndromes,[68] infancy,[69] altered digitoxin metabolism[70] and rare instances of digitalis antibodies.[54,71]

Current evidence indicates that susceptibility to digitalis toxic arrhythmias is increased in certain types of heart disease. Electrical toxicity is probably more frequent in the presence of acute myocardial infarction and chronic coronary artery disease than in normally perfused hearts.[31] Furthermore, patients with advanced ventricu-

lar failure from any cause are more prone to digitalis arrhythmias than are those with less severe dysfunction.[32] In subjects with a normal heart and in children with heart disease, A-V conduction disturbances occur more often than do tachyarrhythmias with glycoside overdosage.[72] In adult patients with latent disease of the A-V node, digitalis can produce heart block before accelerated activity of ectopic pacemakers.[31] There is increased frequency of cardiac toxicity in patients with chronic pulmonary disease, probably related to systemic arterial hypoxemia.[32] In addition, hypokalemia,[41] hypomagnesemia,[73] hypercalcemia,[74] alkalosis,[75] hypothyroidism[76] and increased myocardial adrenergic activity[77] predispose to digitalis-provoked tachyarrhythmias. The special problem of the precipitation of ventricular tachyarrhythmias attributable to digitalis after elective countershock to convert supraventricular arrhythmias[78-80]—even in the absence of digitalis toxicity prior to electrical discharge—is discussed and its proper management delineated in chapter 23 on antiarrhythmic agents.

Although digitalis is probably capable of producing every type of cardiac arrhythmia, certain abnormalities occur more frequently than others[57-63,31-83] (Figure 15). Two of three rhythm disorders are premature ventricular systoles; particularly characteristic are bigeminy and multifocal ectopic beats. Manifestations of A-V block appear in about one-third of patients with digitalis-induced arrhythmias. Less common but more indicative of digitalis toxicity are paroxysmal atrial tachycardia with block, junctional (A-V nodal) tachycardia, A-V dissociation in which the ventricular pacemaker exhibits a faster frequency than the atrial rate without block, sinoatrial arrest, sinoatrial block, ventricular tachycardia and ventricular fibrillation. Bidirectional ventricular tachycardia is particularly characteristic of severe digitalis overdose and results from alterations in intraventricular conduction, junctional tachycardia with aberrant intraventricular conduction or, on rare occasions, alternating ventricular pacemakers.[61] The incidence of atrial fibrillation due to digitalis toxicity is higher than is commonly appreciated. Thus, slow regular ventricular rates induced by digitalis in the treatment of atrial fibrillation might be due to complete heart

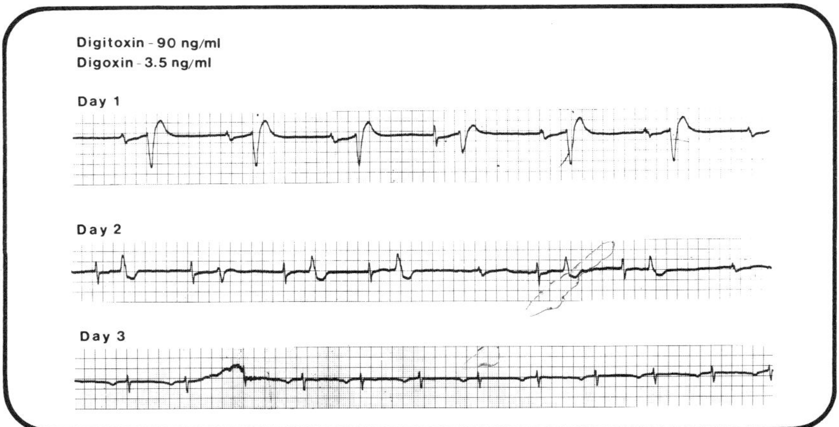

FIGURE 15. Sequential daily electrocardiograms (precordial monitor lead) from a 67 year old patient after self-administered intentional overdose of oral digitoxin. The excessive dose of digitoxin resulted in, in addition to a toxic serum level of digitoxin (90 ng/ml), a toxic serum level of digoxin (3.5 ng/ml) due to metabolism of digitoxin. Cardiac rhythm progressed from sinus bradycardia (day 1), to idioventricular rhythm with bigeminy (day 2) and finally to normal sinus rhythm (day 3). Successful treatment consisted of prophylactic temporary pacemaker ventricular overdrive.

block or drug-prolonged concealed conduction of fibrillatory waves into the A-V junction.

Since no specific cardiac arrhythmia is absolutely pathognomonic of digitalis excess, the diagnosis of glycoside toxicity is not based entirely on electrocardiographic evidence. A number of factors must be taken into account—the onset and duration of action, metabolism and excretion of the digitalis preparation employed and the predisposing background to glycoside sensitivity—as well as the electrocardiographic features and disappearance of the arrhythmia when the drug is withdrawn.[84] A spectrum of electrophysiologic manifestations resulting from digitalis administration is observed on the standard electrocardiogram, beginning with ST-T wave changes that often accompany the salutary contractile effects of the drug and ending with ectopic impulses and conduction disturbances considered to be evidence of digitalis excess.[85] Isolated prolongation of the P-R interval is not considered a toxic manifestation; reducing conduction velocity and prolonging the functional refractory period in the A-V node is beneficial in decreasing the rapid ventricular rate observed with supraventricular tachycardias and atrial fibrillation. In congestive heart failure, the slowing of sinus tachycardia by digitalis is attributable to improvement of impaired hemodynamics and accompanying sympathetic withdrawal—not to a direct or vagal action of the drug upon the sinus pacemaker.[3,4,13,86] However, when extrasystoles are isolated or occur in runs, or when it is concluded that advanced A-V block is being produced by the glycosides, digitalis toxicity should be recognized and appropriate management of these electrical disorders instituted.

Treatment of Toxicity

Although glycoside toxicity can be reversed with digitalis antibodies in dogs,[87–89] no practical specific antidote is currently available for the too common problem of digitalis intoxication in patients. However, special advantages pertain to the use of potassium,[41] diphenylhydantoin,[90] lidocaine,[91] propranolol,[92] bretylium[93] and cardiac pacing.[94] Although the administration of potassium or antiarrhythmic drugs after the onset of electrical toxicity in experimental animals can suppress digitalis-induced tachyarrhythmias, studies in our laboratories have shown that the accumulated dose of digitalis at which these arrhythmias become refractory and fatal is not increased by this treatment.[94] Similarly, ventricular overdrive pacing begun at the onset of ouabain-provoked

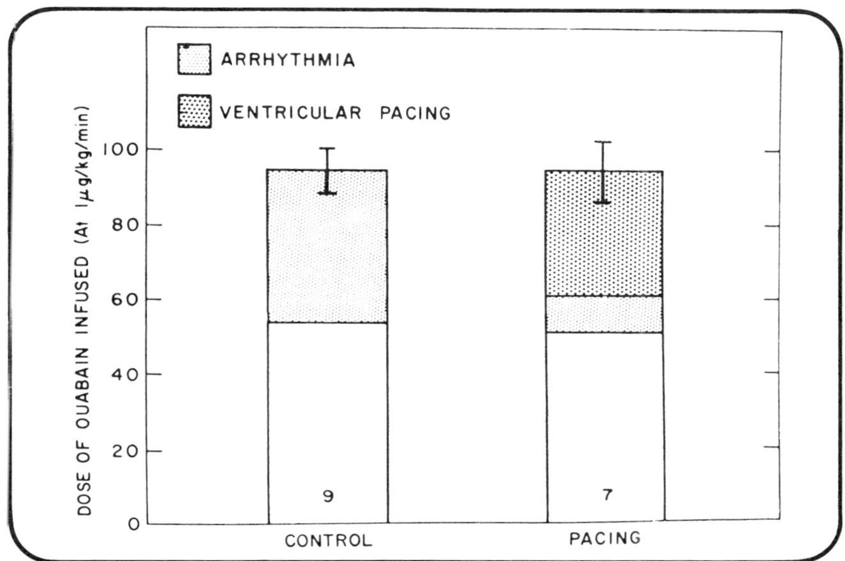

FIGURE 16. Cumulative doses of ouabain required to produce arrhythmias and death in control animals and in dogs in which electrical pacing of the ventricle was carried out at the onset of arrhythmias. (Reprinted by permission from Mason et a .[4])

tachyarrhythmias transiently overcame these rhythm disorders, but the maximal tolerated dose of ouabain prior to death was not altered compared with that in control animals receiving digitalis in the same manner[94] (Figure 16).

In clinical practice, however, digitalis is discontinued at the onset of toxicity, and antiarrhythmic measures are employed to suppress ectopic activity until the glycoside is excreted or metabolized. Any hypokalemia should, of course, be corrected. Even in the absence of hypokalemia, potassium should be administered whenever ventricular irritability is present, since ventricular arrhythmias are related to intracellular potassium loss, potassium delays further binding of the glycosides to the myocardium, and the cation has the antiarrhythmic effect itself of reducing diastolic depolarization of ectopic pacemakers.[95]

Although both quinidine and procainamide are useful in reducing increased automaticity produced by digitalis, these antiarrhythmic drugs may induce or worsen A-V block. In using procainamide for ventricular tachyarrhythmias, it may become necessary to discontinue the drug because of the development of excessive widening of the QRS complex. Continued suppression of the arrhythmia can be obtained by adding lidocaine or diphenylhydantoin without exacerbating the conduction delay, while increasing depression of ectopic automaticity.[90,91]

Lidocaine is more effective than procainamide or quinidine in the treatment of digitalis-induced ventricular tachycardias[96] and is reported not to affect the conduction velocity in the A-V node and the ventricular myocardium.[91] Diphenylhydantoin is particularly useful for premature ventricular contractions associated with digitalis toxicity, since this antiarrhythmic drug depresses enhanced ventricular automaticity without affecting intraventricular conduction. Diphenylhydantoin also tends to reverse the glycoside-induced prolongation of A-V conduction. Diphenylhydantoin has been shown to dissociate the inotropic and arrhythmic actions of digitalis,[97] thus depressing digitalis-induced tachyarrhythmias without diminishing the contractile effects of the glycoside. In addition, diphenylhydantoin can terminate supraventricular tachycardias induced by digitalis,[98] whereas lidocaine has not been as useful in these conditions.

Quinidine, procainamide, lidocaine and diphenylhydantoin are useful in terminating ectopic impulses resulting from disorders of either impulse formation or conduction, since each of the drugs diminishes diastolic depolarization—thereby reducing automaticity—and alters conduction velocity and the refractory period. However, since quinidine and procainamide depress conduction velocity and lengthen the refractory period, whereas lidocaine and diphenylhydantoin shorten the refractory period, these latter two drugs may be effective when procainamide and quinidine are not; the reverse may also be true.

Propranolol is particularly effective in the treatment of certain digitalis-induced tachyarrhythmias,[92] and current evidence suggests that the beta-adrenergic blocking action, rather than the direct membrane effect of the agent, is most important in this regard.[99,100] Although propranolol is useful in the treatment of both supraventricular and ventricular arrhythmias due to digitalis toxicity, it has been most successful in terminating premature ventricular extrasystoles.[92] In patients who have digitalis-induced atrial tachycardia with A-V block, propranolol usually has restored sinus rhythm, although depressed nodal conduction has been exacerbated.[92] Thus, diphenylhydantoin is preferable to propranolol in the initial treatment of glycoside-induced atrial tachycardia with block. Since propranolol, the quinidine-like drugs and potassium diminish conduction velocity, their use appears to be limited to supraventricular and ventricular extrasystoles and tachycardias unassociated with serious degrees of A-V block. In patients with digitalis-induced paroxysmal supraventricular arrhythmias with or without A-V block, propranolol can be used to slow rapid ventricular rate by decreasing the atrial rate or by reducing the conduction velocity and increasing the functional refractory period of of the A-V node. Bretylium also has been reported to be useful in digitalis-provoked ventricular tachyarrhythmias.[93,101]

A new approach in the treatment of digitalis toxicity is the use of cholestyramine, which diminishes the absorption and enterohepatic circulation of digitoxin.[102] Although a specific antidote is not clinically available at this time for reversal of digitalis intoxication, the recent development of an immunologic technique for the preparation of specific antibodies to digitalis preparations offers an experimental direct approach to this problem. Glycoside-induced rhythm disorders in experimental animals have been reversed and fatal arrhythmias prevented after administration of these antibodies by the functional removal of digitalis from the myocardium.[87-89]

Electrical pacemaker ventricular overdrive by electrode catheter has been successful in suppressing digitalis-induced ventricular tachyarrhythmias.[94] However, neither ventricular pacing nor potassium alters the maximal tolerated dose of digitalis before the development of fatal arrhythmias.[94] More important is that rapid ventricular pacing with a single electrical stimulus effectively overcomes serious digitalis-induced arrhythmias. Although the total fatal dose of digitalis is not changed by electrical pacing, digitalis is discontinued at the onset of toxicity, and antiarrhythmic drugs in addition to ventricular overdrive are employed to suppress ectopic activity until the glycoside is metabolized or excreted. Ventricular pacing should not be utilized as the initial approach in the treatment of digitalis-induced ventricular tachycardias; rather, it should be employed only when standard measures fail, since digitalis lowers the threshold for spontaneous repetitive ventricular extrasystoles in response to pacemaker stimuli.[79] The administration of diphenylhydantoin to suppress automaticity without encouraging reentry mechanisms mediating ectopic tachycardias might eliminate the electrical hazard of provoking spontaneous arrhythmias.[103]

Rapid right atrial pacing has been reported to be a useful means of terminating supraventricular tachycardias due to digitalis toxicity without enhancing the tendency for glycoside-provoked ventricular tachyarrhythmias.[104] Although paired electrical ventricular pacing has been shown to be an effective means of overcoming digitalis-induced arrhythmias in experimental animals,[105] this technique has not been used clinically because of the danger of inducing ventricular fibrillation. Precordial electrical countershock is contraindicated in the presence of digitalis toxicity since there is an increased propensity for glycoside-related ventricular fibrillation after electroshock.[78-80]

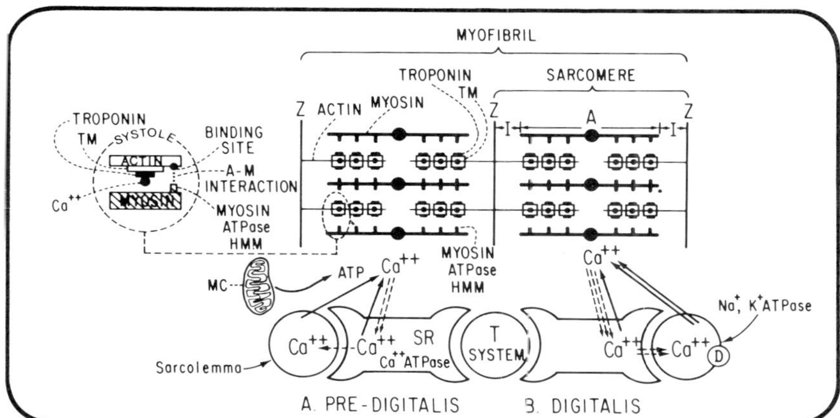

FIGURE 17. Schematic diagram of the substructure within a cardiac cell demonstrating the proposed subcellular mechanism of the contractile stimulating action of digitalis. A-M = actin-myosin; D = digitalis receptor site in the sarcolemma membrane (Na+, K+–ATPase); HMM = heavy meromyosin; MC = mitochondria; SR = sarcoplasmic reticulum; TM = tropomyosin. For further explanation, see text. (Reprinted by permission from Mason.[84])

In the management of digitalis-induced conduction abnormalities with advanced degrees of heart block and slow ventricular rate, it is important to discontinue the drug and consider protective therapy. Since potassium itself prolongs impulse conduction and lengthens refractory period in the A-V node,[106] the cation is usually not given in this manifestation of digitalis toxicity. Atropine may be effective in terminating A-V block induced by excessive vagal action of digitalis.[61] Isoproterenol has the disadvantage of increasing ventricular ectopic activity in the presence of toxic levels of digitalis.[61] Cardiac stimulation with an endocardial electrode catheter has been used successfully in the management of digitalis-induced ventricular asystole with complete heart block.

Subcellular Actions

Concerning the subcellular mechanism of the positive contractile property of digitalis, present evidence suggests that the glycosides act on the sarcolemma cell membrane to stimulate calcium influx,[107–111] thereby enhancing the process of excitation-contraction coupling by providing a greater quantity of calcium to the contractile proteins, which results in a more forceful contraction. Consideration of the ultrastructure of heart muscle is useful in under-

standing the presently-held concepts of the subcellular actions of digitalis.[112] Within the cardiac cell, the proteins actin and myosin are arranged in overlapping filaments to constitute sarcomeres—the basic functional units comprising the longitudinal myofibrils. The cardiac cell is covered externally by its electrically excitable cell membrane—the sarcolemma—which makes deep invaginations into the cell to constitute the transverse tubular or T system (see Figure 1 in chapter 23 on antiarrhythmic agents). Internal to the superficial membranes is a second membrane system that is entirely intracellular—the sarcoplasmic reticulum. Sodium, potassium and calcium fluxes between the outside and inside of the cell take place across the sarcolemma-T system, and the sarcoplasmic reticulum is important in intracellular calcium transport. The T system allows digitalis to reach readily the sarcoplasmic reticulum in the vicinity of the contractile proteins throughout the entire cardiac cell without requiring exit of the drug from the interstitial medium. Indeed, the site of action of radioactive digitalis has been specifically located within the T system adjacent to the sarcoplasmic reticulum.[113]

Figure 17 is a diagrammatic representation of the interior of a cardiac cell showing the structures just described. The three circles on the bottom half of the figure represent the T system;

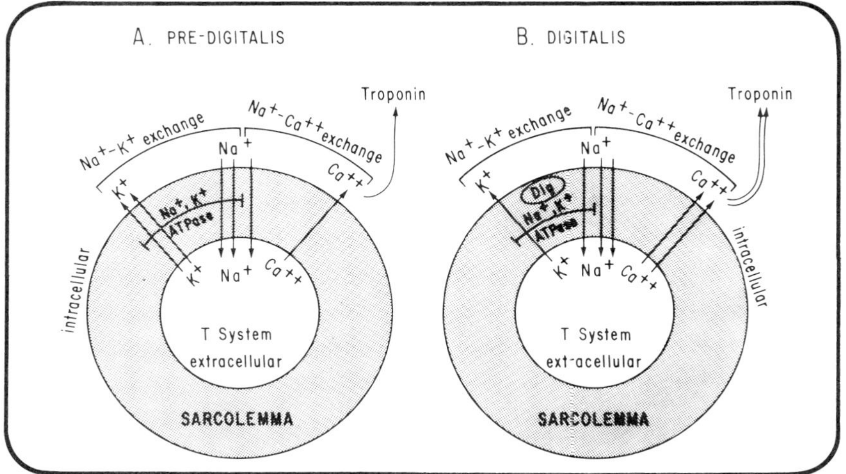

FIGURE 18. Schematic diagram of digitalis effects on the movement of Ca^{++} across the superficial cardiac cell membrane (sarcolemma-transtubular-T system). Dig = digitalis binding site (Na^+, K^+-ATPase receptor) in the sarcolemma. For further explanation, see text. (Reprinted by permission from Mason.[84])

inside these circles is the interstitial medium and outside them is the intracellular space. The sarcoplasmic reticulum is shown abutting the T system. On the top half of the figure, two sarcomeres are shown with their overlapping movable thin actin filaments and stationary thick myosin filaments. In addition to the contractile proteins actin and myosin, juxtaposed to actin are two modulator proteins, troponin and tropomyosin, which inhibit actin-myosin interaction during diastole.

Linkage of electrical excitation of the superficial membranes (sarcolemma-T system) to mechanical contraction of the sarcomere is achieved by delivery of calcium to troponin—the calcium receptor for the contractile apparatus—by trans-T system influx of calcium immediately after depolarization and intracellular shift of calcium from the sarcoplasmic reticulum (depicted by the solid arrows in the bottom left of Figure 17). The combination of calcium with troponin activates the contractile process by releasing troponin-tropomyosin inhibition of actin-myosin binding (shown in the broken circle in the upper left of Figure 17). Contraction occurs by myosin ATPase-regulated cyclic interactions between the actin-myosin linkages with the development of force and shortening. ATP energy for operation of the contractile machinery is supplied by the mitochondria.

With relaxation, calcium shifts from troponin to the sarcoplasmic reticulum, with some of this calcium moving to the extracellular space (indicated by the broken arrows in the bottom left of Figure 17).

Concerning the operation of digitalis within this subcellular framework, recent studies have shown that the drug binds to a specific sarcolemma-T system receptor thought to be sodium, potassium-ATPase (Na^+, K^+–ATPase),[108–111] the activity of which the glycoside characteristically inhibits (depicted in the lower right of Figure 17). This results in increased trans-T membrane calcium influx (shown by the solid arrows in the lower right of the figure), thereby providing a greater quantity of calcium to the contractile proteins and consequently a more forceful contraction.

Considerable investigation has been directed toward elucidation of how digitalis augments calcium influx across the superficial membranes. The mechanism proposed by Langer[110] is formulated in Figure 18, although the matter has not yet been completely settled. In Figure 18, the circles are the sarcolemma-T system with the center the extracellular space and outside the intracellular space. Prior to administration of digitalis on the left of the figure, Na^+, K^+–ATPase in the membrane normally pumps sodium out and potassium into the cell. This sodium-potassium exchange system is coupled with a sodium-calcium exchange system in the membrane which transports some sodium out of the cell in exchange for some calcium brought into the cell. Normally the mechanism for sodium-potassium is more active than is that for sodium-calcium.

On the right of Figure 18, digitalis depresses the activity of Na^+, K^+–ATPase with consequent diminished activity of the sodium-potassium exchange system. This causes an increase in intracellular sodium, which results in greater activity of sodium-calcium transport with consequent augmentation of calcium influx to the contractile proteins and a more forceful systole. In addition, a result of digitalis-induced depression of Na^+, K^+–ATPase is loss of potassium from the cardiac cell, which appears to be related to the electrical toxic effects of the glycosides.

Summary

It has become quite clear that the fundamental therapeutic action of digitalis is stimulation of ventricular contractile state. The expression of this increase in contractility is dependent on the integrity of cardiocirculatory status at the time the glycoside is administered. Thus, as a result of interplay between direct and indirect cardiac and vascular effects, variable and even opposite effects on cardiac output, peripheral circulatory dynamics and myocardial oxygen consumption can take place. Highlights of the recent advances in improved understanding of the digitalis glycosides include:

(1) Its fundamental therapeutic action in congestive heart failure is stimulation of depressed contractile state.

(2) The direct vasoconstrictor action is overridden by an indirect decrease in systemic vascular resistance resulting from sympathetic withdrawal accompanying use of the agent in congestive heart failure.

(3) Positive inotropic action directly elevates myocardial oxygen consumption and is overridden by indirect decreases in ventricular size and tension that reduce cardiac oxygen needs with digitalis therapy in heart failure.

(4) Improvement in cardiac function is inconsistent in congestive heart failure due to acute myocardial infarction.

(5) Therapeutic digoxin concentration is usually 1 to 2 ng/ml of serum; 90 percent of cases of toxicity occur with concentrations above 2 ng/ml.

(6) Increased sensitivity to toxicity accompanies hypokalemia, hypothyroidism, hypomagnesemia, hypercalcemia, alkalosis, hypoxia and ischemic and primary myocardial diseases.

(7) Oral digoxin is 80 percent absorbed; the total oral digitalizing dose is 2 mg.

(8) Oral daily maintenance doses of digoxin achieve therapeutic concentrations in 7 to 10 days.

(9) Renal insufficiency is the most frequent predisposition to digoxin toxicity.

(10) Electrophysiologic effects include increased automaticity, reduced conduction velocity and decreased refractoriness.

(11) Treatment of digitalis tachyarrhythmias is carried out with potassium, diphenylhydantoin, idocaine, propranolol, bretylium and cardiac pacing.

(12) The relation between therapeutic dose and contractile response is linear.

(13) Pretreatment with potassium delays binding of digitalis to myocardial receptors (Na^+, K^+–ATPase); potassium therapy has relatively little effect on digitalis already bound to the heart.

(14) Electrical toxicity is related to potassium loss from myocardium.

(15) The positive inotropic property is due to increased calcium influx by glycoside action on cardiac cell membrane.

The fundamental positive inotropic property of digitalis now appears to rest upon an intracellular influx of calcium produced by action of the drug on the cardiac cell membrane. In contrast, transmembrane fluxes of sodium and potassium underlie the electrical properties of the glycoside. Promising directions for future research include clarification of the digitalis receptor and further definition of the subcellular contractile and toxic mechanisms of the agent. Finally, it is apparent that thorough knowledge of the hemodynamic and cellular actions of the glycosides is essential for their proper application in patients.

Acknowledgment: This work was supported in part by Research Program Project Grant HL-14780 and Training Grant HL-5901 from the National Heart and Lung Institute, National Institutes of Health.

The authors gratefully acknowledge the technical assistance of Leslie J. Silvernail.

References

1. **Bloomfield RA, Rapoport B, Milnor JP, et al:** Effects of cardiac glycosides upon dynamics of circulation in congestive heart failure; ouabain. J Clin Invest 27:588, 1948

2. **Ferrer MI, Conroy RJ, Harvey RM:** Some effects of digoxin upon the heart and circulation in man. Digoxin in combined left and right ventricular failure. Circulation 21:372, 1960

3. **Mason DT, Braunwald E:** Digitalis: new facts about an old drug. Amer J Cardiol 22:151, 1968

4. **Mason DT, Spann JF, Zelis R:** New developments in the understanding of the actions of the digitalis glycosides. Progr Cardiovasc Dis 6:443, 1969

5. **Mason DT, Spann JF Jr, Zelis R, et al:** Alterations of hemodynamics and myocardial mechanics in patients with congestive heart failure: pathophysiologic mechanisms and assessment of cardiac function and ventricular contractility. Progr Cardiovasc Dis 12:507, 1970

6. **Mason DT:** Regulation of cardiac performance in clinical heart disease: interactions between contractile state, mechanical abnormalities and ventricular compensatory mechanisms. Amer J Cardiol 32:437, 1973

7. **Braunwald E, Bloodwell RD, Goldberg LI, et al:** Studies on digitalis. IV. Observations in man on the effects of digitalis preparations on the contractility of the nonfailing heart and on total vascular resistance. J Clin Invest 40:52, 1961

8. **Mason DT, Braunwald E:** Studies on digitalis. IX. Effects of ouabain on the nonfailing human heart. J Clin Invest 42:1105, 1963

9. **Sonnenblick EH, Williams JF, Glick G, et al:** Studies on digitalis. XV. Effects of cardiac glycosides on myocardial force-velocity relations in the nonfailing heart. Circulation 34:532, 1966

10. **Mason DT:** Usefulness and limitations of the rate of rise in intraventricular pressure (dp/dt) in the evaluation of myocardial contractility in man. Amer J Cardiol 23:516, 1969

11. **Capone RJ, Mason DT, Amsterdam EA, et al:** Digitalis in mitral stenosis with normal sinus rhythm: studies of left atrial contractility and cardiac hemodynamics. Circulation 46 suppl II:75, 1972

12. **Mason DT:** The cardiovascular effects of digitalis in normal man. Clin Pharmacol Ther 7:1, 1966

13. **Mason DT, Braunwald E:** Studies on digitalis. X. Effects of ouabain on forearm vascular resistance and venous tone in normal subjects and in patients in heart failure. J Clin Invest 43:532, 1964

14. **Beiser GD, Epstein SE, Stampfer M, et al:** Studies on digitalis. XVIII. Effects of ouabain on the hemodynamic response to exercise in patients with mitral stenosis in normal sinus rhythm. New Eng J Med 278:131, 1968

15. **Mason DT, Spann JF, Zelis R, et al:** Comparison of the contractile state of the normal, hypertrophied, and failing heart in man. In, Cardiac Hypertrophy (Alpert NR, ed). New York, Academic Press, 1971, p 433

16. **Braunwald E:** Control of myocardial oxygen consumption: physiologic and clinical considerations. Amer J Cardiol 27:416, 1971

17. **Covell JW, Braunwald E, Ross J Jr, et al:** Studies on digitalis. XVI. Effects on myocardial oxygen consumption. J Clin Invest 45:1535, 1966

18. **Coleman HN:** Role of acetylstrophanthidin in augmenting myocardial oxygen consumption: relation of increased O_2 consumption to changes in velocity of contraction. Circ Res 21:487, 1967

19. **Maroko PR, Kjekshus LK, Sobel BE, et al:** Factors influencing infarct size following experimental coronary occlusion. Circulation 43:67, 1971

20. **Watanabe T, Covell JW, Maroko PR, et al:** Effects of increased arterial pressure on the severity of myocardial ischemia in the acutely depressed heart. Amer J Cardiol 30:371, 1972

21. **Amsterdam EA, Huffaker HK, DeMaria A, et al:** Hemodynamic effects of digitalis in acute myocardial infarction and comparison with furosemide. Circulation 46 suppl II:113, 1972

22. **Amsterdam EA, Choquet Y, Lenz J, et al:** Attenuation of positive inotropic action of digitalis by hypoxia and comparison with isoproterenol. Circulation 46 suppl II:124, 1972

23. **Hopkins BE, Taylor RR, Henderson C, et al:** Myocardial digoxin concentrations in myocardial infarction. In, Proceedings of Fifth Asian-Pacific Congress of Cardiology, Singapore, 1972, p 246

24. **Amsterdam EA, Kamiyama T, Rendig S, et al:** Differential regional contractile actions of digitalis in experimental myocardial infarction. Clin Res 22:257A, 1974

25. **Doherty JE, Flanigan WJ, Murphy ML, et al:** Tritiated digoxin. XIV. Enterohepatic circulation, absorption, and excretion studies in human volunteers. Circulation 42: 867, 1970

26. **Doherty JE:** Digitalis glycosides: pharmacokinetics and their clinical implications. Ann Intern Med 79:229, 1973

27. **Doherty JE, Perkins WH, Flanigan WJ:** The distribution and concentration of tritiated digoxin in human tissues. Ann Intern Med 66:116, 1967

28. **Marcus FI, Burkhalter L, Cuccia C, et al:** Administration of tritiated digoxin with and without a loading dose: a metabolic study. Circulation 34:865, 1966

29. **Caldwell JH, Greenberger NY:** Interruption of enterohepatic circulation of digitoxin by cholestyramine. I. Protection against lethal digitoxin intoxication. J Clin Invest 50:2626, 1971

30. **Doherty JE, Perkins WH:** Studies with tritiated digoxin in human subjects after intravenous administration. Amer Heart J 63:528, 1962

31. **Smith TW, Haber E:** Digoxin intoxication: the relationship of clinical presentation to serum digoxin concentration. J Clin Invest 49:2377, 1970

32. **Beller GA, Smith TW, Abelmann WH, et al:** Digitalis intoxication: a prospective clinical study with serum level correlation. New Eng J Med 284:989, 1971

33. **Jelliffe RW, Buell J, Kalaba R:** Reduction of digitalis toxicity by computer-assisted glycoside dosage regimens. Ann Intern Med 77:891, 1972

34. **Bloom PM, Nelp WB:** Relationship of the excretion of tritiated digoxin to renal function. Amer J Med Sci 251:133, 1966

35. **Ewy GA, Groves BM, Ball MF, et al:** Digoxin metabolism in obesity. Circulation 44:810, 1971

36. **Ewy GA, Kapadia GG, Yao L, et al:** Digoxin metabolism in the elderly. Circulation 39:449, 1969

37. **Williams JF Jr, Klocke FJ, Braunwald E:** Studies on digitalis. XIII. Comparison of the effects of potassium on the inotropic and arrhythmia-producing actions of ouabain. J Clin Invest 45:346, 1966

38. **Klein M, Nejad NS, Lown B, et al:** Correlation of the electrical and mechanical changes in the dog heart during progressive digitalization. Circ Res 29:635, 1971

39. **Mason DT, Lee G, Peng CL, et al:** The digitalis inotropic dose-response curve: demonstration of linearity and attenuation by potassium. Circulation 46 suppl II:30, 1972

40. **Lee G, Peng CL, Mason DT, et al:** Similarity of the inotropic time course of differing digitalis preparations in isolated cardiac muscle. Circulation 46 suppl II:31, 1972

41. **Mason DT, Zelis R, Lee G, et al:** Current concepts and treatment of digitalis toxicity. Amer J Cardiol 27:546, 1971

42. **Cohn KE, Kleiger RE, Harrison DC:** Influence of potassium depletion on myocardial concentration of tritiated digoxin. Circ Res 20:473, 1967

43. **Goldsmith C, Kapadia GG, Nimmo L, et al:** Correlation of digitalis intoxication with myocardial concentration of tritiated digoxin in hypokalemic and normokalemic dogs. Circulation 40 suppl III:92, 1969

44. **Prindle KH Jr, Skelton CL, Epstein SE, et al:** Influence of extracellular potassium concentration on myocardial uptake and inotropic effect of tritiated digoxin. Circ Res 28:337, 1971

45. **Morgan LM, Binnion PF:** The distribution of H-digoxin in normal and acutely hyperkalaemic dogs. Cardiovasc Res 4:235, 1970

46. **Goldman RH, Coltart DJ, Friedman JP, et al:** The inotropic effects of digitalis in hyperkalemia: relation to Na$^+$-ATPase. Circulation 48:830, 1973

47. **Matsui H, Schwartz A:** Mechanism of cardiac glycoside inhbition of the (Na$^+$ K$^+$)-dependent ATPase from cardiac tissue. Biochim Biophys Acta 151:655, 1968

48. **Allen JC, Schwartz A:** Further therapeutic implications of potassium-digitalis interaction with the transport enzyme, Na$^+$, K$^+$-ATPase. Circulation 44 suppl II:134, 1971

49. **Mason DT, Zelis R, Amsterdam EA, et al:** Mechanisms of digitalis arrhythmias: electrophysiologic and myocardial subcellular considerations. In, Cardiac Arrhythmias (Dreifus L, Likoff W, ed). New York, Grune & Stratton, 1973, p 491

50. **Rosen MR, Gelband H, Merker C, et al:** Mechanisms of digitalis toxicity: effects of ouabain on phase four of canine Purkinje fiber transmembrane potentials. Circulation 47:681, 1973

51. **Watanabe Y, Dreifus LS:** Interactions of lanatoside C and potassium on atrioventricular conduction in rabbits. Circ Res 27:931, 1970

52. **Massumi RA, Amsterdam EA, Zelis R, et al:** The digitalis glycosides: contractile and electrophysiologic actions, clinical indications, precautions, and toxicity. Semin Drug Treat 2:221, 1972

53. **Smith TW, Butler VP Jr, Haber E:** Determination of therapeutic and toxic serum digoxin concentrations by radioimmunoassay. New Eng J Med 281:1212, 1969

54. **Butler VP Jr:** Digoxin: immunologic approaches to measurement and reversal of toxicity. New Eng J Med 283:1150, 1970

55. **Oliver GC Jr, Parker BM, Brasfield DL, et al:** The measurement of digitoxin in human serum of radioimmunoassay. J Clin Invest 47:1035, 1968

56. **Smith TW:** Ouabain-specific antibodies: immunochemical properties and reversal of Na$^+$, K$^+$-activated adenosine triphosphotase inhibition. J Clin Invest 51:1583, 1972

57. **Castellanos A Jr, Ghafour AA, Soffer A:** Digitalis-induced arrhythmias: recognition and therapy. In, Cardiovascular Therapy (Breast AN, ed). Philadelphia, FA Davis, 1969, p 108

58. **Gaffney TE, Lipicky RJ:** The cardiac pharmacology of digitalis and of antiarrhythmic and antihypertensive drugs. In, Clinical Cardiopulmonary Physiology, third edition (Gordon BL, Carleton RA, Faber LP, ed). New York, Grune & Stratton, 1969, p 91

59. **Stone JM, Fisch C:** Digitalis toxicity: a review. J Indiana Med Ass 62:459, 1969

60. **Chou T-C:** Digitalis-induced arrhythmias. Mod Treatm 7:96, 1970

61. **Fisch C, Knoebel SB:** Recognition and therapy of digitalis toxicity. Progr Cardiovasc Dis 13:71, 1970

62. **Church G, Schamroth L, Schwartz NL, et al:** Deliberate digitalis intoxication. A comparison of the toxic effects of four glycoside preparations. Ann Intern Med 57:946, 1962

63. **Dreifus LS, McKnight EH, Katz M, et al:** Digitalis intolerance. Geriatrics 18:494, 1963

64. **Lindenbaum J, Mellow MH, Blackstone MO, et al:** Variation in biologic availability of digoxin from four preparations. New Eng J Med 285:1344, 1971

65. **Smith TW:** Contribution of quantitative assay technics to the understanding of the clinical pharmacology of digitalis. Circulation 46:118, 1972

66. **Doherty JE:** Determinants of digitalis dosage. J Arkansas Med Soc 66:121, 1969

67. **Doherty JE, Perkins WH:** Digoxin metabolism in hypo- and hyperthyroidism: studies with tritiated digoxin in thyroid disease. Ann Intern Med 64:489, 1966

68. **Heizer WD, Smith TW, Goldfinger SE:** Absorption of digoxin in patients with malabsorption syndromes. New Eng J Med 285:257, 1971

69. **Robinson SJ:** Digitalis therapy in infants and children. J Pediat 56:536, 1960

70. **Solomon HM, Reich SD, Spirt N, et al:** Interactions between digitoxin and other drugs in vitro and in vivo. Ann NY Acad Sci 179:362, 1971

71. **Young RC, Nachman RL, Horowitz HI:** Thrombocytopenia due to digitoxin: demonstration of antibody and mechanisms of action. Amer J Med 41:605, 1966

72. **Levine OR, Somlyo AP:** Digitalis intoxication in premature infants. J Pediat 61:70, 1962

73. **Seller RH, Cangiano J, Kim KE, et al:** Digitalis toxicity and hypomagnesemia. Amer Heart J 79:57, 1970

74. **Nola GT, Pope S, Harrison DC:** Assessment of the synergistic relationship between serum calcium and digitalis. Amer Heart J 79:499, 1970

75. **Warren MC, Gianelly RE, Cutler SL, et al:** Digitalis toxicity. II. The effect of metabolic alkalosis. Amer

Heart J 75:358, 1968

76. **Frye RL, Braunwald E:** Studies on digitalis. III. The influence of triiodothyronine on digitalis requirements. Circulation 23:376, 1961

77. **Waxman MB, Chan HK, Heimbecker RO:** Influence of variations in sympathetic drive on digitalis tolerance. Clin Res 19:763, 1971

78. **Lown B:** Electrical reversion of cardiac arrhythmias. Brit Heart J 29:469, 1967

79. **Lown B, Cannon RL III, Rossi MA:** Electrical stimulation and digitalis drugs: repetitive response in diastole. Proc Soc Exp Biol Med 126:698, 1967

80. **Hughes JL, Mansour E, Salel AF, et al:** Elective conversion of atrial fibrillation: relation of energy level, digitalis and lidocaine to post-shock rhythm. Amer J Cardiol 26:639, 1970

81. **Mason DT, Braunwald E:** Mechanisms of action and therapeutic uses of cardiac drugs. In, Modern Trends in Pharmacology and Therapeutics (Fulton WFM, ed). New York, Appleton-Century-Crofts, 1967, p 112

82. **Mason DT, Braunwald E:** Digitalis and related preparations. In Cardiovascular Disorders (Brest AN, Moyer JH, ed). Philadelphia, FA Davis, 1968, p 383

83. **Pick A, Igarashi M:** Mechanisms, differential diagnosis and clinical significance of digitalis-induced arrhythmias. In, Digitalis (Fisch C, Surawicz B, ed). New York, Grune & Stratton, 1969, p 148

84. **Mason DT:** Recent advances in digitalis pharmacology and therapeutics. Ann Intern Med 80:520, 1974

85. **Fisch C, Stone JM:** Recognition and treatment of digitalis toxicity. In, Ref 83, p 162

86. **Mason DT, Spann JF Jr, Zelis R, et al:** Mechanisms of action of digitalis glycosides. In, The Art and Science of Cardiovascular Therapy (Russek H, ed). Baltimore, Williams & Wilkins, 1971, p 11

87. **Schmidt DH, Butler VP Jr:** Reversal of digoxin toxicity with specific antibodies. J Clin Invest 50:1738, 1971

88. **Mandel WJ, Bigger JT Jr, Butler VP Jr:** The electrophysiologic effects of low and high digoxin concentrations on isolated mammalian cardiac tissue: reversal by digoxin-specific antibody. J Clin Invest 51:1378, 1972

89. **Smith TW:** Ouabain-specific antibodies: immunochemical properties and reversal of Na$^+$, K$^+$-Activated adenosine triphosphatase inhibition. J Clin Invest 51:1583, 1972

90. **Damato AN:** Diphenylhydantoin: pharmacological and clinical use. Progr Cardiovasc Dis 12:1, 1969

91. **Bigger JT Jr, Heissenbuttel RH:** The use of procainamide and lidocaine in the treatment of cardiac arrhythmias. Progr Cardiovasc Dis 11:515, 1969

92. **Gibson D, Sowton E:** The use of beta-adrenergic receptor blocking drugs in dysrhythmias. Progr Cardiovasc Dis 12:16, 1969

93. **Amsterdam EA, Mansour E, Hughes JL, et al:** Present status of glucagon and bretylium tosylate. In, Changing Concepts in Cardiovascular Disease (Russek H, Zohman B, ed). Baltimore, Williams & Wilkins, 1972, p 215

94. **Zelis R, Mason DT, Spann JF Jr, et al:** Effects of ventricular stimulation and potassium administration on digitalis-induced arrhythmias. Amer J Cardiol 25:428, 1970

95. **Fisch C, Greenspan K, Knoebel SM, et al:** Effect of digitalis on conduction of the heart. Progr Cardiovasc Dis 6:345, 1964

96. **Hilmi KI, Regan TJ:** Relative effectiveness of antiarrhythmic drugs in treatment of digitalis-induced ventricular tachycardia. Amer Heart J 76:365, 1968

97. **Helfant RH, Scherlag BJ, Damato AN:** Protection from digitalis toxicity with the prophylactic use of diphenylhydantoin sodium: an arrhythmic-inotropic dissociation. Circulation 36:119, 1967

98. **Conn RD:** Diphenylhydantoin sodium in cardiac arrhythmias. New Eng J Med 272:277, 1965

99. **Coltart DJ, Gibson DG, Shand DG:** Plasma propranolol levels associated with suppression of ventricular ectopic beats. Brit Med J 1:490, 1971

100. **Seides SF, Josephson ME, Batsford WP, et al:** The electrophysiology of propranolol in man. Amer Heart J 88:733, 1974

101. **Bacaner MB:** Treatment of ventricular fibrillation and other acute arrhythmias with bretylium tosylate. Amer J Cardiol 21:530, 1968

102. **Caldwell JH, Greenberger NY:** Cholestyramine enhances digitalis excretion and protects against lethal intoxication. J Clin Invest 49:16a, 1970

103. **Helfant RH, Scherlag BJ, Damato AN:** Diphenylhydantoin prevention of arrhythmias in the digitalis-sensitized dog after direct-current cardioversion. Circulation 37:424, 1968

104. **Lister J, Cohen L, Bernstein W, et al:** Treatment of supraventricular tachycardia by rapid atrial stimulation. Circulation 38:1044, 1968

105. **Frommer PL, Robinson BF, Braunwald E:** Studies on digitalis-induced arrhythmias. J Pharmacol Exp Ther 151:1, 1965

106. **Fisch C, Knoebel SB, Feigenbaum H, et al:** Potassium and the monophasic action potential, electrocardiogram, conduction and arrhythmias. Progr Cardiovasc Dis 8:387, 1966

107. **Nayler WG:** Calcium exchange in cardiac muscle: a basic mechanism of drug action. Amer Heart J 73:379, 1967

108. **Schwartz A, Allen JC, Harigaya S:** Possible involvement of cardiac Na$^+$, K$^+$-adenosine triphosphatase in the mechanism of action of cardiac glycosides. J Pharmacol Exp Ther 168:31, 1969

109. **Lee KS, Klaus W:** The subcellular basis for the mechanism of inotropic action of cardiac glycosides. Pharmacol Rev 23:193, 1971

110. **Langer GA:** Effects of digitalis on myocardial ionic exchange. Circulation 46:180, 1972

111. **Smith TW, Wagner J Jr, Markis JE, et al:** Studies on the localization of the cardiac glycoside receptor. J Clin Invest 51:1777, 1972

112. **Mason DT:** Mechanisms of cardiac contraction: structural, biochemical and functional relations in the normal and diseased heart. In, Pathologic Physiology, fifth edition. (Sodeman WA Jr, Sodeman WA, ed). Philadelphia, WB Saunders, 1974, p 206

113. **Sonnenblick EH, Spotnitz HM, Spiro D:** Role of the sarcomere in ventricular function and the mechanism of heart failure. Circ Res 15 suppl II:70, 1964

Chapter 21

Ventricular Afterload-Reducing Agents in Congestive Heart Failure Therapy

Richard R. Miller, MD, FACC
David O. Williams, MD
Anthony N. DeMaria, MD, FACC
Ezra A. Amsterdam, MD, FACC
Dean T. Mason, MD, FACC

Facilitation of ventricular emptying leading to enhancement of stroke volume is the fundamental objective of therapy for heart failure consequent to cardiac dysfunction. Conventional treatment of congestive heart failure primarily has focused on increasing ventricular stroke volume and cardiac output through use of direct positive inotropic agents and concomitant diuretic therapy. In patients with coronary heart disease in whom refractory pump failure principally results from impairment and loss of myocardial contractile units, an increase in inotropic state of the remaining functioning heart muscle may insufficiently enhance cardiac performance, although some rise in stroke volume is often effected. Moreover, the powerful inotropic stimulus provided by cardiotonic agents may increase overall myocardial oxygen demands,[1] which is potentially detrimental in clinical ischemic heart disease.

In contrast to elevating low stroke output by direct inotropic stimulation in heart failure, reducing impedance to left ventricular ejection by administration of systemic arteriolar dilator drugs provides a unique therapeutic mechanism for the augmentation of pump performance by increasing ventricular emptying, while also diminishing myocardial oxygen requirements ($M\dot{V}O_2$).[2-16] Furthermore, concomitant systemic venodilation reduces ventricular preload with attendant salutary effects on pulmonary congestion and additional lowering of $M\dot{V}O_2$.[16-28] It is the purpose of this chapter to delineate the interactions and influences of the peripheral circulatory determinants of left ventricular performance, to clarify and compare the mechanisms of actions of the important vasodilator agents recently found clinically useful in the management of pump failure, and to elucidate the effects of ventricular unloading on the pump and mechanical properties of ventricular performance and myocardial energetics in clinical cardiac disease.

Peripheral Circulatory Determinants of Cardiac Function

It has become increasingly apparent that peripheral circulatory factors induce major alterations of central hemodynamics;[9,11,29] moreover, the influence of changes in systemic arterial and venous dynamics on cardiac performance assumes greatest importance in the critical setting of impaired ventricular function.[5,6,16] The princi-

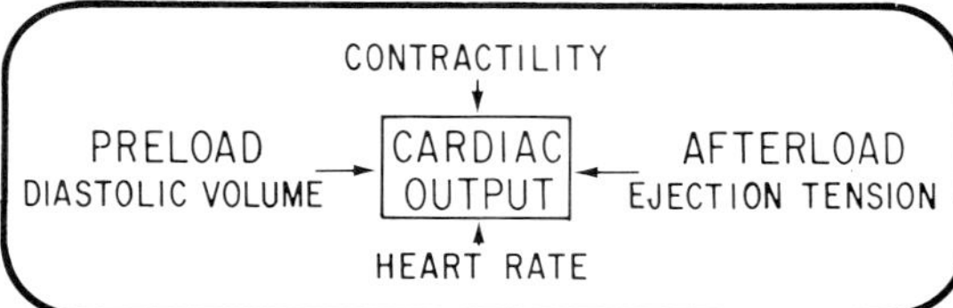

FIGURE 1. Diagrammatic representation of the four principal determinants of cardiac output.

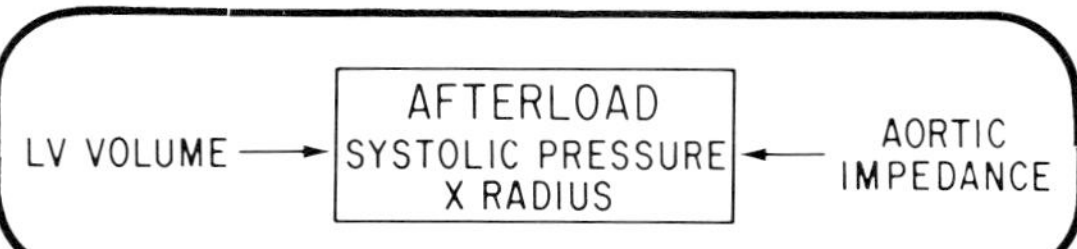

FIGURE 2. Diagrammatic representation of the two major determinants of left ventricular afterload.

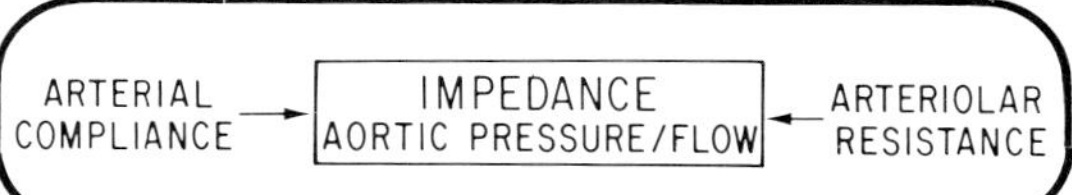

FIGURE 3. Diagrammatic representation of the two major determinants of aortic impedance.

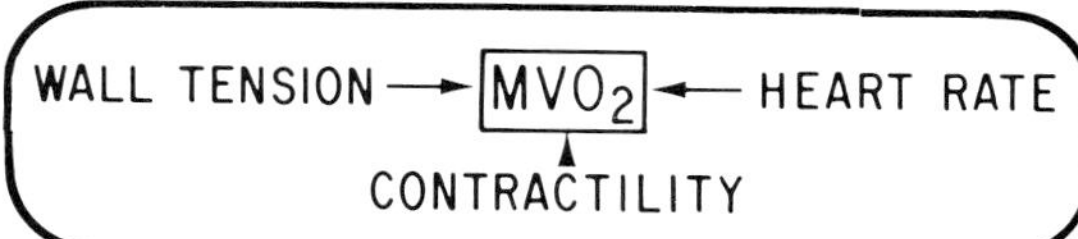

FIGURE 4. Diagrammatic representation of the three major determinants of myocardial oxygen requirements ($M\dot{V}O_2$).

pal peripheral vascular determinants of cardiac function are (1) venomotor changes that prominently alter ventricular preload or end-diastolic fiber length and (2) arterial resistance alterations that regulate the impedance to left ventricular ejection, which primarily governs ventricular afterload or the ventricular tension developed during contraction (Figure 1).

Preload: Interventions that influence ventricular preload do so by effecting an absolute change in intravascular volume, by redistributing intravascular volume, by altering end-systolic volume through changes in myocardial contractility or changes in ejection impedance and by varying ventricular diastolic compliance. Thus, preload may be reduced by di-

uresis, venodilation, enhancement of ejection fraction and increased ventricular stiffness.

Afterload: As with ventricular filling (preload), several factors influence afterload and impedance to left ventricular outflow. The load or tension that the left ventricle must develop to eject stroke volume constitutes ventricular afterload. Afterload is defined in Figure 1 as the wall tension during left ventricular ejection. In this discussion, the afterload of the left ventricle is considered in terms of wall tension or total force per unit of ventricular circumferential length (product of pressure and radius) and, therefore, independent of wall thickness—in contradistinction to wall stress or force per unit of cross-sectional wall area (product of pressure and radius divided by wall thickness), which is reduced by wall thickening resulting from ventricular hypertrophy. The two principal determinants of afterload are shown in Figure 2; tension during ejection is the integrated product of systolic pressure and radius of the ventricle, according to the Laplace formula. In turn, systolic pressure is related to the impedance to blood flow in the aorta, and the radius of the chamber is related to left ventricular volume (Figure 2).

Impedance: Impedance to left ventricular ejection is the instantaneous relation between the rate of change in aortic pressure and aortic flow[30] (Figure 3). Left ventricular outflow impedance is governed primarily by the compliance (relation of pressure to flow) in the large arteries and by total peripheral vascular resistance (the rate of runoff from the systemic arterial tree), which is determined principally by the radius or cross-sectional area of the systemic arteriolar beds (Figure 3). In addition, aortic impedance is related to blood viscosity and intraarterial volume. Of these factors regulating impedance, systemic arteriolar tone or resistance is the most important and the variable most subject to modification by pharmacologic vasodilation. In addition, it should be reemphasized that variations in impedance to ejection that are characteristic of different degrees of systolic mechanical ventricular overloading due to various types of structural heart disease largely account for the differences in cardiac performance among the various forms of chronic hemodynamic overloading (see Figure 8 in chapter 9 on regulation of cardiac performance).

Energetics: In the presence of impaired ventricular performance, elevation of outflow impedance results in reductions in the extent and rate of fiber shortening and in ejection fraction, with consequent elevation of left ventricular filling pressure.[31] Thus, stroke volume must be maintained at increased energy costs due to the increase in intramyocardial wall tension according to the Laplace relation[31-33] (Figure 4). An additional factor causing an increase in myocardial energy consumption is the duration of systolic wall tension.[33] In severe pump failure —particularly that due to coronary heart disease —elevations of impedance and afterload, which are inherent consequences of the heart failure state[29,34,35] result in a further increase in myocardial energy demand. This rise in $M\dot{V}O_2$ leads to additional ischemia and continued impairment of pump function, causing greater sympathetic-induced elevation of peripheral vascular resistance with resultant increases in ventricular afterload and preload. Thus, a progressively deleterious cycle adversely affecting myocardial oxygen needs and pump performance is set in motion by cardiovascular compensatory mechanisms that attempt to maintain cardiocirculatory integrity. Systemic vasodilation therapy that produces reductions in both afterload and preload may interrupt this potentially harmful chain of events while augmenting cardiac output, diminishing pulmonary congestion and improving myocardial energetics.[16]

Nitroprusside

The well established hypotensive action of nitroprusside is the result of direct peripheral vascular relaxation independent of sympathetic innervation.[36,37] The pharmacologically active component of nitroprusside is the nitroso (NO) group, which is chemically similar to the nitrite (NO_2) group common to all of the clinically useful nitrates.[38] Despite the chemical similarity of nitroprusside and the nitrates, nitroprusside is a more potent vasodilator, and the important quantitative differences in the relative clinical actions of nitroprusside and the nitrates on the systemic arterial and venous systems are of substantial therapeutic significance in heart failure therapy, as described in this chapter.

To determine the peripheral circulatory sites of vasodilation induced by nitroprusside, its effects on an isolated vascular bed were quantified by the techniques of forearm strain-gauge plethysmography,[39] which allowed determination of blood flow, vascular resistance and venous tone in the forearm of patients with chronic left ventricular dysfunction.[16] Both forearm arteriolar resistance and venous tone were reduced by nitroprusside infusion (Figure 5). In addition, total peripheral vascular resistance was diminished[16] (Figure 5). Therefore, alterations in left ventricular pump and mechanical function produced by nitroprusside occur secondary to cardiac unloading due to the primary direct dilator actions of the agent on the systemic arteriolar and venous beds.

Consequent to venodilation, pooling of blood in the peripheral veins diminishes venous return to the heart, thereby decreasing left ventricular end-diastolic volume and pressure. The resultant reduction in ventricular preload produces variable effects on myocardial pump function that are importantly related to the level to which left ventricular end-diastolic pressure (LVEDP) is decreased by nitroprusside.[5,7,16] Accordingly, with the clinical use of nitroprusside therapy, when markedly elevated LVEDP was lowered to levels that remained somewhat above normal and near the beginning of the plateau of the depressed ventricular function curve, the nitroprusside-induced decline in total systemic vascular resistance allowed lowered stroke volume to be augmented (Figure 6), with systemic pressure diminishing mildly and heart rate remaining essentially unchanged[16] (Figure 7). Conversely, when LVEDP was lowered to less than 12 mm Hg (the upper limit of normal LVEDP), cardiac output was not altered or decreased because ventricular preload was reduced to a position on the ascending limb of the ventricular function curve;[16] thus, the decrease in preload offset the reduction in impedance when preload was not maintained at the upper limits of normal (Figure 6).

The importance of an optimally elevated left ventricular filling pressure combined with reduction in impedance is further exemplified by carrying out volume expansion during nitroprusside infusion[16] (Figure 8). In patients who exhibited a reduction in LVEDP to less than 12 mm Hg and a simultaneous decrease in stroke

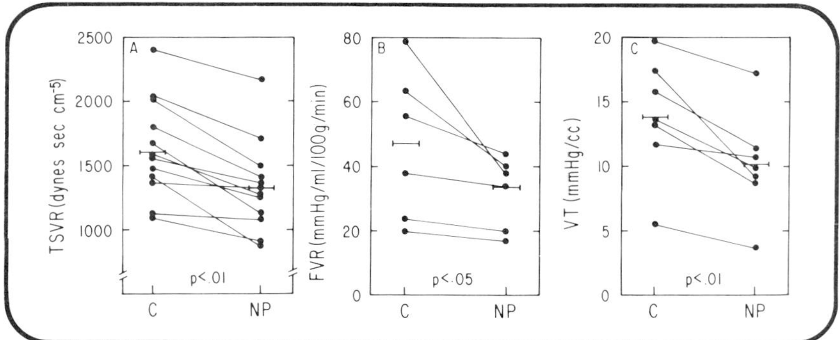

FIGURE 5. Effects of nitroprusside on (**A**) total systemic vascular resistance (TSVR), (**B**) forearm vascular resistance (FVR) and (**C**) venous tone (VT). (Reproduced by permission from Miller et al.[16])

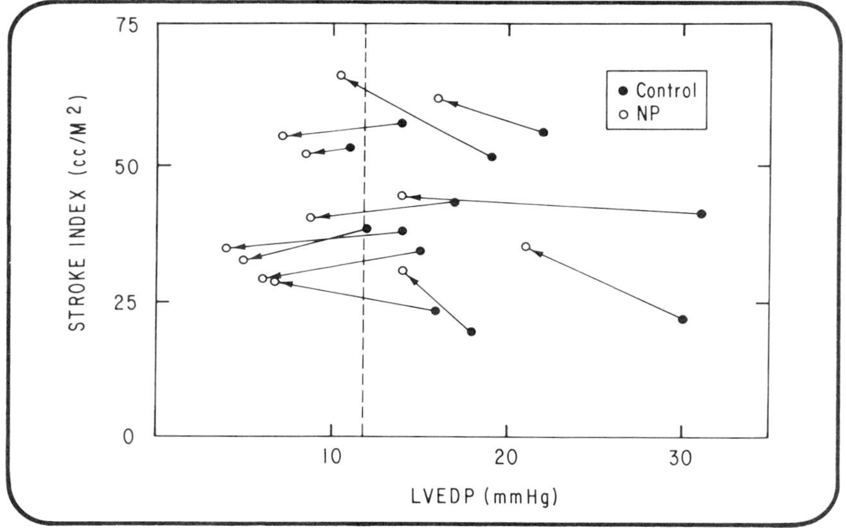

FIGURE 6. Relation between left ventricular end-diastolic pressure (LVEDP) and stroke index before and during nitroprusside infusion. **Dashed line** indicates upper limit of normal for LVEDP. (Reproduced by permission from Miller et al.[16])

index with administration of nitroprusside alone, volume expansion by dextran administration combined with constant nitroprusside infusion resulted in a return of LVEDP to slightly elevated levels with a substantial rise in stroke index to values considerably above control.[16] Therefore, it is apparent that nitroprusside produces maximal pump performance in ventricular dysfunction when elevated LVEDP is reduced to levels that are somewhat above normal. Through careful adjustment of ventricular unloading by reducing impedance with nitro-

prusside and increasing preload with volume expansion when LVEDP falls below the upper limit of normal, maximal enhancement of stroke volume and cardiac output is achieved.[16] Previous reports[40,41] on the benefit of volume expansion alone in acute myocardial infarction have indicated that LVEDP levels of 15 to 18 mm Hg usually allow optimal elevation of lowered cardiac output without producing pulmonary congestion.

In addition, nitroprusside infusion results in substantial augmentation of ejection fraction in

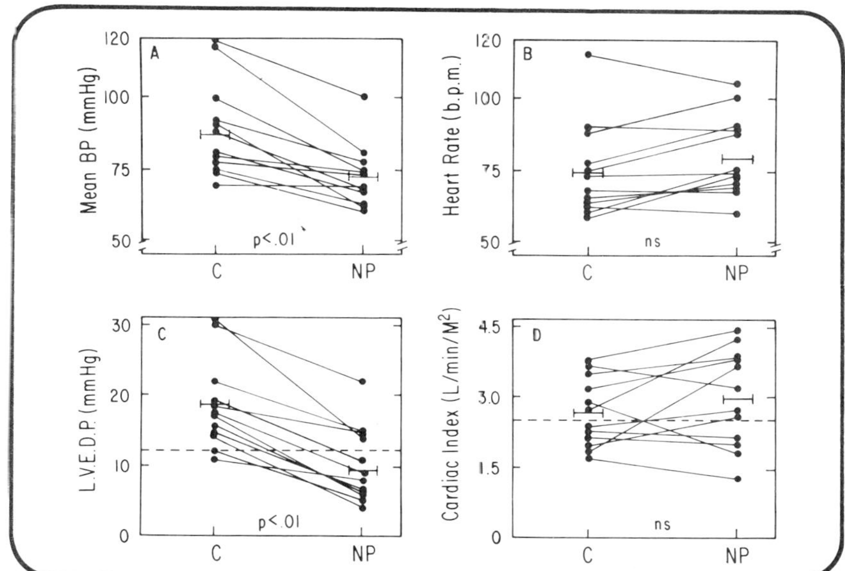

FIGURE 7. Effects of nitroprusside (NP) on **(A)** mean arterial pressure (BP), **(B)** heart rate, **(C)** left ventricular end-diastolic pressure (LVEDP) and **(D)** cardiac index. bpm = beats/min; C = control; ns = not significant. **Dashed lines** indicate upper limit of normal LVEDP **(C)** and lower limit of normal cardiac index **(D).** (Reproduced by permission from Miller et al.[16])

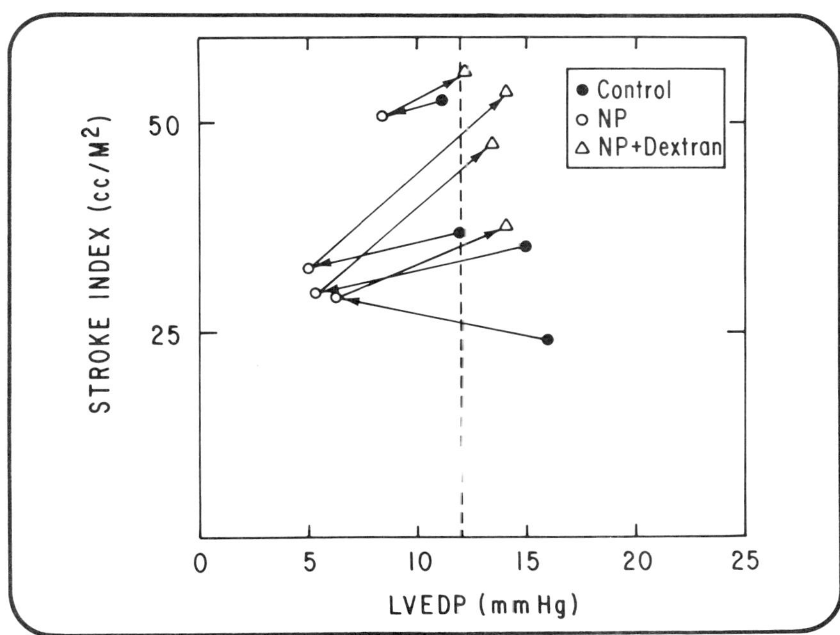

FIGURE 8. Effect of dextran infusion on the relation between LVEDP and stroke index during nitroprusside administration. **Dashed line** indicates upper limit of normal for LVEDP. (Reproduced by permission from Miller et al.[16])

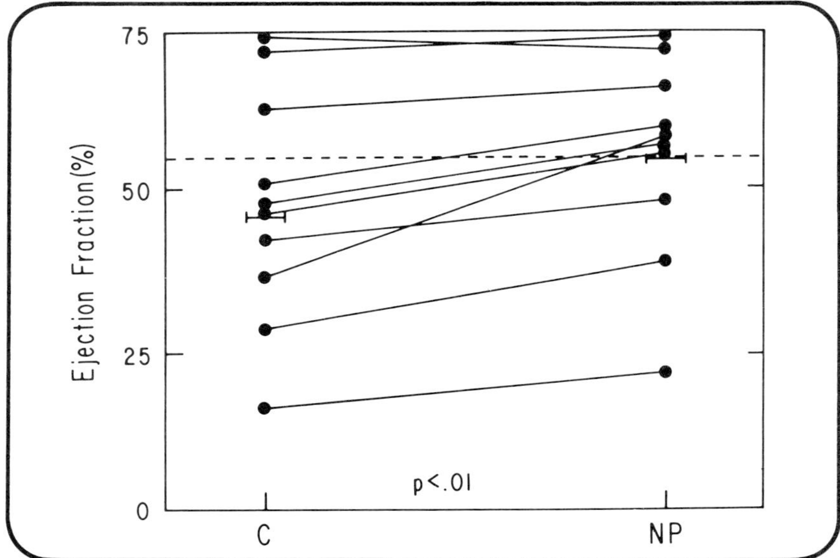

FIGURE 9. Effect of nitroprusside on left ventricular ejection fraction. **Dashed line** indicates lower limit of normal for ejection fraction. (Reproduced by permission from Miller et al.[16])

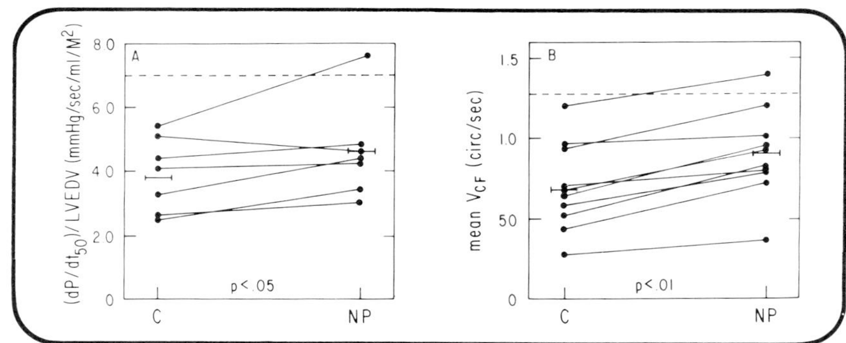

FIGURE 10. Effects of nitroprusside on an isovolumic index of left ventricular contractility **(A)** and an ejection index of contractility **(B).** (dP/dt$_{50}$)/LVEDV = rate of ventricular pressure rise (dP/dt) at 50 mm Hg developed pressure normalized for left ventricular end-diastolic volume index (LVEDV); mean V$_{CF}$ = mean velocity of circumferential fiber shortening. **Dashed Lines** indicate lower limits of normal. (Reproduced by permission from Miller et al.[16])

patients in whom this variable is depressed[7,16] (Figure 9). Furthermore, ejection fraction is not lowered in patients with normal control values. In the presence of severely abnormal hemodynamics—very high LVEDP with low stroke volume in ischemic heart disease—nitroprusside increases ejection fraction principally by producing a decline in impedance to ejection that predominates over the decrease in preload.[16] In contrast, there is little change in ejection fraction in patients with only mild to moderate elevation above control LVEDP, since filling pressures become normal with nitroprusside; consequently, stroke volume and cardiac output are unaltered in these patients because the decline in impedance is equally counterbalanced by the decrease in preload.[16]

Although nitroprusside possesses no direct

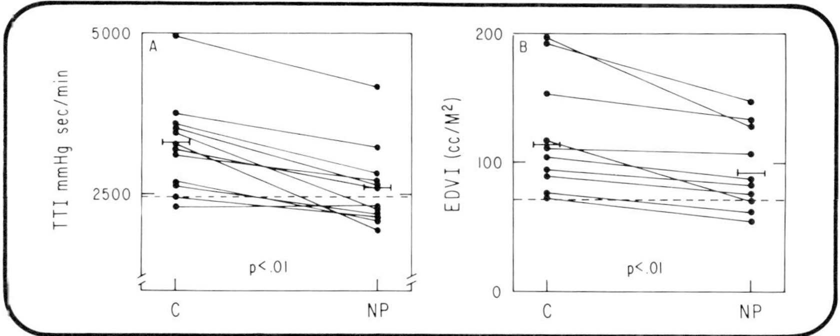

FIGURE 11. Effects of nitroprusside on two indexes of myocardial oxygen consumption (MV̇O₂). **A,** tension time index (TTI); **B,** end-diastolic volume index (EDVI). **Dashed** **lines** represent upper limits of normal. (Reproduced by permission from Miller et al.[16])

inotropic properties in experimental papillary muscles,[6] there are increases in the isovolumic index of contractility, (dP/dt₅₀)/LVEDP, and the ejection index of contractility, V̄CF, during nitroprusside infusion in clinical coronary heart disease[16] (Figure 10). It is likely that these modest increases in contractile state are the result of mild reflex sympathetic discharge due to a slight decline in arterial pressure and/or a decrease in ventricular ischemia resulting from reduced myocardial oxygen requirements. Although this indirect increase in contractility probably contributes somewhat to the improvement in ventricular function caused by nitroprusside, the major salutary actions of the agent on cardiac performance are the result of reduced ventricular loading.[16]

Concerning the effect of nitroprusside on myocardial energetics, unloading of the ventricle by systemic vasodilation decreases both the end-diastolic volume (Figure 11) and systemic arterial pressure (Figure 7), thereby decreasing ventricular wall tension—the principal determinant of MV̇O₂.[16] In terms of the major factors governing myocardial oxygen requirements, the decline in wall tension that lowers MV̇O₂ is essentially unopposed, since heart rate is unaltered (Figure 7) and contractile state is only minimally affected (Figure 10). The overall reduction of the principal determinants of MV̇O₂ produced by nitroprusside is reflected by diminution of the ventricular tension time index[16] (Figure 11). In contrast to positive inotropic drugs, which raise MV̇O₂ directly,[1] and beta ad-

renergic blocking agents, which depress both contractile state and MV̇O₂,[42,43] nitroprusside is unique in its ability to enhance ventricular function while lowering myocardial oxygen requirements.[16]

In patients with cardiac dysfunction, the overall mechanical unloading effect of nitroprusside on cardiac performance is dependent on the hemodynamic setting in which the agent is administered[16] (Figure 6). When ventricular function is minimally impaired, stroke output is usually unaltered or slightly reduced while LVEDP falls, since preload is reduced to the same extent as is impedance to ejection with a leftward shift onto the ascending limb of the ventricular function curve. However, when ventricular function is moderately to markedly abnormal, stroke index and cardiac output rise concomitant with a decrease in LVEDP. Therefore, in the presence of severe left ventricular dysfunction with marked elevation of LVEDP, nitroprusside reduces ejection impedance more than it diminishes preload in terms of stroke output, since the ventricle remains operative at the elevated filling pressures on the flat portion of its Frank-Starling curve. Thus, the relatively flattened nature of the depressed ventricular function curve characteristic of markedly impaired contractile state allows reduction in impedance produced by nitroprusside to be expressed hemodynamically as a rise in stroke output with decreased LVEDP.[16] In patients with only mildly to moderately increased LVEDP in whom reduction in ventricular contractility is not marked, lowered stroke output can be improved by combining nitroprusside with volume expansion to keep the ventricle preloaded at the top of the ascending limb of its function curve[16] (Figure 8).

Phentolamine

The vasodepressor agent phentolamine is an alpha adrenergic blocking agent that is chemically related to tolazoline and histamine.[44] In addition to alpha adrenergic blockade, its potent vasodilating properties are also related to direct vascular smooth muscle relaxation.[45] Alpha receptor blockade and direct dilation due to phentolamine have been described in both the systemic arterial and venous beds.[34,46]

Concerning the use of phentolamine in cardiac pump failure, the agent has been shown to improve abnormal hemodynamics and lower $M\dot{V}O_2$ in patients with acute myocardial infarction.[2–4,6,10,15] Mean arterial pressure, systemic vascular resistance and elevated left ventricular filling pressure are lowered while stroke volume is increased and heart rate is unaltered in patients with severe ventricular dysfunction. However, as with nitroprusside,[5,6,12,16] the effects of phentolamine on stroke volume are influenced by the level of left ventricular filling pressure prior to administration of the agent.[6] In patients with minimal elevations of left ventricular preload, phentolamine produced a slight reduction in stroke index when LVEDP decreased below the upper limit of normal.

Although it is apparent that both nitroprusside and phentolamine principally exert their influences on left ventricular function through reductions in both ejection impedance and filling pressure, quantitative comparisons of the actions of these agents on these two loading variables have been carried out.[47] Each agent was infused separately in patients with coronary heart disease who had mild elevations of LVEDP to reduce mean systemic arterial pressure by 15 mm Hg, with the sequence of administration of nitroprusside and phentolamine alternated between patients. Phentolamine increased cardiac index and heart rate concomitant with reductions in LVEDP and systemic vascular resistance while stroke index was unchanged.[47] In contrast, nitroprusside infusion in the same patients did not alter cardiac index

while stroke index was decreased, heart rate was increased, and systemic vascular resistance was reduced slightly. The reduction in afterload relative to the decrease in preload was greater with phentolamine than with nitroprusside.[47] Therefore, nitroprusside produced a relatively greater effect on left ventricular preload than did phentolamine, causing a greater leftward shift of the ventricle on its function curve. In these patients in whom the left ventricle was operating at the top of the ascending limb of the function curve, decline in stroke volume resulted from the greater leftward shift produced by nitroprusside than by phentolamine. Further, in contrast to phentolamine, vasodepressor-induced reflexes with nitroprusside infusion may compete with the direct vasodilator action of the agent,[47] thereby limiting reduction in ejection impedance.

From these observations, comparison of phentolamine with nitroprusside reveals that phentolamine exerts less dilation on the venous capacitance bed, resulting in smaller reduction in left ventricular preload for a given reduction in impedance. Therefore, phentolamine appears to be more effective than is nitroprusside alone in elevating cardiac output in patients in whom the left ventricle does not remain fully preloaded at the function curve apex. Conversely, phentolamine infusion for extended periods is impractical clinically because of the expense of the large doses required for persistent vasodilation.

Nitroglycerin

The principal cardiovascular action of sublingual nitroglycerin is direct relaxation of smooth muscle in the systemic venous system,[18,21,23,27,28] thereby increasing the distensibility of the systemic venous capacitance bed—that is, reducing peripheral venous tone (Figures 12 and 13) —with consequent pooling of blood volume in the systemic capacitance system and diminished venous return to the heart. In addition to predominant venodilation, the sublingual nitrate exerts a relatively mild direct systemic arteriolodilator action, manifested regionally by a decline in forearm vascular resistance and elevation of forearm blood flow,[18] associated with a modest decrease in systemic blood pressure but

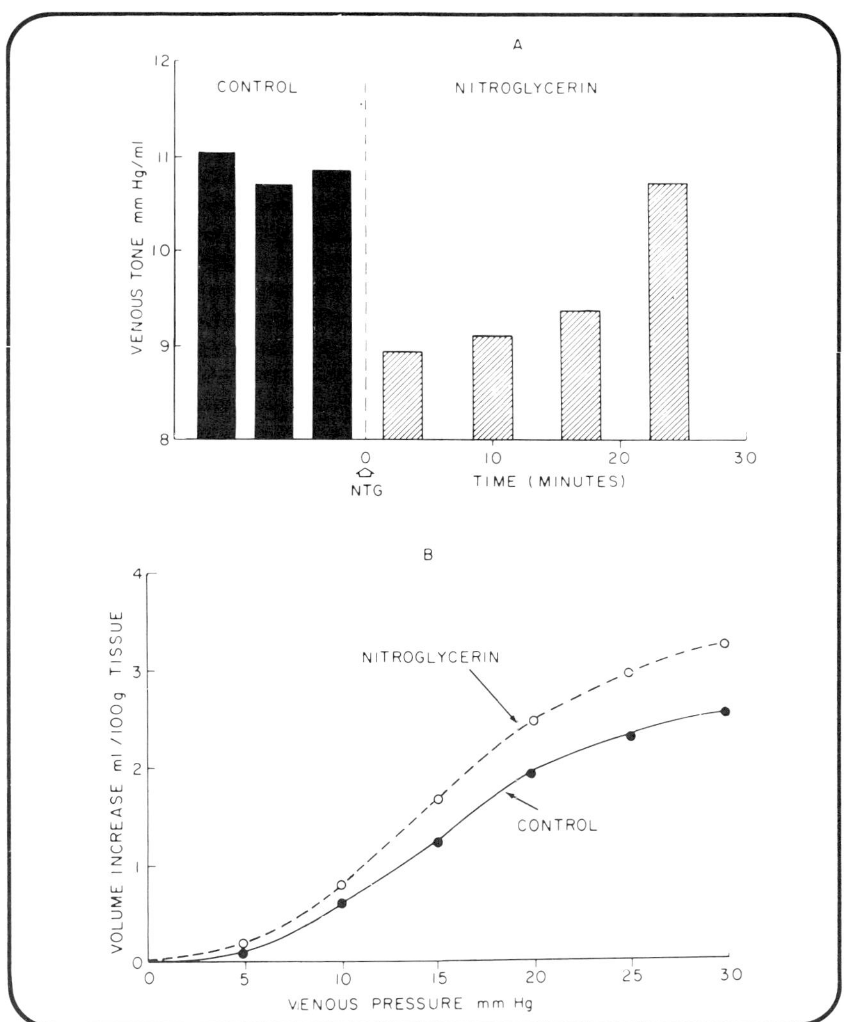

FIGURE 12. A, venous tone measurements carried out by an equilibration method 2 minutes after inflation of a forearm venous occlusion cuff. The **solid bars** represent 3 values during the control period. The **cross-hatched bars** represent measurements made at various time intervals after administration of 0.9 mg of nitroglycerin. **B,** relationship between venous pressure and forearm volume increases, determined by the stepwise occlusion equilibration method, during the control period and after nitroglycerin. (Reproduced by permission from Mason and Braunwald.[8])

inconsistently accompanied by a reduction in total peripheral vascular resistance.[17,27,28,48,49] Thus, the major therapeutic effect of nitroglycerin—that of lowering myocardial oxygen requirements—is accomplished principally through reduction of venous return to the heart, which results in decreases in left ventricular size and intramyocardial wall tension, thereby diminishing ventricular preload and $M\dot{V}O_2$. Also,

the direct systemic arteriolodilation contributes to the lowering of $M\dot{V}O_2$ by diminishing systolic intraventricular pressure, which results in decreased left ventricular afterload.

When a nitrate enters the circulation relatively slowly, such as after sublingual nitroglycerin, its direct dilator action on the systemic veins dominates over that on peripheral arterioles,[18,23] since cardiac output and stroke volume are re-

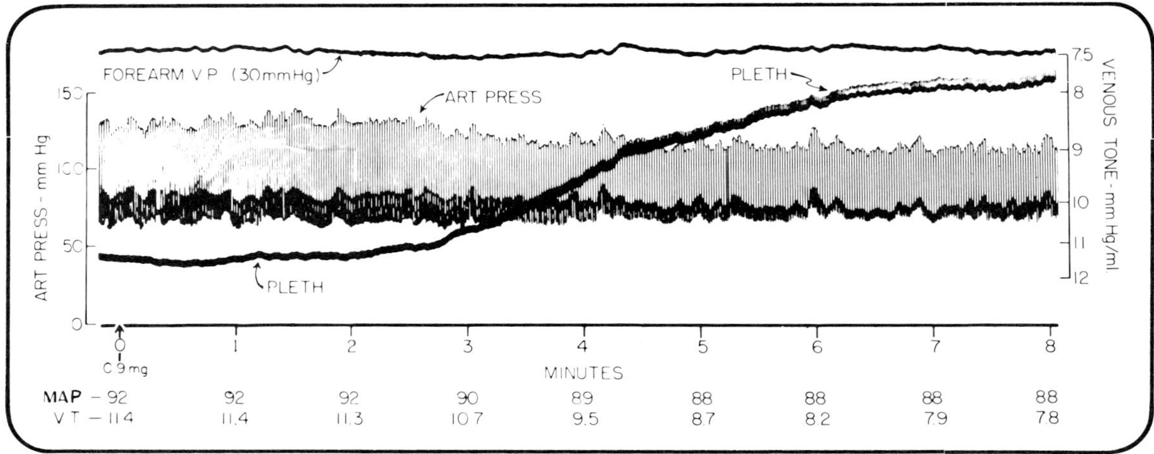

FIGURE 13. Plethsmographic tracing in a normal subject in whom forearm venous tone was determined by an equilibration method in which venous pressure was held constant while venous volume was allowed to vary. Forearm circumference (venous volume) was measured continuously before and after the administration of nitroglycerin. Note that after nitroglycerin the forearm circumference increased, while forearm venous pressure was held constant at 30 mm Hg, signifying that dilation of the capacitance vessels had occurred. Art press = phasic systemic arterial pressure. (Reproduced by permission from Mason and Braunwald.[18])

duced in normal subjects[18,19,21,23,26,27,48] and in patients with acute and chronic coronary heart disease.[17,19,21,22,24,48,50,51] In contrast, when the nitrate gains the circulatory system rapidly, such as with inhaled amyl nitrite, the marked vasodepressor effect caused by profound systemic arteriolodilation, as well as the hyperventilation and anxiety occurring with this agent, leads to intense adrenergic discharge with resultant reflex venoconstriction overriding the direct dilator property of the nitrate on the venous bed[18,23] (Figures 14 and 15). Thus, inhaled amyl nitrite produces an elevation of cardiac output while heart size declines, due to a marked reduction in left ventricular afterload with the rapid rise of nitrate concentration in the blood.

Since the principal action of sublingual nitroglycerin is peripheral venodilation, ventricular size should be diminished after administration of the agent. Recently, it has been possible to document reduction in left ventricular endocardial dimensions by echocardiography after sublingual nitroglycerin[27] (Figure 16); this nitroglycerin-induced decrease in heart size is consonant with results of other workers.[21,24,26,52] Sublingual nitroglycerin depresses cardiac function—shown by declines in stroke volume and

cardiac output—due to its predominant effect of reducing ventricular preload in both normal subjects and patients with coronary heart disease.[27,28] No significant decrease in total systemic vascular resistance was observed, although slight reductions occurred in the majority of individuals.[27,28]

The consistent preload-reducing property of sublingual nitroglycerin was clearly demonstrated by its greater diminution of end-diastolic volume than reduction of end-systolic volume, accompanied by the fall in stroke volume[27] (Figure 17). Thus, in regard to pump performance, the sublingual organic nitrate reduces ventricular preload relatively more than afterload. Interestingly, sublingual nitroglycerin did not consistently lower total systemic vascular resistance, and these observations are in agreement with previous investigations suggesting that the predominant action of the sublingual agent is on the systemic venous bed.[18,23] The administration of nitroglycerin in intact patients elicits reflex sympathetic activity due to the agent's vasodepressor action, thereby resulting in increased heart rate. This increase in sympathetic activity with nitroglycerin also produces slight augmentation of cardiac con-

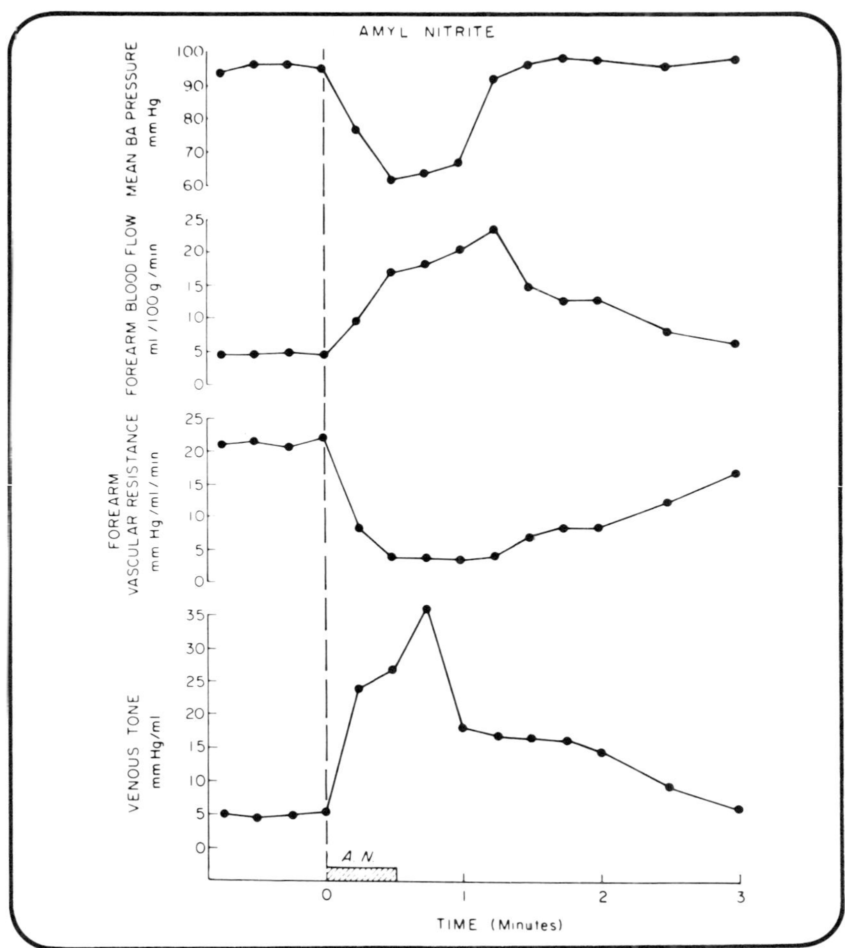

FIGURE 14. Serial changes in forearm vascular dynamics before and after inhalation of amyl nitrite in a normal subject. (Reproduced by permission from Mason et al.[23])

tractility[53] (Figure 18). The principal preload reduction caused by sublingual nitroglycerin is the predominant effect of the agent in terms of the major factors regulating $M\dot{V}O_2$. The venodilator action of nitroglycerin provides an immediately responsive peripheral circulatory mechanism for its antianginal effect through reduction of $M\dot{V}O_2$. Therefore, relief of myocardial ischemic pain by nitroglycerin is considered to be primarily the result of reduced myocardial oxygen demands rather than an increase in lowered myocardial perfusion via the diseased coronary vessels.[23,51]

Because of the profound ventricular unloading properties of nitroglycerin, it has been suggested by some workers that the agent might be useful in the treatment of pump dysfunction in acute myocardial infarction.[54] Recent clinical evaluation in our laboratories has shown that sublingual nitroglycerin resulted in a rapid decline in left ventricular filling pressure in acute myocardial infarction and this reduction was more pronounced in patients with the greatest elevation of filling pressure prior to administration of the nitrate[28] (Figure 19). Concomitantly, mean systemic arterial pressure fell substantially

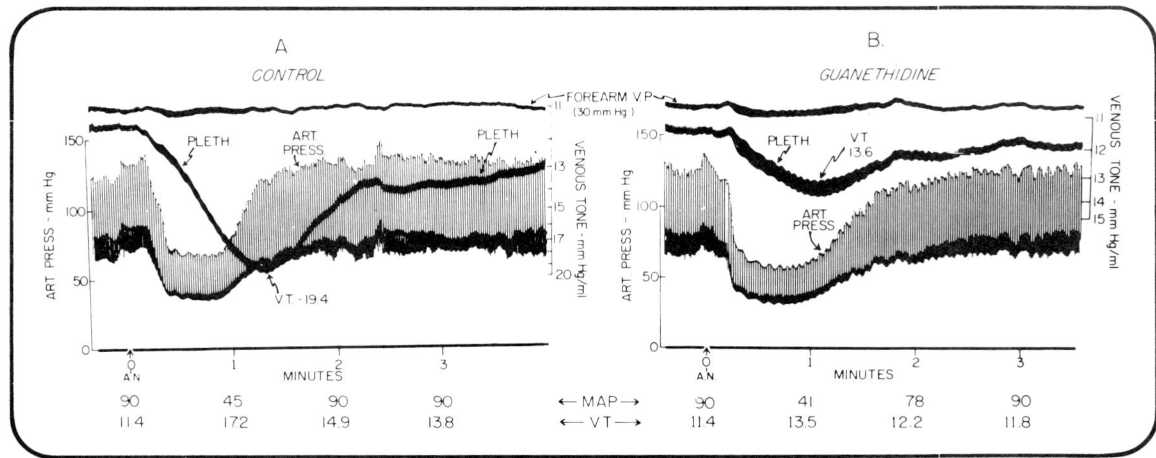

FIGURE 15. Recordings of arterial and venous pressures and forearm circumference after amyl nitrite inhalation in a normal subject. Venous tone was determined by the same equilibration method explained in the legend to Figure 13. **A,** during the control period; **B,** after guanethidine. After adrenergic blockade (**B**) amyl nitrite decreased forearm volume considerably less than during the control period (**A**), indicating that venoconstriction was markedly diminished. (Reproduced by permission from Mason and Braunwald.[18])

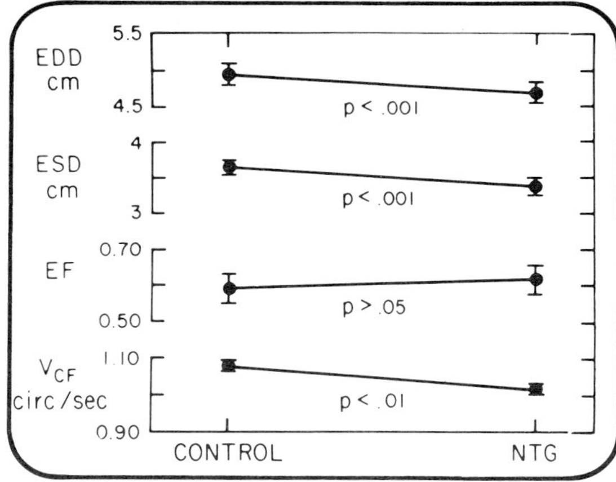

FIGURE 16. Average values for end-diastolic dimension (EDD), end-systolic dimension (ESD), ejection fraction (EF) and mean fiber shortening rate (V_{CF}) in circumferences per second before and after the administration of nitroglycerin in coronary patients. (Reproduced by permission from DeMaria et al.[27])

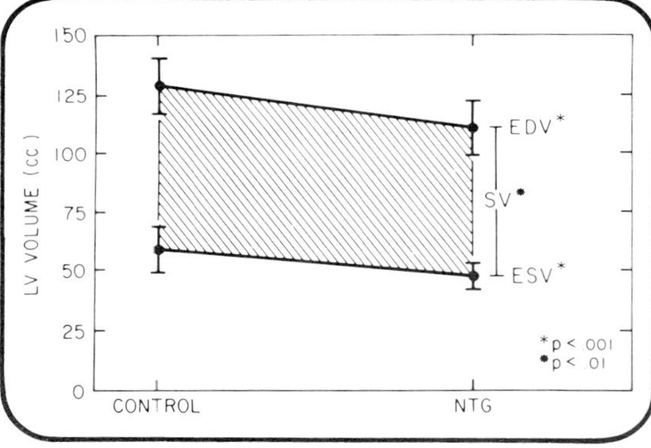

FIGURE 17. Average values of left ventricular (LV) volumes and stroke volume (SV) before and after the administration of nitroglycerin. Since end-diastolic volume (EDV) decreased more than end-systolic volume (ESV), stroke volume was diminished with nitroglycerin. (Reproduced by permission from DeMaria et al.[27])

(Figure 20) while there was little or no change in heart rate. Pump performance was worsened by nitroglycerin in the patients with acute myocardial infarction as evidenced by the decline in cardiac index in those with elevated LVEDP, as well as in the patients without abnormal filling pressure (Figure 21). Since the total peripheral vascular resistance was not changed by nitroglycerin, the decline in blood pressure was the result of reduced cardiac output in these patients.[28]

These clinical observations of the hemody-

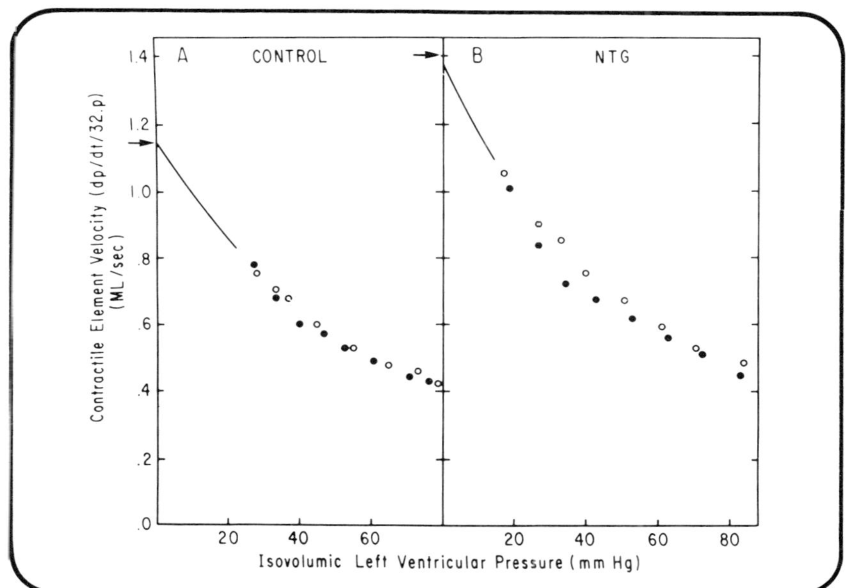

FIGURE 18. Left ventricular (LV) pressure-velocity curves before **(A)** and after **(B)** the sublingual administration of 0.6 mg of nitroglycerin (NTG). Contractile element velocity was calulated from two sequential beats denoted by the **solid** and **closed circles** as the ratio of dp/dt to 32 times the corresponding instantaneous (LV) pressure. The **arrows** indicate extrapolation of the curves to zero load. This maximal unloaded contractile element velocity (Vmax) is taken as an index of myocardial contractility. (Reproduced by permission from Zelis et al.[53])

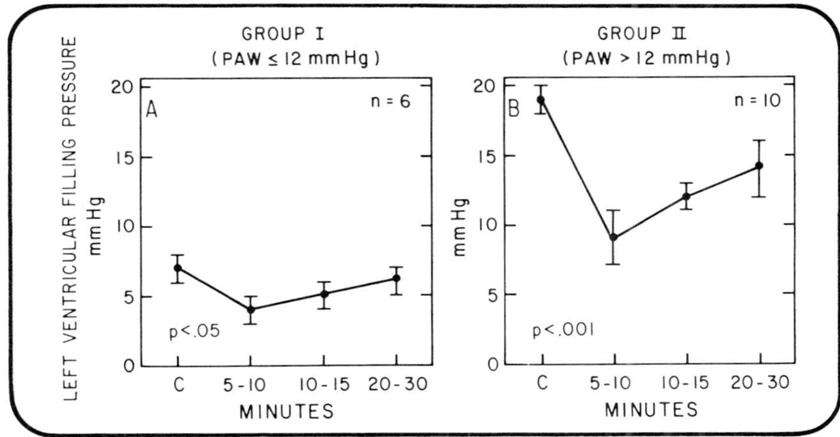

FIGURE 19. Clinical effects of sublingual nitroglycerin on left ventricular filling pressure, measured as mean pulmonary artery wedge pressure (PAW), in acute myocardial infarction in **(A)** those with pre-nitroglycerin PAW less than 12 mm Hg and **(B)** those with pre-nitroglycerin PAW above 12 mm Hg. (Reproduced by permission from Williams et al.[20])

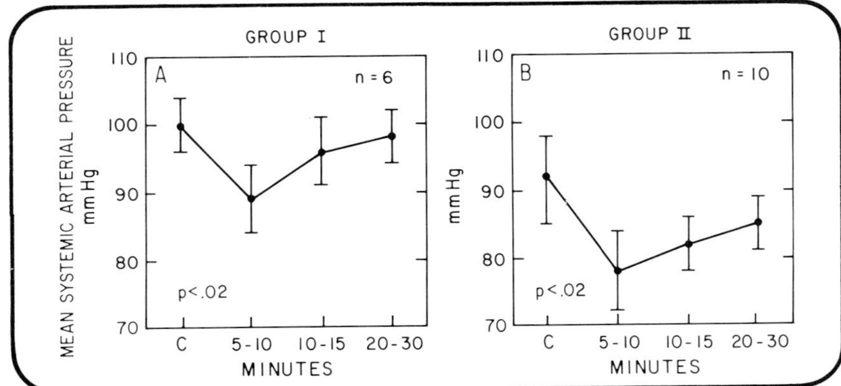

FIGURE 20. Clinical effects of sublingual nitroglycerin on mean systemic arterial pressure in acute myocardial infarction in **(A)** those with pre-nitroglycerin PAW below 12 mm Hg and **(B)** those with pre-nitroglycerin PAW above 12 mm Hg. (Reproduced by permission from Williams et al.[28])

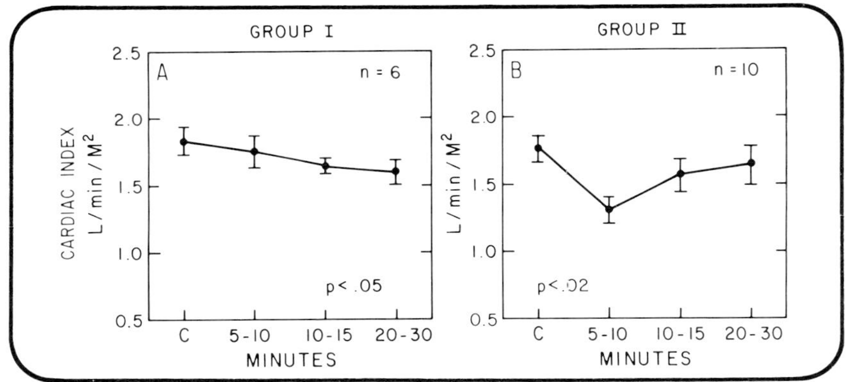

FIGURE 21. Clinical effects of sublingual nitroglycerin on cardiac index in acute myocardial infarction in **(A)** those with pre-nitroglycerin PAW less than 12 mm Hg and **(B)** those with pre-nitroglycerin PAW above 12 mm Hg. (Reproduced by permission from Williams et al.[28])

namic effects of nitroglycerin administered during the acute phase of myocardial infarction do not support the use of the sublingual nitrate to increase cardiac output and enhance pump performance in this condition.[28] Rather, nitroglycerin may result in the deleterious effect of further diminishing the lowered cardiac output in acute myocardial infarction. Our investigations indicate that sublingual nitroglycerin acts principally as a ventricular preload-reducing agent in acute coronary pump dysfunction with attendant reduction of cardiac output[28]—similar to its primary action of decreasing venous return to the heart in patients with chronic coronary heart disease and in normal subjects. Further-

more, this agent did not produce an observable decline in total peripheral vascular resistance in patients with acute myocardial infarction, and thus, nitroglycerin does not diminish impedance to ventricular ejection in these patients. In addition, the lack of total systemic arteriolar dilation with sublingual nitroglycerin in acute coronary heart disease is consistent with previous observations in patients with chronic coronary disease and in normal subjects. Although nitroglycerin has the ability to relieve pulmonary vascular congestion rapidly, the degree of decrease in left ventricular filling pressure is unpredictable and often results in some decline in cardiac output.

Concerning the effects of nitroglycerin on myocardial oxygen consumption in acute myocardial infarction, the decrease in left ventricular filling pressure and mean systemic arterial pressure with little increase or no change in heart rate suggest that myocardial oxygen requirements are reduced.[28] Thus, nitroglycerin in this condition might reduce ischemic pain and extent of necrosis, as well as diminish frequency of ventricular tachyarrhythmias and increase ventricular fibrillation threshold;[55] the ability of nitroglycerin to limit ischemia and improve electrical stability is enhanced by simultaneous administration of methoxamine to maintain arterial blood pressure.[25] Conversely, the decrease in cardiac index and reduced diastolic coronary perfusion pressure may attenuate the beneficial lowering of myocardial oxygen demand. In contrast to the effects of nitroglycerin, the impedance-lowering effect of nitroprusside allows improvement in pump output with concomitant preload reduction, affording diminution of myocardial ischemia and potential protection against ventricular rhythm disorders.

Clinical Application of Ventricular Unloading Drugs

From the foregoing observations concerning the actions of nitroprusside, nitroglycerin and phentolamine, a number of important conclusions can be formulated regarding the comparative effects and relative therapeutic value of these cardiac unloading agents in specific clinical conditions. Peripheral vasodilator therapy appears to be useful in four principal types of complications related to left heart disease as the result of actions of these agents effecting: (1) decreases in ventricular ischemia, angina pectoris and infarct size by reducing $M\dot{V}O_2$; (2) elevations of lowered cardiac output and cardiac performance by decreasing impedance to ventricular ejection; (3) decreases in elevated LVEDP, pulmonary congestion and dyspnea by lowering elevated LVEDP; and (4) reduction of ventricular tachyarrhythmic disorders by improving myocardial electrical stability. The transformation of the direct peripheral vascular relaxing properties of the vasodilator drugs into the hemodynamic alterations produced and the ventricular preload and afterload effects

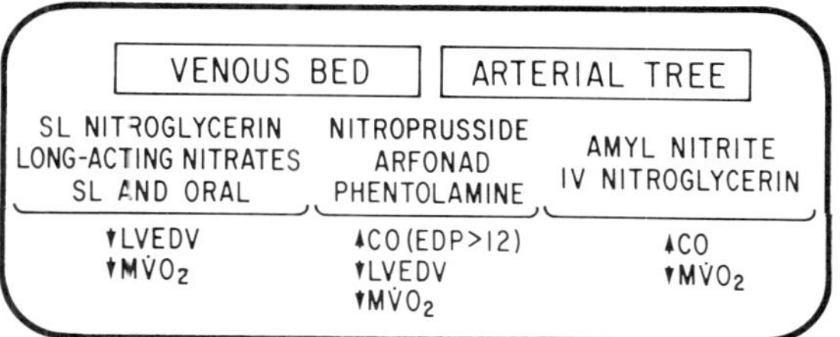

FIGURE 22. Diagram of the spectrum of actions of systemic vasodilator agents on the peripheral arterial tree and systemic venous bed. CO = cardiac ouput; EDP = LVEDP; IV = intravenous; SL = sublingual.

achieved is primarily dependent on the interplay between two major factors: (1) the relative dilator effect of the agents on the systemic venous bed compared with that on the systemic arterial tree (the reduction of venous return versus the decrease in aortic impedance)[47,56] (Figure 22) and (2) the configuration of the Frank-Starling function curve and the position on it at which the ventricle operates (Figure 23), which are controlled by the cardiocirculatory status when the vasodilator agent is administered.

Intravenous infusion of nitroprusside is begun at a low dose of 0.25 μg/kg/min (15 μg/min) with constant monitoring of intraarterial blood pressure and LVEDP as pulmonary artery end-diastolic or pulmonary capillary wedge pressure. The infusion rate of nitroprusside is regulated to lower the LVEDP to 15 to 18 mm Hg without a marked decrease in systemic blood pressure. With arterial systolic pressure kept above 95 to 105 mm Hg, the average infusion rate is about 65 μg/min (range, 15 to 150 μg/min). Determinations of cardiac output and systemic arterial resistance should be carried out frequently. Nitroprusside exerts potent vasodilator effects of similar magnitude on both the systemic arteriolar and venous beds.[16] In the failing heart—with filling pressure markedly elevated and the left ventricle operative far to the right on the plateau of its depressed and flattened Frank-Starling curve—the combined nitroprusside-induced balanced impedance and preload reductions are beneficially translated hemodynamically into enhancement of depressed cardiac output and diminution of elevated LVEDP with concomitant lowering of increased $M\dot{V}O_2$[16] (Figures 6 and 22 through 24). Optimal preload can be

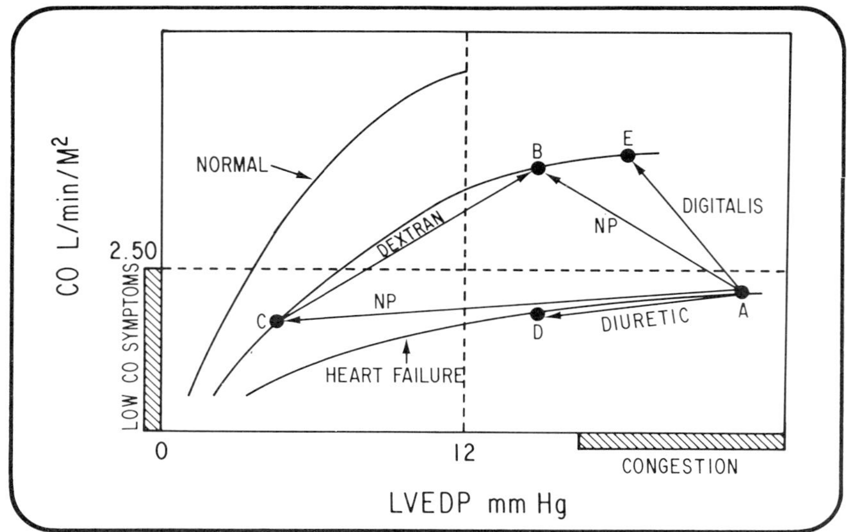

FIGURE 23. Relationship between cardiac output (CO) and left ventricular end-diastolic pressure (LVEDP) in a normal subject **(left curve)** and a patient with congestive heart failure **(right curve).** Point A indicates the point of operation of the dysfunctioning left ventricle in CHF. The **intermediate curve** is the improved relation between CO and LVEDP after digitalis (point E), nitroprusside (NP) to above LVEDP of 12 mm Hg (point B), and NP to below LVEDP of 12 mm Hg (point C) with the addition of dextran (point B). It should be pointed out that the improvement from point A on the low-est ventricular function curve to point B on the intermediate ventricular function curve after NP is not the result of increased contractility; rather, it is due to the enhanced relation between CO and LVEDP that the reduction of impedance to left ventricular ejection by NP affords. Point D on the CHF curve is the LVEDP after diuretic therapy. The **horizontal broken line** indicates the lower limit of normal for CO, and the **vertical broken line** indicates the upper limit of normal of LVEDP. Congestion = pulmonary congestion.

maintained, when necessary, by increasing blood volume with rapid infusion of 300 to 500 cc of low molecular weight dextran or saline solution (Figures 8 and 23). The ganglionic blocking agent trimethaphan (Arfonad®) also possesses balanced peripheral arterial and venous dilatory properties similar to those of nitroprusside;[57] consequently, trimethaphan has the same favorable effects on cardiac pump function as has nitroprusside,[57,58] with the added potential advantage that trimethaphan does not allow reflex increases in heart rate.[57]

In contrast to nitroprusside, sublingual nitroglycerin acts primarily to dilate only the systemic venous bed. Therefore, the nitrate-effected predominant preload reduction often results in an unfavorable decline of cardiac output (Figure 21), while producing transiently the useful relief of LVEDP and $M\dot{V}O_2$ elevations.[23,27,28] The short duration of the vasodilator action of sublingual nitroglycerin (about 15 to 30 min-utes) can be extended to approximately 1 to 4 hours with the use—instead of sublingual nitroglycerin—of sublingual isosorbide dinitrate,[59,60] oral sustained release nitroglycerin,[61,62] oral isosorbide dinitrate[60,63] or cutaneously applied nitroglycerin ointment.[64,65] Although nitrate tolerance appears to develop in some patients chronically taking oral long-acting nitrates,[66,67] this problem has been inconsistently observed[68] and may be incomplete in those patients demonstrating the phenomenon.[67] Tolerance to nitrates has not been a clinical problem in patients receiving only sublingual nitroglycerin or the long-acting nitrates.

Prolonged relief of pulmonary congestion can be provided by diuretics (Figure 23). Substantial reduction of markedly elevated LVEDP can be achieved with these agents without lowering cardiac output,[69] provided ventricular filling pressure is not lowered below the upper limit of normal by decreased blood volume. The decrease in LVEDP produced by certain diuretics is also due in part to a mild venodilator action possessed by many of these agents such as the thiazides[70] and furosemide.[71] In addition, the relief of acute pulmonary congestion by intravenous morphine appears to be related partly to indirect systemic venodilation produced by the process of central nervous system sympatholysis.[72]

Intravenous infusion of phentolamine is begun at a low dose of 0.1 mg/min. Hemodynamic monitoring is performed as with nitroprusside. The range of effective phentolamine infusion is between 0.1 and 2 mg/min. Phentolamine, in contrast to nitroprusside[15] and nitroglycerin,[28] produces a principal decrease in ventricular impedance.[47,56] Consequently, in heart failure with markedly elevated LVEDP, phentolamine appears to result in a relatively greater increase in cardiac output for a given decrease in LVEDP than does nitroprusside.[47] This observation is consonant with the finding that, in the presence of mildly increased LVEDP, phentolamine results in a decline in filling pressure while cardiac output is maintained.[47]

In regard to ventricular filling pressure, LVEDP is reduced more by nitroglycerin than by nitroprusside and more by nitroprusside than by phentolamine. Concerning myocardial oxygen requirements, $M\dot{V}O_2$ appears to be decreased relatively equally by nitroglycerin, nitroprusside and phentolamine. It is emphasized that, of these three vasodilator agents, only nitroprusside and phentolamine have the unique ability to improve cardiac output and LVEDP while simultaneously decreasing $M\dot{V}O_2$.[16,28] Sublingual nitroglycerin, therefore, does not enhance pump performance but does provide a means of rapidly lowering elevated ventricular filling pressure and excessive $M\dot{V}O_2$ for the prompt relief of pulmonary congestion and ischemic pain in instances in which reduction in stroke output is not deleterious.[28] In summary, due to differential relaxing actions on the peripheral arterial and venous circulations with resultant dissimilar ventricular unloading effects, each of the three vasodilator agents is clinically useful in treating dyspnea and angina pectoris, but only nitroprusside and phentolamine are of value in improving cardiac pump output.

The clinical usefulness of parenteral vasodila-

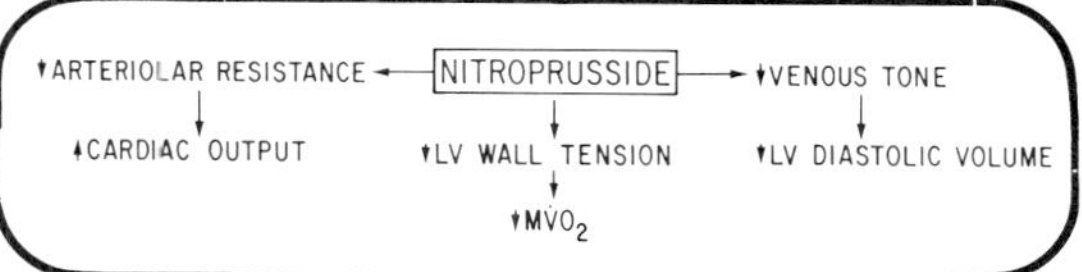

FIGURE 24. Diagrammatic representation of the salutary effects of nitroprusside vasodilator therapy in congestive heart failure. LV = left ventricular.

tor therapy in the management of congestive cardiac failure was initially recognized in hypertensive heart disease,[36,37] a condition in which intravenous hydralazine, trimethaphan and diazoxide have been successful in rapidly lowering elevated peripheral vascular resistance.[37] Vasodilator agents are also beneficial for the treatment of left ventricular dysfunction in acute myocardial infarction associated with hypertension.[10] In addition, nitroprusside and phentolamine are clinically valuable in the therapy of heart failure complicating acute myocardial infarction with normal blood pressure.[5,15,73] More recently, nitroprusside has been shown to be of substantial benefit in the management of congestive heart failure in patients with chronic coronary heart disease.[16]

In mitral regurgitation due to papillary muscle dysfunction in cardiomyopathies and in acute or chronic coronary heart disease, nitroprusside infusion has afforded marked hemodynamic improvement.[7] Reduced forward stroke volume is increased concomitant with reduction in regurgitant fraction, the prominent magnitude of V waves in the left atrium is reduced, elevated left ventricular filling pressure is lowered, and increased total systemic vascular resistance is diminished. Nitroprusside-induced reduction of impedance to ejection allows a greater portion of the total left ventricular stroke volume to be delivered downstream, thereby diminishing the regurgitant volume and the left artrial V wave amplitude (Figure 25). In addition, systemic venous relaxation produced by nitroprusside principally decreases the ventricular filling pressure and further reduces the size of the V wave in the left atrium. The regurgitant volume also is diminished, in part, by improvement of ventricular and papillary muscle energetics, as well as by diminution in ventricular chamber size leading to amelioration of distorted papillary muscle geometry.

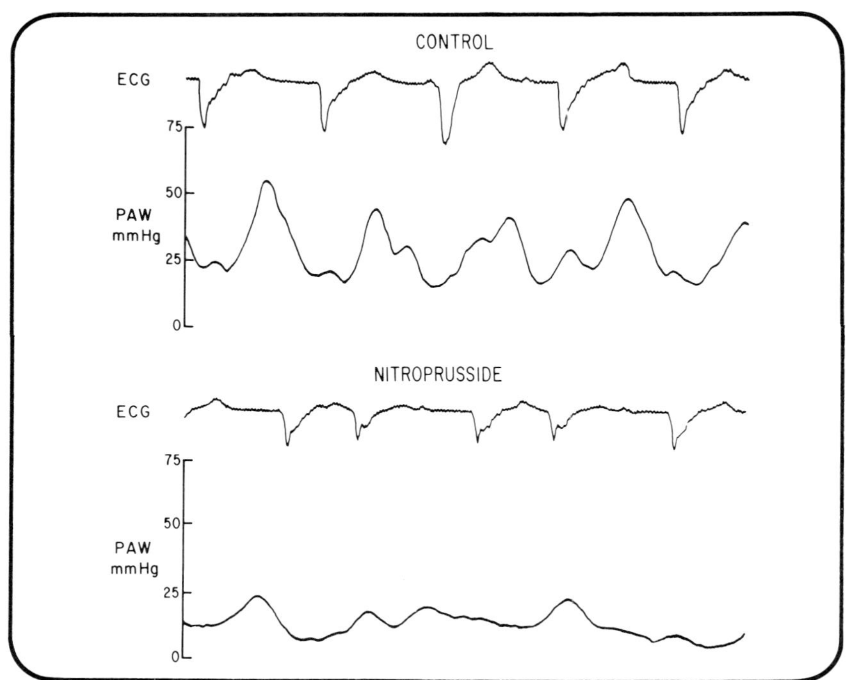

FIGURE 25. Phasic left atrial pressure, represented as pulmonary capillary wedge pressure (PAW), before **(top)** and after **(bottom)** nitroprusside systemic vasodilator ther-apy in a patient with sudden, severe mitral regurgitation due to acute myocardial infarction.

Similar in mechanism, nitroprusside recently has been shown to reduce the magnitude of left-to-right shunting across interventricular septal defects occurring in acute myocardial infarc-tion. Thus, in acquired ventricular septal defects with pulmonary and left ventricular volume overloads and critically lowered cardiac output, the decrease in systemic arterial resistance pro-duced by nitroprusside increases forward stroke volume, thereby diminishing left-to-right shunt-ing and decreasing pulmonary congestion. Further reduction of pulmonary artery hyper-tension is provided by its systemic venodilator action. In addition, nitroprusside has been of special value in improving impaired cardiac function in severe aortic regurgitation.[47]

Combined Nitroprusside-Dopamine Therapy

Additional improvement of abnormal pump performance is achieved by the simultaneous administration of a positive inotropic agent with nitroprusside infusion. We have shown that di-rect augmentation of cardiac contractility by dopamine increases lowered cardiac output to a greater extent than that obtained with nitroprus-side alone in patients with cardiomyopathies and in acute myocardial infarction. Further, we have found the combined use of dopamine with nitroprusside to be salutary in patients with de-pressed ventricular function states in the early postoperative period after coronary revascular-ization.

Combined Nitroprusside-Counterpulsation Therapy

In left ventricular pump failure due to coro-nary heart disease, a potential hazard of sys-temic vasodilation is reduction in coronary per-fusion consequent to decline in aortic diastolic pressure. Thus, further reduction of coronary blood flow may extend the area of myocardial ischemia and necrosis with resultant additional left ventricular pump dysfunction. Aortic dia-

	Nitrites	Propranolol	Tolamolol	CSNS	Exercise Training
1. Afterload					
a. systolic pressure	↓	variable	↓	↓↓	↓
b. preload	↓↓	↑	↑	variable	↑
2. Contractility	↑*	↓	↓	↓	variable
3. Heart Rate	↑*	↓↓	↓↓	↓	↓

FIGURE 26. Effects of different medical means antianginal therapy on the three principal determinants of left ventricular myocardial oxygen consumption (MV̇O₂). By reducing overall MV̇O₂, these modalities relieve myocardial ischemic pain by the mechanisms shown. CSNS = carotid sinus nerve stimulator; * = indirect reflex stimulation; large arrows = major effects; small arrows = minor effects.

stolic pressure augmentation provided by intraaortic balloon pumping or external counterpulsation[13] coupled with the systemic vasodilator action of nitroprusside allows improvement of coronary diastolic perfusion concomitant with reduction in ventricular outflow impedance. This combination of therapeutic modalities offers decided hemodynamic and cardiac metabolic advantages in the particularly difficult condition of left ventricular failure in acute and chronic coronary occlusive disease with normal, or sometimes even reduced, systolic blood pressure.

Limitation of Myocardial Infarct Size and Reduction of Tachyarrhythmias

Improved understanding of the hemodynamic-related determinants that govern myocardial oxygen consumption[1] (Figure 4) and the successful clinical extension of this knowledge to the treatment of angina pectoris[51] (Figure 26) have led to considerable interest in the application of a variety of therapeutic modalities to limit the extent of ischemia and necrosis in acute myocardial infarction.[75,76] Thus, increased MV̇O₂ induced by isoproterenol-augmented contractility, elevation of heart rate and methoxamine-induced hypertension enlarge the areas of myocardial ischemia and necrosis in experimental coronary occlusion.[75,76] Further, propranolol, counterpulsation, nitroglycerin, steroids, glucose-potassium-insulin, mannitol and hyaluronidase protectively affect experimental infarct size.[75,76] Recently, the clinical efficacy of reducing MV̇O₂ to modify the quantity of acute myocardial necrosis and ischemia has been shown by serum creatine phosphokinase analysis,[77] precordial electrocardiographic ST segment mapping[78-81] and central hemodynamic measurements[81,82] after propranolol administration and systemic vasodilator therapy with nitroglycerin, nitroprusside and trimethaphan. Finally, elevation of MV̇O₂ by an atropine-induced excessive increase in heart rate may occasionally provoke ventricular tachyarrhythmias in acute coronary disease,[83] whereas reduction of MV̇O₂ by nitroglycerin with maintenance of arterial blood pressure appears to improve ventricular electrical instability in both experimental and clinical coronary occlusion.[55]

Summary

The clinical application of peripheral vasodilator drugs to reduce left ventricular afterload constitutes a new approach in the clinical treatment of congestive heart failure. There are two principal mechanisms by which systemic vasodilator agents can diminish left ventricular wall tension during systole (ventricular afterload). First, these agents may reduce systemic vascular resistance, decreasing aortic impedance to left ventricular ejection; thus, the left ventricle is capable of a greater stroke volume and cardiac output. Since low cardiac output usually increases to the same extent that elevated peripheral vascular resistance decreases, there is little or no decline in systemic arterial blood pressure, accompanied by minimal if any increase in heart rate.

Second, peripheral vasodilator drugs may also relax vascular smooth muscle in the systemic venous bed, causing peripheral pooling of blood with diminished venous return to the heart. Consequently, left ventricular filling pressure (LVEDP) and end-diastolic volume (ventricular preload) are reduced and pulmonary congestion is relieved. In additon, myocardial oxygen requirements ($M\dot{V}O_2$) are reduced by the decrease in left ventricular wall tension during contraction, due to the peripheral vasodilator-induced decreases in ventricular volume and aortic impedance. Thus, the major objectives of treatment in many forms of acute and chronic congestive heart failure may be achieved by systemic vasodilator therapy that lowers left ventricular afterload: (1) an increase in low cardiac output; (2) a decrease in elevated ventricular filling pressure with relief of pulmonary congestion; (3) a reduction of myocardial oxygen requirements with decreased ventricular ischemia; with (4) little or no alteration in systemic blood pressure and heart rate.

The principal vasodilator drugs currently in clinical use for the reduction of ventricular afterload (nitroprusside, phentolamine, nitroglycerin and trimethaphan) exert differential actions on the peripheral arterial and venous beds. Nitroprusside and trimethaphan produce balanced relaxing effects on systemic arteriolar and venous smooth muscle, thereby resulting in increased cardiac output and decreased LVEDP and $M\dot{V}O_2$. Phentolamine has a greater effect on the arterial tree than on the peripheral venous bed, thus increasing cardiac output relatively more than it lowers LVEDP. In contrast, the action of sublingual nitrates is nearly entirely exerted on the systemic venous system, thereby lowering LVEDP and $M\dot{V}O_2$ while cardiac output may decline or remain unchanged.

Acknowledgment: This work was supported in part by Research Program Project Grant HL-14780 from the National Heart and Lung Institute, National Institutes of Health.

The authors gratefully acknowledge the technical assistance of Robert Kleckner, Arthur Lewis and Leslie J. Silvernail.

References

1. **Braunwald E:** Control of myocardial oxygen consumption: physiologic and clinical considerations. Amer J Cardiol 27:416, 1971
2. **Gould L, Zahir M, Ettinger S:** Phentolamine and cardiovascular performance. Brit Heart J 31:154, 1969
3. **Majid PA, Sharma B, Taylor SH:** Phentolamine for vasodilator treatment of severe heart failure. Lancet 2:719, 1971
4. **Perret CI, Poli S, Enrico JF:** Phentolamine for vasodilator treatment of severe heart failure. Lancet 2:978, 1971
5. **Franciosa JA, Guiha NH, Limas CJ, et al:** Improved left ventricular function during nitroprusside infusion in acute myocardial infarction. Lancet 1:650, 1972
6. **Chatterjee K, Parmley WW, Ganz W, et al:** Hemodynamic and metabolic responses to vasodilator therapy in acute myocardial infarction. Circulation 48:1183, 1973
7. **Chatterjee K, Parmley WW, Swan HJC, et al:** Beneficial effects of vasodilator agents in severe mitral regurgitation due to dysfunction of subvalvular appartus. Circulation 48:684, 1973
8. **Cohn JN:** Vasodilator therapy for heart failure. Circulation 48:5, 1973
9. **Cohn JN:** Blood pressure and cardiac performance. Amer J Med 55:351, 1973
10. **Kelly DT, Delgado CE, Taylor DR, et al:** Use of phentolamine in acute myocardial infarction associated with hypertension and left ventricular failure. Circulation 47:729, 1973
11. **Mason DT:** Regulation of cardiac performance in clinical heart disease. Amer J Cardiol 32:437, 1973
12. **Guiha NH, Cohn JN, Mikulic E, et al:** Treatment of refractory heart failure with infusion of nitroprusside. New Eng J Med 291:587, 1974
13. **Parmley WW, Chatterjee K, Charuzi Y, et al:** Hemodynamic effects of noninvasive systolic unloading (nitroprusside) and diastolic augmentation (external counterpulsation) in patients with acute myocardial infarction. Amer J Cardiol 33:819, 1974
14. **Rowe GG, Henderson RN:** Systemic and coronary hemodynamic effects of sodium nitroprusside. Amer Heart J 87:83, 1974
15. **Walinsky P, Chatterjee K, Forrester J, et al:** Enhanced left ventricular performance with phentolamine in acute myocardial infarction. Amer J Cardiol 33:37, 1974
16. **Miller RR, Vismara LA, Zelis R, et al:** Clinical use of sodium nitroprusside in chronic ischemic heart disease: effects on peripheral vascular resistance and venous tone and on ventricular volume, pump and mechanical performance. Circulation 51:328, 1975
17. **Christensson B, Karietors T, Westling H:** Hemodynamic effects of nitroglycerin in patients with coronary heart disease. Brit Heart J 27:511, 1965
18. **Mason DT, Braunwald E:** The effects of nitroglycerin and amyl nitrite on arteriolar and venous tone in the human forearm. Circulation 32:755, 1965
19. **Hoeschen RJ, Bousvaros GA, Klassen GA, et al:** Hemo-

dynamic effects of angina pectoris, and of nitroglycerin in normal and anginal subjects. Brit Heart J 28:221, 1966

20. **Frick MH, Balcon R, Cross D, et al:** Hemodynamic effects of nitroglycerin in patients with angina pectoris studied by an atrial pacing method. Circulation 37:160, 1968

21. **Williams JF, Glick G, Braunwald E:** Studies on cardiac dimensions in intact unanesthetized man: effects of nitroglycerin. Circulation 32:767, 1967

22. **Lee SJK, Sung KK, Zaragoza AJ:** Effects of nitroglycerin on left ventricular volumes and wall tension in patients with ischemic heart disease. Brit Heart J 32:790, 1970

23. **Mason DT, Zelis R, Amsterdam EA:** Actions of the nitrites on the peripheral circulation and myocardial oxygen consumption: significance in the relief of angina pectoris. Chest 59:296, 1971

24. **Chlong NA, West RO, Parker JO:** Influence of nitroglycerin on myocardial metabolism and hemodynamics during angina induced by atrial pacing. Circulation 45:1044, 1972

25. **Smith ER, Redwood DR, McCarron WE, et al:** Coronary artery occlusion in the conscious dog: effects of alterations in arterial pressure produced by nitroglycerin, hemorrhage, and alpha-adrenergic agonists on the degree of myocardial ischemia. Circulation 47:51, 1973

26. **Burggraf GW, Parker JO:** Left ventricular volume changes after amyl nitrite and nitroglycerin in man as measured by ultrasound. Circulation 49:136, 1974

27. **DeMaria AN, Vismara LA, Auditore K, et al:** Effects of nitroglycerin on left ventricular cavitary size and cardiac performance determined by ultrasound in man. Amer J Med 57:754, 1974

28. **Williams DO, Amsterdam EA, Mason DT:** Hemodynamic effects of nitroglycerin in acute myocardial infarction: decrease in ventricular preload at the expense of cardiac output. Circulation 51:421, 1975

29. **Mason DT, Spann JF, Zelis R, et al:** Alterations of hemodynamic and myocardial mechanics in patients with congestive heart failure: pathophysiologic mechanisms and assessment of cardiac function and ventricular contractility. Prog Cardiovasc Dis 12:507, 1970

30. **Mills CJ, Gabe IJ, Gault JH, et al:** Pressure-flow relationships and vascular impedance in man. Cardiovasc Res 4:405, 1970

31. **Graham TP, Covell JW, Sonnenblick EH, et al:** Control of myocardial oxygen consumption: relative influence of contractile state and tension development. J Clin Invest 47:375, 1968

32. **McDonald RH, Taylor RR, Cingoloni NE:** Measurement of myocardial developed tension and its relation to oxygen consumption. Amer J Physiol 211:667, 1966

33. **Skelton CL, Sonnenblick EH:** Myocardial energetics. In, Cardiac Mechanics (Mirsky I, Ghista DN, Sandler H, ed). New York, John Wiley & Sons, 1974, p 113

34. **Zelis R, Mason DT, Braunwald E:** A comparison of the effects of vasodilator stimuli on peripheral resistance vessels in normal subjects and in patients with congestive heart failure. J Clin Invest 47:960, 1968

35. **Zelis R, Mason DT:** Compensatory mechanisms in congestive heart failure: the role of the peripheral resistance vessels. New Eng J Med 282:962, 1970

36. **Schlant RC, Tsagaris TS, Robertson RJ:** Studies on the acute cardiovascular effects of intravenous sodium nitroprusside. Amer J Cardiol 9:51, 1962

37. **Bhatia SK, Frohlich ED:** Hemodynamic comparison of agents useful in hypertensive emergencies. Amer Heart J 85:367, 1973

38. **Palmer RF, Lasseter KC:** Sodium nitroprusside. New Eng J Med 292:294, 1975

39. **Mason DT, Braunwald E:** Effects of guanethidine, reserpine and methyldopa on reflex venous and arterial constriction in man. J Clin Invest 43:1449, 1964

40. **Russell RO, Rackley CE, Pombo J, et al:** Effects of increasing left ventricular filling pressure in patients with acute myocardial infarction. J Clin Invest 49:1539, 1970

41. **Crexells C, Chatterjee K, Forrester JS, et al:** Optimal level of filling pressure in the left side of the heart in acute myocardial infarction. New Eng J Med 289:1263, 1973

42. **Wolfson S, Heinle RA, Herman MV, et al:** Propranolol and angina pectoris. Amer J Cardiol 18:345, 1966

43. **Liang C, Hood WB Jr:** The myocardial depressant effect of beta-receptor blocking agents. Circ Res 35:272, 1974

44. **Hecht HH, Crandall R, Samuels AJ:** Adrenergic blockade in man by a new imidazole derivative C-7337. Fed Proc 9:283, 1950

45. **Taylor SH, Sutherland GR, MacKenzie MB, et al:** The circulatory effects of intravenous phentolamine in man. Circulation 31:741, 1965

46. **Abboud FM, Schmid PE, Eckstein JW:** Vascular responses after alpha adrenergic blockade. J Clin Invest 47:1, 1968

47. **Williams DO, Hilliard GK, Cantor SA, et al:** Comparative mechanisms of ventricular unloading by systemic vasodilator agents in therapy of cardiac failure: nitroprusside versus phentolamine. Amer J Cardiol 35:177, 1975

48. **Gorlin R, Brachfeld N, MacLeod C, et al:** Effect of nitroglycerin on the coronary circulation in patients with coronary artery disease or increased left ventricular work. Circulation 19:705, 1959

49. **Bernstein L, Friesinger GC, Lichtlen PR, et al:** The effect of nitroglycerin on the systemic and coronary circulation in man and dogs. Circulation 33:107, 1966

50. **Najmi M, Griggs DM, Kasparian H, et al:** Effects of nitroglycerin on hemodynamics during rest and exercise in patients with coronary insufficiency. Circulation 35:46, 1967

51. **Mason DT, Spann JF Jr, Zelis R, et al:** Physiologic approach to the treatment of angina pectoris. New Eng J Med 281:1225, 1969

52. **Parker JO, West RO, DiGiorgi S:** The effect of nitroglycerin on coronary blood flow and the hemodynamic response to exercise in coronary artery disease. Amer J Cardiol 27:59, 1971

53. **Zelis R, Amsterdam EA, Mason DT:** Alterations in ventricular contractility produced by nitroglycerin in man. Amer J Cardiol 26:667, 1970

54. **Gold HK, Leinback RC, Sanders CA:** Use of sublingual nitroglycerin in congestive failure following acute myocardial infarction. Circulation 46:839, 1972

55. **Kent KM, Smith ER, Redwood DR, et al:** Beneficial electrophysiologic effects of nitroglycerin during acute myocardial infarction. Amer J Cardiol 33:513, 1974

56. **Miller RR, Vismara LA, Williams DO, et al:** Mechanisms of ventricular unloading in heart failure: comparative effects of nitroglycerin, nitroprusside and phentolamine on cardiac function and peripheral circulation. Circulation 52 suppl II: 76, 1975

57. **Williams DO, Hilliard GK, Merwin R, et al:** Impedance reduction with trimethaphan (Arfonad) for pump failure complicating coronary heart disease. Clin Res 23:215A, 1975

58. **Kouchoukos NT, Sheppard LC, Kirklin JW:** Effects of alterations in arterial pressure on cardiac performance early after open intracardiac operations. J Thorac Cardiovasc Surg 64:563, 1972

59. **Russek HI:** Propranolol and isosorbide dinitrate synergism in angina pectoris. Amer J Cardiol 21:44, 1968

60. **Mantle JA, Russell RO Jr, Moraski RE, et al:** Isosorbide dinitrate and nitroglycerin for the relief of congestive heart failure postmyocardial infarction. Amer J Cardiol 35:155, 1975

61. **Capone R, Mason DT, Amsterdam EA, et al:** A comparison of the action of short and long-action nitrites on the peripheral circulation. Clin Res 20:204, 1972

62. **Amsterdam EA, Awan N, Tonkon M, et al:** Sustained reduction of elevated left ventricular filling pressure in cardiac failure by oral sustained nitroglycerin. Circulation 52 suppl II:154, 1975

63. **Franciosa JA, Mikulic E, Cohn JN, et al:** Hemodynamic effects of orally administered isosorbide dinitrate in patients with congestive heart failure. Circulation 50:1020, 1974

64. **Reichek N, Goldstein RE, Redwood DR, et al:** Sustained effects of nitroglycerin ointment in patients with angina pectoris. Circulation 50:348, 1974

65. **Awan N, Miller RR, Vismara LA, et al:** Enhanced exercise performance by nitroglycerin paste and relation to simultaneous modifications in cardiac dynamics and peripheral circulation in coronary patients. Circulation (in press)

66. **Schelling JL, Lasagna L:** A study of cross-tolerance to circulation effects of organic nitrates. Clin Pharmacol Ther 8:256, 1967

67. **Zelis R, Mason DT:** Demonstration of nitrite tolerance: attenuation of the venodilator response to nitroglycerin by the chronic administration of isosorbide dinitrate. Circulation 40, suppl III:221, 1969

68. **Lee G, Mason DT, Reese L, et al:** Absence of the induction of cross nitrate tolerance to the antianginal effects of sublingual nitroglycerin by chronic oral isosorbide dinitrate: demonstration by exercise testing. Clin Res 24:85A, 1976

69. **Amsterdam EA, Huffaker HK, DeMaria A, et al:** Hemodynamic effects of digitalis in acute myocardial infarction and comparison with furosemide. Circulation 46 suppl II:113, 1972

70. **Conway J:** A vascular abnormality in hypertension. Circulation 27:520, 1963

71. **Dikshit K, Vyden JK, Forrester JS, et al:** Renal and extrarenal hemodynamic effects of furosemide in congestive heart failure after myocardial infarction. New Eng J Med 288:1087, 1973

72. **Zelis R, Mansour EJ, Capone RJ, et al:** The cardiovascular effects of morphine: the peripheral capacitance and resistance vessels in human subjects. J Clin Invest 54:1247, 1974

73. **Angel J, DeMaria A, Amsterdam EA, et al:** Alterations in left ventricular size and performance induced by sodium nitroprusside in myocardial infarction patients: evaluation by echocardiography. Clin Res 24:80A, 1976

74. **Miller RR, Vismara LA, Williams DO, et al:** Improved hemodynamics and reduced regurgitant volume in severe aortic insufficiency by ventricular unloading with nitroprusside. Circulation 52 suppl II:218, 1975

75. **Maroko PR, Kjekshus JK, Sobel BE, et al:** Factors influencing infarct size following experimental coronary artery occlusions. Circulation 43:67, 1971

76. **Maroko PR, Braunwald E:** Modification of myocardial infarction size after coronary occlusion. Ann Intern Med 79:720, 1973

77. **Shell WE, Sobel BE:** Protection of jeopardized ischemic myocardium by reduction of ventricular afterload. New Eng J Med 291:481, 1974

78. **Maroko PR, Libby P, Covell JW, et al:** Precordial S-T segment elevation mapping: an atraumatic method for assessing alterations in the extent of myocardial ischemic injury: the effects of pharmacologic and hemodynamic interventions. Amer J Cardiol 29:223, 1972

79. **Awan N, Amsterdam E, Tonkon M, et al:** Clinical effects of nitroprusside on extent of ischemic injury and pump function in acute myocardial infarction: assessment by precordial ST mapping and cardiac catheterization. Circulation 52 suppl II:154, 1975

80. **Awan N, Amsterdam EA, Vera Z, et al:** Clinical effects of nitroglycerin on extent of ischemic injury in acute myocardial infarction assessed by precordial ST segment mapping. Circulation 52 suppl II:154, 1975

81. **Miller RR, Vismara LA, Williams DO, et al:** Effects of ventricular unloading by nitroprusside on myocardial energetics and coronary blood flow in patients with ischemic heart disease. Circulation 52 suppl II:217, 1975

82. **Amsterdam EA, Hilliard G, Williams DO, et al:** Hemodynamic effects of propranolol in acute myocardial infarction. Circulation 48 suppl IV:138, 1973

83. **Massumi RA, Mason DT, Amsterdam EA, et al:** Ventricular fibrillation and tachycardia after intravenous atropine for treatment of bradycardias. New Eng J Med 287:336, 1972

Chapter 22

Myocardial Infarction Shock
Mechanisms and Management

Ezra A. Amsterdam, MD, FACC
Anthony N. DeMaria, MD, FACC
James L. Hughes, MD
Edward J. Hurley, MD, FACC
Arthur J. Lurie, MD
David O. Williams, MD
Richard R. Miller, MD, FACC
Dean T. Mason, MD, FACC

Cardiogenic shock is a syndrome of extreme impairment of circulatory function resulting from severe, primary derangement of cardiac pump performance. Although—as in congestive heart failure—it is characterized by inadequate perfusion of vital organ systems, depression of cardiac and circulatory function is of a greater degree in shock; in contrast to congestive heart failure, untreated shock is generally incompatible with survival beyond several hours. Cardiogenic shock may be the clinical culmination of end-stage function of any disease of the heart, but it is most typically related to acute myocardial infarction. It characteristically presents as an abrupt, catastrophic complication of myocardial infarction and is approached mainly from this perspective in the following discussion.

Clinical Significance of Shock in Myocardial Infarction

Although significant progress has been achieved in reducing mortality from acute myocardial infarction in the past decade, this has largely been the result of aggressive treatment and prevention of life-threatening arrhythmias by innovative pharmacologic and electrical means, as implemented by the coronary intensive care unit approach. Current medical management has lowered hospital mortality in acute myocardial infarction by one-third, from approximately 30 percent to less than 20 percent.[1] Cardiogenic shock, which occurs in approximately 15 percent of patients with myocardial infarction, accounts for the greatest proportion of this mortality. The system of intensive coronary care has had little effect in improving survival in this syndrome. At present, mortality in acute myocardial infarction complicated by shock remains 80 to 100 percent and approximates 50 percent when associated with severe congestive failure.[2-4] These figures contrast with mortality rates lower than 10 percent when myocardial infarction is uncomplicated[5] and commonly lower than 20 percent when it is accompanied by signs of only mild left heart failure.[6]

Pathophysiology of Myocardial Infarction Shock

Myocardial Factors: The fundamental physiologic defect in myocardial infarction shock is depression of myocardial contractility consequent to loss of functioning cardiac muscle.[4,7,8] Marked impairment of cardiac pump function results with severely reduced perfusion of all organ systems. The diagnosis of cardiogenic shock is made when clinical evidence of severe low cardiac output state secondary to myocardial infarction is present, including (1) documentation of acute myocardial infarction; (2) evidence of hypotension (systolic blood pressure lower than 80 mm Hg), oliguria (less than 30 ml of urine per hour), diaphoresis, cyanosis and altered sensorium; (3) persistence of shock syndrome after elimination of arrhythmias, abolition of pain, administration of oxygen and a trial of volume expansion. The inadequate functional performance of the heart is usually manifested by severe derangement of all parameters of cardiac pump function, such as systemic blood pressure, cardiac output, stroke output, cardiac work, stroke work and left ventricular ejection fraction with resultant elevation of left ventricular filling pressure.[3,4,7-12] Although these hemodynamic variables may be abnormal in the presence of uncomplicated myocardial infarction, the degree of impairment is considerably greater in the shock state.[2,7-12] Heart failure in acute myocardial infarction is usually characterized by clinical manifestations of pulmonary congestion.[4,5] Derangement of the underlying hemodynamic function may be marked in cardiac failure, but it is quantitatively of lesser degree than in shock.[4,5] Arterial hypoxemia is a consistent finding in cardiogenic shock[13] as well as in uncomplicated infarction[14] and may be related to pulmonary congestion or ventilation-perfusion imbalance, or both.

Depression of cardiac performance in acute myocardial infarction is, as a rule, directly related to the extent of myocardial damage. Thus, the anatomic basis for the extremely depressed cardiac function in the great majority of patients with myocardial infarction shock is the extensive loss of cardiac muscle. Whereas uncomplicated myocardial infarction is usually associated with relatively small quantitative damage, myocardial destruction in shock involves at least 40 percent, and usually more, of the ventricle, as documented by postmortem studies.[4,15,16] Angiographic evaluation of the left ventricle, which we have performed in patients with acute myocardial infarction, has provided in vivo confirmation of these pathologic findings.[10] When shock accompanies acute myocardial infarction, left ventriculography usually demonstrates severe asynergy of a massive proportion of left ventricular myocardium, in contrast to the more modest involvement in uncomplicated infarction[10] (see Figure 7 in chapter 11 on function of the hypoxic myocardium). The magnitude of the loss of left ventricular muscle in cardiogenic shock explains, to a large extent, the failure of conventional therapeutic approaches in this syndrome.

The extensive ventricular damage associated with cardiogenic shock represents cumulative, past and present myocardial loss. Total nonviable myocardial mass in this setting may be comprised, in variable proportions, of old and new areas of infarction as well as recent extension of infarction.[16] The essential factor resulting in shock is net loss of critical mass of left ventricular muscle—whether it evolves over an extended period from multiple, separate infarctions or occurs acutely from a single, massive infarction.

The mechanical complications of acute myocardial infarction may also exacerbate the depression of intrinsic cardiac function resulting from infarction. Acute ventricular septal rupture, mitral regurgitation and a large paradoxically expansile or dyskinetic segment of myocardium may critically overload an injured ventricle and further impair pump performance.

Coronary Collateral Vessels: The role of the coronary collateral circulation in ischemic heart disease is controversial. Although these vessels classically have been considered to have a protective effect on the myocardium[17] and experimental studies indicate enhancement of coronary blood flow by these auxiliary channels,[18–20] recent investigations have produced variable findings in both chronic coronary heart disease and myocardial infarction.[21–32] Postmortem studies demonstrating lack of any relation between collateral vessels and the presence and extent of myocardial infarction[33] are at variance with earlier conclusions indicating a protective effect of collaterals against infarction.[17] However, in patients with myocardial infarction who underwent acute angiographic evaluation, we recently correlated the presence of collateral vessels with reduced frequency of complications.[34] Hemodynamic dysfunction, incidence of shock and mortality were greater in patients without collaterals than in those with collaterals. In the former group, shock developed in 71 percent (10 of 14) and mortality was 57 percent (8 of 14); in contrast, in the latter group of 6 patients, there was no shock and all patients survived.

Many aspects of collateral vessel function in man remain uncertain, including the determinants of and capacity for blood flow in these channels. However, their documented ability— albeit limited—to augment human regional myocardial perfusion[25] suggests a potential for maintenance of local cell viability in myocardial infarction and a critical reduction in extent of damage that may be sufficient to avert shock in some patients.

Extramyocardial Factors: Although cardiac pump dysfunction in acute myocardial infarction is principally related to the quantity of myocardium lost, other factors may also be operative in some patients. Hypovolemia and impaired reflex sympathetic vasoconstriction in response to reduced systemic blood pressure may be important factors in circulatory failure accompanying myocardial infarction. The occurrence of these conditions in the presence of reduced myocardial contractility and loss of contractile units resulting from acute myocardial infarction—in themselves insufficient to cause shock—may further impair hemody-

namic function and thereby play a role in the genesis of the shock syndrome.

Hypovolemia: Hypovolemia has been documented in myocardial infarction shock.[35] Hypovolemia of absolute or relative degree deprives the injured ventricle of the beneficial hemodynamic effect of the Starling mechanism. Thus, impairment of circulatory function due to depression of intrinsic cardiac capacity may be exacerbated by coexisting hypovolemia. The effect on cardiac performance is represented by a low point on an already depressed ventricular function curve (Figure 1). Hypovolemia in patients with acute myocardial infarction may be related to previous or current diuretic therapy, inadequate fluid intake or replacement, emesis, diarrhea, fever or hyperventilation. In addition, alpha adrenergic stimulation by endogenous catecholamines or exogenous sympathomimetic agents may produce preferential, intense constriction of postcapillary arteriolar sphincters that results in loss of plasma volume by transudation of fluid to the extravascular space.[36] Severe hypoxia or acidosis may result in loss of structural or functional integrity in the microcirculation with consequent escape of intravascular fluid.

Impaired Vasoconstrictor Response: Impairment of sympathetic reflex vasoconstriction in acute myocardial infarction has been demonstrated experimentally[37–39] and clinically.[40] In experimental myocardial infarction, this effect has been noted even in the presence of systemic hypotension[37–39] and has been attributed to inhibition of vasoconstriction[37,38,41] and competitive vasodilation[39] produced by inhibitory reflexes from receptors in the myocardium. It has been suggested that these receptors are activated by chemical[41] or mechanical[42] stimuli arising in injured cardiac muscle and mediated by vagal[43] or sympathetic[44] afferent pathways. This physiologic defect has serious potential in acute myocardial infarction. Most patients with myocardial infarction have extensive coronary artery disease;[45,46] thus, coronary blood flow is dependent on maintenance of perfusion pressure within a relatively narrow range, since the normal autoregulatory function of the coronary circulation is impaired in the presence of obstructive coronary disease.[47,48] Inability to maintain blood pressure by compensating for reduced

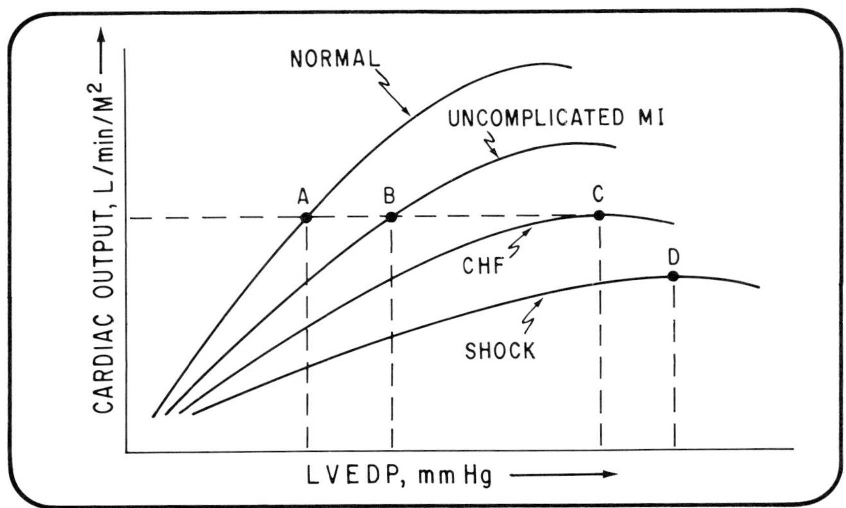

FIGURE 1. Ventricular function curves relating left ventricular performance (stroke work, stroke volume or cardiac output) to left ventricular filling pressure. Normally, the curve is relatively steep. In acute myocardial infarction (MI), the curve falls, indicating depressed left ventricular function. In acute MI with congestive heart failure (CHF), the ventricular function curve is more depressed than in uncomplicated acute MI. In acute MI shock, the markedly depressed function curve indicates severe impairment of left ventricular performance. Points A, B and C all represent the same cardiac output, but each is at a different level of left ventricular end-diastolic pressure (LVEDP) shown by the vertical broken lines. In cardiogenic shock, despite operation of left ventricle at the apex of its depressed function curve (point D) with marked elevation of LVEDP, cardiac output adequate to sustain life cannot be delivered and hypotension results. (Reproduced by permission from Mason et al.[161])

stroke volume with elevation of peripheral vascular resistance may thus result in increased myocardial ischemia and necrosis with further deterioration of hemodynamic function.

When these physiologic alterations are associated with myocardial infarction shock, it may not be strictly cardiogenic—in that depression of intrinsic myocardial function is not the singular cause. Although shock in acute myocardial infarction can be directly related to the foregoing derangements in only a relatively small proportion of patients, these conditions, which may not be readily appreciated clinically, are emphasized since they are usually responsive to appropriate medical management—in contrast to the characteristically refractory state of true cardiogenic shock.

Other extramyocardial factors may also be involved in the genesis of hypotension and circulatory failure when superimposed on only moderate intrinsic cardiac dysfunction in acute myocardial infarction. These include tachy- or bradyarrhythmias, hypoxemia of noncardiac etiology, unmitigated pain and iatrogenic causes—for example, drugs such as morphine, which depress cardiorespiratory function, and diuretic agents, the overzealous use of which can produce hypovolemia. Diagnostic evaluation should also include the search for concurrent or alternative causes for the shock syndrome such as cardiac tamponade, aortic dissection, pulmonary embolism, septicemia, hemorrhage or abdominal catastrophe.

Clinical Findings

Predisposing Factors: In addition to the high mortality (80 to 100 percent) and not infrequent occurrence (15 percent) of shock in myocardial infarction, certain other clinical findings are noteworthy. Although patients with acute myocardial infarction in whom shock develops may be slightly older than those without shock, no differences have been found in prevalence of other predisposing factors such as prior myocardial infarction, cardiac failure, angina pectoris or hypertension.[3,4] Patients with and without shock also had similar intervals between onset of symptoms and hospital admission and similar drug therapy prior to occurrence of shock.[3] However, although there was no difference in the quantity of myocardium involved by previous myocardial infarctions in the two groups, the magnitude of recent infarction was significantly greater in the patients with shock.[16] Total mass of left ventricular tissue involved by infarction, therefore, was far greater in the patients with shock (51 percent of left ventricle) than in those without shock (23 percent of the left ventricle).

Time of Onset of Shock: Although the onset of shock after infarction is variable—ranging from immediate to one week or more—it usually occurs early. Several studies have demonstrated that the syndrome developed in one-half of shock patients within 24 hours and in two-thirds at 36 hours,[3] in one-third within 24 hours and in one-half in less than 3 days,[16] and in three-fourths within 28 hours.[4] Further, the majority of patients in whom shock develops have clinically evident hemodynamic dysfunction on admission, ranging from mild cardiac failure to shock. It is also apparent from these data that late development of shock is not unusual in myocardial infarction. This has been attributed to continuing or new ischemic injury to the myocardium, to be discussed.

Duration of Shock: Cardiogenic shock is usually fatal within a short period. Among 73 patients in shock, Killip and colleagues[3] noted 65 percent mortality in 24 hours and a median survival time of 10.2 hours. In a second study of 21 patients with cardiogenic shock, all of whom died, the group was divided into 12 (57 percent) with rapid death (duration of shock, less than 24 hours; mean, 12 hours) and 9 (43 percent) with prolonged shock (duration of shock, more than 24 hours; mean, 88 hours).[16]

Extension of Infarction: It has been proposed that progression or extension of infarction is an important mechanism in the destruction of myocardial tissue sufficient to produce cardiogenic shock.[4,16] Of 22 shock patients, 18 had had extension of recent infarct, which was temporally associated with onset of shock in a number of them.[16] However, infarct extension has also been considered the result rather than the

cause of shock.[15] In regard to the possibility that progression of infarction does contribute to the pathogenesis of cardiogenic shock, it is significant that this process may not be manifested clinically. In one study, symptoms and electrocardiographic evidence were usually absent, diagnosis in most cases being established by postmortem dating of infarct zones.[16] Therapeutic interventions to interrupt extension of infarction must be based on recognition of this process, which may be enhanced by newer diagnostic techniques such as precordial ST segment mapping and myocardial infarct scanning that may provide more sensitive analysis of alterations in the myocardium than conventional methods allow (Figure 2). Recent data are encouraging in this regard in demonstrating superiority of precordial ST segment mapping over standard electrocardiography in the detection of extension of infarction.[49]

Significance of Infarct Location: Although infarct size is uniformly acknowledged to be the major factor responsible for the development of shock in acute myocardial infarction,[4,15,16,50] opinions vary as to the significance of infarct location. No relation between the presence of shock and the location of infarction has been noted in a number of studies.[3,15,50,51] In contrast, recent investigations have provided substantial evidence that derangement of cardiac pump function is greater and the occurrence of shock more frequent in anterior infarction than in inferior. This finding stems from anatomic and physiologic factors involving the relation of relative myocardial mass to coronary artery distribution. The left coronary system predominates in the human heart in terms of total mass of myocardium and left ventricle supplied. Further, in the majority of instances the left anterior descending artery supplies a greater quantity of left ventricular myocardium than is supplied by either the right or left circumflex artery.[32,52] The left anterior descending artery perfuses the left ventricular free wall, apex and interventricular septum. The left circumflex artery supplies the lateral wall of the left ventricle and contributes variably to the supply of its inferior wall. In approximately 10 percent of hearts it provides the major supply to this area. The left ventricular distribution of the right coronary artery varies reciprocally with that of the circumflex artery

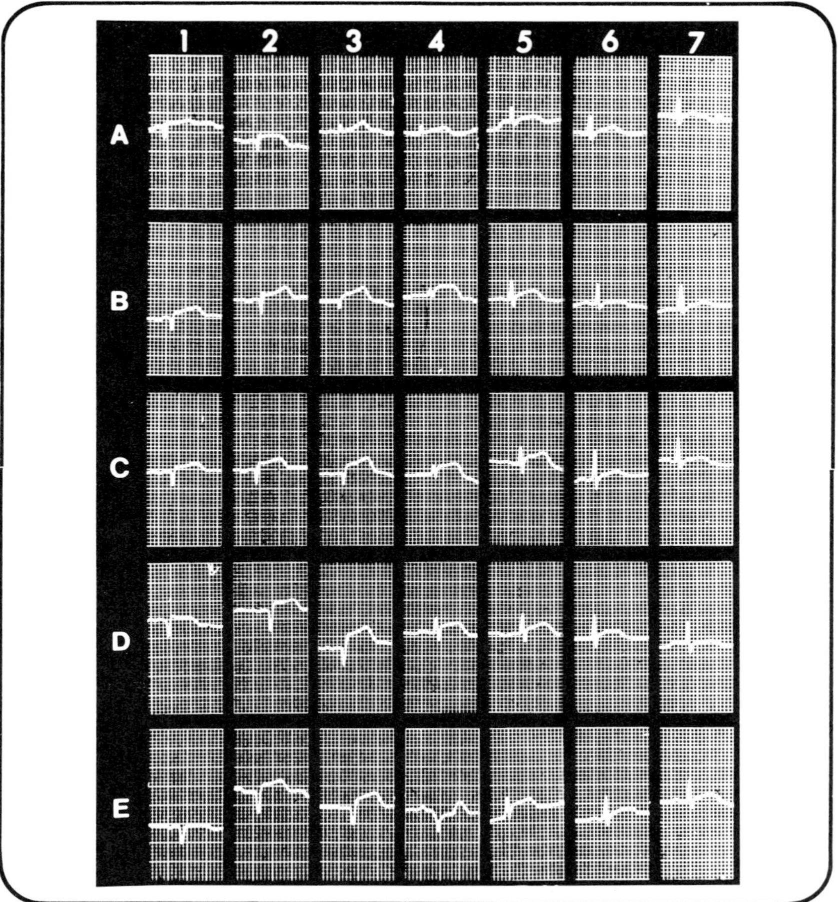

FIGURE 2. Precordial electrocardiographic ST segment map in a patient with acute anterior myocardial infarction, utilizing 35 precordial leads (5 horizontal rows of 7 adjacent leads). The course of ischemic injury is followed by serial determination of the number of ST segments that are elevated (NST), the sum of ST segment elevation (ΣST) and the average ST segment rise per lead demonstrating ST segment elevation ($\overline{ST}$). For orientation with the standard precordial 6-lead ECG. D_{1-4} corresponds to V_{1-4} and E_5 and E_6 correspond to V_5 and V_6. The pre-nitroglycerin control blanket showed ΣST 61 mm, NST 27 leads and $\overline{ST}$ 2.3 mm lead. The illustration shown was made after sublingual nitroglycerin: ΣST 49 mm, NST 23 and $\overline{ST}$ 1.5 mm, indicating that the area and intensity of ischemic injury were reduced with lowering of myocardial oxygen needs by the nitrate.

and involves the inferior wall and inferior aspect of the septum. It contributes the major portion of the blood supply to the inferior left ventricular wall in about 90 percent of human hearts. Anterior infarction, as localized electrocardiographically, is related to occlusive disease of the anterior descending artery and usually involves a relatively large quantity of left ventricular muscle. By contrast, inferior infarction results from disease of the right coronary artery in the great majority (approximately 90 percent) of instances and is thereby usually associated with substantially less myocardial damage.

Recent studies have supported the more serious consequences of anterior compared with inferior infarction in terms of ventricular function. Consistent findings have resulted from both clinical and hemodynamic investigation of this question in both stable coronary heart dis-

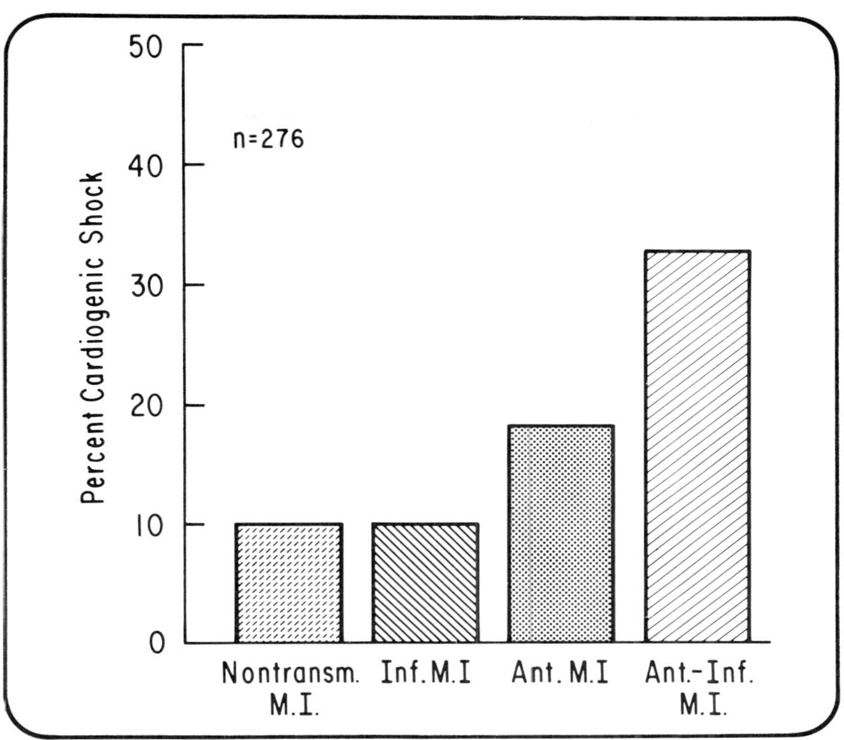

FIGURE 3. Prevalence of shock in acute myocardial infarction (MI) (shown as percent of patients with acute MI) in relation to electrocardiographic infarct location. Shock is most frequent in combined anterior-inferior (ant-inf) infarction. Prevalence in anterior (ant) infarction is approximately twice as great as that in inferior (inf) and nontransmural (nontransm) infarction. n = total number of patients with acute MI.

ease and acute myocardial infarction. Further, our studies and those of others indicate that within broad limits the electrocardiogram identifies and localizes left ventricular asynergy,[53] provides a quantitative estimate of its extent[53] and bears a consistent relation to left ventricular functional status.[52,54–59] Thus, the presence of pathologic Q waves correlates closely with left ventricular asynergy, the site of which is localized by the electrocardiogram. In addition to Q waves, other electrocardiographic abnormalities such as convex ST segment elevation and T wave inversion are associated not only with the presence of left ventricular aneurysm, as classically described, but also with asynergy of considerably greater extent than is observed when these ST-T wave abnormalities are not present.[53]

We have found a substantially greater incidence of shock in anterior myocardial infarction than in either inferior or nontransmural infarction[57] (Figure 3). Rackley and colleagues have demonstrated similar results.[59] In both series, differential frequency of shock relative to electrocardiographic infarct location paralleled the more severe hemodynamic dysfunction associated with combined anterior-inferior and anterior infarction compared with inferior and nontransmural infarction (Figure 4). Indeed, we have been impressed with the high proportion of patients with inferior and nontransmural infarction who demonstrate normal hemodynamic function during the acute phase of infarction. Electrocardiographic evidence of combined anterior-inferior infarction is associated with the most severely impaired function and highest frequency of shock, a finding consistent with pathologic data previously noted relating extent of involved myocardium to functional derangement.[57] Further, even in the presence

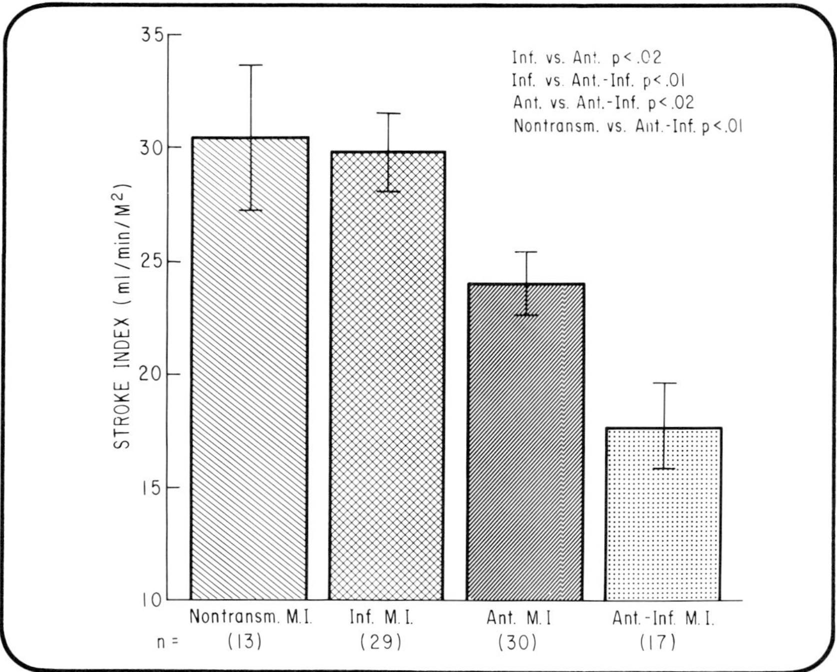

FIGURE 4. Stroke work index related to electrocardiographic location of acute myocardial infarction (MI). Stroke index is most impaired in combined anterior-inferior (ant-inf) infarction and markedly reduced in anterior (ant) infarction compared with inferior (inf) and nontransmural (nontransm) infarction. n = number of patients with given location of acute MI.

of similar baseline hemodynamics in acute infarction, evaluation by volume loading and resultant ventricular function curves has demonstrated diminished performance in anterior compared with inferior infarction[57] (Figure 5), an observation also noted by Gunnar and colleagues.[60] On the basis of this experience, the occurrence of shock in inferior or nontransmural infarction suggests the not infrequent association of additional etiologic factors such as a mechanical complication of infarction—rupture of papillary muscle, septum or ventricular wall (Figure 6)—or intercurrent illness.

Electrocardiographic location of previous myocardial infarction in patients with chronic coronary heart disease yields similar results regarding ventricular function. Extent and severity of left ventricular asynergy[53] and pump dysfunction are more severe in anterior infarction than in inferior[54,56] and most impaired in combined anterior-inferior infarction.[57] These angiographic studies have added a further dimension to the investigation of this question. We have found that infarct location per se is not the critical factor determining ventricular performance. When extent of involvement by previous infarction is equivalent, as assessed by the percentage of left ventricular perimeter with abnormal contractile motion, function is similar regardless of infarct location.[54,56] The consistent difference in hemodynamic dysfunction associated with infarct location is related to the finding that anterior infarction is usually quantitatively greater than inferior,[53,54,56] a result of involvement of the anterior descending coronary artery in the former and the right or circumflex coronary vessel in the latter.

Physiologic Basis of Therapy

The rapidly expanding scope of therapy for myocardial infarction complicated by severe cardiac pump failure, including diverse pharmacologic agents, mechanical circulatory assist

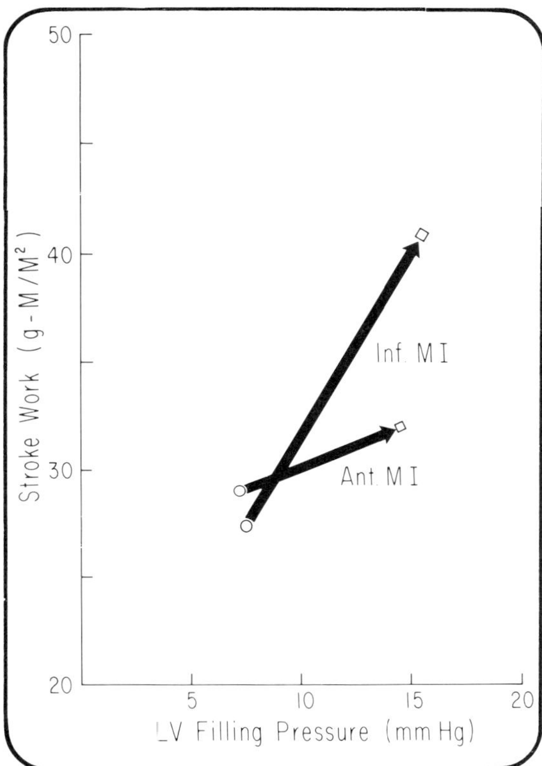

FIGURE 5. Effect of plasma volume expansion on left ventricular (LV) function (stroke work) in acute myocardial infarction. Although function prior to volume expansion is similar in the two groups, this intervention of increasing preload (elevation of LV filling pressure) with rapid dextran infusion resulted in substantial enhancement of left ventricular performance in inferior infarction (inf MI arrow) but little change in stroke work in anterior infarction (ant MI arrow), indicating more depression of left ventricular function in the latter than in the former group of patients.

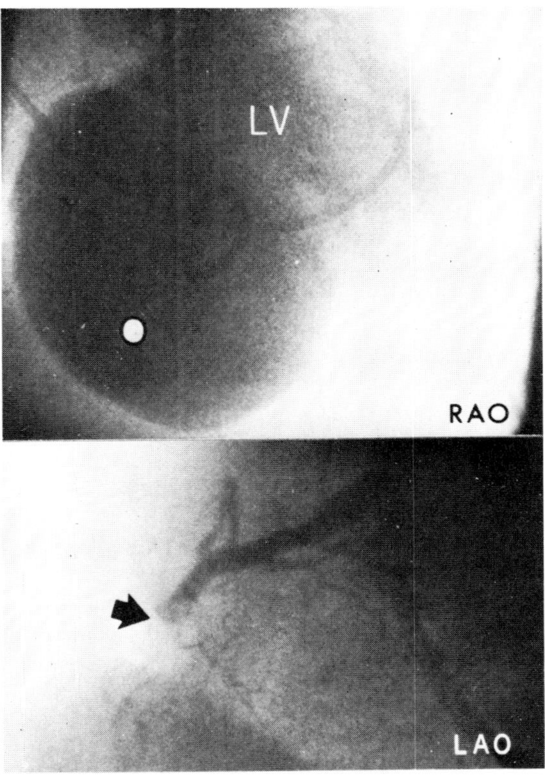

FIGURE 6. Left ventricular (LV) angiogram **(top)** (right anterior oblique position; RAO) and right coronary arteriogram **(bottom)** (left anterior oblique position; LAO) in a patient with intractable cardiac failure associated with acute inferior myocardial infarction related to total occlusion **(arrow)** of the right coronary artery. Angiography revealed rupture of the free inferior left ventricular wall indicated by opacification of a large area (the center of which is indicated by the **open circle**) beyond the inferior left ventricular border. Adhesion of pericardium to myocardium throughout the circumference of the rupture produced a false aneurysm. (Reproduced by permission from Mason et al.[162])

and direct cardiac surgery, has substantially enhanced therapeutic potential in this syndrome. However, rational, effective and safe use of these potent treatment alternatives is based on appropriate patient selection. Because the indications for differing types of therapy may be quite specific in relation to the pattern of altered physiology, proper application of treatment is essential both to achieve maximal efficacy and to avoid deleterious effects. Thus, selection of therapy involves, in each case, a systematic approach to patient assessment, including evaluation of clinical status, quantitative definition of hemodynamic function and estimation of prognostic class.

Structure and Function of Infarct Area: Consideration of the structural and pathophysiologic aspects of myocardial infarction provides an understanding of the mechanisms of the effects produced by current therapeutic modalities. Myocardial infarction results in a zone of central necrosis surrounded by an area of ischemia, in turn surrounded by relatively normal or uninvolved tissue.[61] The central zone is irreversibly damaged—in some instances, extensively enough to preclude survival with any form of therapy. However, in the absence of this extreme, the region of greatest potential for influencing survival—and, thus, of principal therapeutic interest—is the acutely ischemic area, which, although depressed, remains viable. The anatomic outcome in the ischemic area is a primary determinant of the clinical course in patients with cardiac function compatible with survival after acute myocardial infarction. Thus, to the extent that the nonlethally injured zone can be influenced toward recovery of structural and functional integrity, left ventricular performance and prognosis may be favorably altered. By contrast, factors promoting ischemia result in increased myocardial injury, further cell death and continued deterioration of ventricular function.

Limitations of Positive Inotropic Agents: A wide spectrum of drugs is currently available for support of the failing myocardium in myocardial infarction shock.[2,62-64.] However, until recently, pharmacologic therapy was principally limited to the conventional positive inotropic drugs—usually sympathomimetic agents.[62,64,65] This approach is capable, in most instances, of at least transiently elevating the blood pressure in myocardial infarction shock and has been suggested to have produced some improvement in survival.[65] However, most studies have indicated that mortality is not significantly affected by such treatment,[3,66-68] remaining at 80 to 90 per cent.[3,68] Indeed, the current multiplicity of these agents and continuing pursuit of more effective forms of pharmacotherapy to some extent reflects their lack of success.

Recent investigations have suggested several bases for the observed failure of traditional drug therapy in myocardial infarction shock:

(1) Experimental studies indicate that the basis for the enhancement of hemodynamic function by positive inotropic drugs is their action upon normal areas of myocardium, since their action on injured myocardium is markedly attenuated.[69-71] The massive degree of myocardial loss that characterizes myocardial infarction shock[3,4,15,16] severely reduces the extent of uninvolved—and, thus, normally responsive—car-

diac muscle upon which a positive inotropic agent can exert its effect. As a result, these agents have a limited potential for significantly improving cardiac function in the large majority of patients with myocardial infarction shock.

(2) Acutely infarcted myocardium is characterized by passive, systolic expansion resulting from the distending force produced by contraction of the uninvolved areas of the ventricle.[72,73] In experimental myocardial infarction, this paradoxical expansion is augmented by positive inotropic agents because of their enhancement of contractile function of normal myocardium with little effect on injured areas. Thus, a significant portion of the stroke volume may be diverted into the expansile area of the ventricle during systole. These factors result in counterproductive dissipation of contractile energy and exacerbation of the already deranged ventricular function.

(3) Recent experimental studies have demonstrated that positive inotropic interventions may augment the intensity and extent of myocardial ischemia in myocardial infarction.[74] This results from their elevation of myocardial oxygen requirements when a concomitant rise in coronary blood flow is precluded by structural restrictions in the coronary arteries. Thus, the zone of ischemia and necrosis may be enlarged.

Modification of Infarct Size: Since development of cardiac pump failure is more closely related to cumulative quantity of myocardium destroyed by both previous and new infarction, it is relevant to consider the therapeutic implications of recent investigations concerned with modification of infarct size. These studies have demonstrated the potential for reduction of ischemia—and, thus, infarct size—by favorable alteration of the cardiac oxygen supply-demand relationship. They are based on the concept that myocardial ischemia and necrosis in coronary heart disease result from an imbalance between myocardial oxygen needs and availability and that myocardial injury can be limited by favorable alteration of this balance.[74-76] Understanding of the regulation of myocardial oxygen consumption and supply is fundamental to this approach.[77] The major determinants of myocardial oxygen consumption are heart rate, myocardial contractile state and intramyocardial tension (directly related to intraventricular pressure and volume). Myocardial oxygen supply is principally related to coronary blood flow, which is governed by mechanical, neural, humoral and metabolic factors normally integrated by exquisitely sensitive autoregulatory mechanisms that modulate coronary vascular resistance—and, thus, coronary blood flow.[48] In coronary artery disease in which these autoregulatory mechanisms are limited in their ability to maintain adequate coronary flow because of the unresponsiveness due to obstructive narrowing in the vessels, mechanical factors assume preeminence. Thus, coronary perfusion pressure as produced by aortic diastolic pressure—normally a primary determinant of coronary blood flow—becomes even more critical and must be maintained within a relatively narrow range because of the diminished capacity of the coronary circulation to compensate for alteration in this factor.[32,48]

Evaluating infarct size in experimental coronary artery occlusion by ST segment alteration obtained from epicardial electrocardiography,[74] myocardial enzyme (creatine phosphokinase) content[74] and microstructural and histochemical analysis,[78] Braunwald, Maroko and colleagues have defined the effects of a variety of interventions in augmenting or diminishing myocardial ischemia and injury.[74-76] Myocardial injury in acute infarction has been increased by isoproterenol, glucagon, ouabain, tachycardia and hypotension. Hypotension reduces myocardial oxygen availability, and the positive inotropic agents and tachycardia increase oxygen requirements beyond supply capacity. Reduction of myocardial injury in experimental infarction has been demonstrated with interventions that (1) decrease myocardial oxygen consumption—beta adrenergic blocking agents, digitalis in the failing heart and ventricular unloading therapy—or (2) increase oxygen supply—coronary artery reperfusion, elevation of coronary perfusion pressure by vasopressors, counterpulsation and a number of metabolic factors such as increased glucose availability and corticosteroid administration.[75,76] On the basis of indirect methods of assessment such as precordial ST segment mapping and enzyme disappearance curves in myocardial metabolic studies, initial clinical application of this approach has been encouraging in suggesting reduction of

myocardial ischemic injury by beta adrenergic blockade,[79,80] nitroglycerin,[81] nitroprusside[82] and lowering of hypertensive pressure,[76] all of which decrease myocardial oxygen demand, and intraaortic balloon counterpulsation (Figure 7), which both reduces myocardial oxygen needs and augments supply. Myocardial revascularization, by increasing oxygen delivery, has produced reversal of acute ischemic ventricular dysfunction.[75,76]

In the context of therapy for myocardial infarction shock, these studies have several significant implications. The theoretical importance of maintaining coronary perfusion pressure in association with positive inotropic therapy is supported, as is simultaneous increase in myocardial oxygen supply and reduction of demand by counterpulsation. In addition—and perhaps of most relevance in relation to shock —attenuation of myocardial injury suggests the therapeutic potential for prevention of the continuing evolution of ischemic damage responsible for shock in many patients in whom the syndrome is not an early complication of infarction. In these patients, in whom cardiac pump function is commonly adequate initially, agents that reduce myocardial oxygen demand, such as beta blocking drugs and nitrates, frequently may be given with beneficial effect and without deleterious results.[79,80,83] However, because such agents do not support and may seriously impair ventricular performance, they have no place in the therapy of established shock. Similarly, a drug such as nitroprusside, which, by its unloading effects, may improve pump performance and reduce ischemic injury in myocardial infarction with congestive failure, is contraindicated in shock associated with significant hypotension because of its hypotensive action. In contrast, counterpulsation, as discussed later, has most advantageous potential in shock in that it supports coronary perfusion pressure by diastolic augmentation and reduces myocardial oxygen demand by systolic pressure unloading. Thus, potential for modification of infarct size must be viewed in terms of the clinical setting. Whereas in uncomplicated infarction with adequate ventricular function, modest negative contractile action or reduction of blood pressure may be associated with a net favorable effect on the balance between myocardial oxygen supply and demand and, thus, reduction of injury, these alterations would contribute to further deterioration in the patient with little or no functional cardiac reserve.

Approach to the Patient

Clinical Evaluation: Early, accurate diagnosis of shock and prompt institution of appropriate treatment are essential in order to maximize therapeutic potential in this syndrome, in which delay exacts an inordinate toll in terms of progressive myocardial damage and functional deterioration. The diagnosis of shock in myocardial infarction is usually, but not always, readily apparent. It is based on evidence of severely reduced tissue perfusion and the clinical manifestations of the underlying marked derangement of cardiac pump function (see page 366). Systolic blood pressure is generally reduced to less than 80 mm Hg—or 40 mm Hg or more below the usual systolic level in the presence of preexisting hypertension. Because of the inaccuracy of sphygmomanometric determination of blood pressure in states of severe vasoconstriction,[84] reliable evaluation is facilitated by measurement of intraarterial pressure. Significant arterial hypoxemia is usually present.

When direct hemodynamic analysis of ventricular function is not available, indirect estimation of circulatory status can be achieved by clinical evaluation. Adequacy of systemic blood flow can be inferred from clinical assessment of renal, cerebral and integumentary status. Inadequate renal blood flow is indicated by oliguria, cerebral hypoperfusion is manifested by altered sensorium, and cold, diaphoretic or cyanotic skin reflects reduced peripheral blood flow and heightened sympathetic drive, the latter a compensatory response to decreased perfusion.

Hemodynamic Evaluation: Therapeutic efficacy in cardiogenic shock is predicated on accurate evaluation of cardiac function, which may now be obtained by direct hemodynamic analysis. This involves cardiac catheterization for determination of left ventricular filling pressure and cardiac output and insertion of a small polyethylene catheter into a systemic artery for accurate measurement of blood pressure. Peripheral vascular resistance may then be calculated. These procedures are facilitated by current techniques that allow right or left ventricular catheterization at bedside with or without fluoroscopic guidance.[85,86] However, left ventricular filling pressure can be determined accurately from pulmonary artery and pulmonary capillary wedge pressures, which are readily obtained by right heart catheterization with a flow-directed catheter.[85] This catheter also allows withdrawal of blood from the central circulation for determination of arterial blood gases and pH and provides a secure route for the administration of drugs.

Central venous pressure, although widely accessible, has distinct disadvantages in the hemodynamic evaluation of patients with myocardial infarction. It provides a measure of right, rather than left, ventricular filling pressure and, thus, may be normal in the presence of considerable elevation of filling pressure of the injured left ventricle.[87] It is also affected by the degree of venoconstriction present. However, central venous pressure has been found useful as a guide to volume expansion[35,60,88] as its alteration during such therapy in myocardial infarction may reflect directional, although not quantitative, changes in left ventricular filling pressure.[35,60] However, even for this purpose, there is controversy based on findings that indicate central venous pressure monitoring may be misleading.[87] Thus, caution must be exercised in utilizing this method.

The diagnosis of cardiogenic shock is made when clinical evidence of low cardiac output state is present (see page 366) and all reversible causes as well as alternative etiologic factors, as previously discussed, have been excluded. When these factors have been eliminated and the severely deranged hemodynamic function persists, direct therapy of circulatory failure is initiated.

Objective Assessment of Prognosis: To obviate delay in identifying patients at high risk of death from cardiac pump failure, a precise, objective means of evaluation is essential. Clinical estimation, although generally useful for classification of patients with acute myocardial infarction, is not sufficiently sensitive to predict the outcome in an individual patient[89] and may differ widely from hemodynamic status.[90] Hemodynamic analysis provides a more direct means of assessing prognosis. Initial studies of quantitative assessment of hemodynamic function in acute myocardial infarction have yielded a high degree of accuracy in predicting survival and mortality related to cardiac pump dysfunction. A small number of variables have been most closely related to prognosis in these studies, which achieved an accuracy of 80 to 100 percent in predicting outcome.[91-98] The factors chiefly utilized were left ventricular stroke work,[92] stroke work index,[91,93,94,98] cardiac index,[93,97] cardiac work[95] and cardiac work index[94,98] alone or in combination with left ventricular filling pressure. Recent innovations that are promising in this regard are noninvasive techniques for estimating extent of myocardial damage—and, thus, prognosis—in acute myocardial infarction. These include serum enzyme disappearance curves[99] and isotopic myocardial scanning.[100]

In our experience utilizing catheterization for assessment of prognosis related to cardiac pump dysfunction in over 200 patients with acute myocardial infarction, cardiac work index of 0.7 kg-M/min/M^2 or more, stroke work index of 11.0 gm-M/M^2 or more and stroke work index/left ventricular filling pressure of 0.5 or above were associated with survival in more than 90 percent of patients.[98] In patients in whom these values were lower, mortality from cardiac pump dysfunction was greater than 85 percent. This information on clinical outlook afforded by hemodynamic assessment allows selection of appropriate treatment in patients with myocardial infarction and provides a rational basis for early institution of recently available aggressive forms of therapy when prognosis is grave.

Therapy of Myocardial Infarction Shock

The goal of therapy in this syndrome is to achieve a cardiac output and perfusion pressure sufficient to meet systemic requirements, support cardiac function and prevent extension of infarction. Advances in diagnostic techniques and therapeutic methods have afforded more specific and systematic treatment of shock and enhanced potential for reduction of the awesome mortality in this syndrome.

Volume Expansion

When cardiogenic shock persists after elimination of all reversible factors, as previously delineated, a trial of volume expansion is usually appropriate.[35,60,62,64,101-104] This in itself may improve cardiac output and blood pressure or, if severe hemodynamic dysfunction persists, will provide optimal plasma volume and left ventricular filling pressure prior to initiation of specific drug or other therapy.

Volume expansion may increase cardiac output by augmenting venous return to the heart, thereby elevating left ventricular filling pressure and end-diastolic fiber length. The enhancement of cardiac pump function follows from the Starling relation, which describes augmented ventricular performance, within limits, with increased end-diastolic fiber length. Although in the presence of injury to the ventricle, as in myocardial infarction, the beneficial effect on ventricular performance after elevation of filling pressure is diminished in comparison with that in the normal state (Figure 1), the increment of improvement may be of critical importance in the patient with cardiac pump failure. Elevation of filling pressure in itself, of course, is not without hazard, and excessive elevation may result in pulmonary congestion or pulmonary edema. Clinical experience has demonstrated that although increases in cardiac output may result from volume expansion, little or no improvement is associated with elevation of left ventricular filling pressure above 20 mm Hg.[102,104] Furthermore, improvement in cardiac output is not an inevitable result of increased left ventricular filling pressure, as has been previously noted in regard to large infarctions resulting in severely diminished cardiac reserve[60] (Figure 5). Volume expansion in this setting results only in increased filling pressure and the potential hazard of pulmonary congestion. Therefore, this form of therapy should be undertaken with caution, especially in the presence of large infarction, and therapeutic response in the individual patient rather than a predetermined level of filling pressure should be regarded as the most prudent guide to volume expansion. Therapeutic efficacy will be evident from the influence of improved hemodynamic function on the readily observable parameters of blood pressure and urine flow, which will increase if cardiac output improves.

On the basis of the preceding factors, volume expansion is most rationally administered in conjunction with accurate assessment of left ventricular filling pressure. This is accomplished by the methods previously described for direct[86] or indirect[85] measurement of left ventricular pressure. A trial of volume expansion is indicated if left ventricular filling pressure is low or even normal. It is accomplished by rapid infusion of one of a number of substances, such as 10 percent dextran 40 (Rheomacrodex®), 6 percent dextran 75 (Macrodex®) or normal saline solution. When the hazard of pulmonary congestion is high or the filling pressure is normal initially, 5 percent dextrose in water can be utilized, although it is not as useful a plasma expander as are the other materials. Initial administration consists of infusion of 100 to 200 ml of fluid relatively rapidly, over 5 to 10 minutes. If a salutary effect occurs (increase in cardiac output, blood pressure or urine flow) without evidence of pulmonary congestion, infusion can be continued to a total of 500 to 1,000 ml over 30 to 60 minutes with care not to exceed a left ventricular filling pressure of 18 to 20 mm Hg. Assessment of the presence or absence of dyspnea and pulmonary rales also guides continuation of fluid administration. If volume expansion produces an increase in filling pressure and no enhancement of function, it is probable that the ventricle cannot respond to an increased volume load. The danger of pulmonary congestion is, therefore, imminent and fluid therapy should not be pursued. If volume expansion results in correction of the deranged hemodynamic status, further therapy may not be required. However, if adequate function is not restored by fluid administration or if elevated filling pressure precludes this approach, further treatment is necessary and consists of utilization of specific pharmacologic agents to enhance depressed ventricular performance.

The necessity of eliminating hypovolemia and attaining optimal left ventricular filling pressure before instituting treatment with cardiac and vasoactive drugs is reemphasized. Administration of these agents after left ventricular function has been maximized by fluid administration increases their efficacy, reduces the required dosage and decreases the hazard of untoward effects. Of course, as previously indicated, because of the not uncommon association of excessive left ventricular filling pressure with myocardial infarction shock, volume expansion is often contraindicated.

Drug Therapy

Despite its limitations, drug therapy retains an important role in the treatment of shock. An enlarged spectrum of differing drugs recently has been reviewed,[2,62-65,103] and increased understanding of pathophysiologic mechanisms has afforded a more rational approach to their use. Further, newer techniques utilizing mechanical cardiac assist and direct cardiac surgery are limited in their availability and applicability.

Augmentation of depressed cardiac output in shock can be effected by several pharmacologic means: (1) as indicated previously, increase in venous return by volume expansion may raise cardiac output; (2) positive inotropic agents may increase cardiac output by enhancing myocardial contractility; most such agents possess a combination of effects on the myocardium and peripheral vasculature; (3) reduction of impedence to left ventricular outflow, or cardiac unloading, may increase cardiac output; this effect is achieved by certain vasodilator agents that diminish left ventricular afterload. As noted previously, maintenance of adequate coronary perfusion pressure is critically important in myocardial infarction shock. In addition to enhancing myocardial function and, thus, improving systemic circulation, support of coronary perfusion is essential for preservation of the ischemic zone surrounding the infarct and prevention of extension of the area of necrosis. Since the vasodilating agents usually reduce blood pressure, their applicability in shock is limited. However, in shock characterized by markedly elevated peripheral vascular resistance and adequate blood pressure, they may be useful.

On the basis of these considerations, the hemodynamic pattern, which is not consistent in cardiogenic shock, is a major determinant in the proper selection of a therapeutic agent. If systolic blood pressure is markedly reduced, a drug with vasoconstrictive as well as positive inotropic effects (for example, norepinephrine or metaraminol) is indicated in order to support coronary blood flow. If peripheral resistance is excessive and blood pressure adequate, however, a vasodilating agent with positive inotropic effects (for example, dopamine) or without inotropic action (nitroprusside) is appropriate.

Catecholamines: The drugs most commonly utilized for cardiogenic shock—and, thus, about which most information is available—are the sympathomimetic agents, which include the catecholamines and certain noncatecholamine drugs with similar structural and pharmacologic properties.[62] The catecholamines are characterized by a benzene ring with two adjacent hydroxyl groups (comprising the catechol nucleus) to which is attached a short carbon chain with an amine group. The noncatecholamine sympathomimetic drugs are structurally similar but lack the distinct catechol nucleus. The catecholamines include both endogenous compounds and synthetic forms. The endogenously produced catecholamines are dopamine, norepinephrine and epinephrine. Of the large number of synthetically produced catecholamines, those of pertinence to this discussion (Table I) are norepinephrine (Levophed®), dopamine (Intropin®), isoproterenol (Isuprel®), epinephrine (Adrenalin®), metaraminol (Aramine®) and mephentermine (Wyamine®).

The effects of adrenergic stimuli are mediated by receptors, the nature of which has not fully been elucidated, in the effector organs. These receptors are termed alpha and beta, and their presence has been postulated in most organs subserved by the adrenergic nervous system. Endogenous catecholamines, synthetic catecholamines, and other sympathomimetic agents can activate these receptors and are therefore adrenergic stimulating agents; other types of chemical agents lacking structural similarity to the catecholamines are without effect at these sites. In the cardiovascular system, both alpha and beta receptors are present in the smooth muscle of blood vessels, and beta receptors are present in the myocardium; there is no evidence of alpha receptors in the myocardium itself. Contraction of smooth muscle of the blood vessels brought about by adrenergic agents, resulting in vasoconstriction, is mediated by alpha receptors in the smooth muscle; relaxation of this tissue, resulting in vasodilation, is mediated by beta receptors. In the heart, beta receptor stimulation increases contractility, heart rate and metabolic activity. Drugs that stimulate the respective adrenergic receptors are termed alpha- or beta-stimulating agents. The actions of an adrenergic drug may stimulate alpha receptors of one organ and beta receptors of another. Norepinephrine activates myocardial beta receptors (cardiac stimulation) and predominantly excites alpha receptors in blood vessel smooth muscle (vasoconstriction).

The effects of the catecholamines on adrenergic receptors can be direct or indirect. The latter refers to the mechanism of action of the catecholamines that in themselves have little or no intrinsic effect on adrenergic receptors and produce their effects by stimulation of release of the stored neurotransmitter norepinephrine from sympathetic nerve terminals. Norepinephrine, epinephrine, dopamine and isoproterenol directly stimulate adrenergic receptor sites. Mephentermine possesses only indirect adrenergic effects and metaraminol acts via both modes (Table I). Whereas the activity of the direct-acting catecholamines is independent of endogenous norepinephrine stores, indirect-acting agents are totally dependent on adequate endogenous norepinephrine stores for their effects. Thus, long-term administration of norepinephrine-depleting drugs (reserpine or guanethidine) or prolonged use of an indirect-acting catecholamine (metaraminol or mephentermine) can markedly limit responsiveness to the latter class of agents because of depletion of norepinephrine from sympathetic nerve terminals.

Norepinephrine and Metaraminol: Norepinephrine and metaraminol, which have quite similar hemodynamic effects, are the two drugs most widely employed in the treatment of cardiogenic shock. Norepinephrine acts directly; metaraminol, as previously noted, acts both directly and by causing norepinephrine release from endogenous stores. These drugs stimulate both alpha and beta adrenergic receptors and thus possess vasoconstrictor and positive inotropic properties. Consequently, they have the potential, in cardiogenic shock, to raise cardiac output and arterial blood pressure simultaneously. However, their actual effects vary with

TABLE I

Cardiovascular Effects of Sympathomimetic Agents

Agent	Positive inotropic effect by stimulation of myocardial beta adrenergic receptors		Increase in PVR by stimulation of arteriolar alpha adrenergic receptors		Decrease in PVR by direct stimulation of arteriolar beta adrenergic receptors	Decrease in systemic arterial resistance by non-adrenergic, direct, dilating effect	Administration
	Direct	Indirect	Direct	Indirect			
Postive inotropic effect; increase in PVR							
Norepinephrine (Levophed)	+		+				9 to 32 mg (4 to 16 ml) of the bitartrate in 1,000 ml of 5 percent dextrose in H_2O; initial rate 1 to 2 μg per minute intravenously
Metaraminol bitartrate (Aramine)	+	+	+	+			50 to 200 mg (5 to 20 ml) in 1,000 ml of 5 percent dextrose in H_2O; initial intravenous rate 1 to 2 μg per minute intravenously; may also be given intramuscularly, 2 to 10 mg
Positive inotropic effect; decrease in PVR							
Isoproterenol hydochloride (Isuprel)	+				+		1 to 5 mg (10 to 50 cc) in 500 ml of 5 percent dextrose in H_2O; initial rate 0.5 to 1.0 μg per minute intravenously
Positive inotropic effect; mixed effect on vascular resistance							
Epinephrine (Adrenalin)	+		+		+		1 to 5 mg (1 to 5 ml) in 500 ml of 5 percent dextrose in H_2O; initial rate 1 to 2 μg per minute intravenously
Dopamine (Intropin)	+		+			+	200 mg (5 ml) in 1,000 ml of 5 percent dextrose in H_2O; initial rate 0.02 to 0.04 mg per minute intravenously
Mephentermine sulfate (Wyamine)		+		+		+	500 to 1,000 mg (16.7 to 33.3 ml) in dextrose in H_2O; initial rate 0.24 to 0.50 mg per minute intravenously; may also be given intravenously, 10 to 30 mg in single injection

PVR = peripheral vascular resistance.

the condition of the individual patient and the dosage employed. With small doses, cardiac output and blood pressure are increased, mainly as a result of predominant beta adrenergic stimulating action on the heart.[105] With large doses, vascular resistance is markedly increased and cardiac output may actually fall, despite the positive inotropic effects of these drugs. Such an adverse effect can also occur with administration of norepinephrine or metaraminol in patients with already excessive peripheral resistance who actually may need reduction in this factor. This inordinate elevation of peripheral resistance may have the deleterious effect of decreasing cardiac output and increasing the metabolic needs of the heart without a proportionate rise in coronary blood flow and myocardial perfusion, resulting in further deterioration of an already injured myocardium.[106] In the treatment of cardiogenic shock with norepinephrine or metaraminol, cardiac output is usually increased with maintenance of systolic blood pressure at 90 to 100 mm Hg.[62,64,105,106] Such an approach maximizes positive cardiac inotropic effects and avoids excessive systemic vasoconstriction, thereby enhancing cardiac output without undue increases in cardiac workload. Therefore, these drugs should be administered in the smallest effective dosage with frequent attempts at withdrawal.

Several undesirable pharmacologic effects may be associated with the use of norepinephrine and metaraminol. Aggravation of oliguria may result from renal artery constriction produced by these drugs. Prolonged therapy may reduce plasma volume because of fluid transudation at the capillary level secondary to post-capillary sphincter constriction.[107] The resultant hypovolemia may exacerbate the shock state to the point of apparent intractability. Indeed, in some instances cardiogenic shock requiring constant therapy with these drugs has been abolished by administration of fluids. The importance is again stressed of the use of minimal effective dosage as well as careful attention to fluid requirements during sustained administration of these vasoconstrictor agents.

Although the hemodynamic actions of norepinephrine and metaraminol are similar, certain differences merit emphasis. As previously noted, metaraminol should be avoided in patients previously treated with catecholamine-depleting drugs. Norepinephrine produces local tissue necrosis on extravasation, an effect not shared by metaraminol, which can be administered intramuscularly as well as intravenously. As with other indirect-acting catecholamines, the effects of metaraminol are somewhat prolonged—lasting up to 20 minutes after administration is discontinued—in comparison with those of norepinephrine, which are more abrupt in onset and cessation.

Mortality in this syndrome remains distressingly high after all forms of medical therapy; thus, it is difficult to substantiate the suggested beneficial effects of these vasopressor-positive inotropic agents on survival because of the grave and multifactorial nature of the problem. However, their use in patients with cardiogenic shock is frequently successful in improving coronary blood flow, systemic blood pressure and cardiac output[65]—the therapeutic goals upon which reduction in mortality is based.

Dopamine: Because of its unique properties (Table I), dopamine possesses several advantages for use in the shock state.[108,109] In addition to its beta adrenergic stimulation in the myocardium, it produces direct, non-adrenergic dilation of the renal, mesenteric, coronary and intracerebral vascular beds and also causes vasoconstriction in skeletal muscle by alpha adrenergic stimulation. Thus, its effect on total peripheral vascular resistance is the net result of its separate actions on the regional circulations. In general, total peripheral vascular resistance is unaltered or mildly reduced, heart rate is not significantly changed, and cardiac output rises. Blood pressure is thus increased as a result of the enhanced cardiac output.[108,109] At high doses, the predominant effect of dopamine is alpha adrenergic stimulation in all vascular beds—and, thus, vasoconstriction.

In patients with coronary artery disease, peripheral resistance is reduced and cardiac output and blood pressure are elevated by dopamine without impairment of overall myocardial energy metabolism.[109,110] In comparative studies of patients with shock, dopamine has produced greater increments in cardiac output and urine flow than has norepinephrine,[109,111] and its potential value in this syndrome is further supported by additional experimental and clinical studies.[64,109] The salutary effects of dopamine on renal blood flow have been of particular importance in oliguric patients with shock.[109] It should be emphasized, however, that because of its peripheral vascular effects, dopamine may not be capable of supporting adequate blood pressure in patients in whom it does not increase cardiac output. Norepinephrine has been required in such patients. The most serious adverse effect of dopamine is ventricular arrhythmias. Hypotension has also occurred—particularly at lower doses—and other side effects include angina, nausea and vomiting.

Isoproterenol: This drug is a relatively pure beta adrenergic agonist (Table I) with potent stimulatory effects on the heart, augmenting contractility and cardiac rate and causing peripheral vasodilation. Cardiac output may, therefore, be significantly increased by its actions. In patients with coronary artery disease who are not acutely ill, isoproterenol has not only increased cardiac output but also raised overall coronary blood flow more than it raised myocardial oxygen demands.[112] Thus, no metabolic evidence of ischemia was present in association with increased myocardial contractility and mechanical effort. The effect of isoproterenol on blood pressure is the net result of its combined actions on cardiac output and systemic vascular resistance. When cardiac output increases in excess of the decrease in peripheral resistance, blood pressure rises. Volume expansion may be necessary with the use of isoproterenol because of the increased vascular capacitance associated with its vasodilatory effects.

Isoproterenol has been found beneficial, in some studies, in the treatment of patients with myocardial infarction shock. Elevations in both cardiac output and blood pressure have been obtained with isoproterenol in patients with cardiogenic shock.[113] The combination of isoproterenol and volume expansion has also been useful in this syndrome. However, further evaluation has demonstrated that its usefulness is largely limited to shock of mild degree. In patients with shock and severe hypotension, the drug has not been beneficial, in some instances having deleterious effects on the clinical course.[64] This is largely due to the substantial increase in myocardial oxygen requirements produced by the drug without a concomitant

rise in coronary blood flow, resulting from the inability of isoproterenol to augment the reduced blood pressure in patients with profound hypotension.[62-65] Indeed, in such situations, isoproterenol may actually further reduce blood pressure. Increased myocardial ischemia and further depression of cardiac pump function as well as ventricular irritability result. Intensified myocardial ischemia after the administration of isoproterenol has been demonstrated experimentally.[74-76] Its role in cardiogenic shock is limited.

Epinephrine: Epinephrine (Table I) acts directly on cardiac beta adrenergic receptors as a potent cardiac stimulant, increasing myocardial contractility and frequency of contraction. Its effect on the peripheral vasculature, however, is mixed since it predominantly affects alpha receptors in some vascular beds (skin, mucosa and kidney) and beta receptors in others (skeletal muscle).[108] These effects are also dose-dependent, the intensity of alpha stimulation increasing with increasing dosage of epinephrine. The net effect of epinephrine on total peripheral vascular resistance is the resultant of its effects on the various regional circulations and, importantly, a function of the dosage utilized. At therapeutic doses, beta adrenergic effects predominate in the peripheral vessels, and total peripheral vascular resistance is reduced. However, constriction is maintained in the renal and cutaneous circulations due to predominant alpha adrenergic effects in these areas. Thus, because of the redistribution of the circulating blood volume, the rise in cardiac output after epinephrine results in increased regional blood flow primarily to skeletal muscle with no enhancement or actual reduction of flow to vital organs such as the kidney. Cardiac arrhythmias, resulting from increased automaticity, are a potential hazard with epinephrine. There has been only limited use and little systematic investigation of epinephrine in the treatment of cardiogenic shock.

Mephentermine: Mephentermine produces release of norepinephrine from sympathetic nerves; thus, its primary actions are similar to those of metaraminol[62,108] (Table I). Its effects on vascular resistance are, however, somewhat complex; in current studies, they have varied with dosage and patient population. In normal subjects, mephentermine increased cardiac output, heart rate and peripheral vascular resistance. In patients with shock, however, large doses of mephentermine have resulted in decreases in peripheral resistance, apparently by a direct non-adrenergic effect on peripheral blood vessels.[109]

Pure Alpha Adrenergic-Stimulating Agents: It is to be noted that those sympathomimetic amines producing alpha adrenergic stimulation and no positive inotropic effect have little or no place in the treatment of cardiogenic shock. Such agents include methoxamine (Vasoxyl®) and phenylephrine (Neo-Synephrine®). Although blood pressure is usually increased by their action, cardiac output is often diminished because of their lack of supportive action on the myocardium while they impose a greater work load—increased peripheral vascular resistance —on the heart. Further cardiac deterioration is the consequence of such a combination of actions. The use of pure alpha adrenergic agonists is rational only in those very uncommon cases of hypotension in which the primary defect is reduced peripheral vascular resistance in the presence of minimal myocardial damage and normal cardiac output.

Other Drugs: The lack of notable success in the treatment of cardiogenic shock with traditional medical therapy has spurred development of differing pharmacologic agents and new application of old ones to this syndrome. Initial therapeutic trials have been carried out with the positive inotropic agents (digitalis and glucagon) and the vasodilator drugs (nitroprusside, phentolamine, phenoxybenzamine, chlorpromazine and corticosteroids).

Digitalis: Because of its demonstrated efficacy in enhancing performance of the failing myocardium and the view that cardiogenic shock is an extreme form of heart failure, the potential role of digitalis in this syndrome has received attention. In addition to its direct, positive inotropic effect, which is unrelated to adrenergic mechanisms, digitalis also produces direct constriction of peripheral arteries. However, when increased cardiac output is associated with digitalis therapy in congestive heart failure, reduction in peripheral vascular resistance occurs as the result of sympathetic withdrawal associated with improved cardiac pump function, which overrides the relatively weak constricting action of the glycoside.[114]

In experimental cardiogenic shock, digitalis has produced beneficial effects on cardiac function.[115] However, similar results have not been forthcoming from clinical studies. Although digitalis has produced inconsistent hemodynamic effects in cardiac failure associated with myocardial infarction,[116–121] the glycoside has been of no benefit in myocardial infarction shock[121,122] and proved potentially deleterious because of its acute vasoconstricting effects.[122] Attenuation of the hemodynamic effects of digitalis in this setting appears to be related to its diminished contractile action on ischemic myocardium, as demonstrated experimentally.[71]

Glucagon: Extensive investigations of glucagon have established that it possesses a positive inotropic effect independent of beta adrenergic receptor stimulation and that it mildly dilates peripheral arteries. Clinical evaluation of its use in patients with severe cardiac pump failure has been disappointing, however, in that significant beneficial effects have not been consistent.[64,123] This may stem from the inability of glucagon to augment contractility in the chronically failing heart. Its positive inotropic action may provide adjunctive therapy in patients with recent onset of cardiac pump dysfunction; however, its role in cardiogenic shock is a limited one.

Vasodilator Drugs: These agents have been demonstrated to improve hemodynamic function in cardiac failure by reduction of left ventricular afterload and preload.[124] They produce no direct inotropic effects; thus, alteration of ventricular function is achieved entirely by their extra-myocardial actions. The relative effects on afterload and preload vary with the individual agents. These drugs are discussed in detail in chapter 21 on afterload-reducing agents and are referred to here only generally.

The vasodilator agents that have received principal attention and application are nitroprusside and phentolamine. They are capable of substantially improving depressed ventricular performance in cardiac failure, as manifested by increased cardiac output and decreased left ventricular filling pressure. These salutary effects are achieved while myocardial oxygen consumption is simultaneously reduced, suggesting potential for limitation of infarct size and also enhancement of intrinsic contractile state by a decrease in ischemia.

Reduction in myocardial oxygen demand is the result of conversion of contractile effort to flow work rather than the metabolically more costly pressure work[77] by the lowering of left ventricular afterload. However, because of this vasodilation and consequent hypotensive effect, these agents have limited use in cardiogenic shock in which, as previously noted, elevation of reduced coronary perfusion pressure is a prime therapeutic requisite. In those cases of shock characterized by extreme vasoconstriction and reduced cardiac output, however, afterload reduction would be rational treatment with potential to raise cardiac output, maintain adequate blood pressure and favorably influence the metabolic status of the mechanically overburdened myocardium.

Other agents with vasodilating action that have received experimental attention and clinical consideration in the treatment of cardiogenic shock are dibenzyline, chlorpromazine and corticosteroids.[62,64] The potential hazards of these agents in this syndrome and the impropriety of their use in the presence of hypotension—when they could produce catastrophic consequences—are reemphasized.

Mechanical Cardiac Assist

The limitations of conventional medical therapy in cardiogenic shock have resulted in innovative therapeutic methods, among the most significant of which is mechanical cardiac assist. This approach is based on the principle of reducing myocardial oxygen demands and increasing coronary blood flow while providing support of the systemic circulation.[125,126] This unique capability has the potential to alleviate myocardial ischemia and injury, thereby reversing hemodynamic deterioration.

In the development of mechanical devices for temporary support of the failing heart, two general approaches have been utilized: (1) modifications of total cardiopulmonary bypass techniques used in open-heart surgery and (2) counterpulsation by phasic alterations of aortic pressure applied synchronously with the cardiac cycle. The bypass approach has included various forms of partial venoarterial pumping

that can be carried out for several hours with or without a membrane oxygenator. Although left heart bypass can be accomplished clinically by a transseptal technique not requiring thoracotomy,[127] these shunt methods usually have not been as feasible or effective in shock after myocardial infarction as they have been as postoperative adjuncts in cardiac surgery.

Intraaortic Balloon Counterpulsation: The second approach of synchronous pressure assistance or arterio-arterial pumping utilizes the concept of counterpulsation, in which—originally designed—blood is withdrawn from the aorta during systole and returned during diastole by a reciprocating pump.[125,126,128] An important advance in the practical application of this approach has been the introduction of intraaortic balloon counterpulsation, which is the most frequently applied of these methods in the treatment of cardiogenic shock. In this system, a balloon attached to a catheter is inserted into the descending thoracic aorta through the femoral artery.[128] Diastolic augmentation of coronary blood flow is achieved by raising the diastolic pressure in the ascending aorta by rapid inflation of the balloon during ventricular relaxation (Figure 7). During subsequent deflation of the balloon in systole, resistance to left ventricular ejection is reduced, ventricular outflow is enhanced, and myocardial oxygen requirements are diminished. Balloon counterpulsation can be carried out safely for several days with little discomfort to the patient.

Results with intraaortic balloon counterpulsation in myocardial infarction shock indicate improvement in cardiac output, increase in mean aortic pressure, augmentation of coronary blood flow and resultant beneficial effects on myocardial metabolism, as reflected in evidence of increased myocardial oxygenation.[126,129] Abnormally elevated myocardial oxygen extraction decreased toward normal, and myocardial lactate production—indicating cellular hypoxia—decreased or shifted to extraction. In some patients with cardiogenic shock, enhanced prognosis is associated with these salutary hemodynamic effects;[126] however, deterioration of pump function often follows discontinuance of circulatory assistance, and few patients with myocardial infarction shock unresponsive to pharmacologic management have

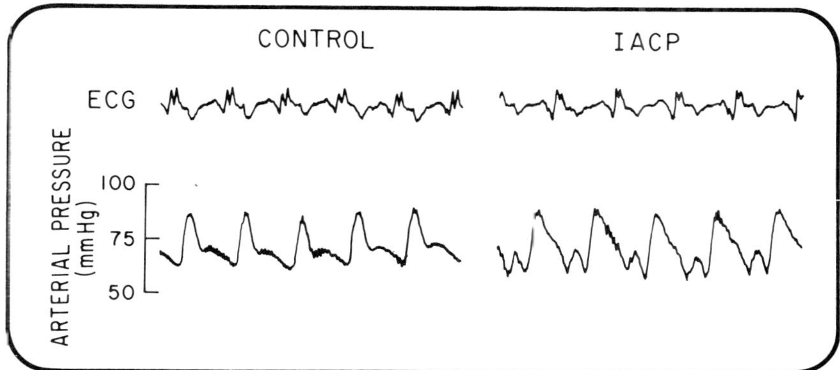

FIGURE 7. Electrocardiogram (ECG) and intraarterial pressure tracings in a patient with acute myocardial infarction shock before (control) and during intraaortic balloon counterpulsation (IACP). Note reduction in systolic pressure and augmentation of diastolic pressure above peak systolic pressure during counterpulsation.

recovered as a result of counterpulsation.[129,130] Prolonging counterpulsation beyond 48 hours in patients who do not demonstrate sufficient improvement within this period to allow withdrawal of mechanical assist does not provide additional benefit in clinical outcome. A major application of counterpulsation in this setting is support of patients during left heart catheterization and selective coronary arteriography in preparation for a definitive surgical procedure.[130,131] Complications of intraaortic counterpulsation have been relatively infrequent and include thromboembolism from the balloon surface (which is avoidable by anticoagulation), trauma to the aorta, arterial insufficiency related to the site of balloon insertion and destruction of blood elements (which has not been a serious problem).[126]

The response of the patient to counterpulsation in the first 24 hours is indicative of the subsequent course and provides the basis for systematic application of this form of therapy.[126,131,132] After 24 hours of counterpulsation, assistance is discontinued and the patient's condition is assessed. If improvement and stability are evident, counterpulsation may be reinstituted for possible further benefit. If reevaluation within 24 hours reveals no additional gains in functional status, gradual discontinuation of counterpulsation is achieved over 24 hours. If, however, further improvement results, continued periods of counterpulsation are undertaken until a stable level of function is achieved. If hemodynamic deterioration ensues after the first 24 hours of assist, counterpulsation is reinstituted for another 24 hours with reassessment after its cessation. Clinical deterioration at this time indicates balloon dependence, and consideration is directed toward evaluation of potential for definitive therapy by cardiac surgery.

External Counterpulsation: Noninvasive external counterpulsation devices have been developed that utilize intermittent external body compression synchronized with the cardiac cycle[125] (Figure 8). These atraumatic external synchronous methods are currently undergoing clinical evaluation. Although preliminary evidence suggests that external counterpulsation may reduce the extent, complications and mortality of uncomplicated myocardial infarction,[133] these devices do not appear to be beneficial in the severe condition of established myocardial infarction shock. One such external counterpulsation device consists of a system of arm and leg cuffs for sequenced pulsation of the extremities. Another technique utilizes the lower body boot or wet suit that hydraulically provides phasic positive and negative ambient pressures in diastole and systole, respectively. External assistance may also be achieved by the technique of body acceleration applied synchronously with the heartbeat (BASH procedure). The patient is abruptly moved in a caudal direction on a shake-bed during cardiac ejec-

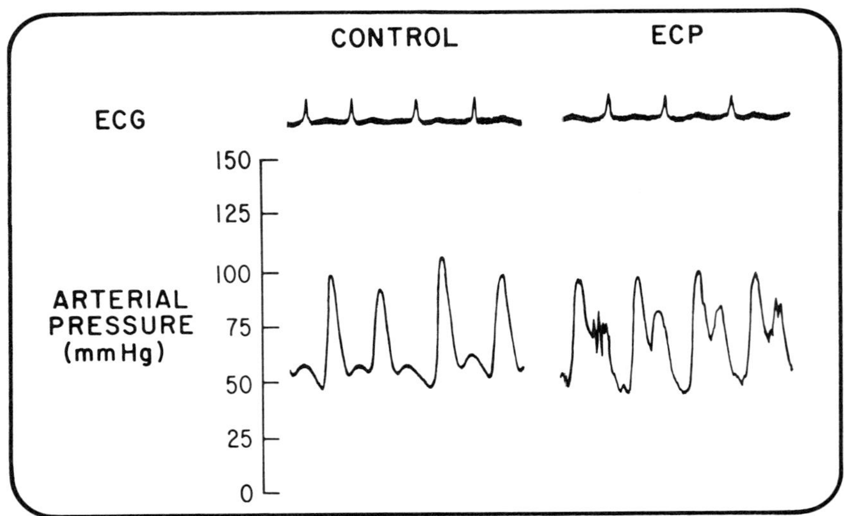

FIGURE 8. Intraaterial pressure in a patient with acute myocardial infarction before (control) and during external counterpulsation (ECP). Note augmentation of diastolic pressure during counterpulsation.

tion, thereby enhancing the delivery of stroke volume from the left ventricle into the ascending aorta.

Cardiac Surgery

In patients in whom the preceding sequence of management is unsuccessful, consideration is given to the potential for direct cardiac surgery to correct any major mechanical defects of the heart resulting from infarction and to restore reversibly injured myocardium in order to enhance cardiac function and reverse the shock syndrome. Because delay in definitive therapy of this syndrome may contribute to irreversible hemodynamic deterioration, it is our approach to initiate early objective determination of prognosis by the means previously described and consider evaluation for cardiac lesions potentially remediable by surgery in patients at high risk of death from pump failure despite the aforementioned forms of therapy.

Current application of cardiac surgery in acute myocardial infarction has evolved as a result of the availability of safe and accurate methods for hemodynamic and angiographic assessment of the status of the left ventricle and coronary arteries coupled with the development of effective techniques for revascularization and repair of the mechanical defects resulting from acute ischemic injury to the ventricle. The surgical procedures successfully utilized in acute myocardial infarction have included coronary artery bypass grafting, repair of ventricular septal defect, mitral valve replacement and infarctectomy singly and in combination for the treatment of cardiac pump failure.[134]

Angiographic Evaluation: Identification of a surgically remediable lesion entails angiographic analysis of the left ventricle and coronary arteries. Although the risk of left ventriculography and selective coronary arteriography would appear to be increased in acute myocardial infarction, recent experience has demonstrated their feasibility and relative safety in these circumstances. Coronary angiography and left ventriculography have been performed safely in cardiogenic shock with the aid of mechanical circulatory assist,[130-132] and we have carried out these procedures in the absence of artificial support devices without an increase in complications.[10] The significance of angiographic evaluation in myocardial infarction shock is reflected in the findings of potentially operable cardiac lesions in a majority of patients, demonstrating the utility of these studies.[132] After identification of such lesions in the suitable patient with refractory shock, emergency corrective surgery is undertaken.

Defects currently considered potentially amenable to corrective cardiac surgery are significant obstructive lesions in the coronary arteries associated with adequate distal patency by coronary artery bypass graft, asynergic segments of myocardium by infarctectomy, acute ventricular septal defect by direct repair and mitral regurgitation by valve replacement. Not uncommonly, a combination of these procedures may be indicated and performed. Although indications for surgery in myocardial infarction have not been definitively established, several factors limit or contraindicate its application in terms of potential for successful results. Impairment of general health by significant extracardiac disease eliminates surgical candidacy. Inadequate distal patency in obstructed coronary arteries precludes bypass grafting. Severe asynergy involving more than 60 percent of the left ventricle has been considered a relative contraindication to surgery[98]—suggesting, however, that even in the group with such extensive myocardial deficiency, some patients may benefit from surgery. This is borne out by our experience with corrective surgery in myocardial infarction shock in which a number of successfully treated patients had left ventricular asynergy involving more than 60 percent of the ventricle and ejection fractions lower than 30 percent.[134] Thus, identification of candidates for surgery currently involves careful, individual patient selection within a framework of general indications and restrictions.

Myocardial Revascularization: The basis for myocardial revascularization in myocardial infarction shock is reversibility of myocardial ischemia—and, thus, of the resulting impairment in ventricular function. Loss of contractile capacity in the ischemic, noninfarcted zone of myocardium associated with infarction has been well documented.[8] Abnormalities of ventricular wall motion resulting from myocardial ischemia, that is, hypokinesis, akinesis or paradoxical systolic expansion,[135] contribute to hemodynamic dysfunction quantitatively according to their extent.[8,54,56] Thus, to the degree that structural and functional integrity can be restored in ischemic, nonlethally injured myocardium, cardiac performance can be enhanced.

Experimental and clinical studies have confirmed the reversibility of ischemic damage and impaired contractile function upon restoration of blood flow to previously ischemic myocardium.[136] In man, direct revascularization of the myocardium by aorto-coronary saphenous vein bypass graft or, less commonly, by direct anastomosis of internal mammary artery to coronary artery[137] is capable of enhancing myocardial function, as demonstrated by objective criteria of contractile performance. After bypass grafting for angina pectoris, improvement has been documented in left ventricular segmental contractile activity of previously asynergic areas[138,139] and in indexes of left ventricular pump function,[134] although this has not been a consistent finding.[140] The salutary effect of coronary artery bypass surgery on ventricular performance during acute myocardial infarction in one of our patients is depicted in Figure 9. After surgery, asynergy was corrected and ejection fraction increased to normal in this patient.

Limited experience with coronary bypass surgery in myocardial infarction shock has demonstrated its feasibility and favorable results when compared with medical therapy for this syndrome. Three groups of investigators[141-143] have reported on a total of 19 patients in whom surgery consisted exclusively of coronary artery bypass grafting; 14 (74 percent) survived operation with reversal of shock and were discharged from the hospital, and there were 11 (58 percent) long-term survivors followed up for as long as 16 months. Single, additional patients have also been reported on, one of whom lived for 2 months.[134]

Since the rationale for myocardial revascularization in myocardial infarction shock is reversal of ischemia and restoration of function, the time during which this can be accomplished successfully is limited by the progressive nature of the infarction process. Coronary bypass surgery in this setting is, therefore, an urgent procedure and has been instituted within 24 hours or less after evidence of hemodynamic deterioration.[141,142] This is in accord with experimental evidence indicating continuing enlargement of

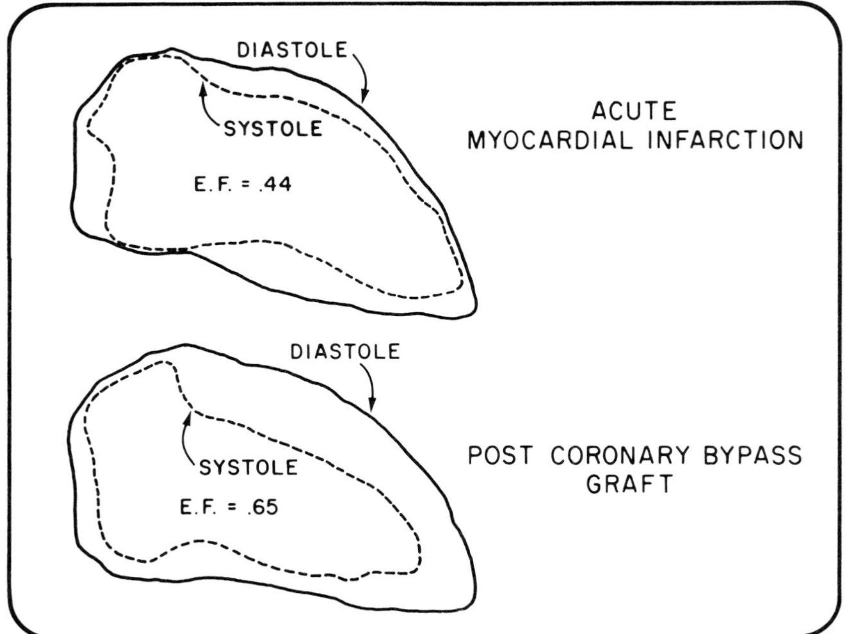

FIGURE 9. Tracings of left ventricular cineangiograms (right anterior oblique view) in a patient with acute myocardial infarction, pump dysfunction and sustained myocardial ischemic pain. Segmental dyssynergy and reduced ejection fraction (EF) **(top)** were markedly improved **(bottom),** and chest pain was relieved by double aortocoronary saphenous vein bypass graft carried out in the early period after acute infarction. (Reproduced by permission from Amsterdam et al.[134])

the necrotic area from ischemic myocardium for 18 hours after myocardial infarction,[61] resulting in a relatively brief period during which injury is reversible. Surgery has been performed with[141,142] and without[143,144] the use of pre- and postoperative mechanical circulatory assist devices. The operative procedure used by different groups has varied, multiple coronary bypass grafts predominating in one series[141] and single grafts in another.[142]

Infarctectomy: The rationale for excision of the acutely infarcted region of myocardium in myocardial infarction shock is based on the deleterious influence of this area on hemodynamic function. As previously noted, this involves more than merely loss of the contribution of the infarcted zone to total ventricular contractile activity. The passive, systolic expansion of acutely infarcted myocardium also may divert stroke volume resulting in reduced cardiac output, increase end-diastolic volume with elevation of myocardial oxygen requirements and augmentation of ischemia, elevate left ventricular end-diastolic pressure producing pulmonary congestion, impair papillary muscle function with consequent mitral valve incompetence and provoke serious arrhythmias from electrically unstable tissue. Studies of infarctectomy in experimental myocardial infarction have demonstrated significant benefit manifested as marked enhancement of defibrillation and resuscitation of acutely infarcted canine hearts, augmentation of left ventricular hemodynamic performance and increase in survival.[144] These effects in experimental myocardial infarction have been obtained with resection of as much as 25 to 30 percent of left ventricular myocardium.[145,146] When infarctectomy exceeds 35 percent of left ventricular muscle mass in experimental infarction, hemodynamic function is severely depressed and incompatible with survival.[147]

Cardiac pump dysfunction becomes manifest in the presence of coronary artery disease and ventricular asynergy when the involved area comprises more than 20 percent of the left ventricle.[148] Although relatively widely applied with considerable success in patients with chronic left ventricular aneurysms,[134] segmental ventricular resection alone has been utilized rarely in the acute phase of myocardial infarction shock. Of two reported cases, there has been one early death and one long-term survival.[149] One patient of ours underwent extensive acute infarctectomy for shock and is well and gainfully employed more than five years after surgery (Figure 10). This case illustrates the magnitude of resection that can be performed. Angiographic evaluation revealed—in addition to the major ventricular asynergy—three-vessel, diffuse, obstructive coronary artery disease, precluding myocardial revascularization.

Although acute infarctectomy as an isolated procedure has been unusual, it has been utilized more commonly in conjunction with other surgical techniques. Of seven patients who underwent simultaneous infarctectomy and coronary artery bypass graft surgery for myocardial infarction shock, there were five early deaths and two long-term survivals.[141] Thus, the long-term success rate in the group of ten patients cited herein is 40 percent, representing a substantial improvement over conservative therapy in cardiogenic shock, which is associated with a mortality approaching 100 percent.

Mitral Valve Replacement for Papillary Muscle Dysfunction: Rupture of a papillary muscle is a relatively rare but catastrophic complication of acute myocardial infarction, having an incidence of approximately 1 percent.[134,150] This lesion results in severe, acute mitral regurgitation with rapid onset of massive pulmonary edema and is associated with mortality of 70 percent within 24 hours and 90 percent at 2 weeks.[150] Quantitation of mitral insufficiency has indicated that in severe valvular incompetence, the regurgitant blood volume may comprise more than half of the total left ventricular stroke volume.[15] This hemodynamic burden, when superimposed on an already injured ventricle, has major significance even in a small infarct and can result in profound failure or shock in a larger infarct. Papillary muscle dysfunction is more common than rupture in acute infarc-

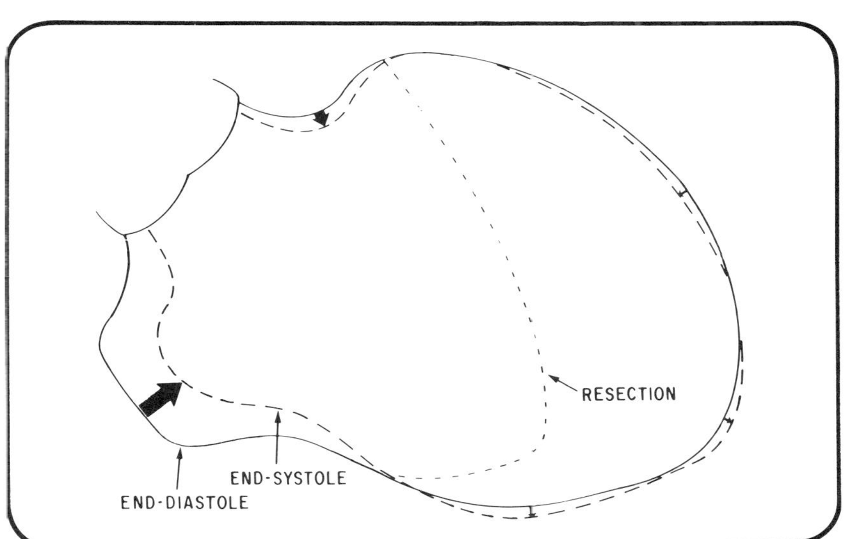

FIGURE 10. Diagrammatic representation of preoperative left ventricular angiogram (right anterior oblique view) in a patient with cardiogenic shock during acute myocardial infarction. The extensive area of dyssynergy involving the apex and anterior free wall was resected as indicated by the **short dashes.** Contraction was relatively well preserved in the basal segments. Recovery followed successful emergency infarctectomy and long-term survival was achieved. (Reproduced by permission from Mason et al.[163])

tion [152] and can produce the entire clinical spectrum of mitral regurgitation, from mild to severe.[153] This lesion is usually associated with papillary muscle ischemia of various degrees and the clinical presentation differs accordingly from that of papillary muscle rupture.[154.]

Papillary muscle rupture most commonly occurs within the first 10 days after acute infarction. It usually is characterized by a loud, holosystolic murmur at the cardiac apex, which may be accompanied by a thrill, but severe mitral regurgitation may occur in myocardial infarction shock in the absence of a murmur.[155] A more common problem is differentiating mitral regurgitation from ventricular septal rupture, for which cardiac catheterization is required. This can be accomplished by right heart catheterization at the bedside. Identification of large "V" waves in the pulmonary capillary wedge pressure (see Figure 25 in chapter 21 on afterload-reducing agents) is consistent with mitral regurgitation, and negative findings on analysis of right ventricular blood oxygen content and indicator dilution curves exclude ventricular septal rupture. If surgery is to be performed, it should be preceded—in all but unusual circumstances —by angiographic evaluation of the left ventricle and coronary arteries to detect any associated operable lesions.

Surgical correction of mitral regurgitation complicating myocardial infarction consists of mitral valve replacement. When surgery can be delayed for several months after infarction, operative risk is markedly reduced. However, as previously noted, circulatory failure is usually extreme in these patients; the great majority die within 24 hours, and survival beyond 2 weeks is uncommon.[150] In these grave circumstances, definitive therapy by surgical correction of the mitral lesion and other potentially operable defects offers the greatest probability of improving prognosis. Although experience with valve replacement in the acute phase of infarction with cardiac pump failure is limited, this procedure has demonstrated its potential for favorably altering the course of this disorder.

Repair of Ventricular Septal Defect: The incidence of rupture of the ventricular septum in acute myocardial infarction is 0.5 to 1.0 percent, and it most frequently occurs during the first 2 weeks.[134] Mortality has been reported as

24 percent within 24 hours; the majority of patients die within 1 week and only 13 percent survive for 2 months.[156] The defect most frequently involves the lower portion of the muscular septum[157] and is usually associated with extensive infarction. The resulting left-to-right shunt is large in most cases, the ratio of pulmonary to systemic flow usually exceeding 2:1.[158] The hemodynamic burden imposed on an infarcted and thereby compromised ventricle produces biventricular failure, pulmonary edema and, commonly, shock. The infarction also commonly produces acute aneurysm of the left ventricle, which increases ventricular dysfunction.

Rupture of the ventricular septum is characterized by abrupt clinical deterioration associated with the sudden onset of a loud holosystolic murmur at the lower left sternal border often accompanied by a thrill. However, a thrill is commonly absent, and the murmur may be most prominent at the cardiac apex—a phenomenon which may be related to infero-apical location of the septal defect.[158] Definitive diagnosis therefore requires right heart catheterization for analysis of right ventricular blood oxygen content and indicator dilution curves (Figure 11). Documentation of the diagnosis should be followed, if circumstances permit, by angiographic evaluation of the left ventricle and coronary arteries for detection of additional, correctable defects.

Repair of the ventricular septal defect consists of surgical closure by suture or prosthetic patch. Because of the frequency of associated major segmental dyskinesis of the left ventricle, infarctectomy is often combined with septal repair.[159] Surgical success has been highest when repair was performed 2 or more months after occurrence of the defect. After septal rupture, vigorous efforts should be directed toward achieving adequate hemodynamic status with conservative management in order to delay operation to a more optimal time. However, as previously noted, marked clinical deterioration is usually abrupt after development of this defect[156] in myocardial infarction, and survival is most often dependent on early, definitive therapy.

The results of surgery for ruptured ventricular septum in those cases in which it must be undertaken in the early, high risk period have been

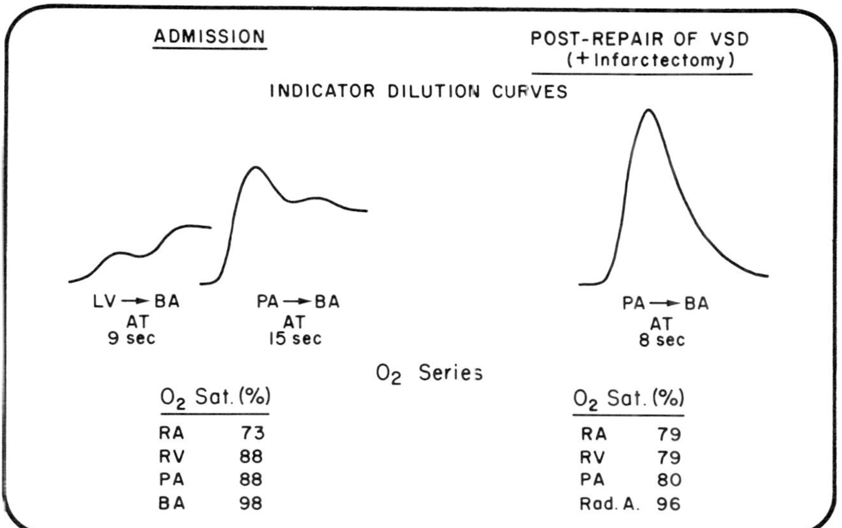

FIGURE 11. Indicator dilution curves (**left**) and oxygen saturation (O₂ Sat.) series (**left**) obtained by right heart catheterization in a 50 year old woman with cardiogenic shock from acute myocardial infarction associated with ventricular septal rupture (VSD). The studies on admission indicated the presence of a left-to-right shunt at the ventricular level with a 2.5:1 pulmonary-to-systemic flow ratio. After repair of the septal defect during the immediate period after acute MI (combined with infarctectomy), there was no evidence of residual shunt as shown by the indicator dilution curves and the oxygen series on the **right.** AT = appearance time; BA = brachial artery; LV = left ventricle; PA = pulmonary artery; RA = right atrium; RV = right ventricle; Rad. A = radial artery. (Reproduced by permission from Amsterdam et al.[134])

encouraging. Review of 35 patients who had surgery 1 to 30 days after septal perforation reveals success in 17 (49 percent) with continuing survival at as long as 29 months.[134] Our recent experience includes two patients who had septal repair by a new double patch technique 6 and 24 hours after rupture and another in whom surgery was performed at 6 days.[160] All are well 9 to 14 months after operation. Figure 11 demonstrates preoperative studies (indicator dilution curves and oxygen series) diagnostic of left-to-right intracardiac shunt at the ventricular level in one of these patients. Combined closure of septal defect and infarctectomy was performed and postoperative studies confirmed successful septal repair. The overall experience with early septal repair in the presence of profound clinical deterioration represents a distinct improvement over conservative treatment and is largely the result of advances in surgical technique allowing corrective procedures in the injured, friable myocardium.[160]

Summary

Shock is a syndrome characterized by severe impairment of circulatory function. It accounts for the major proportion of hospital mortality in acute myocardial infarction and is chiefly related to extensive loss of left ventricular muscle, although extra-myocardial factors may be contributory. Quantitative hemodynamic evaluation allows accurate assesment of prognosis related to cardiac pump dysfunction in acute myocardial infarction and provides a physiologic basis for rational application of available modes of treatment. Therapy consists of pharmacologic agents, mechanical circulatory assist and surgery to correct mechanical cardiac defects related to the infarction. The goal of treatment is to reduce myocardial ischemia, limit infarct size and enhance circulatory function. Positive inotropic agents may increase myocardial ischemic injury because of the increase in myocardial oxygen demands that they produce while a concomitant rise in oxygen supply is precluded by coronary obstructive disease. Mechanical circulatory assist has the capacity to enhance cardiac performance while simultaneously reducing myocardial ischemia by decreasing left ventricular afterload and increasing coronary blood flow. Evaluation for surgically correctable cardiac defects is initiated in appropriate patients when shock is refractory to medical management and mechanical circulatory assist. Systematic application of a widening range of therapeutic alternatives provides the potential for prevention of myocardial infarction shock and reduction of mortality when it occurs.

Acknowledgment: This work was supported in part by Research Program Project Grant HL 14780 and Training Grant HL 05901 from the National Heart and Lung Institute, National Institutes of Health, and Research Grants from the Golden Empire Chapter of the American Heart Association.

The authors gratefully acknowledge the technical assistance of Martie Wood, Robbie Brocchini, Robert Kleckner and Leslie Silvernail.

References

1. **Lown B, Klein MD, Herber PI:** Coronary and pre-coronary care. Amer J Med 46:705, 1969
2. **Swan HJC, Forrester JS, Danzig R, et al:** Power failure in acute myocardial infarction. Progr Cardiovasc Dis 12:568, 1970
3. **Scheidt S, Ascheim R, Killip R:** Shock after acute myocardial infarction. Amer J Cardiol 26:556, 1970
4. **Weber KT, Ratshin RA, Janicki JS, et al:** Left ventricular dysfunction following acute myocardial infarction. A clinicopathologic and hemodynamic profile of shock and failure. Amer J Med 54:697, 1973
5. **Wolk MJ, Scheidt S, Killip T:** Heart failure complicating acute myocardial infarction. Circulation 45:1125, 1972
6. **Killip T, Kimball JT:** Treatment of myocardial infarction in a coronary care unit. Amer J Cardiol 20:457, 1967
7. **Swan HJC, Forrester JS, Diamond G, et al:** Hemodynamic spectrum of myocardial infarction and cardiogenic shock. A conceptual model. Circulation 45:1097, 1972
8. **Amsterdam EA:** Function of the hypoxic myocardium: experimental and clinical aspects. Amer J Cardiol 32:461, 1973
9. **Gunnar RM, Pietras RJ, Stavrakos C, et al:** The physiologic basis for treatment of shock associated with myocardial infarction. Med Clin N Amer 51:69, 1967
10. **Amsterdam EA, Choquet Y, Bonanno JA, et al:** Correlative hemodynamic and angiographic studies in acute coronary syndromes. Clin Res 21:232, 1973
11. **Karliner JS, Ross J:** Left ventricular performance after acute myocardial infarction. Progr Cardiovasc Dis 13:374, 1971
12. **Gunnar RM, Loeb HS, Pietras RJ, et al:** Hemodynamic measurements in a coronary care unit. Progr Cardiovasc Dis 11:29, 1968
13. **Mackenzie GJ, Taylor SH, Fleney DC, et al:** Circulatory and respiratory studies in myocardial infarction and cardiogenic shock. Lancet 2:825, 1964
14. **Loeb HS, Chuquima R, Sinno MZ, et al:** Effects of low flow oxygen on hemodynamics and left ventricular function in patients with uncomplicated acute myocardial infarction. Chest 60:352, 1971
15. **Page DL, Caulfield JB, Kastor JA, et al:** Myocardial changes associated with cardiogenic shock. New Eng J Med 285:133, 1971
16. **Alonso DR, Scheidt S, Post M, et al:** Pathophysiology of cardiogenic shock. Quantification of myocardial necrosis: clinical, pathologic and electrocardiographic correlations. Circulation 48:588, 1973
17. **Zoll PM, Wessler S, Schlesinger MJ:** Interarterial coronary anastomoses in the human heart, with particular reference to anemia and relative cardiac anoxia. Circulation 4:797, 1951
18. **Chimoskey JE, Szentivanyi M, Zakheim R, et al:** Temporary coronary occlusion in conscious dogs: collateral flow and electrocardiogram. Amer J Physiol 212:1025, 1967
19. **Haft JI, Damato AN:** Measurement of collateral blood flow after myocardial infarction in the closed-chest dog. Amer Heart J 77:641, 1969
20. **Elliot EC, Bloor CM, Jones EL, et al:** Effect of controlled coronary occlusion on collateral circulation in conscious dogs. Amer J Physiol 220:857, 1971
21. **Bjork L:** Angiographic demonstration of collaterals to the coronary arteries in patients with angina pectoris. Acta Radiol (Diagn) (Stockholm) 8:305, 1969
22. **Amsterdam EA, Most AS, Wolfson S, et al:** Relation of degree of angiographically documented coronary artery disease to mortality. Ann Intern Med 72:780, 1970
23. **Helfant RH, Vokonas PS, Gorlin R:** Functional importance of the human coronary collateral circulation. New Eng J Med 284:1277, 1971
24. **Miller RR, Mason DT, Salel A, et al:** Determinants and functional significance of the coronary collateral circulation in patients with coronary artery disease. Amer J Cardiol 29:281, 1972
25. **Smith SC, Gorlin R, Herman MV, et al:** Myocardial blood flow in man: effects of coronary collateral circulation and coronary artery bypass surgery. J Clin Invest 10:2556, 1972
26. **Amsterdam EA, Vismara L, Miller RR, et al:** Relationship of ventricular ectopic rhythms to angiographically defined coronary artery disease. Clin Res 21:233, 1973
27. **Miller RR, Amsterdam EA, Zelis R, et al:** Determinants

and functional significance of the coronary collateral circulation in ischemic heart disease. In, Cardiovascular Disease (Russek HI, ed). Baltimore, University Park Press, 1974, p 75

28. **Amsterdam EA, Miller RR, Hughes JL, et al:** Pathophysiology of angina pectoris. In, Atherosclerosis and Coronary Heart Disease (Likoff W, Segal BL, Insull W Jr, et al, ed). New York, Grune & Stratton, 1972, p 178

29. **Carroll RJ, Verani MS, Falsetti HL:** The effect of collateral circulation on segmental left ventricular contraction. Circulation 50:709, 1974

30. **Banka VS, Bodenheimer MM, Helfant RH:** Determinants of reversible asynergy. Circulation 50:714, 1974

31. **Levin DC:** Pathways and functional significance of the coronary collateral circulation. Circulation 50:831, 1974

32. **Amsterdam EA, Miller RR, Foley DH, et al:** Pathophysiology and treatment of coronary artery disease. In, The Peripheral Circulation (Zelis R, ed). New York, Grune & Stratton, 1975, p 363

33. **Snow PJD, Jones AM, Daber KS:** Coronary disease: a pathological study. Brit Heart J 17:503, 1955

34. **Williams DO, Amsterdam EA, Hughes JL, et al:** Importance of coronary collaterals in acute myocardial infarction: relation to pump function. Circulation 49 and 50 suppl III:108, 1974

35. **Loeb HS, Pietras RJ, Tobin JR Jr, et al:** Hypovolemia in shock due to acute myocardial infarction. Circulation 40:653, 1969

36. **Finnerty FA Jr, Bucholz JH, Guilkauden RL:** The blood volumes and plasma protein during levarterenol-induced hypertension. J Clin Invest 37:425, 1958

37. **Agress CM, Rosenberg MJ, Jacobs HI, et al:** Protracted shock in the closed chest dog following coronary embolization with graded microspheres. Amer J Physiol 170:536, 1952

38. **Toubes DB, Brody MJ:** Inhibition of reflex vasoconstriction after experimental coronary embolization in the dog. Circ Res 26:211, 1970

39. **Hanley HG, Costin JC, Skinner NS:** Differential reflex adjustments in cutaneous and muscle vascular beds during experimental coronary artery occlusion. Amer J Cardiol 27:513, 1971

40. **Hughes JL, Amsterdam EA, Mason DT, et al:** Abnormal peripheral vascular dynamics in patients with acute myocardial infarction: diminished reflex arteriolar constrict on. Clin Res 19:321, 1971

41. **Constantin L:** Extracardiac factors contributing to hypotension during coronary occlusion. Amer J Cardiol 11:205, 1963

42. **Sleight P, Widdicombe JG:** Action potentials in fibers from receptors in the epicardium and myocardium of the dog's left ventricle. J Physiol (London) 181:235, 1966

43. **Kezdi P, Misra SN, Kordenat RK, et al:** The role of vagal afferents in acute myocardial infarction. Amer J Cardiol 26:642, 1970

44. **Brown AM:** Excitation of afferent cardiac sympathetic nerve fibers during myocardial ischemia. J Physiol (London) 190:35, 1967

45. **Blumgart HL, Schlesinger MJ, Davis D:** Studies in the relationship of the clinical manifestations of angina pectoris, coronary thrombosis and myocardial infarction to pathologic findings. Amer Heart J 19:1, 1940

46. **Amsterdam EA, Bogren H, Baker WL, et al:** Dynamic analysis of left ventricular pathoanatomy in the acute phase of myocardial infarction. Clin Res 22:139A, 1974

47. **Braunwald E:** Acute myocardial infarction with shock: physiological, pharmacological and clinical considerations. In, Symposium on Coronary Heart Disease (Blumgart HL, ed). New York, American Heart Association, 1968, p 110

48. **Berne RM:** Regulation of coronary blood flow. Physiol Rev 44:1, 1964

49. **Reid PR, Taylor DR, Kelly DT, et al:** Myocardial-infarct extension detected by precordial ST-segment mapping. New Eng J Med 290:123, 1974

50. **Buja LM, Roberts WC:** The coronary arteries and myocardium in acute myocardial infarction shock. In, Shock in Myocardial Infarction (Gunnar RM, Loeb HS, Rahimtoola SH, ed). New York, Grune & Stratton, 1974, p 1

51. **Watson A, Hackel DB, Estes EH:** Acute coronary occlusion and the "power failure" syndrome. Amer Heart J 79:613, 1970

52. **Ratshin RA, Massing GK, James TN:** The clinical significance of the location of acute myocardial infarction. In, Myocardial Infarction (Corday E, Swan HJC, ed). Baltimore, Williams & Wilkins, 1973, p 77

53. **Miller RR, Amsterdam EA, Bogren HG, et al:** Electrocardiographic and cineangiographic correlations in assessment of the location, nature and extent of abnormal left ventricular segmental contraction in coronary artery disease. Circulation 49:447, 1974

54. **Olson HG, Miller RR, Amsterdam EA, et al:** Determinants of pump dysfunction in coronary artery disease: importance of extent, site and pattern of abnormal left ventricular segmental contraction. Clin Res 22:293, 1974

55. **Hamby RI, Hoffman I, Hilsenrath J, et al:** Clinical, hemodynamic and angiographic aspects of inferior and anterior myocardial infarctions in patients with angina pectoris. Amer J Cardiol 34:513, 1974

56. **Miller RR, Olson HG, Vismara LA, et al:** Determinants of pump dysfunction following myocardial infarction: importance of location, extent and pattern of abnormal left ventricular segmental contraction. Clin Res 22:293A, 1974

57. **Hughes JC, Salel AF, Massumi RA, et al:** The electrocardiogram as a predictor of ventricular function and cardiogenic shock in acute myocardial infarction. Circulation 44 suppl II:179, 1971

58. **Russell RO, Hunt D, Rackley CE:** Left ventricular hemodynamics in anterior and inferior myocardial infarction. Amer J Cardiol 26:658, 1970

59. **Ratshin RA, Rackley CE, Russell RO:** Hemodynamic evaluation of left ventricular function in cardiogenic shock complicating myocardial infarction. Circulation 45:127, 1972

60. **Loeb HS, Rakintoola SH, Rosen KM, et al:** Assessment of ventricular function after acute myocardial infarction by plasma volume expansion. Circulation 47:720, 1973

61. **Cox JL, McLaughlin VW, Flowers NC, et al:** The ischemic zone surrounding acute myocardial infarction. Its morphology as detected by dehydrogenase staining. Amer Heart J 76:650, 1968

62. **Amsterdam EA, Massumi RA, Zelis R, et al:** Evaluation and management of cardiogenic shock. II. Drug therapy. Heart and Lung 1:663, 1972

63. **Gunnar RM, Loeb HS:** Use of drugs in cardiogenic shock due to acute myocardial infarction. Circulation 45:211, 1972

64. **Kuhn LA:** The treatment of cardiogenic shock. II. The use of pressor agents in the treatment of cardiogenic shock. Amer Heart J 74:725, 1967

65. **Kuhn LA:** Changing treatment of shock following acute myocardial infarction—a critical evaluation. Amer J Cardiol 20:757, 1967

66. **Binder MJ:** Effect of vasopressor drugs on circulatory dynamics in shock following myocardial infarction. Amer J Cardiol 16:834, 1965

67. **Shubin H, Weil MH:** The treatment of shock complicating acute myocardial infarction. Progr Cardiovasc Dis 10:30, 1967

68. **Smith HJ, Oriol A, Morch J, et al:** Hemodynamic studies in cardiogenic shock: treatment with isoproterenol and metaraminol. Circulation 35:1084, 1967

69. **Puri PS, Bing RJ:** Effect of drugs on myocardial contractility in the intact dog and in experimental myocardial infarction. Amer J Cardiol 21:866, 1968

70. **Serur JR, Urschel CW:** Attenuation of inotropic interventions by myocardial ischemia. Cardiovasc Res 7:458, 1973

71. **Amsterdam EA, Kamiyama T, Rendig S, et al:** Differential regional contractile actions of digitalis in experimental myocardial infarction. Clin Res 22:257A, 1974

72. **Tennant R, Wiggers CJ:** The effect of coronary occlusion on myocardial contraction. Amer J Physiol 112:351, 1935

73. **Tatooles CJ, Randal WC:** Local ventricular bulging after acute coronary occlusion. Amer J Physiol 201:451, 1961

74. **Maroko PR, Kjekshus JK, Sobel BE, et al:** Factors influencing infarct size following experimental coronary artery occlusions. Circulation 43:67, 1971

75. **Maroko PR, Braunwald E:** Modification of myocardial infarction size after coronary occlusion. Ann Intern Med 79:720, 1973

76. **Braunwald E, Maroko PR:** The reduction of infarct size—an idea whose time (for testing) has come. Circulation 50:206, 1974

77. **Sonnenblick EH, Skelton CL:** Oxygen consumption of the heart: physiological principles and clinical implications. Mod Conc Cardiovas Dis 40:9, 1971

78. **Maroko PR, Libby P, Sobel BE, et al:** The effect of glucose-insulin-potassium infusion on myocardial infarction following experimental coronary artery occlusion. Circulation 45:1160, 1972

79. **Maroko PR, Libby P, Covell JW, et al:** Precordial ST segment mapping: an atraumatic method for assessing alterations in the extent of myocardial ischemic injury. The effects of pharmacologic and hemodynamic interventions. Amer J Cardiol 29:223, 1972

80. **Pelides LJ, Reid DW, Thomas M, et al:** Inhibition by beta-blockade of the ST segment elevation after acute myocardial infarction in man. Cardiovasc Res 6:295, 1972

81. **Gold HK, Leinbach RC, Sanders CA:** Use of sublingual nitroglycerin in congestive failure following acute myocardial infarction. Circulation 46:839, 1972

82. **Miller RR, Vismara LA, Williams DO, et al:** Effects of ventricular unloading by nitroprusside on myocardial energetics and coronary blood flow in patients with ischemic heart disease. Circulation 52 suppl II:217, 1975

83. **Williams DO, Amsterdam EA, Mason DT:** Hemodynamic effects of nitroglycerin in acute myocardial infarction: decrease in ventricular preload at the expense of cardiac output. Circulation 51:421, 1975

84. **Cohn JN:** Blood pressure measurement in shock. Mechanisms of inaccuracy in auscultatory and palpatory methods. JAMA 199:972, 1967

85. **Swan HJC, Ganz W, Forrester J, et al:** Catheterization of the heart in man with use of a flow directed balloon-tipped catheter. New Eng J Med 283:447, 1970

86. **Cohn JN, Khatri IM, Hamosh P:** Bedside catheterization of the left ventricle. Amer J Cardiol 25:66, 1970

87. **Forrester JS, Diamond G, McHugh TJ, et al:** Filling pressures in the right and left sides of the heart in acute myocardial infarction: a reappraisal of central venous pressure monitoring. New Eng J Med 285:190, 1971

88. **Cohn JN:** Monitoring techniques in shock. Amer J Cardiol 26:565, 1970

89. **Thompson PL, Sloman G:** Acute myocardial infarction: predictors of arrhythmias and shock. Ann Clin Res 3:377, 1971

90. **Ramo BW, Myers N, Wallace AG, et al:** Hemodynamic findings in 123 patients with acute myocardial infarction on admission. Circulation 42:567, 1970

91. **Prakash R, Forrester J, Parmley WW, et al:** Prognostic implications of left ventricular stroke work index in acute myocardial infarction. Clin Res 20:391, 1972

92. **Parmley WW, Diamond G, Tomoda H, et al:** Clinical evaluation of left ventricular pressures in myocardial infarction. Circulation 45:358, 1972

93. **Weber KT, Ratshin RA, Janicki JS, et al:** Left ventricular dysfunction following acute myocardial infarction. Amer J Med 54:697, 1973

94. **Price J, Amsterdam EA, Miller RR, et al:** Prognosis in acute myocardial infarction assessed by left heart catheterization. Circulation 48 suppl IV:204, 1973

95. **Scheidt S, Fillmore S, Ascheim R, et al:** Objective assessment of prognosis after acute myocardial infarction. Circulation 41 suppl III:196, 1970

96. **DaLuz P, Afifi AA, Liu V, et al:** Objective index of hemodynamic status for quantitation of severity and prognosis of shock complicating myocardial infarction. Amer J Cardiol 29:259, 1972

97. **Amsterdam EA, DeMaria AN, Wood M, et al:** Accurate assessment of prognosis in acute myocardial infarction by hemodynamic evaluation. Clin Res 23:170A, 1975

98. **Mundth ED, Buckley MJ, Daggett WM, et al:** Surgery for complications of acute myocardial infarction. Cir-

culation 45:1279, 1972

99. **Sobel BE, Bresnahan GF, Shell WE, et al:** Estimation of infarct size in man and its relation to prognosis. Circulation 46:640, 1972

100. **Zaret BL, Pitt B, Ross RS:** Determination of the site, extent and significance of regional ventricular dysfunction during acute myocardial infarction. Circulation 45:441, 1972

101. **Allen HN, Danzig R, Swan HJC:** Incidence and significance of relative hypovolemia as a cause of shock associated with acute myocardial infarction. Circulation 35 suppl II:50, 1967

102. **Russell RO Jr, Rackley CE, Pombo J, et al:** Effects of increasing left ventricular filling pressure in patients with acute myocardial infarction. J Clin Invest 49:1539, 1970

103. **Amsterdam EA, Massumi RA, Zelis R, et al:** Evaluation and management of cardiogenic shock. I. Approach to the patient. Heart and Lung 1:402, 1972

104. **Crexells C, Chatterjee K, Forrester JS, et al:** Optimal filling pressure in the left side of the heart in acute myocardial infarction. N Eng J Med 289:1263, 1973

105. **Diamond G, Forrester J, Danzig R, et al:** Acute myocardial infarction in man. Comparative hemodynamic effects of norepinephrine and glucagon. Brit Heart J 33:290, 1971

106. **Yurchak PM, Rolett EC, Cohen LS, et al:** Effects of norepinephrine on the coronary circulation in man. Circulation 30:180, 1964

107. **Nies AS, Melmon KL:** The rational management of cardiogenic shock. Cardiovasc Clin 1:65, 1969

108. **Goldberg LI, Talley RC:** Current therapy of shock. Advances Intern Med 17:363, 1971

109. **Goldberg LI:** Dopamine—clinical uses of an endogenous catecholamine. New Eng J Med 291:707, 1974

110. **Amsterdam EA, Bonanno J, Mansour E, et al:** Effects of dopamine on hemodynamics and myocardial metabolism in patients with coronary artery disease. Clin Res 20:202, 1972

111. **Loeb HS, Winslow EBJ, Rahimtoola SH, et al:** Acute hemodynamic effects of dopamine in patients with shock. Circulation 44:163, 1971

112. **Krasnow N, Rolett EL, Yurchak PM, et al:** Isoproterenol and cardiovascular performance. Amer J Med 37:514, 1964

113. **Smith HJ, Oriol A, March J, et al:** Hemodynamic studies in cardiogenic shock: treatment with isoproterenol and metaraminol. Circulation 35:1084, 1967

114. **Mason DT:** Digitalis pharmacology and therapeutics: recent advances. Ann Intern Med 80:520, 1974

115. **Marano AJ Jr, Kline HJ, Cestero J, et al:** Hemodynamic effects of oubain in experimental acute myocardial infarction with shock. Amer J Cardiol 17:327, 1966

116. **Malmcrona R, Schroder G, Werko L:** Haemodynamic effects of digitalis in acute myocardial infarction. Acta Med Scand 180:55, 1966

117. **Balcon R, Hoy J, Sowton E:** Haemodynamic effects of rapid digitalization following acute myocardial infarction. Brit Heart J 30:373, 1968

118. **Hodges M, Friesinger GC, Riggins RCK, et al:** Effects of intravenously administered digoxin on mild left ventricular failure in acute myocardial infarction in man. Amer J Cardiol 29:749, 1972

119. **Rahimtoola SH, Sinno MZ, Chuquimia R, et al:** Effects of ouabain on impaired left ventricular function in acute myocardial infarction. New Eng J Med 287:527, 1972

120. **Amsterdam EA, Huffaker HK, DeMaria A, et al:** Hemodynamic effects of digitalis in acute myocardial infarction and comparison with furosemide. Circulation 46 suppl II:113, 1972

121. **Rahimtoola SH, Loeb HS, Gunnar RM:** Digitalis in myocardial infarction. In Ref 50, p 157

122. **Cohn JN, Tristani FE, Khatri IM:** Cardiac and peripheral vascular effects of digitalis in clinical cardiogenic shock. Amer Heart J 78:318, 1969

123. **Amsterdam EA, Mansour EJ, Hughes JL, et al:** Present status of glucagon and bretylium tosylate. In, Changing Concepts in Cardiovascular Disease (Russek H, Zohman B, ed). Baltimore, Williams & Wilkins, 1972, p 215

124. **Chatterjee K, Swan HJC:** Vasodilator therapy in acute myocardial infarction. Mod Conc Cardiovasc Dis 43:119, 1974

125. **Amsterdam EA, Massumi RA, Zelis R, et al:** Evaluation and management of cardiogenic shock. III. The roles of cardiac surgery and mechanical assist. Heart and Lung 2:122, 1973

126. **Mueller H, Giannelli S Jr, Ayres SM:** Mechanical cardiac assistance in shock following acute myocardial infarction. In, Ref 50, p 229

127. **Dennis C, Carlens E, Senning A, et al:** Clinical use of a cannula for left-heart bypass without thoracotomy: experimental protection against fibrillation by left-heart bypass. Ann Surg 156:623, 1962

128. **Lesch M:** Assisted circulation in the treatment of shock complicating acute myocardial infarction. Cardiovasc Clin 3:22, 1971

129. **Scheidt S, Wilner G, Mueller H, et al:** Intra-aortic balloon counterpulsation in cardiogenic shock. New Eng J Med 288:979, 1973

130. **Willerson JT, Curry GC, Watson JT, et al:** Intraaortic balloon counterpulsation in patients in cardiogenic shock, medically refractory left ventricular failure and/or recurrent ventricular tachycardia. Amer J Med 58:183, 1975

131. **Leinbach RC, Mundth ED, Dinsmore RE, et al:** Selective coronary and left ventricular cine angiography during intraaortic balloon assist for cardiogenic shock. Amer J Cardiol 26:644, 1970

132. **Leinbach RC, Gold HK, Dinsmore RE, et al:** The role of angiography in cardiogenic shock. Circulation 47 suppl III:95, 1973

133. **Messer JV, Willerson JT, Loeb HS, et al:** Evaluation of external pressure circulatory assist in acute myocardia infarction. Clin Res 23:197A, 1975

134. **Amsterdam EA, Miller RR, Mason DT:** Surgery for acute myocardial infarction. In, Ref 50, p 257

135. **Herman MV, Heinle RA, Klein MD, et al:** Localized disorders in myocardial contraction. Asynergy and its role in congestive heart failure. New Eng J Med 277:222, 1967

136. **Maroko PR, Libby P, Ginks WR, et al:** Coronary artery

reperfusion. I. Early effects on local myocardial function and the extent of myocardial necrosis. J Clin Invest 51:2710, 1972

137. **Spencer RC, Green GE, Tice DA, et al:** Bypass grafting for occlusive disease of the coronary arteries: report of experience with 195 patients. Ann Surg 173:1029, 1971

138. **Chatterjee K, Swan HJC, Parmley WW, et al:** Depression of left ventricular function due to acute myocardial ischemia and its reversal after aortocoronary saphenous-vein bypass. New Eng J Med 286:1117, 1972

139. **Amsterdam EA, DeMaria AN, Markson W, et al:** Effect of myocardial revascularization on left ventricular contractile function and factors influencing results of surgery. Clin Res 22:256A, 1974

140. **Wilson WS:** Aortocoronary bypass surgery. II. An updated review. Heart and Lung 3:435, 1974

141. **Sanders CA, Mortimer JB, Leinbach RC, et al:** Mechanical circulatory assistance. Current status and experience with combining circulatory assistance, emergency coronary angiography and acute myocardial revascularization. Circulation 45:1292, 1972

142. **Keon WJ, Bedard P, Shankar KR, et al:** Experience with emergency aortocoronary bypass grafts in the presence of acute myocardial infarction. Circulation 47 suppl III:151, 1973

143. **Abbas SZ, Shankar KR, Cohen G, et al:** Medical versus surgical management of cardiogenic shock. Amer J Cardiol 29:250, 1972

144. **Heimbecker RO:** Surgery for massive myocardial infarction. Prog Cardiovasc Dis 11:338, 1969

145. **Glass BA, Carter RL, Albert HM, et al:** Excision of myocardial infarcts. Arch Surg 97:940, 1968

146. **Kaiser GA, Waldo AL, Bowman FO, et al:** The use of ventricular electrograms in the surgery for coronary artery disease and its complications. Ann Thorac Surg 10:153, 1970

147. **Stein M, Cordell AR:** Arrhythmias and left ventricular efficiency following infarction and infarctectomy. Arch Surg 99:802, 1969

148. **Klein MD, Herman MV, Gorlin R:** A hemodynamic study of left ventricular aneurysm. Circulation 35:614, 1967

149. **Buckley MJ, Mundth ED, Daggett WM, et al:** Surgical therapy for early complications of myocardial infarction. Surgery 70:814, 1971

150. **Sanders RJ, Neuberger KT, Ravin A:** Rupture of papillary muscles: occurrence of rupture of posterior muscle in posterior myocardial infarction. Dis Chest 31:316, 1957

151. **Miller GAH, Kirklin JW, Swan JHC:** Myocardial function and left ventricular volumes in acquired valvular insufficiency. Circulation 31:374, 1965

152. **Heikkila J:** Mitral incompetence complicating acute myocardial infarction. Brit Heart J 29:162, 1967

153. **Burch GE, DePasquale NP, Phillips JH:** The syndrome of papillary muscle dysfunction. Amer Heart J 75:399,1968

154. **Burch GE, DePasquale NP, Phillips JH:** Clinical manifestations of papillary muscle dysfunction. Arch Intern Med 112:112, 1963

155. **Forrester JS, Diamond G, Freedman S, et al:** Silent mitral insufficiency in acute myocardial infarction. Circulation 44:877, 1971

156. **Sanders RJ, Kern WH, Blount SG Jr:** Perforation of the interventricular septum complicating myocardial infarction. Amer Heart J 51:736, 1956

157. **Swithinbank JM:** Perforation of the interventricular septum in myocardial infarction. Brit Heart J 21:562, 1959

158. **Selzer A, Gerbode F, Kerth WJ:** Clinical hemodynamic and surgical consideration of rupture of the ventricular septum after myocardial infarction. Amer Heart J 78:598, 1969

159. **Kitamura S, Mendez H, Kay JH:** Ventricular septal defect following myocardial infarction. J Thorac Cardiovasc Surg 61:186, 1971

160. **Iben A, Miller R, Amsterdam E, et al:** Successful immediate repair of acquired ventricular septal defect and survival in patients with acute myocardial shock using a new double patch technique. Chest 66:665, 1974

161. **Mason DT, Amsterdam EA, Miller RR, et al:** Cardiogenic shock in acute myocardial infarction. In, The Acute Cardiac Emergency (Eliot R, ed). Mt. Kisco, New York, Futura Publishing, 1972, p 135

162. **Mason DT, Amsterdam EA, Miller RR, et al:** Recent advances in pathophysiology and therapy of myocardial infarction shock. In Ref 27, p 143

163. **Mason DT, Amsterdam EA, Miller RR, et al:** Consideration of the therapeutic roles of pharmacologic agents, collateral circulation and saphenous vein bypass in coronary artery disease. Amer J Cardiol 28:608, 1971

Chapter 23

Antiarrhythmic Agents
Clinical Pharmacology and Therapeutics

Dean T. Mason, MD, FACC
Anthony N. DeMaria, MD, FACC
Ezra A. Amsterdam, MD, FACC
Louis A. Vismara, MD, FACC
Richard R. Miller, MD, FACC
Zakauddin Vera, MD
Rashid A. Massumi, MD, FACC

The ability to identify and successfully treat arrhythmias represents one of the major advances in the management of clinical heart disease in recent years. This remarkable progress has stimulated great interest in the basic understanding and application of antiarrhythmic agents in patients. The mechanisms of action and therapeutic applications of the antiarrhythmic drugs are best understood in light of their electropharmacology—that is, their effects upon the electrophysiologic properties of cardiac muscle. In this chapter, attention is initially focused upon the fundamental electrical characteristics of myocardial tissue responsible for the genesis and conduction of the normal cardiac impulse, the subcellular events that underlie these characteristics and the pathophysiologic alterations responsible for arrhythmias. Proceeding within this basic framework, the electropharmacologic properties of each of the antiarrhythmic agents and the clinical benefits derived from their actions are considered. Finally, this review provides a concise discussion of the clinical approach to the management of the specific disorders of cardiac rhythm using the available therapeutic antiarrhythmic armamentarium, delineating the relative roles of the individual drugs and the modalities of electrical pacing and direct current cardioversion.

Basic Cardiac Electrophysiology

When the normal pacemaker impulse is released from the sinoatrial node, excitation of the cardiac chambers takes place in an orderly sequence by spread of the stimulating current throughout specialized automatic fibers in the atria, atrioventricular node and ventricular Purkinje network. When the pacemaker impulses reach the individual myocardial cell, electrical excitation of the entire fiber occurs rapidly via its superficial membrane system. The superficial membrane consists of the external sarcolemma covering the cell surface and its extensive transverse tubular invaginations, termed the sarcotubular or T system (Figure 1). The sarcotubules consist of deep extensions of the sarcolemma into the cardiac cell. In addition, the intercalated disks between cardiac cells are derivatives of the superficial membrane system. The inter-

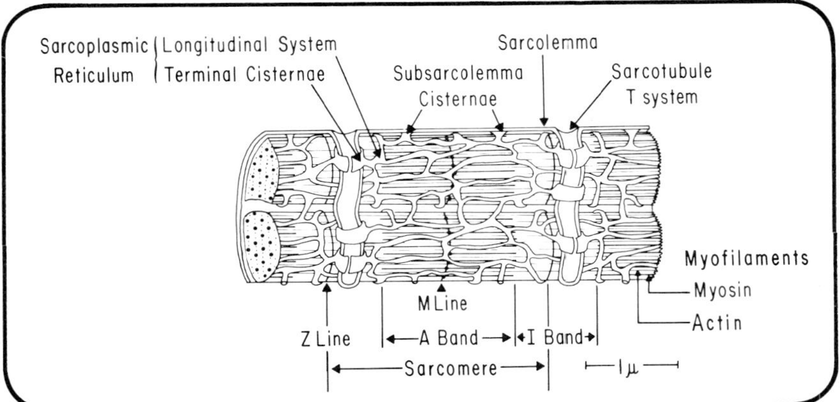

FIGURE 1. Diagram of the ultrastructure of a myocardial cell showing the relationships between the superficial (sarcolemma and sarcotubules) and intracellular (sarcoplasmic reticulum) membrane systems. The fundamental mechanical unit within the cell is the sarcomere comprising the contractile proteins action and myosin. (Reproduced by permission from Mason et al. In, Pathologic Physiology, fifth edition; Sodeman WA Jr, Sodeman WA, ed. Philadelphia, Saunders, 1974, p 206)

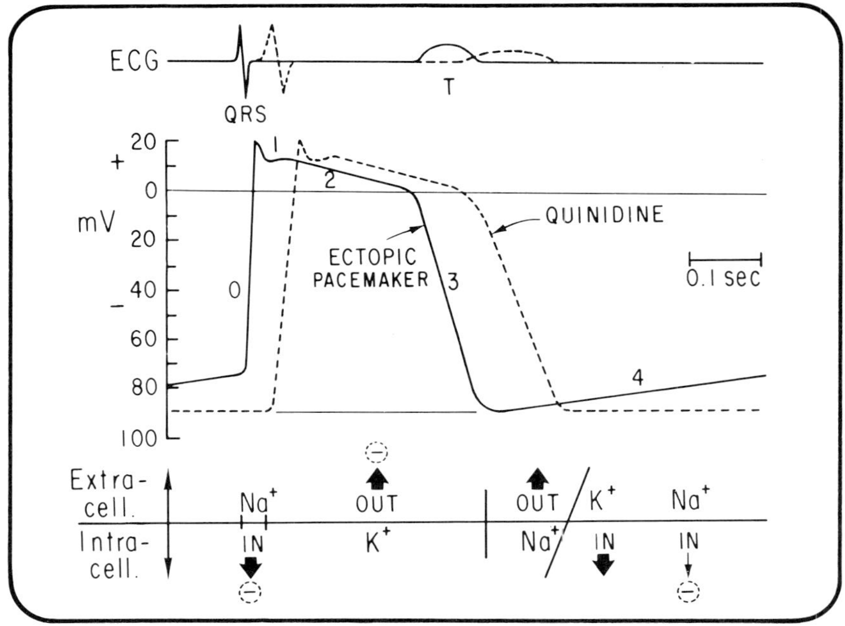

FIGURE 2. Diagram of the transmembrane electrical potential **(middle),** electrocardiogram **(top)** and transmembrane cation movements **(bottom)** of a spontaneously depolarizing automatic cardiac cell **(solid line)** and after quinidine **(broken line). Top,** QRS wave occurs at time of depolarization and T wave during the final phase of repolarization. **Middle,** 0 = depolarization; 1, 2 and 3 = phases of repolarization; 4 = resting period exhibiting diastolic depolarization prior to quinidine; mV = millivolts. **Bottom,** the **horizontal line** represents the cell membrane and the **arrows** indicate the transmembrane flux of sodium (Na⁺) and potassium (K⁺) ions during depolarization, repolarization and resting period. At onset of resting period, active exit (↑) of Na⁺ extracellularly (extracell) is accompanied by active entrance (↓) of K⁺ intracellularly (intracell). During remainder of resting period, diastolic depolarization takes place with passive Na∓ movement into the cell. The size of **arrows** is directly related to large or small movement of cations. The effects of quinidine on these cation movements are shown by the sign within the **broken circles.** (Reproduced by permission from Mason et al.[21])

calated disks and sarcotubular membranes provide pathways for swift transmission of the depolarizing impulses that electrically excite adjacent fibers and the internal membrane system, the intracellular sarcoplasmic reticulum, with subsequent activation of the sarcomere contractile machinery.

Understanding of the electrophysiologic properties of myocardial tissue has been markedly enhanced by the ability to record electrical potentials from within the cardiac cell by means of a microelectrode directly impaled into the myocardium. Such an intracellular action potential is demonstrated in Figure 2. As can be seen, during the diastolic phase of the cardiac cycle (designated phase 4) a voltage difference across the cell membrane (termed the resting potential) is maintained with negative intracellular potential of approximately 90 millivolts (mv). It is currently accepted that this transmembrane voltage difference represents the differential concentrations of potassium (K^+) and sodium (Na^+) ions in the intracellular and extracellular fluid. It appears that an active transport pump mechanism supported by adenosine triphosphatase (ATPase) is responsible for maintaining K^+ concentration within the cell at approximately 30 times the concentration in extracellular fluid and concurrently maintaining extracellular Na^+ at a concentration much greater than that intracellularly. This results in the voltage differential observed.

Automaticity: As illustrated in Figure 2, in many cardiac cells of the specialized conducting system (sinus node, atrial conduction pathways, lower region of the atrioventricular node and the His-Purkinje system), diastolic transmembrane voltage difference is not static but pursues a gradual decrease in membrane potential toward 0 mv, presumably due to alteration in function of the active pump mechanism. The ionic events responsible for diastolic depolarization consist of decreased outward current of K^+ in the presence of continued slow inward leakage of Na^+, resulting in accumulation of Na^+ intracellularly.[2] This diastolic depolarization continues until a point is reached (termed threshold potential) when a self-propagated wave of complete depolarization occurs, represented by phase 0, or the spike action potential. The capacity for phase 4 depolarization is termed automaticity and is a property of automatic or pacemaker cells. At any given moment, the cell or group of fibers comprising the cardiac pacemaker is that having the greatest slope of phase 4 depolarization and is normally located in the sinoatrial node.[3]

Conduction Velocity: The mechanism responsible for the self-sustained wave of complete depolarization that occurs at threshold is related to marked increased in Na^+ conductance across the cell membrane. The influx of Na^+ is a passive process not requiring energy utilization and may be related to activation of either available Na^+ carriers or electrostatically controlled fast-membrane channels (pores). At threshold potential, membrane permeability to Na^+ ions increases approximately 100 times and large amounts enter the cell, resulting in an intense inward current that thereby inscribes the spike action potential (Figure 2). It is the rate of rise of the spike action potential that determines conduction velocity. In the sinoatrial and atrioventricular nodes, the fast-channel for Na^+ is thought to be absent; instead, slow inward currents of Na^+ and Ca^{++} appear to predominate in these tissues.[4-6] The phase 0 spikes of the sinoatrial node, atria and atrioventricular node are collectively represented on the surface electrocardiogram as the P wave duration and PR interval, whereas phase 0 in the ventricles is appreciated as the QRS duration.

Refractoriness: The massive influx of Na^+ during the spike action potential causes the intracellular voltage to approach Na^+ equilibrium potential of approximately $+20$ mv or more. During repolarization, negative intracellular potential equal to the resting transmembrane voltage difference is reestablished. Although repolarization is divided into three stages, phases 1, 2 and 3 (Figure 2), the major portion is accomplished during phase 3 and is the result of passive efflux of K^+ ions out of the cell. Influx of Cl^- accounts for phase 1 repolarization.[2] During phase 2, a small inward movement of Ca^{++} takes place through a slow-channel mechanism that is believed to be important in the process of excitation-contraction coupling.[7] The process of repolarization determines duration of the action potential and is represented electrocardiographically by the QT interval. The duration of the action potential is directly related to duration of the refractory period of cardiac muscle (Figure 3), which may be defined as the minimal

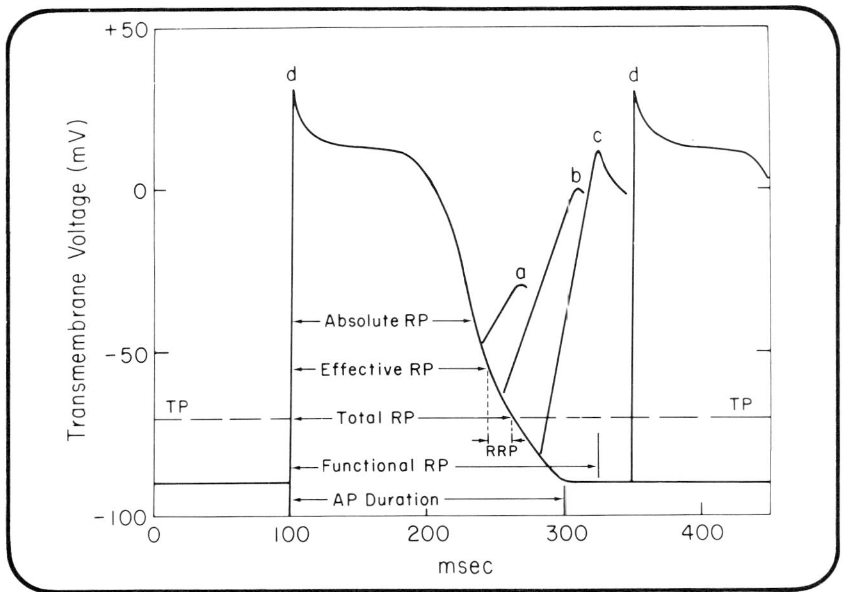

FIGURE 3. Diagram of the transmembrane electrical potential of a non-automatic cardiac cell demonstrating that the maximal rate of complete depolarization depends on the action potential at the moment of excitation. Electrical Vmax is least (a) at low level of membrane potential and becomes progressively greater as intracellular negativity is increased (b, c and d). Absolute refractory period (RP) = interval during which no stimulus evokes an action potential; effective RP = time when a strong stimulus results in a weak action potential that is unable to be propagated to adjacent muscle; relative refractory period (RRP) = time interval during which suprathreshold stimulation produces a propagated action potential; total (relative) RP = period that ends when the stimulus for causing a propagated action potential reaches threshold potential (TP); functional RP = full recovery time (FRT) which terminates when TP stimulation induces a propagated impulse without increased delay in electrical Vmax; AP duration = recorded action potential duration.[1] A supernormal period exists between the end of the relative RP and FRT termination during which a subthreshold stimulus may excite the fiber.[10] (Reproduced by permission from Mason et al. Drugs 5:261, 1973)

interval between the points at which two adequate stimuli will result in propagated responses.[8]

Responsiveness: An additional major electrophysiologic property of cardiac muscle of importance to the understanding of electropharmacology of antiarrhythmic drugs has been termed membrane responsiveness.[9] It has been demonstrated that conduction velocity—as determined by the maximal rate of rise, or maximal dv/dt, of the phase 0 spike action potential (electrical Vmax)—is dependent in part upon the level of negative intracellular potential at the moment at which the fiber is excited. This is illustrated in Figure 3, which shows that the maximal rate of rise of phase 0 increases as the fiber returns to progressively more negative intracellular potential at the moment of excitation. When this relation is plotted for the entire length of time from the end of the absolute re-

fractory period to completion of repolarization, an S-shaped curve is obtained, as shown in Figure 4. It is evident that responsiveness is also an important electrophysiologic property since it contributes to the ability of a fiber to respond to a stimulus, and when response occurs, responsiveness partially determines conduction velocity, stimulation potential for neighboring fibers and tendency to undergo blockage. When the resting potential is raised (greater negative charge intracellularly), the rate of complete spontaneous depolarization is increased, while excitability is reduced. Furthermore, since alterations in the time course of the spike action potential influence refractory period, a mechanism is defined in which automaticity, excitability, responsiveness, conduction velocity and refractoriness are interrelated, with each of these properties regulated to a certain extent by changes occurring in any one of them.[11]

Mechanisms of Tachyarrhythmias

Although the pathophysiologic mechanisms responsible for the genesis of cardiac arrhythmias are not completely defined, it is generally agreed that arrhythmias arise as the result of either disorders of impulse formation or disorders of impulse conduction, or a combination of both processes.[11–13]

Automaticity Disorders: Disorders of impulse formation are manifested by ectopic pacemaker activity discharging irregularly or rhythmically in specialized conductive tissue other than the sinoatrial node (Figure 2). It is assumed that production of such ectopic impulses involves a defect in the normal mechanism of automatic function—that is, abnormal acceleration of spontaneous phase 4 diastolic depolarization. In addition, other mechanisms appear to cause disordered automatic function, such as after-potentials or sustained depolarization from ischemic myocardium.[12] It is obvious that disorders of impulse formation are best treated with drugs that have the ability to suppress spontaneous phase 4 diastolic depolarization.

Reentry Disorders: Disorders of impulse conduction, commonly referred to as reentry disturbances, are probably the more common of the two mechanisms of arrhythmias. It is known that the most distant portions of the Purkinje network arborize into multiple branches at their junction within the ventricular myocardium, providing the anatomic and physiologic substrate for retrograde activation of adjacent pathways.[14] An impulse conduction abnormality requires the presence of a localized area of unidirectional functional block that establishes circular micro- or macrocellular impulse movements of the reentry or reciprocal excitation type. As demonstrated in Figure 5, an impulse that normally traverses branches *a* and *b* may undergo unidirectional block in pathway *b* with subsequent retrograde activation via pathway *c*, thereby allowing the wavelet to reenter the regional conduction system consisting of limbs *a*, *c* and *b*. Unidirectional block can result from a region of partial depolarization caused by localized disease. In addition, the mechanism of unidirectional block may involve inactivation of Na^+ fast-membrane channels by the antegrade impulse, thereby leading to an area of slow con-

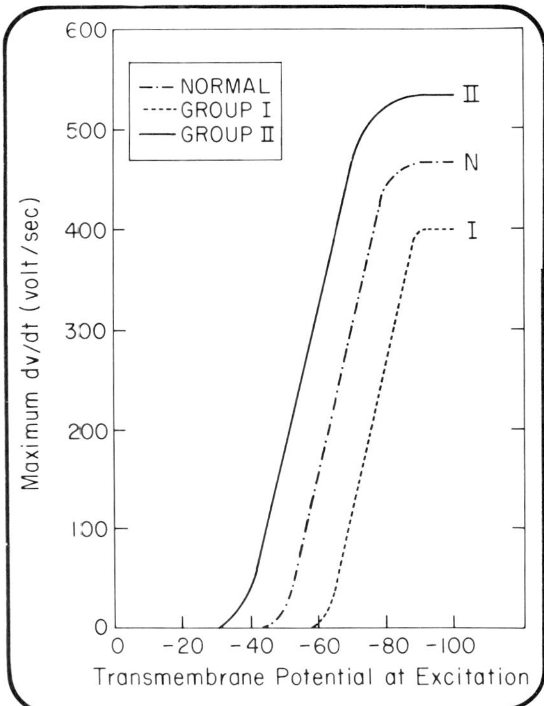

FIGURE 4. Diagram showing membrane responsiveness of the relation between maximal dv/dt and transmembrane potential at excitation. This relationship is shifted to the right by Group I antiarrhythmic drugs and to the left by Group II agents. (Reproduced by permission from Mason et al. Drugs 5:261, 1973)

duction in which the fibers become dependent upon Na^+ and Ca^{++} inward-current slow-channels for sufficient depolarization to propagate the retrograde impulse.[4,6] Conduction velocity and duration of refractory period are the electrophysiologic properties most critical in arrhythmias of the reentrant type, and pharmacologic intervention is based upon alteration of these two properties.[15]

In routine clinical practice it is usually not possible to determine whether an arrhythmia represents a disorder of impulse formation or impulse conduction. Intracardiac electrography may sometimes be useful in estimating the mechanism responsible, and a fixed coupling interval between a normal beat immediately preceding the ectopic beat is highly suggestive of the reentrant type of mechanism. However,

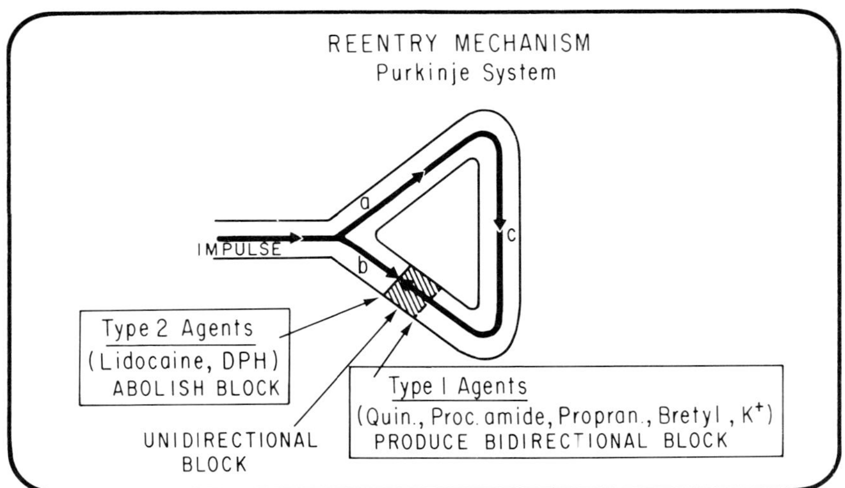

FIGURE 5. Diagram of reentry mechanism in Purkinje tissue showing the circus pattern of reciprocol excitation responsible for tachyarrhythmias due to abnormal impulse conduction. The impulse entering the Purkinje system normally branches and transverses pathways a and b. However, in reentrant disorders, the area of localized unidirectional block does not allow passage of the antegrade impulse in path b, thereby leading to establishment of the reentrant circus of impulse movement from pathway a to c and retrograde through path b. The zone of unidirectional block in pathway b allows retrograde conduction but not forward conduction. The continuity of the circus wavelet is terminated by Group (type) I agents producing complete localized block, and by Group (type) II drugs abolishing the antegrade block. bretyl. = bretylium tosylate; quin. = quinidine; proc. amide = procainamide; propran. = propranolol. (Reproduced by permission from Mason et al.[102])

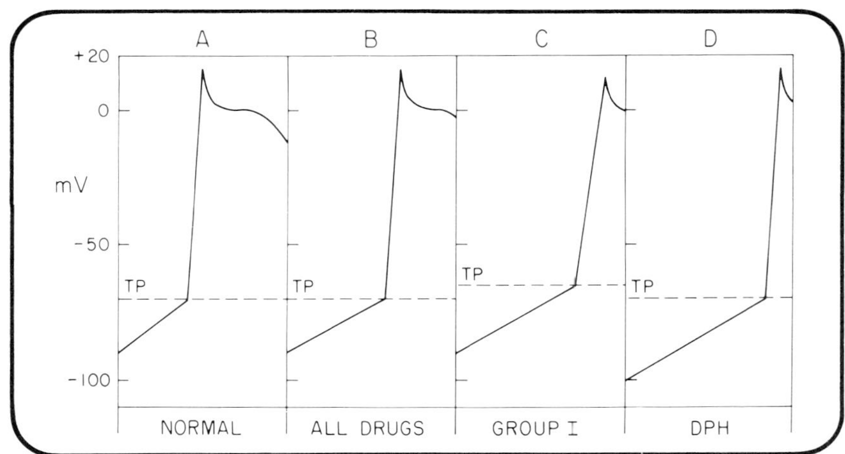

FIGURE 6. Diagram of a pacemaker cardiac cell **(A)** showing mechanisms of action of antiarrhythmic drugs in reducing automaticity and thereby slowing rate of fiber excitation. **B,** all antirrhytmic drugs decrease rate of diastolic depolarization; **C,** diastolic cycle length is also extended by Group I agents by raising excitation threshold (lowering threshold potential at which complete depolarization occurs); **D,** diphenylhydantoin prolongs the resting period in part by increasing maximal diastolic intracellular negativity. TP = threshold potential **(broken line).** (Reproduced by permission from Mason et al. Drugs 5:261, 1973)

identical arrhythmias on the scalar electrocardiogram may result from disparate mechanisms in different patients—or even in the same patient at different times. Therefore, at present, with few exceptions, an antiarrhythmic drug cannot be selected simply on the basis of its effects on electrophysiologic properties relative to a known clinical tachyarrhythmic mechanism. Rather, a planned, systematic, empirical approach must be employed, in which trial is undertaken of an antiarrhythmic drug known usually to be successful in abolishing a specific tachyarrhythmia in a certain condition, although other drugs or combinations of agents might prove to be necessary. Further, it is usually not possible by routine clinical means to know which electrophysiologic property of the antiarrhythmic agents is producing the salutary action in the termination of clinical disorders of cardiac rhythm.

Mechanisms of Antiarrhythmic Action

It is evident from the foregoing discussion that in the presence of disorders of heart rhythm, certain electrophysiologic properties of cardiac tissue may be altered with potential antiarrhythmic benefit. It is the purpose of this section to elucidate these electrical characteristics, to discuss the modes in which they may be changed and to consider the therapeutic agents known to possess such abilities. It is highly reasonable to believe that antiarrhythmic agents derive their salutary actions from the electrophysiologic effects they exert in normal cardiac tissue, although the precise mechanisms by which they terminate tachyarrhythmias are not definitely established in the majority of rhythm disorders in diseased myocardium.

Automaticity: Derangements in the normal mechanism of automaticity—that is, spontaneous phase 4 diastolic depolarization—are believed to underlie disorders of impulse formation. Therefore, the ability to prolong the interval required for phase 4 depolarization to reach threshold potential and result in a propagated action potential is clearly of therapeutic benefit in these situations—provided, of course, that this effect is selectively more intense upon the ectopic focus. This may be accomplished in several ways (Figure 6A). The most obvious

method of delaying threshold, and therefore decreasing the frequency of pacemaker discharge, is to diminish the rate at which spontaneous diastolic depolarization occurs (Figure 6B). The cycle length can also be prolonged by increasing the absolute voltage differential required to reach threshold potential. A shift in threshold potential toward 0 mv, as shown in Figure 6C, and an increase in the maximal diastolic potential reached, as illustrated in Figure 6D, widen the cycle length. Suppression of rate of phase 4 depolarization is a property of all antiarrhythmic agents. In addition, diphenylhydantoin has been demonstrated to increase maximal diastolic potential, and quinidine, procainamide and propranolol shift threshold potential toward 0 mv.[8]

Conduction Velocity: Conduction velocity is a critical factor in tachyarrhythmias of the reentrant variety.[12] As stated previously, unidirectional functional block is a requisite condition for these circular arrhythmias. This unidirectional block and its resultant ectopic rhythm may be abolished either by increasing conduction velocity in affected tissue—and, thus, overcome the block—or by decreasing conduction velocity—and, in so doing, convert unidirectional to bidirectional block (Figure 5). In addition, the timing of the reciprocal impulse is critical for reentry; it must arrive late enough to avoid refractoriness in the blocked pathway, but early enough to precede the next antegrade impulse. In atrial, ventricular and His-Purkinje tissue, lidocaine and diphenylhydantoin do not alter or may have the ability to increase conduction velocity,[16-19] whereas quinidine, procainamide, propranolol and bretylium decrease conduction velocity.[13,20,21] There may be slight vagolytic acceleration of atrioventricular nodal conduction accompanying low doses of quinidine. Of importance is the fact that the increase in atrioventricular conduction exhibited by diphenylhydantoin and lidocaine is accentuated in the presence of depressed conduction in this structure.[8] Recent study of the effects on cardiac membrane of the antiarrhythmic agent verapamil has suggested an additional mechanism for the termination of reentrant tachycardias.[22] Since this drug possesses the special property of depressing slow-channel Ca^{++} transport into cardiac cells, it appears that its antiarrhythmic efficacy is due to suppression of reentrant disorders that result from the dependency of the area of unidirectional block upon this slow-channel mechanism for the development of action potentials. In this manner, verapamil converts unidirectional to bidirectional block, thereby abating reexcitation loops caused by imbalance between fast- and slow-membrane depolarization responses.

Refractory Period: The duration of the refractory period plays a role analogous to that of conduction velocity in regard to reentrant arrhythmias. Thus, decreasing refractoriness may eliminate unidirectional block, whereas increasing refractoriness may produce bidirectional block (Figure 5). In addition, in disorders of automaticity, an increase in the refractory period with subsequent prolongation of the duration of the action potential may increase cycle length —and, thus, decrease the discharge rate of an ectopic focus. A distinction is made concerning changes in refractory period. Certain agents, such as quinidine and procainamide, increase the refractory period by prolonging repolarization. In addition, these agents—by virtue of their effects on membrane responsiveness—prolong the functional refractory period out of proportion to the duration of the action potential. In contrast, lidocaine and diphenylhydantoin decrease the durations of repolarization, action potential and refractory period. However, these agents do not decrease the functional refractory period to the same extent as they decrease the duration of the action potential. Therefore, lidocaine and diphenylhydantoin share with quinidine and procainamide the property of increasing functional refractoriness relative to the duration of action potential.[13]

Membrane Responsiveness: Inasmuch as the conduction velocity of an impulse for any level of membrane potential at the time of stimulation is a property of membrane responsiveness, it is obvious that alterations in membrane responsiveness have effects upon reentrant arrhythmias identical to alterations in conduction velocity. Thus, as shown in Figure 4, the S-shaped curve describing membrane responsiveness can be altered to either the left or right. If the curve is altered to the right, conduction velocity, as represented by maximal rate of rise of spike action potential, will be decreased at any level of membrane potential, and conversion of unidirectional block to bidirectional block will be enhanced. Quinidine, procainamide and propranolol produce such a shift.[8] In contrast, if the membrane responsiveness curve is shifted to the left, conduction velocity is enhanced, and unidirectional block may be eliminated. Diphenylhydantoin and lidocaine have been observed to exert this effect.[16,18] In addition to influencing conduction velocity, membrane responsiveness also affects amplitude and duration of action potential at extremes of membrane potentials. Therefore, responsiveness may alter functional refractory period, as previously discussed.

Excitability: Excitability is a term that has led to much confusion and generally has been used to describe the least amplitude of an electrical stimulus necessary to produce excitation of the cell at a given point in the cardiac cycle. It has been possible to demonstrate small alterations in excitability in response to several antiarrhythmic agents. However, since a propagating action potential, which is the normal stimulus to excitation, has many times the amplitude necessary, it has been thought that important antiarrhythmic actions are not mediated via alterations in this property.

Classes of Antiarrhythmic Agents

From the foregoing considerations, antiarrhythmic agents can be generally divided into two major classes as a result of their effects upon electrophysiologic properties of myocardial cells. It is of interest that differences between classes are not necessarily related to chemical structure and, indeed, some agents share greater similarity of chemical structure with drugs of the opposite class than with those of their own.

Group I Drugs: Drugs in the first group—quinidine, procainamide, propranolol, bretylium and potassium—are characterized by depression of normal electrophysiologic properties. These agents decrease conduction velocity, prolong the duration of the action potential and refractory period and diminish diastolic depolarization and membrane responsiveness (Figure 5). Quinidine[23] and procainamide[24] are the prototype agents of Group I, and propranolol, although differing in several aspects, is usually considered a Group I agent.[25-27] Potassium also shares these properties.[28,29]

Group II Drugs: In contrast, drugs in the second group —lidocaine and diphenlhydantoin— are characterized by facilitation of normal electrophysiologic activity relative to conduction and refractoriness. Thus, Group II agents result in no change or even acceleration of conduction velocity, reduction of action potential duration and refractoriness, decrease in diastolic depolarization and no change or an increase in membrane responsiveness (Figure 5). Diphenylhydantoin[16,30-33] and lidocaine[18,24] are the prototypes of this group.

It is emphasized that both groups share two important characteristics; they (1) decrease the rate of spontaneous phase 4 diastolic depolarization and (2) increase the functional refractory period in relation to action potential duration. Group I agents additionally decrease automaticity by shifting threshold potential toward 0 mv. In general, Group I agents are useful in both supraventricular and ventricular arrhythmias,[21,24] whereas Group II agents have their major utility in arrhythmias of ventricular origin and those originating from digitalis toxicity.[24,33-35] The beta adrenergic receptor-blocking agents such as propranolol and practolol[38] particularly suppress supraventricular arrhythmias and control ventricular rate in these disorders, although they are also efficacious in tachyarrhythmias due to digitalis intoxication. Bretylium tosylate[19,39-42] and potassium [28,29,43] share some properties of both groups of agents.

Certain theoretic considerations can be advanced for the expected efficacy of either group in specific clinical arrhythmias. However, quite different electrophysiologic mechanisms may be operative in diseased myocardium and it is possible that antiarrhythmic agents may have different actions on abnormal myocardium.[44,45] Therefore, antiarrhythmic therapy continues to be based somewhat on reasoned trial and error, although combinations of agents may now be selected more rationally than in the past.

Specific Antiarrhythmic Agents

Quinidine: Quinidine is considered to be the prototype of antiarrhythmic drugs and has held a position of prime importance in the management of arrhythmias since its first utilization by Wenkebach and Frey in 1918. Quinidine is the dextro-isomer of quinine and shares all its pharmacologic properties, although the electrical effects of quinidine upon myocardial cells are of greater magnitude than are those of quinine.[8] Although numerous attempts have been made to relate the antiarrhythmic activity of quinidine to its chemical structure, none has wholly succeeded and this area remains incompletely understood. Current evidence indicates that quinidine is principally concentrated in the cell membrane and exerts its fundamental antiarrhythmic effect at that location. Radioautographic studies have shown that the unchanged drug itself binds to the lipoprotein of the cell membrane (sarcolemma-sarcotubular system), which apparently hinders membrane cation transport.[23] In this manner, quinidine modifies the cation flux during both action and resting phases of the membrane potential, and this effect is translated into alterations of cardiac fiber electrophysiology (Figure 7).

In the case of the resting potential, quinidine diminishes Na^+ entry into the cell and thereby depresses phase 4 diastolic depolarization[46,47] (Figures 2 and 7). In addition, quinidine shifts the intracellular threshold potential toward 0 mv (Figure 6C). These two actions have the effect of diminishing spontaneous frequency of pacemaker tissues and thus depressing automaticity. In addition, this combined direct effect results in reduction of impulse formation in the sino-atrial node, and in denervated preparations relative bradycardia occurs. However, quinidine also possesses an indirect anticholinergic action that acts to increase sinoatrial rate. Thus, in the intact organism, this vagolytic effect usually counteracts the direct effect; therefore, no change or even a slight acceleration of the sinus rate occurs in the presence of therapeutic blood levels of quinidine.[23] However, in the presence of quinidine toxicity,[48] the direct depressive effect predominates, resulting in loss of impulse formation in the normal pacemaker and other automatic tissues, which is manifested initially by absent P waves and finally by ventricular standstill.

Quinidine, when bound to the cell membrane, decreases transmembrane permeability to passive influx of Na^+ ions during the spike

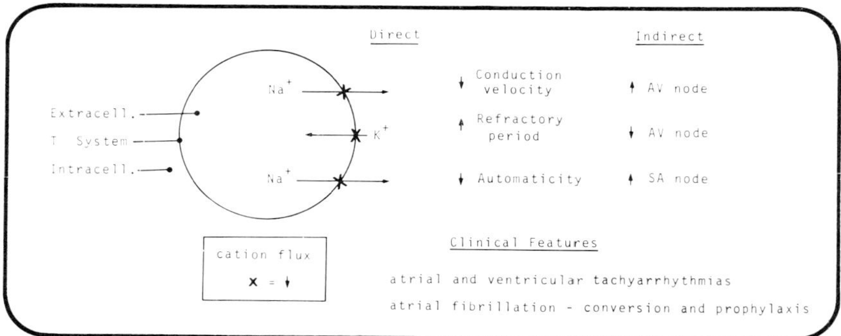

FIGURE 7. Diagram of the subcellular actions of quinidine and procainamide. The alterations of transmembrane cation fluxes underlying the direct electrophysiologic effects of these drugs are demonstrated. Also shown are the indirect anticholinergic effects of the drugs on electrophysiologic properties. The principal useful clinical features of the agents are listed. The **large circle** represents the transverse tubular cell membrane (T system) across which the movements of sodium and potassium are shown by the **arrows.** X = diminished transmembrane movement of cations. Within the circle is the extracellular space and outside the circle is the sarcoplasm. In reference to electrophysiologic properties, ● = increase and x = decrease. AV = atrioventricular node; SA = sinoatrial node. (Reproduced by permission from Mason et al.[40])

action potential (Figures 2, 5 and 7). This action results in a reduced rate of rise of the spike potential, thereby slowing the process of phase 0 depolarization, which diminishes conduction velocity. Also, quinidine-induced depression of conduction velocity contributes to prolongation of the duration of the action potential. Electrical Vmax is reduced by quinidine to a greater extent in ectopic pacemaker tissue than in the sinoatrial node and other normally automatic fibers.

The effects of quinidine upon the refractory period are complex—representing a composite of its direct and anticholinergic actions and also depending on the specific cardiac tissue involved. Quinidine reduces membrane permeability to passive K⁺ efflux during phase 3 repolarization, thereby prolonging the durations of the action potential and refractory period by this direct effect[49,50] (Figures 2, 5 and 7). In addition, by virtue of its ability to decrease membrane responsiveness, quinidine also prolongs the functional refractory period in relation to the action potential duration. Quinidine also exerts an anticholinergic action on the refractory period in the supraventricular structures innervated by the vagus. Since the effects of vagal stimulation shorten the refractory period of atrial muscle and increase that of the atrioventricular node without influence on ventricular cells, the

overall action of quinidine in the intact organism prolongs the refractory period markedly in the atria, increases refractory period in the ventricles to a lesser extent and decreases refractoriness in the atrioventricular node. The combination of slower atrial wavelets with fewer impulses exhibiting decremental conduction in the atrioventricular node, together with increased atrioventricular nodal conduction velocity, is believed to be the cause of sudden acceleration of ventricular rate sometimes seen in atrial flutter and fibrillation with qunidine. This potentially adverse effect has prompted the common practice of using digitalis before beginning quinidine therapy in atrial tachyarrhythmias.

Quinidine acts to reduce membrane responsiveness by decreasing conduction velocity and amplitude of the propagated action potential at any level of resting potential (Figure 4). This mechanism results in alterations referable both to conduction velocity and to prolongation of the functional refractory period in relation to the duration of the action potential. Indeed, since some studies have demonstrated that therapeutic concentrations of quinidine prolong the functional refractory period with little or no prolongation of action potential, it has been suggested that lengthening of the functional refractory period alone may adequately explain the therapeutic actions of quinidine in certain arrhythmias due to reentrant mechanisms.

These electrophysiologic effects of quinidine result in predictable alterations in the surface electrocardiogram. Reduction of conduction velocity is appreciated as prolongation of the QRS complex, whereas extension of the duration of the action potential results in proportionate increase in the QT interval. Alterations of sinus rate and PR interval are variable and a function of the interaction of indirect vagolytic and direct depressant effects of the drug.

Quinidine is almost completely absorbed from the gastrointestinal tract with peak plasma levels being reached 1 to 2 hours after a single oral dose.[8] Intramuscular administration of quinidine results in essentially the same interval before peak plasma concentration is achieved; however, peak levels have been found to be somewhat lower when this route is utilized. Although intravenous quinidine can rapidly achieve therapeutic plasma concentrations, there has been relatively little experience with this route of administration due to potential production of severe hypotension. Of the absorbed quinidine, 80 percent is bound to serum albumin.[8] Circulating quinidine is quickly taken up by body tissues, including the myocardium, so that a large tissue-to-plasma gradient is established within a few minutes. Quinidine is primarily metabolized by the liver with a half-life of 2 to 3 hours. Therapeutic plasma levels range between 3 and 7 μg/ml.

Quinidine toxicity may occur in several forms. Anaphylaxis has occured with quinidine administration, prompting some physicians to administer initially small test doses. Also, quinidine occasionally forms a complex with platelets capable of evoking an antibody response and subsequent thrombocytopenia. This thrombocytopenia is usually corrected by drug withdrawal. Gastrointestinal symptoms, especially diarrhea, are very common with quinidine administration, but if mild, they need not interfere with administration of the agent. Cinchonism—with tinnitus, headache and blurring of vision—may occur and appears to be dose-related. The most frequent serious toxic effects of quinidine are upon the electrical properties of the heart. Plasma concentrations of quinidine above 8 mg/L may result in conduction block in the si-

noatrial and atrioventricular nodes and in the Purkinje system.[51] Alternately, ventricular ectopic beats leading to ventricular tachycardia or ventricular fibrillation may occur. On the electrocardiogram, the QRS duration correlates best with plasma levels of quinidine, and the traditional approach is to decrease dosage if the QRS complex becomes prolonged by 50 percent or more of its pre-drug value.

Procainamide: Procainamide, differing from procaine by replacement of the ester linkage with an amide, has proved to be an efficacious antiarrhythmic agent. Although less extensive experience has been gained with procainamide than with quinidine, it appears that procainamide possesses all of the electrophysiologic effects of quinidine[24,52] (Figures 6C and 7). Procainamide diminishes automaticity, decreases conduction velocity, increases the duration of the action potential—and, thereby, the refractory period—and increases refractory period in relation to duration of the action potential via a decrease in membrane responsiveness (Figure 4). Moreover, the mechanisms of action of procainamide in abolishing arrhythmias due to disorders of both impulse formation (Figure 2) and conduction (Figure 5) are identical to those of quinidine. Although many clinicians have favored the use of procainamide for ventricular tachyarrhythmias and quinidine for rapid atrial disorders, the effectiveness of the two drugs appears to be essentially the same in both situations—with allowance for differences in dose.

From these observations, both procainamide and quinidine are relatively potent, wide-spectrum, antiarrhythmic agents. Further, it is important to realize that the electrophysiologic effects of procainamide and quinidine are additive; therefore, the administration of procainamide after large doses of quinidine carries with it the same risk of electrical toxicity as would the administration of additional quinidine. However, in certain conditions of potential or procainamide-induced QRS prolongation, it may be useful to combine agents of the two different antiarrhythmic groups—for example, diphenylhydantoin with procainamide.[33]

Procainamide, like quinidine, is almost completely absorbed from the gastrointestinal tract. It may safely be administered intravenously if given slowly in 100 mg increments every 5 min-

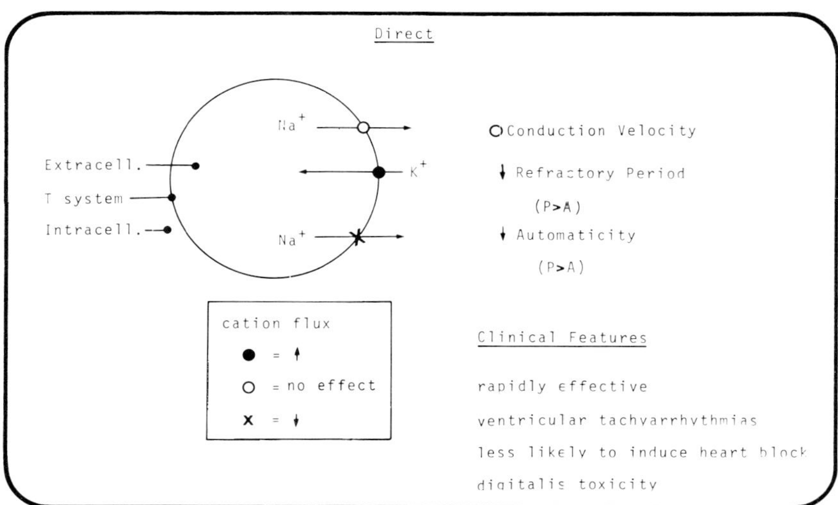

FIGURE 8. Diagram of the subcellular actions of lidocaine. Format and abbreviations as in Figure 7. (Reproduced by permission from Mason et al.[40])

utes until the desired effect is achieved, adverse electrical reaction is noted or a total dose of 1,000 mg is reached—whichever occurs first. Unlike quinidine, procainamide is only minimally bound to plasma proteins,[53] is largely excreted unchanged in the urine and also is hydrolysed by plasma esterases, although to a much lesser extent than is its base, procaine. Therapeutic plasma levels are 3 to 8 μg/ml.

Cardiac electrical toxicity to procainamide resembles, as would be expected, that to quinidine. Of special note is the syndrome resembling systemic lupus erythematosus (SLE) that has been reported to occur in almost one-third of patients on prolonged procainamide therapy of over 2 g daily.[54,55] Despite the arthralgias, fever and pleuritis, renal and cerebral involvement are not observed in procainamide-induced SLE. The syndrome usually resolves after withdrawal of the drug.

Lidocaine: Lidocaine is a local anesthetic that resembles procainamide in chemical structure but differs markedly in its electrophysiologic effects. Although there are few data available regarding the subcellular mechanisms modulating the electrical actions of lidocaine, the fact that these actions differ from those of quinidine and procainamide have led to the postulation that lidocaine influences the trans-membrane flux of Na+ and K+ ions in a manner somewhat opposite that of the other two agents. Since little effect on the electrophysiologic function of the atria and sinoatrial and atrioventricular nodes is usually observed, it appears that lidocaine does not significantly alter membrane cation exchange in these structure. Further, conduction per se is usually not altered in the ventricles, indicating that lidocaine does not influence Na+ entrance during excitation in this area. Also in contrast to quinidine and procainamide, lidocaine enhances K+ exit during repolarization in the ventricles, thus shortening the action potential duration (Figure 5 and 8).

Like quinidine and all other antiarrhythmic drugs, lidocaine depresses Na+ influx during diastole, thereby diminishing automaticity. In addition, it alters membrane responsiveness in Purkinje tissues so that conduction velocity and amplitude are increased for any membrane potential at the time of excitation[18] (Figure 4). This property therefore confers upon lidocaine the ability to increase conduction velocity in the ventricles under certain conditions.[18] Finally, since ventricular action potential duration is shortened more than responsiveness is enhanced, lidocaine increases the duration of functional refractory period relative to the duration of action potential.

Thus, lidocaine differs fundamentally from quinidine and procainamide in electrophysiologic properties. Although it depresses diastolic depolarization and automaticity in the Purkinje network and increases the functional refractory period relative to action potential duration, lidocaine is unlike quinidine and procainamide in that it usually has no effect on, or enhances, conduction velocity and increases membrane responsiveness. Therefore, lidocaine may be effective when quinidine and procainamide are not, and the reverse may also be true. Inasmuch as the electrophysiologic effects of lidocaine are primarily limited to ventricular myocardium, its major utility is in abolishing ventricular arrhythmias. In addition, since lidocaine usually has no effect upon, or occasionally accelerates, atrioventricular nodal conduction velocity, it is a preferred agent in the treatment of digitalis-induced ventricular arrhythmias.[56] Also, lidocaine is not useful in atrial fibrillation and may have the unwanted effect of increasing ventricular response in this disorder. As would be expected, usually lidocaine is virtually without effect upon the surface electrocardiogram.

Lidocaine administration is limited to the parenteral route and, in practice, is nearly always given intravenously, resulting in rapid plasma concentrations. Adequate blood levels are also achieved with intramuscular administration.[57] Lidocaine is minimally bound to plasma proteins and is primarily concentrated in the tissues. It is metabolized rapidly in the liver so that the half-life of a single injection is very short, ranging from 15 to 30 minutes.[58] Therefore, lidocaine is usually administered by an initial intravenous bolus injection followed by constant intravenous infusion. In the therapeutic range of 1 to 5 μg/ml. plasma concentrations of lidocaine are directly related to infusion rate.

The popularity of lidocaine as an antiarrhythmic agent is attributed to its rapid beneficial action and its relative freedom from cardiac toxicity. In recommended dosage, lidocaine toxicity is infrequently seen in the absence of hepatic disease, although its plasma concentration time-curve is greater in patients with congestive heart failure than in normal patients.[59] Toxicity is essentially limited to central nervous system aberrations including progressive drowsiness, paresthesias, muscle twitching, disorientation and convulsions with progressively elevated plasma levels.[60] Although respiratory arrest has been reported, cardiac electrical toxicity has been rare.

Diphenylhydantoin: Diphenylhydantoin is structurally related to the barbiturates and possesses electrophysiologic properties different from those of quinidine and procainamide. It appears to act on the cell membrane to enhance Na^+ influx during depolarization and K^+ efflux during repolarization (Figures 4, 9 and 10). Thus, like lidocaine, diphenylhydantoin has the electrophysiologic effects on atrioventricular nodal and Pukinje tissues of increasing or not altering conduction velocity, and membrane responsiveness is elevated (Figure 4) to a relatively lesser degree than action potential duration is shortened.[16] Thus, unlike quinidine and procainamide, diphenylhydantoin often enhances atrioventricular conduction and occasionally increases intraventricular conduction.[30,32] Diphenylhydantoin also decreases automaticity, not only by decreasing diastolic depolarization, but also by increasing maximal diastolic depolarization[8] (Figure 6D).

Diphenylhydantoin has found its greatest clinical application in the treatment of digitalis-induced ventricular arrhythmias.[33,61] Like lidocaine, diphenylhydantoin depresses digitalis-enhanced ventricular automaticity without adversely affecting intraventricular conduction while tending to reverse glycoside-prolonged atrioventricular conduction. Diphenylhydantoin has also been shown to exert a protective effect against ventricular arrhythmias that may occur after synchronized direct current electrical cardioversion in the presence of digitalis sensitization.[62] Further, diphenylhydantoin has been demonstrated to dissociate the positive inotropic and electrical toxic effects of the digitalis glycosides, thus depressing glycoside-induced arrhythmias without altering its enhancement of myocardial contractility.[31] In addition to its role in ventricular arrhythmias, diphenylhydantoin has been useful in supraventricular tachycardias, primarily in the area of digitalis toxicity. The possibility should be recognized of increased ventricular response in supraventricular tachycardias due to the ability of diphenylhydantoin to increase atrioventricular nodal conduction.

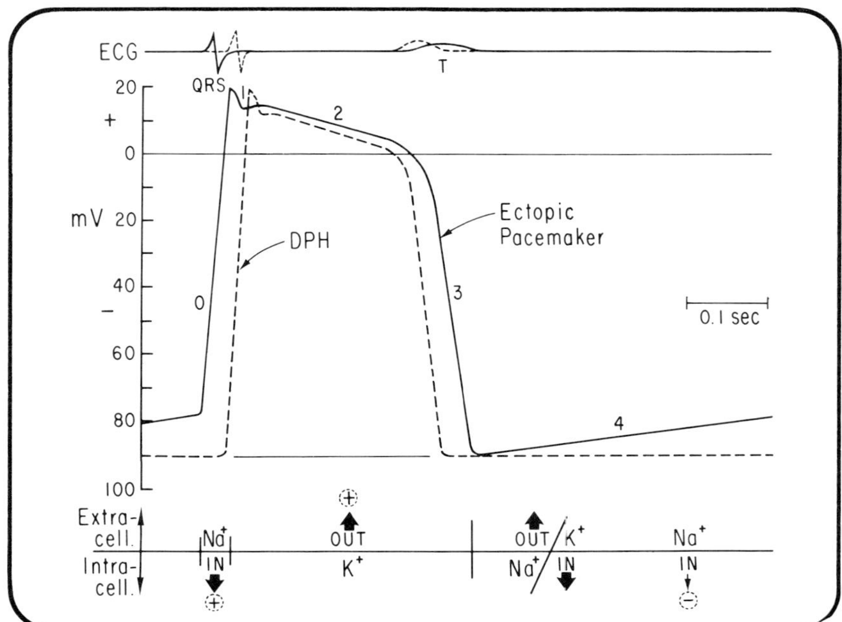

FIGURE 9. Diagram of transmembrane electrical potential **(middle)**, electrocardiogram **(top)** and transmembrane cation movements **(bottom)** of a spontaneously depolarizing automatic cardiac fiber **(solid line)** and after diphenylhydantoin (DPH) **(broken line).** Format and abbreviations as in Figure 2. (Reproduced by permission from Mason et al.[102])

Oral administration of diphenylhydantoin results in essentially complete absorption, although 12 hours may be required to achieve peak plasma concentration.[63] Therapeutic plasma concentrations (10 to 20 μg/ml) can easily be maintained orally, and the delay in achieving an initial salutary level may be reduced by an oral loading dose. Diphenylhydantoin may also be administered parenterally and is typically given by intravenous bolus injections of 100 mg every 5 minutes in a regimen similar to that for procainamide when it is important to abolish tachyarrhythmias abruptly. Diphenylhydantoin is usually not given by constant intravenous infusion due to the high incidence of phlebitis caused by its alkaline diluent. Once administered, diphenylhydantoin is avidly bound by body tissues, especially fat and liver, leading to large gradients between concentrations in these tissues and plasma concentrations. It is largely metabolized in the liver, where it is conjugated to glucuronic acid and subsequently excreted in the urine. Of potential importance is that in addition to hepatic impairment, concurrent administration of other drugs,

notably isoniazid,[64] may also inhibit diphenylhydantoin metabolism.

Diphenylhydantoin toxicity is uncommon when the agent is administered carefully in small incremental doses.[65,66] However, when large intravenous doses have been given, diphenylhydantoin has exhibited the paradoxical effect of producing atrioventricular block, and bradycardia and cardiac arrest have been reported—apparently due to marked depression of diastolic depolarization and automaticity.[33,66] Like lidocaine, diphenylhydantoin in large doses can produce central nervous system toxicity and may lead to progressive drowsiness and obtundation. Although diphenylhydantoin has produced marked hypotension, this has been attributable to too large or rapidly administered doses of the agent or to the presence of underlying severe cardiac decompensation. Also, similar to lidocaine, diphenylhydantoin has little effect upon the electrocardiogram, although it may shorten the QT interval.

Propranolol: Propranolol, the prototype beta adrenergic receptor-blocking agent, possesses considerable efficacy in the management of car-

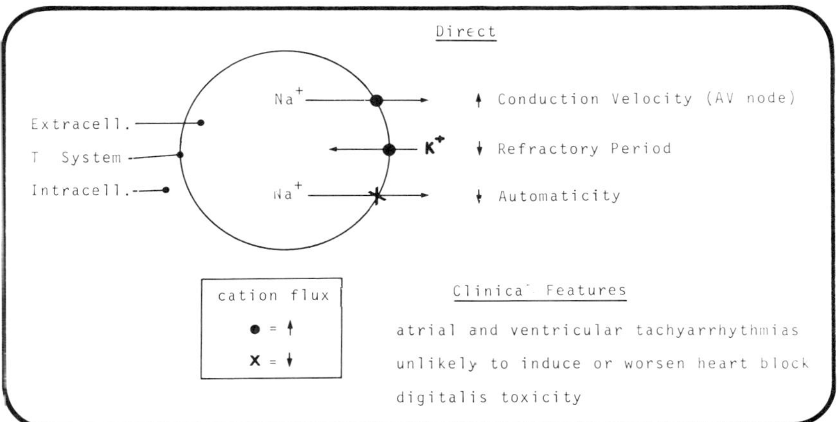

FIGURE 10. Diagram of the subcellular actions of diphenylhydantoin. Format and abbreviations as in Figure 7. (Reproduced by permission from Mason et al.[40])

diac rhythm disorders. The antiarrhythmic properties of propranolol are now considered to result principally from inhibition of adrenergic stimulation of the heart, since its direct membrane-mediated action upon the electrophysiology of the myocardium appears of relatively lesser importance with concentrations of the drug achieved clinically.[67,68] Since sympathetic stimulation increases automaticity by increasing phase 4 depolarization in automatic fibers, enhances conduction velocity and shortens the refractory period, especially in supraventricular tissues,[25] propranolol can reverse these effects by beta adrenergic receptor blockade.[27] The direct membrane effects of propranolol decrease diastolic Na^+ leak into the cell, reduce Na^+ conductance intracellularly during the spike action potential and increase K^+ extrusion from the cell during repolarization (Figures 5, 6 and 11). These combined antiadrenergic and direct effects result in decreased automaticity and conduction velocity, and refractoriness is increased while the functional refractory period is prolonged relative to the duration of action potential.[26] Since some studies have shown that the refractory period in supraventricular tissue is directly reduced by propranolol, the membrane actions of the agent are considered intermediate between those of quinidine and diphenylhydantoin.

The following classification of beta-blocking drugs comprises the more widely studied agents of potential clinical importance and those illus-

trative of a particular subclass.[69,70] (Table I). Class 1 is characterized by beta blockers with direct membrane activity and beta sympathomimetic activity. Dichloroisoproterenol produces marked beta stimulation and is designated subclass 1A.[71] Unlike a pure competitive beta blocker, it also has a residual intrinsic stimulant action on beta receptors, which renders it of little clinical value. In contrast, pronethalol,[72] alprenolol[73] and oxprenolol[74] have considerably less beta sympathomimetic activity and are subclassified 1B. The first of the 1B drugs, pronethalol, shown to be beneficial in the control of angina pectoris, arrhythmias and the adverse cardiocirculatory effects of thyrotoxicosis, was found to induce lymphoid tumors in mice and therefore was withdrawn from clinical trial in this country. Oxprenolol and alprenolol have undergone extensive clinical investigation and are effective in the same settings as is pronethalol. Class 2 beta blockers are characterized by membrane activity without intrinsic sympathomimetic activity. Propranolol, the prototype, is the beta blocker most widely studied and clinically applied. The class 3 drugs have some intrinsic beta sympathomimetic activity but no membrane activity. Pindolol, one of this group, alleviates angina pectoris and cardiac arrhythmias, although it is less potent than is propranolol. The class 4 agents possess neither direct membrane nor beta-stimulating activities. Sotalol is the member of this class that has received most attention.[75] It has antiarrhythmic

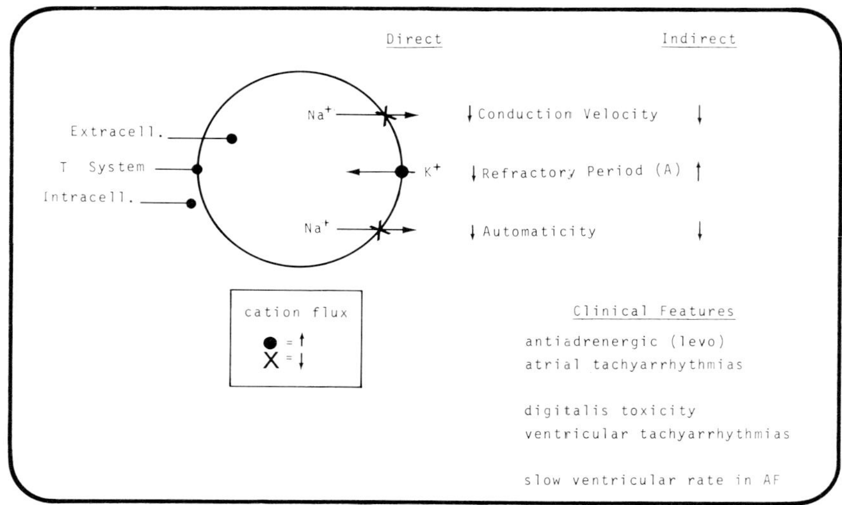

FIGURE 11. Diagram of the subcellular actions of propranolol. Format and abbreviations as in Figure 7. A = atrial conductive tissue; AF = atrial fibrillation. (Reproduced by permission from Mason et al.[102])

actions with less depression of cardiac pump activity than has propranolol.

The drugs in the important class 5 category exert selective blockade on beta receptors in specific tissues. These drugs are now receiving considerable experimental and clinical attention because of their potential salutary effects with less hazard of concomitant extracardiac beta-blocking action than noted with agents in the other classes of beta blockers. Practolol has been the most widely studied[38,76] and is reported to relatively selectively block beta receptors in the heart (beta$_1$ receptors) while sparing beta receptors in the smooth muscle of bronchi and blood vessels (beta$_2$ receptors). Thereby a therapeutic advantage is obtained in the management of tachyarrhythmias and angina pectoris in clinical settings such as chronic obstructive airway disease and cardiac pump dysfunction. Practolol does not appear to directly depress myocardial contractility but may selectively block beta receptors affecting the heart rate. However, it has recently been reported that the chronic use of practolol may be associated with a psoriasiform rash and ocular changes; therefore, this agent has been withdrawn from clinical use. The more recently developed agent, tolamolol, possesses selective beta$_1$-blocking action similar to that of practolol[77–80] without its skin or eye problems.

The beta adrenergic receptor-blocking and direct membrane effects of propranolol can be related to its stereoisomeric forms. As commonly available, propranolol consists of a racemic mixture of dextro- and levorotatory forms. Dextro-propranolol has little beta-blocking action when compared with levo-propranolol and is less effective against catecholamine-induced tachyarrhythmias, whereas levo-propranolol has the same direct membrane activity as dextro-propranolol.[27,69,81,82] This differential property has provided improved understanding of the mechanism of antiarrhythmic action of propranolol in various conditions. Thus, tachyarrhythmias precipitated by sympathetic discharge induced by exercise, emotion or anesthesia are antagonized by levo-propranolol but not by dextro-propranolol, indicating that the primary antiarrhythmic modality is beta blockade.[83] Although pretreatment with large doses of dextro-propranolol prevents ouabain-induced arrhythmias in experimental animals,[81,84] levo-propranolol is more effective in treating digitalis-induced tachyarrhythmias in patients.[85]

Propranolol, like diphenylhydantoin, is particularly effective in the treatment of digitalis-induced arrhythmias. Although propranolol is useful in the treatment of both supraventricular and ventricular arrhythmias due to digitalis toxicity, it has had greatest success in eradicating

TABLE I
Classification of Beta Adrenergic-Blocking Drugs

Class	Generic Name	Trade Name	Beta Blockade Relative Potency	Selectivity			Beta Stimulation	Membrane Activity
				B_1 Heart	B_2 Arterioles	B_2 Bronchi		
1	Dichloroisoproterenol	DCI	0.1	2+	+	+	3+	+
	Pronethalol	Alderlin	0.1	2+	+	+	2+	+
	Oxprenolol	Trasicor	2.0	2+	+	+	2+	+
	Alprenolol	Aptine	1.0	2+	+	+	2+	+
2	Propranolol	Inderal®	1.0	2+	3+	3+	0	+
3	INPEA	Pindolol	0.04	2+	+	2+	+	0
4	Sotalol	MJ-1999	0.1	2+	+	+	0	0
5	Practolol	ICI 50,172	0.5	2+	0	0	+	0
	Tolamolol	UK 6558	1.0	2+	0	0	0	0

premature ventricular extrasystoles. It has usually restored normal sinus rhythm in patients with digitalis-induced atrial tachycardia with atrioventricular block, but exacerbation of depressed nodal conduction has occurred.[27] It appears that although the direct membrane action causes reversion to sinus rhythm, the beta-blocking action may reduce atrioventricular nodal conduction. For this reason, many clinicians believe that diphenylhydantoin is preferable to propranolol in the initial treatment of digitalis-induced atrial tachycardia with block. Since electrical cardioversion may result in fatal ventricular arrhythmias in the presence of digitalis toxicity,[86] either agent is preferable to electro-shock in the management of glycoside-provoked tachyarrhythmias.

Propranolol has, however, been more effective in the treatment of supraventricular rhythm disorders in the absence of cardiac glycoside toxicity, although it retains beneficial actions in instances of non-digitalis ventricular tachyarrhythmias.[27] Propranolol has been particularly successful in converting paroxysmal atrial tachycardia to normal sinus rhythm and in slowing discharge from the ectopic supraventricular focus. It has also been effective in suppressing atrial tachycardias associated with the Wolff-Parkinson-White syndrome. In addition to its role in suppressing or converting supraventricular arrhythmias, propranolol, via beta adrenergic receptor blockade, has been valuable in reducing ventricular response in these situations. This effect is mediated by reduced conduction and increased functional refractory period in the atrioventricular node with decreased transmission of impulses to the ventricles. This decrease in atrioventricular nodal conduction has been shown to be additive to that of digitalis; therefore, the addition of propranolol is beneficial in certain patients with atrial fibrillation and flutter in whom the ventricular rate cannot be controlled with digitalis alone. Concerning sinus rate, propranolol is able to abolish exercise-induced increases in heart rate and to reduce sinus tachycardia due to hyperthyroidism and some states of excessive anxiety. Finally, propranolol is useful in maintaining sinus rhythm after electrical cardioversion alone or in combination with quinidine.[87–89]

The pharmacokinetic properties of propranolol are beginning to become known.[90] Propranolol is well absorbed from the intestine, an oral dose producing peak plasma concentrations in 1 to 2 hours. It is avidly metabolized and cleared by the liver. The active metabolite, 4-hydroxy-propranolol, which has beta-blocking properties itself, is formed only after oral—not after intravenous—administration. Thus, the beta-blocking effect of a given plasma concentration of propranolol may be greater after oral than after intravenous administration. Since hepatic hydroxylation of propranolol may vary substantially among individuals, the plasma concentration of the same dose of the drug can vary widely after oral administration in different patients. The plasma half-life of propranolol is relatively short—2 to 3 hours after intravenous and 4 to 6 hours after oral administration. Relatively large and frequent doses may be necessary to maintain tissue equilibrium at the beta receptor site, and difficulties are evident in correlating the degree of beta blockade with plasma concentrations of propranolol. Therapeutic plasma levels are considered to be 50 to 100 ng/ml.

Intravenously administered propranolol leads to a decrease in heart rate, reduction in myocardial contractile force and depression of cardiac output. The effect on arterial blood pressure is variable, depending upon the rate of administration. When the drug is given rapidly, the blood pressure may decline as a result of a decrease in the cardiac output. When it is administered slowly, there is little change in the blood pressure. Responses to adrenergic stimuli are altered after propranolol administration, resulting in partial or complete inhibition of sympathetic nerve stimulation and of the action of exogenously administered catecholamines on the heart. Tachycardia resulting from increased sympathetic activity or elevated circulating catecholamines is attenuated or blocked. It is important to bear in mind that the magnitude of cardiocirculatory changes induced by beta blockade are directly related to the background level of sympathetic activity prior to administration. Thus, congestive heart failure may be provoked by beta blockade in patients with heart disease who require increased basal sympathetic activity as a compensatory mechanism for maintaining cardiac function. The intravenous dose of propranolol for complete beta adrenergic blockade with no chronotropic, inotropic or vasodilator responses to isoproterenol is approximately 0.1 mg per kg of body weight. After this dose of propranolol, the cardiac stimulatory effects of norepinephrine and epinephrine are abolished, but the blood pressure may be raised moderately by the unopposed alpha constrictor effect of these catecholamines.

Catecholamine administration causes an increase in circulating free fatty acids through accelerated lipolysis, as well as a rise in the blood glucose level as a result of increased glycogenolysis.[91] Beta blockade inhibits these effects. The increase in nonesterified fatty acids seen immediately after exercise is reduced by beta blockade. This effect is noteworthy because of the possible role of nonesterified fatty acids resulting in arrhythmias and sudden death in coronary disease. In liver disease with a lack of hepatic glycogen, the inhibition of sympathetically mediated stimulation of glycogenolysis in skeletal muscle may exacerbate hypoglycemia. Beta blockade may prevent clinical mainfestations of hypoglycemia such as tachycardia and sweating. Recovery of blood glucose after insulin administration may also be delayed.

It is important that the dosage of propranolol be carefully individualized according to the clinical effect desired while avoiding adverse reactions. Starting doses should be 10 to 20 mg orally 3 or 4 times daily, before meals and at bedtime. The amount of drug should be gradually increased until an optimal response is obtained. The total effective daily dosage may vary between 80 and 400 mg in angina pectoris.[36] With cautious administration, it is usually possible to use the drug effectively in most patients with cardiac disease without congestive heart failure. Concomitant therapy with digitalis or diuretics may permit the use of propranolol in the presence of some cardiac dysfunction. The dosage for effective control of tachyarrhythmias may be substantially less than that needed for antianginal action—40 to 240 mg daily. For the immediate treatment of life-threatening arrhythmias, propranolol is given intravenously, 1 to 3 mg in 5 minutes initially, the total dosage not to exceed 6 to 7 mg.

Propranolol toxicity is principally related to its beta adrenergic receptor-blocking property. Removal of cardiac beta adrenergic receptor stimulation lowers blood pressure and myocardial contractility and reduces heart rate, while removal of beta adrenergic receptor stimulation in bronchial smooth muscle may produce bronchoconstriction. Severe propranolol toxicity may result in progressive bradycardia leading to cardiac asystole. Isoproterenol is the appropriate antagonist and should be administered in large doses if necessary. In addition, intravenous glucagon should be effective in propranolol toxicity, since glucagon increases the activity of adenylate cyclase in the presence of beta adrenergic receptor blockade.[92]

There have been reports of myocardial infarc-

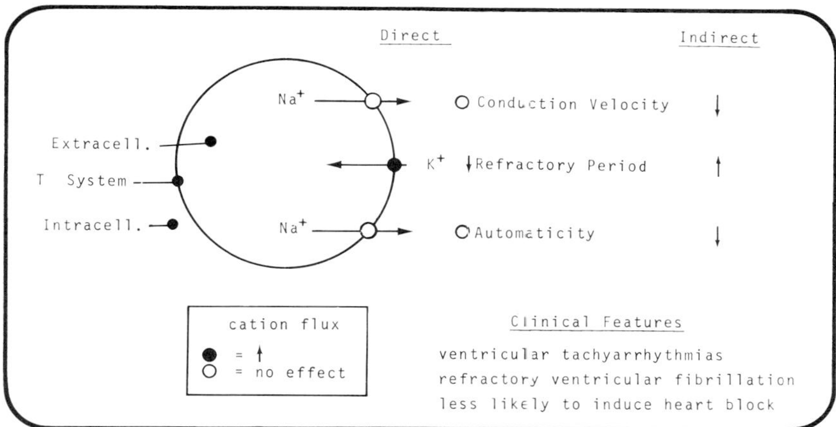

FIGURE 12. Diagram of the subcellular actions of brety-lium tosylate. Format and abbreviations as in Figure 7. (Reproduced by permission from Mason et al.[102])

tion and sudden death after rapid withdrawal of large doses of beta blockers in patients with coronary disease and angina pectoris.[93] Therefore, these drugs always should be withdrawn gradually in patients with coronary atherosclerosis. The notion that mortality in coronary artery bypass surgery is related to the preoperative administration of propranolol has led some clinicians to conclude that it should be discontinued at least 2 weeks prior to operation. However, recent investigation has shown that propranolol disappears from left atrial tissue and plasma in patients undergoing coronary bypass surgery in 36 to 48 hours.[94] Therefore, 48 hours is sufficient for complete recovery from adverse cardiac pump effects of orally administered propranolol. In instances in which the use of propranolol is advantageous for its antianginal or antiarrhythmic actions, it may be administered up to the time of surgery; emergency operation should not be delayed in a patient taking propranolol.

Bretylium: Bretylium tosylate, an adrenergic neuron-blocking agent developed for use in hypertension, has recently been evaluated in the treatment of cardiac arrhythmias.[41] Although mechanisms of its antiarrhythmic actions are still under investigation, present evidence indicates that the principal benefit of bretylium in abating tachyarrhythmias is primarily due to its antiadrenergic properties, rather than to direct effects of the drug[19] (Figure 12). Parenteral bre-

tylium initially causes release of norepinephrine from sympathetic nerve endings, followed by its prolonged antiadrenergic action that prevents further discharge of neurotransmitter from sympathetic nerve endings. The initial release of norepinephrine appears to account for the transient increase in automaticity by bretylium.[19,41,95,96] Concerning direct effects of bretylium, it has been reported to decrease both action potential duration and functional refractory period, and there is evidence that it improves conduction velocity by membrane hyperpolarization. From these considerations, the antiadrenergic action of bretylium appears capable of terminating certain reentrant arrhythmias (Figure 5) and possibly disorders of automaticity, especially those resulting from adrenergic influences producing non-uniform recovery or temporal dispersion of electrophysiologic activity. Furthermore, the direct effect of the agent of decreasing refractoriness may be useful in abolishing reentrant arrhythmias.

Although experimental studies have demonstrated promising results in ventricular tachyarrhythmias,[39,41,42,97] bretylium is currently reserved for therapeutic use in ventricular arrhythmias that are unresponsive to conventional therapy. On occasion, the drug has enabled successful electroversion and permanent abolition of ventricular fibrillation, which could not be accomplished by countershock alone or by countershock in combination with other an-

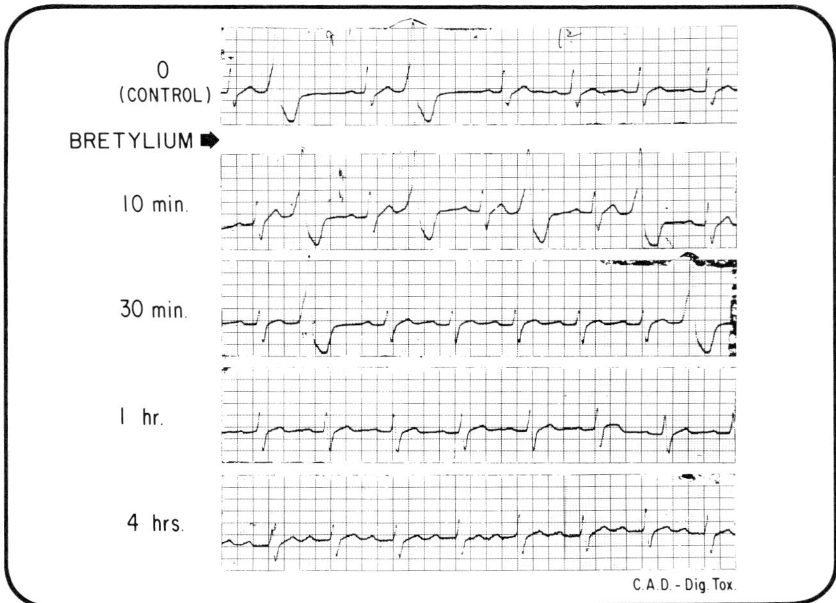

FIGURE 13. Effects of intravenous bretylium (5 mg/kg) on multiple paroxysmal ventricular contractions (PVC) induced by digitalis toxicity **(top panel)** in a patient with coronary artery disease. The frequency of PVC increased 10 minutes after bretylium **(second panel).** The extrasystoles were completely abated at 1 and 4 hours on the ECG tracings. (Reproduced by permission from Amsterdam et al.[42])

tiarrhythmic drugs.[41,95,98] In these serious situations, bretylium is administered parenterally in doses of 5 mg/kg or more and repeated hourly until the arrhythmia is controlled or until hypotension or electrical or gastrointestinal side-effects appear. Gastrointestinal absorption is inefficient after oral administration, amounting to less than half the dose administered by the administered by the oral route.

The relatively frequent occurrence of potentially serious side-effects has hampered the elevation of parenteral bretylium to the status of a first-line antiarrhythmic drug. A fall in systemic blood pressure—particularly with the patient in the upright position—is common due to the drug's antiadrenergic action, although severe hypotension requiring vasopressor therapy has not been a problem when the patient remains supine.[42,95] In addition, because of the early discharge of norepinephrine from adrenergic terminals, ventricular electrical irritability is often increased prior to the onset of bretylium's prolonged antiarrhythmic effect, which ranges from 4 to 12 hours after injection (Figure 13).

Potassium: Potassium may exert antiarrhythmic effects that are useful in certain clinical settings. The electrophysiologic properties of potassium are complex and often depend on the speed of administration and the serum concentration of the cation and the type of cardiac tissue involved.[28,99] Elevation of potassium concentration within the normal range reduces conduction velocity and shortens the refractory period. Further, automaticity may be diminished, especially in ectopic ventricular pacemakers, but this action is variable since the resting membrane potential is elevated while diastolic depolarization is reduced.[28] In general, each of these potassium-induced alterations of electrophysiologic properties is greater in Purkinje tissue and the nonconductive fibers of the myocardium, particularly in the atrium, than in the atrioventricular and sinoatrial nodes and the atrial conductive fibers.[28] Thus, intraventricular block with widening of the QRS duration is more likely than atrioventricular block after potassium administration. Concerning the automaticity of the sinoatrial node, potassium usually exerts a mild direct depressant effect that is counter-balanced by an indirect parasympathomimetic action, and thereby no change in heart rate occurs.[28]

It is important to remember that the antiarrhythmic drugs are often ineffective in the presence of certain abnormalities of the humoral background in which the agents are administered, such as hypokalemia, hypoxia and disorders of acid-base regulation. Correction of these abnormalities may restore sinus rhythm even without the use of antiarrhythmic drugs. [24,99,100] The influence of hypokalemia in predisposing to digitalis toxicity is well recognized.[34,101,102]

On occasion, it is advantageous to use the antiarrhythmic properties of potassium in patients in whom the serum concentration of the cation is normal. In the management of tachyarrhythmias after cardiac operations, elevation of the serum potassium concentration by 0.5 to 1.5 mEq/L or to the upper limits of normal may be effective with or without antiarrhythmic drugs.[99] Potassium should not be used in this manner in the presence of atrioventricular block, since nodal conduction may be further impaired by the cation.

New Antiarrhythmic Agents: The oral antianginal agent perhexiline has also been shown to possess important antiarrhythmic properties.[103-106] The principal antiarrhythmic action of this drug in isolated automatic myocardial tissues appears to be diminution of diastolic depolarization in Purkinje fibers.[104] In addition, the agent has a quinidine-like effect manifested by slowing of sinus rate, prolongation of conduction time and widening of refractory period.[105] In intact canine studies in our laboratories, intravenous perhexiline did not affect intraatrial, transnodal or intraventricular conduction intervals.[106] Oral therapy has reduced the frequency of ventricular tachyarrhythmias with minimal side-effects in patients with chronic coronary artery disease.[103]

Verapamil has been shown to be clinically effective—particularly in abolishing supraventricular tachycardias due to atrioventricular nodal reetrant disorders.[22,107] There has been considerable interest in this agent because of its special mechanism of altering electrophysiologic properties of automatic myocardial fibers.[107] Verampamil depresses conduction ve-

locity, lowers action potential amplitude and suppresses complete depolarization by its inhibition of slow transmembrane inward Ca++ movements.[108] This effect is most pronounced in the atrioventricular node since the action potential of this structure is uniquely dependent on slow inward currents.[22]

The agent 17-monochloroacetyl-ajmaline has been demonstrated to abolish experimental and clinical supraventricular and ventricular tachyarrhythmias.[108-111] The agent exerts quinidine-like membrane effects and also possesses anticholingergic activity.[110] The antiarrhythmic actions of 17-monochloroacetyl-ajmaline that are of special interest include direct membrane depression of electrophysiologic properties with greater prolongation of intraatrial and atrioventricular nodal conduction times than of His-Purkinje conduction time.[111] Thus, ajmaline appears to be particularly effective in supraventricular tachycardias.[110,111]

The clinical efficacy of disopyramide phosphate, a new oral antiarrhythmic agent, has been shown in long-term studies in patients.[112] The drug diminishes the frequency of all types of premature cardiac ectopic depolarizations. Importantly, this salutary effect includes decreases in the frequency of episodic ventricular tachycardia (Figure 14) and complicated ventricular extrasystoles (multifocal, paired, R on T, and greater than 5 per minute) (Figure 15) that are considered especially prone to provoke ventricular fibrillation and thereby lead to sudden death.[112] The agent possesses quinidine-like actions of diminution of conduction velocity and prolongation of action potential duration with vagolytic properties.[113,114] With oral administration, the drug is well tolerated clinically and has not worsened ventricular pump performance in patients with cardiac dysfunction prior to its administration.[112] Furthermore, intravenous administration of disopyramide phosphate in patients with chronic coronary heart disease resulted in only minimal, transient decrease in myocardial mechanical function.[115]

Therapeutic Considerations

Judicious management of disorders of cardiac rhythm is fundamentally based on accurate identification of the nature of the arrhythmia

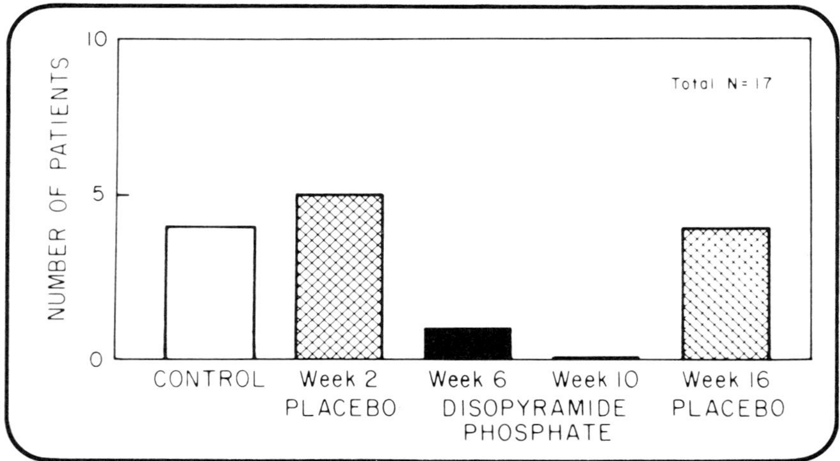

FIGURE 14. Occurrence of episodic ventricular tachycardia as determined by portable electroocardiographic monitoring in patients with chronic coronary artery disease. Ventricular tachycardia was noted in 9 patients during placebo monitoring but in only 1 patient during active drug therapy (p < 0.05). (Reproduced by permission from Vismara et al.[112])

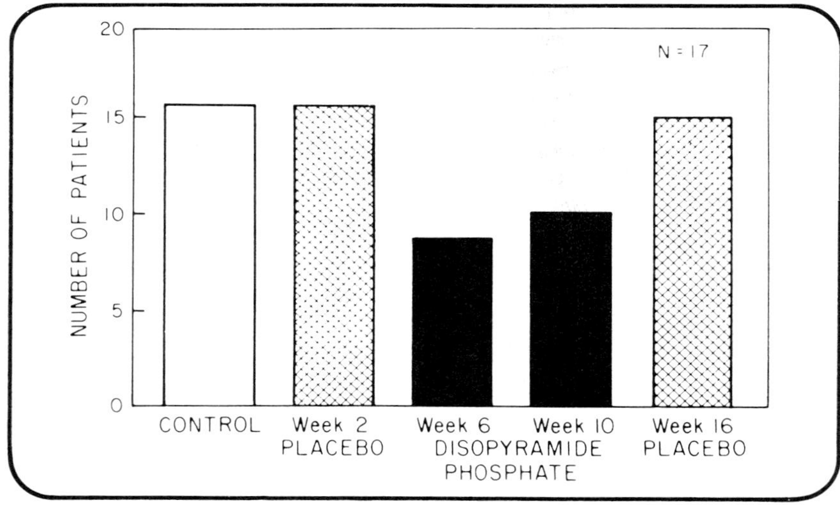

FIGURE 15. Prevalence of complicated ventricular ectopic depolarizations in control, placebo and disopyramide phosphate therapy periods. Significant reduction (p <0.05) of these extrasystoles occurred during active drug administration. (Reproduced by permission from Vismara et al.[112])

and the clinical setting in which it is operative. Indeed, precise definition of certain rhythm disturbances may be more difficult than therapeutic control itself, but it is essential to keep in mind that failure of drug therapy may represent erroneous diagnosis of the type of arrhythmia involved. Further, in the modern era of hospital-based monitors and outpatient continuous tape recorders demonstrating a high frequency of rhythm aberrations in patients, it is important to consider carefully the relative benefits and risks of antiarrhythmic agents. Some rhythm and conduction disorders that are relatively benign in ambulatory patients without abnormal car-

TABLE II
Usual Doses of Antiarrhythmic Agents

	Group I Agents					Group II Agents	
	Quinidine	Procainamide	Propranolol	Bretylium	Potassium	Lidocaine	Diphenylhydantoin
Parenteral	Gluconate; IM: 0.2-0.4 g; IV: 25 mg/min; <800 mg total	IM: 250-500 mg; IV: 100 mg, every 5 min; <1,000 mg total	IV: 1-3 mg initially; <0.1 mg/kg total	IM/IV: 5 mg/kg initially; <15 mg/kg total; Maintenance: 3-5 mg/kg every 4-12 hours	Chloride; IV: 3 g (40 mEq) >2 hours	IV: 50-100 mg every 5 min; <350 mg total; Maintenance: 1-4 mg/min IV	IV: 100 mg every 5 min; <1,000 mg total
Oral	Sulphate; 0.2-0.4 g every 3–6 hours	250-270 mg every 3-6 hours	10-30 mg every 6-8 hours	300-600 mg every 6-12 hours	Chloride; 1-3 g every 6-8 hours		100 mg every 6 hours

IM = intramuscular; V = intravenous.

diac performance may be poorly tolerated hemodynamically in other patients with disturbed pump function—even potentially life-threatening in the presence of acute myocardial infarction. However, the relative toxicity of antiarrhythmic agents tends to be enhanced in advanced heart disease with congestive failure.

In the treatment of tachyarrhythmias, it is generally prudent to administer adequate doses of one antiarrhythmic drug of choice to allow its thorough trial without producing toxic effects before substituting or adding a different agent.[116] Table II lists the usual doses of these agents employed in clinical practice.[21] In the following discussion, a concise approach to the clinical management of cardiac tachyarrhythmias is formulated using the drugs delineated in the preceding portion of this chapter. The special problem of digitalis toxicity is considered more fully in the foregoing chapter on the digitalis glycosides.

Supraventricular Tachyarrhythmias: In the management of supraventricular tachyarrhythmias, the initial objective is to achieve control of the ventricular rate if necessary and then, if possible, to restore normal sinus rhythm.[40] If these arrhythmias exert a relatively marked adverse effect on pump function or provoke myocardial ischemic pain after their acute onset, prompt termination of the rhythm disturbance is indicated, usually by precordial direct current shock. Conversely, if the supraventricular disorder is well tolerated, drug therapy can be directed toward control of the ventricular response rate—with conversion to normal sinus

rhythm achieved during this therapeutic process or accomplished later by electroversion.

Atrial Premature Systoles: Premature atrial contractions are commonly observed in adults without apparent heart disease; in this setting, they ordinarily require no therapy and have a benign prognosis. In contrast, in the presence of elevated atrial pressures and volume such as with mitral stenosis, active disease of atrial muscle such as after myocardial infarction or certain generalized metabolic disorders such as thyrotoxicosis, premature atrial contractions are harbingers of atrial fibrillation. In addition, premature atrial contractions are considered potential forerunners of the return of supraventricular tachycardia, flutter or fibrillation in patients with previous episodes of these disorders. In these abnormal situations, outpatient therapy is usually carried out with quinidine in oral doses ranging from 200 to 400 mg every 6 hours. Effective alternatives are procainamide, digitalis and propranolol. Digitalis is often used as the agent of choice in acute myocardial infarction.

Atrial Tachycardia: Atrial tachycardia is frequently encountered and results from a reentrant pathway through the atrioventricular node or, probably less commonly, a rapidly discharging ectopic atrial focus. This arrhythmia frequently occurs in episodes and is termed paroxysmal atrial tachycardia. As emphasized previously, the therapeutic approach to an acute attack is largely governed by the effects of this disorder on cardiocirculatory function. Since patients who experience paroxysmal atrial tachycardia often have no evidence of organic heart disease, they frequently tolerate rapid ventricular rates without hemodynamic difficulty.

Initially, conversion to normal sinus rhythm is attempted by means of vagal stimulation, carotid sinus massage, vagomimetic agents such as edrophonium or reflex vagal stimulation by pressor agents such as phenylephrine. Edrophonium is given intravenously in a 5 to 10 mg bolus. Phenylephrine, 0.5 to 1 mg, is administered intravenously. If these measures are unsuccessful, 1 to 2 mg of propranolol may be administered intravenously every 5 minutes to a total dose of 0.1 mg/kg of body weight if necessary. Other therapy that can be utilized includes rapid digitalization, intravenous procainamide, intramuscular quinidine and rest with sedation. Also, rapid atrial pacing delivered by a temporary transvenous electrode catheter can terminate paroxysmal atrial tachycardia.[117] In severe circumstances with hemodynamic deterioration due to paroxysmal atrial tachycardia, the arrhythmia can rapidly be converted to normal sinus rhythm by direct current electrical cardioversion.

Between acute episodes, prophylaxis can be achieved with oral digitalis, quinidine, procainamide or propranolol maintenance therapy. Recently, refractory repetitive episodes of incapacitating atrial tachycardia have been treated successfully by rapid atrial pacing delivered through a patient-controlled, permanently implanted coronary sinus pacemaker.[118] Some cases of recurrent atrial tachycardia accompanying the Wolff-Parkinson-White sydrome have responded favorably to surgical division of the anomalous pathway.[119]

Atrial Flutter: Atrial flutter is a less common arrhythmia that is characterized by a more rapid atrial rate than that of atrial tachycardia, usually in the presence of atrioventricular block. Management again is determined by the hemodynamic status of the patient, although atrial flutter is relatively resistant to drug therapy. If there is no evidence of circulatory embarrassment, many clinicians favor the initial administration of digitalis. The response to digitalis is variable; no change may result, or the glycoside may change the flutter to atrial fibrillation, increase atrioventricular block or convert the arrhythmia to normal sinus rhythm. If normal sinus rhythm

is not achieved with digitalis, quinidine, procainamide or propranolol may be added. If these pharmacologic measures are unsuccessful or if the arrhythmia is hemodynamically disabling, direct current cardioversion is applied. Indeed, atrial flutter responds so consistently to cardioversion—often at low energy levels—that electroshock is being utilized more frequently as the primary therapeutic modality.

Atrial Fibrillation: In atrial fibrillation, there are rapid disordered wavelets of atrial depolarization that are blocked to various degrees in the atrioventricular node, thereby producing an irregular ventricular rate response. In addition to possible diminution of cardiac pump function referrable to rapid heart rate, atrial fibrillation results in loss of the contribution of atrial contraction to ventricular filling.[120] Atrial fibrillation may also prove detrimental because of the production of systemic emboli. Usually the ventricular response in atrial fibrillation can easily be controlled with digitalis.

In the few patients in whom the glycoside alone does not adequately control heart rate, small doses of propranolol may be added with considerable salutary effect.[20] In many instances, digitalis may convert atrial fibrillation to normal sinus rhythm, particularly if fibrillation is of recent onset. In addition, therapeutic serum concentrations of quinidine may convert atrial fibrillation to normal sinus rhythm in many patients. Since quinidine may slow the atrial rate in atrial flutter and fibrillation, thus decreasing the number of impulses that are blocked in the atrioventricular node, and increases conduction through the atrioventricular node by vagolysis, more rapid ventricular response may occasionally occur in atrial flutter and fibrillation. To counteract this potential increase in heart rate, digitalis is usually given before quinidine therapy is begun in atrial fibrillation and flutter. Also, the glycoside is usually continued after normal sinus rhythm is achieved to guard against rapid ventricular rate if atrial fibrillation or flutter recurs.

In the majority of patients with atrial fibrillation, the major therapeutic decision is whether or not to electively apply direct current electrical cardioversion. Electrical cardioversion is a highly effective means of restoring normal sinus rhythm. However, in many patients, atrial fibrillation subsequently recurs.[121] Our standard procedure is to attempt electroversion at least once in most patients with atrial fibrillation in whom no contraindications are present. Factors militating against cardioversion include recent systemic embolization, slow ventricular response without drug therapy, intolerance to quinidine and procainamide and, often, advanced age in patients without cardiac dysfunction whose ventricular rate is well controlled by digitalis. In patients with rapid hemodynamic failure due to atrial fibrillation, immediate direct current conversion is recommended. Electroversion in fibrillation is also particularly indicated in chronic heart failure and in those in whom ventricular rate cannot be controlled by digitalis. The efficacy and safety of direct current cardioversion renders forceful attempts at chemical cardioversion imprudent at the present time, although prophylactic maintenance therapy with quinidine or procainamide is mandatory after electroshock-induced normal sinus rhythm.

Ventricular Tachyarrhythmias: One of the principal accomplishments in cardiovascular medicine in the past decade has been the ability to detect and successfully treat life-threatening ventricular arrhythmias. Although the most dramatic benefits have been noted in patients with acute myocardial infarction who reach the hospital, it is anticipated that the identification of patients who have chronic coronary artery disease with risk of lethal arrhythmias will enable the salutary application of appropriate antiarrhythmic agents on a long-term basis.[122] It is emphasized that the correction of systemic hypoxia and any electrolyte or acid-base abnormalities may, in themselves, successfully eliminate cardiac arrhythmias and these disturbances should be normalized prior to the institution of antiarrhythmic drug therapy.[100] In addition, tachyarrhythmias may sometimes be related to abnormal heart rate itself or cardiac pump dysfunction, and these arrhythmias can be abated by rectifying the underlying cause.

The decrease in mortality of 50 percent in acute myocardial infarction in intensive coronary care units of certain medical centers has chiefly been the result of aggressive management of prelethal and otherwise lethal ventricular arrhythmias.[123] Concerning potentially lethal dysrhythmias in myocardial infarction, attention has been focused on the important role of premature ventricular contractions in initiating fatal ventricular tachycardia and ventricular fibrillation.[124] It is currently standard practice to intitiate treatment for premature ventricular contractions when they occur at a rate greater than 5 per minute, are multifocal, appear in salvos or arise during the vulnerable period at the peak of the T wave.

In critical situations such as in acute myocardial infarction in which it is desired to quickly suppress potentially malignant forms of premature ventricular contractions of recent origin, intravenous lidocaine is the agent of choice due to its rapid effectiveness and low propensity for toxicity.[102] Usually 100 mg is given as a slow bolus, which may be repeated every 5 minutes to a total of 5 mg/kg. If the premature ventricular contractions are abolished, a constant intravenous drip is utilized at a rate up to 4 mg/minute and titrated to the smallest dose that controls the arrhythmia. Sustained abolition of premature ventricular contractions with procainamide is then generally employed.

Intravenous procainamide is the agent usually substituted if lidocaine therapy is unsuccessful.[24] Recent studies have shown procainamide to be as effective as lidocaine in terminating premature ventricular contractions without greater electrical or hemodynamic toxicity in myocardial infarction.[125] Procainamide is administered by bolus of 100 mg every 5 minutes until the arrhythmia is eliminated—or to a total of 1 g. Long-term suppression of premature ventricular contractions is subsequently accomplished by intravenous drip of procainamide—and finally by oral therapy. If these agents are ineffective, intravenous propranolol may be tried or diphenylhydantoin added. Parenteral bretylium has been useful when all other agents have failed.[42] Alternatively, temporary cardiac pacing with overdrive suppression of ventricular arrhythmias with antiarrhythmic drugs added may be the most efficacious therapy.[126] Recently there has been considerably discussion concerning the role of prophylactic antiarrhythmic drugs given to all patients hospitalized with acute myocardial infarction even without active rhythm disorders.[127] Although the frequency of ventricular tachyarrhythmias is reduced, mortality remains unaltered. Therefore, it is generally believed that prophylaxis is unnecessary in the hospital in the absence of premature ventricular contractions when cardiac monitoring and intensive care are available.

Outpatient management of frequent premature ventricular contractions is usually achieved with oral quinidine or procainamide. Also, propranolol or diphenylhydantoin may be effective. To help overcome the enormous and difficult problem of sudden death, patient self-administration of lidocaine intramuscularly has been suggested as a potential approach.[57] There has been considerable debate as to possible adverse effects of parenteral atropine used similarly for its conceivable benefits in this prehospital situation.[128,129]

In the treatment of ventricular tachycardia, immediate precordial direct current electroshock is the procedure of choice due to the high propensity of ventricular tachycardia to deteriorate into ventricular fibrillation. After electroconversion to normal sinus rhythm, long-term suppression of ventricular tachycardia is carried out by administration of either lidocaine, quinidine, procainamide or diphenylhydantoin. If ventricular tachycardia is recurrent despite these agents, prophylaxis can be attempted with propranolol, bretylium or pacemaker ventricular overdrive and suppressive drugs. Precordial electroshock is administered immediately in ventricular fibrillation, and cardiopulmonary resuscitation measures of closed-chest cardiac massage and intubation-ventilatory support with intravenous sodium bicarbonate are necessary if direct current conversion is not successful. The intravenous administration of the preceding antiarrhythmic drugs—particularly bretylium—may sometimes allow successful electroversion in refractory ventricular tachycardia and fibrillation.[42]

Electroconversion: The greatest recent achievement in the management of tachyarrhythmias has been the development of electric countershock for the effective and safe treatment of supraventricular and ventricular arrhythmias. Originally introduced in the form of alternating current generating devices for immediate treatment of ventricular fibrillation,[130,131] this method has been extended in the past few years to the elective and emergency control of supraventricular and ventricular tachycardias,

as well as fibrillation, by direct current instruments that are capable of producing high-voltage pulses of brief duration applied to the external precordium.[132] The electrical impulse is delivered at the onset of the QRS wave to avoid the vulnerable period of the ventricle during which a suitable stimulus might produce ventricular fibrillation.[133] The mechanism of action of electroshock is derived from the ability of the high-current pulse to depolarize all cardiac tissues, thereby terminating all impulse wavelets, followed by the resumption of electrical activity of the heart predominated by the normal pacemaker tissue. Use of direct current electroshock has reestablished normal sinus rhythm in 94 percent of patients with atrial fibrillation, 97 percent with atrial flutter, 70 percent with atrial tachycardia with or without block and 98 percent of those with ventricular fibrillation.[98,134]

Prior to elective countershock, the patient is given a maintenance dose of an antiarrhythmic drug, usually quinidine, so that a sufficient blood level is achieved to reduce the possibility of recurrence of the arrhythmia after electrical reversion to normal sinus rhythm.[135] Continued prophylaxis with quinidine or procainamide is required to maintain normal sinus rhythm. Since only 1 percent of patients with atrial fibrillation who receive chronic anticoagulant therapy have systemic or pulmonary emboli at the time of cardioversion compared with 7 percent of those not receiving anticoagulants,[136] it is probably wise to administer anticoagulants for a few weeks before electroconversion in patients with a history of embolic episodes.

In the past, maintenance doses of digitalis were reduced or discontinued in patients without glycoside toxicity prior to elective electroconversion in view of the possibility of serious ventricular arrhythmias attributable to digitalis after use of electrical shock. However, the preferred present practice is to continue the drug because of the risk of problems related to exacerbation of heart failure and return of rapid ventricular rate in atrial fibrillation prior to conversion due to insufficient glycoside, and to use small amounts of electrical energy at the time of cardioversion. In this regard, it has been shown that the incidence of ventricular tachyarrhythmias can be reduced after conversion of supra-

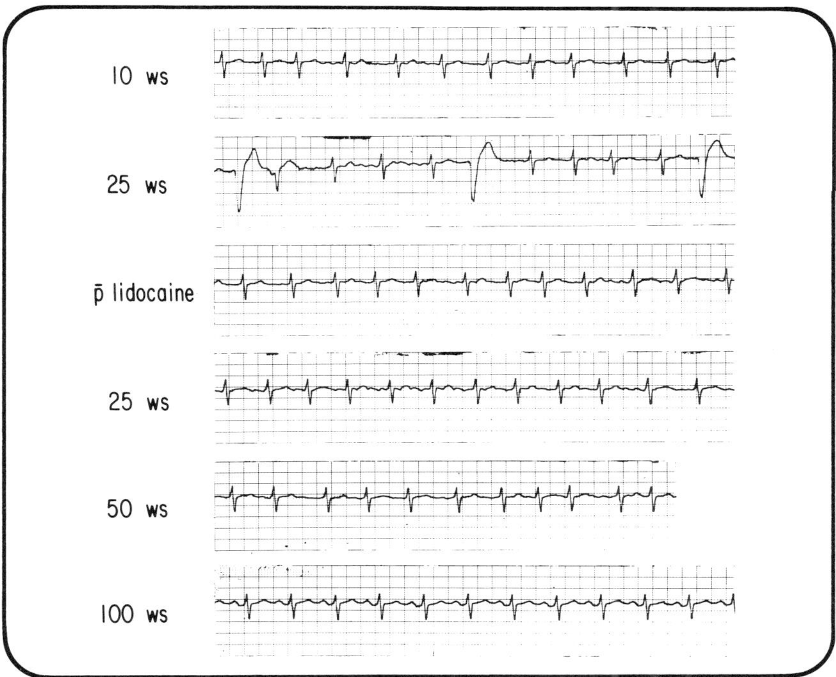

FIGURE 16. Sequence of initially small, incrementally increasing levels of direct current (DC) in cardioversion of atrial fibrillation (AF) in presence of maintenance digitalis in patient with congestive heart failure. In **top panel,** AF persists after 10 watt-seconds (ws) of countershock. After 25 ws in **second panel,** AF remains, now with paroxysmal ventricular contractions, which are abolished after lidocaine (p̄) administration **(third panel).** AF still is not terminated after repeated 25 ws discharge **(fourth panel)** and 50 ws countershock **(fifth panel).** Finally in the **last panel,** normal sinus rhythm is restored after 100 ws DC discharge. (Reproduced by permission from Mason et al.[102])

ventricular arrhythmias in the presence of digitalis, if the shock energy is at a low level[98,137] (Figure 16). The prophylactic administration of diphenylhydantoin in this situation has been reported to be useful. In an attempt to explain the occurrence of digitalis-induced ventricular irritability after electroversion in patients receiving therapeutic doses of digitalis, it has been suggested that the amount of discharge energy required to produce ventricular tachycardia is reduced in the digitalized heart[138] and that the electrical discharge causes K+ loss from the myocardium, thereby promoting glycoside toxicity.[139] An alternate mechanism is that cardiotoxicity to digitalis is reduced in atrial fibrillation, thereby allowing a greater tolerable maintenance dose and that after conversion the tolerable level of digitalis is reduced and leads to supraventricular and ventricular irritability.[140]

Electrical Pacing: An important advance in the acute and chronic treatment of refractory ventricular tachycardia with or without atrioventricular block is the method of electrical ventricular overdrive.[126] In the absence of block, atrial or ventricular stimulation can be employed.[141] In the method of overdrive of the idioventricular focus, the electrical stimulus is delivered at a more rapid rate than the frequency of the ectopic ventricular impulse, thereby suppressing the ectopic pacemaker. Further, with the ventricular rate maintained by electrical stimulation, antiarrhythmic drugs may be given to suppress the ectopic focus and allow the faster electrical rate to be diminished. In addition, the frequency of the electrical rate may often be reduced to a rate even slower than that of the original ectopic pacemaker since the faster rate of the electrical pacemaker itself is capable of depressing the slope of diastolic depolarization of the ectopic pacemaker.[142]

The use of atropine to increase heart rate and thereby to abolish ventricular extrasystoles in patients without atrioventricular block is similar in concept to electrical pacemaker overdrive. Right atrial stimulation at very fast rates has been effective clinically in the acute treatment of refractory atrial flutter[143] and in the chronic suppression of refractory paroxysmal atrial tachycardia. Another pacing method that has been reported useful in refractory paroxysmal atrial tachycardia is patient-controlled electrical stimulation of the carotid sinus nerves.[144] Although paired electrical stimulation of the ventricle—by its action of prolonging the refractory period—had been shown to be an effective means of overcoming ventricular tachycardia in experimental animals,[145] the method has not been used clinically because of the hazard of inducing ventricular fibrillation.

Surgical Procedures: When it is absolutely necessary to control life-threatening tachyarrhythmias that are refractory to medical therapy, operative intervention—other than cardiac pacemaker implantation—can be considered in certain specific situations. In the case of serious, refractory supraventricular disorders, surgical division of the anomalous pathway in the Wolff-Parkinson-White syndrome[119] and the carotid sinus nerve pacemaker[144] have been pointed out previously. Further, operative division of the atrioventricular node may be carried out and the ventricular rate controlled by implantation of a permanent ventricular pacemaker in disabling, intractable, recurrent paroxysmal atrial tachycardia.[146]

In refractory ventricular tachycardias, bilateral thoracic sympathectomy has been performed in conjunction with implantation of a permanent epicardial pacemaker to prevent recurrence.[141] In medically manageable ventricular tachycardia in acute ischemic heart disease, surgical revascularization alone by saphenous vein bypass of coronary stenosis has been successful in a few carefully selected patients. In refractory ventricular tachycardias with acute myocardial ischemia considered to be caused by coronary spasm without angiographically documented atherosclerotic stenosis, the innovative approach of cardiac autotransplantation

to produce autonomic denervation and permanent ventricular pacemaker insertion has achieved abolition of the ventricular tachycardia and relief of angina in a few patients. Operative excision of aneurysmal ventricular segments to remove the ectopic focus and thereby abolish refractory ventricular tachycardia has been successful in several patients with acute or chronic coronary heart disease.[147] Finally, the concept of a permanently implanted ventricular pacemaker capable of accomplishing spontaneous defrillation of ventricular tachycardia is undergoing experimental development.[148]

Hemodynamic Effects of Antiarrhythmic Agents

The antiarrhythmic drugs are capable of exerting important effects on the contractile state of the myocardium. Immediately after phase 0 electrical excitation is an inward influx of Ca^{++} during the phase II plateau of the action potential,[7] thereby raising the Ca^{++} concentration in the cytoplasm adjacent to the contractile proteins during the period of excitation-contraction coupling. The presence of Ca^{++} in the region of these myofilaments is intimately associated with the initiation of the contractile process, and when this cation exceeds a critical level in the presence of ATP and myofibrillar ATPase, contraction is activated. Agents that alter this influx of Ca^{++} or the activity of sarcoplasmic reticulum Ca^{++} pump ATPase appear capable of influencing the intensity of the contractile process.[149] Since certain of the antiarrhythmic drugs bind to the sarcolemma cell membrane and thereby appear to influence the transmembrane movement of cations, a unified concept is suggested for the actions of these drugs on the electrophysiologic and contractile properties of the muscle fiber—altered Na^+ and K^+ fluxes regulate the electrical properties and depression of Ca^{++} movements reduces the inotropic state.

It is generally accepted that depression of cardiac contractility and the action of vasodilation are direct adverse properties of large doses of each of the widely employed antiarrhythmic agents.[150-155] These unfavorable actions have been assumed also to occur with smaller doses, and as a result, there has been hesitancy to use them in patients with cardiac disease. Recently, it has been shown that the relatively small doses of these drugs that are used initially to control cardiac arrhythmias usually have minimal contractile actions and cardiocirculatory effects in patients with compensated heart disease.[156] Thus, cardiac contractility, cardiac output and left ventricular end-diastolic pressure have not been altered significantly by the intravenous administration of 50 to 100 mg of lidocaine (Figure 17), 100 mg of procainamide, 100 mg of diphenylhydantoin or 1 mg of propranolol. In addition, systemic arterial pressure and total peripheral vascular resistance have not been changed significantly.[156] Although depression of cardiac contractility and pump activity should be anticipated with more than small doses of these drugs in patients with severe cardiac decompensation and with larger amounts of these agents in patients with compensated heart disease, relatively small doses of antiarrhythmic drugs often exert a favorable corrective action on rhythm disorders and these beginning amounts can be administered cautiously for their potential salutary action when indicated, without major fear of depression of cardiocirculatory integrity in patients with heart disease. Also, correction of abnormal rate and rhythm in itself leads to improvement in hemodynamic function.

The hemodynamic effects of large doses of procainamide appear to be similar to those of quinidine—direct depression of cardiac contractility and vasodilation.[151] When intravenous treatment is necessary, many clinicians prefer the use of procainamide rather than quinidine because of the supposedly greater incidence of severe cardiac failure and hypotension associated with quinidine. However, taking into account the small dissimilarity in dose, it appears that adverse electrophysiologic and hemodynamic properties of the two agents are essentially identical. The cardiocirculatory effects of lidocaine appear to be the same, except for temporal course of action, as those produced by quinidine and procainamide.[125,154,155] Large doses of lidocaine reduce cardiac contractility and dilate the peripheral resistance vessels in experimental animals. The hemodynamic effects of diphenylhydantoin, as with lidocaine, appear to be a transient depressant action on myocardial contractility and direct vasodilator

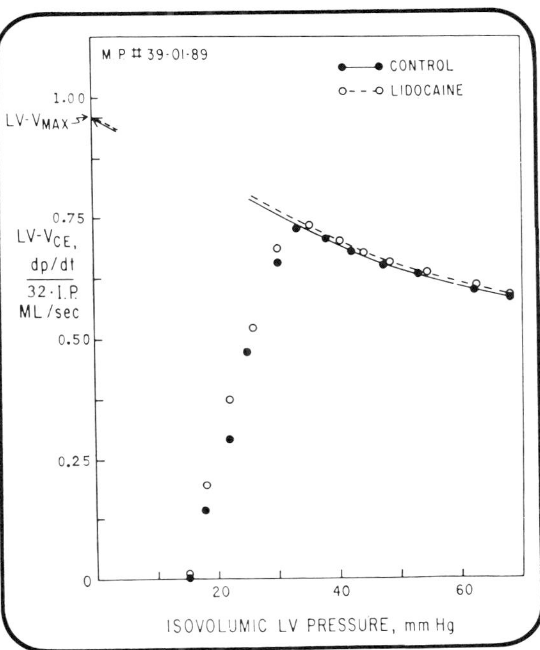

FIGURE 17. Pressure-velocity relation of the left ventricle (LV) during isovolumic contraction before (**solid dots and lines**) and after (**open dots and broken lines**) 50 mg of intravenous lidocaine in a patient with idiopathic myocardiopathy. Contractile element velocity (V_{CE}) of the left ventricle was determined as the instantaneous relation of the rate of rise of intraventricular pressure (dp/dt) to the product of total isovolumic intraventricular pressure (IP) and the series elastic constant. The curves were constructed by relating V_{CE} to total isovolumic pressure at 5 msec intervals from the onset of LV contraction to the opening of the aortic valve. As shown by the **arrows,** extrapolation of the segment of the pressure-velocity curves to zero pressure provides determination of maximal V_{CE} (Vmax), the independent numerical measure of contractility. ML/sec = muscle lengths per second. (Reproduced from Mason et al.[21])

action, which are dose-related.[150,152,153] These actions generally are insignificant when standard doses of the drug are administered slowly intravenously, but they can become important if large doses are administered rapidly.

Propranolol is more likely to produce deleterious hemodynamic actions than are the other antiarrhythmic drugs.[153,157] The sudden reduction of sympathetic support of the failing heart and circulation may lead to the rapid progression of dyspnea and hypotension. It is currently believed that the negative inotropic effect of propranolol is principally the result of beta blockade, and that the direct membrane depressing action of the agent is relatively unimportant in this regard in clinically meaningful doses.[158,159] Concerning the subcellular mechanism of the negative inotropic action of propranolol due to beta adrenergic receptor blockade, the drug inhibits the activity of the superficial membrane enzyme adenylate cyclase and thereby reduces the intracellular formation of cyclic adenosine monophosphate (AMP), the intracellular substance that has been suggested as governing beta adrenergic receptor enhancement of myocardial contractility by stimulation of the sarcoplasmic reticulum.[160]

Concerning cardiac contractility, bretylium is unique among the antiarrhythmic drugs since it does not possess a direct negative inotropic effect.[41,161,162] In fact, bretylium produces an initial transient increase in contractility by its direct action of norepinephrine release.[41] However, the prolonged indirect antiadrenergic action of bretylium leads to reduced sympathetic activity throughout the entire cardiocirculation, which results in reduced pump performance and diminished blood pressure, especially orthostatic, due to vasodilation and loss of reflex integrity.

Summary

In the clinical application of antiarrhythmic drugs, a thorough knowledge of their pharmacologic effects greatly aids in the more rational selection of the drug or combination of drugs in terms of expected benefits, favorable additive actions and contraindications. Each of the agents (1) depresses disorders of rapid impulse formation (repetitive ectopic pacemaker activity) by reducing diastolic depolarization and thereby diminishing automaticity and (2) inhibits disorders of impulse conduction (reentry tachyarrhythmias) by altering conduction velocity and refractory period and thereby interrupting reciprocal excitation pathways. Concerning unidirectional block perpetuating reentry mechanisms, Group I drugs (quinidine, procainamide, propranolol, bretylium and potassium) produce bidirectional block by slowing conduction velocity, whereas Group II drugs (lidocaine and diphenylhydantoin) abolish localized block by enhancing conduction velocity. In addition to depressing automaticity, agents in both groups increase functional refractoriness relative to action potential duration due to alterations in membrane responsiveness. Quinidine and procainamide directly prolong refractory period; in contrast, lidocaine, diphenylhydantoin and propranolol directly reduce this period. Both propranolol and bretylium possess powerful antiadrenergic actions, whereas quinidine and procainamide produce anticholinergic effects. Accompanying their antiarrhythmic actions, quinidine, procainamide and propranolol worsen atrioventricular block, whereas this property in the atrioventricular node usually is not influenced by lidocaine and is accelerated by diphenylhydantoin. Quinidine and procainamide are broad-spectrum antiarrhythmic drugs that are effective in both supraventricular and ventricular tachyarrhythmias, and propanolol and diphenylhydantoin are useful in supraventricular and ventricular disorders. Propanolol is particularly efficacious against supraventricular arrhythmias, and diphenylhydantoin is more beneficial in disturbances of ventricular rhythm. Lidocaine has little action in atrial diorders but markedly suppresses ventricular irritability. Bretylium may successfully terminate refractory ventricular rhythm abnormalities. Diphenylhydantoin, propranolol, lidocaine and potassium possess the most favorable electrophysiologic properties for correction of tachyarrhythmias due to digitalis toxicity.

Clinical management of cardiac tachyarrhythmias is fundamentally founded on precise determination of their nature and the clinical condition in which they occur, together with knowledge of the mechanisms of action and pharmacodynamics of the antiarrhythmic drugs and understanding of the related electrical therapeutic modalities. The initial objective in the therapy of supraventricular tachyarrhythmias is control of ventricular rate and then restoration of normal sinus rhythm. In general, supraventricular disorders are treated with digitalis, vagal stimulation, quinidine, procainamide, propranolol and direct current electroshock. Ventricular tachyarrhythmias are managed with lidocaine, procainamide, quinidine, propranolol, diphenylhydantoin, bretylium, direct current electroshock and electrical pacemaker ventricular overdrive. In general, antiarrhythmic agents have depressant effects on cardiac contractility that are related to dose, speed of administration and extent of myocardial disease. In addition, these agents reduce peripheral vascular resistance. However, the negative inotropic action and vasodilator effect are usually minimal or absent in the small beginning doses used to control tachyarrhythmias. The fundamental subcellular actions of antiarrhythmic agents appear to occur as a consequence of their influence on the cardiac cell membranes, and in this manner, altered transmembrane fluxes of Na^+ and K^+ ions underline their electrophysiologic effects and changes in Ca^{++} movement mediate their contractile properites.

Acknowledgment: This work was supported in part by Research Program Project Grant HL-14780 from the National Heart and Lung Institute, National Institutes of Health.

The authors gratefully acknowledge the technical assistance of Leslie J. Silvernail.

References

1. **Hoffman BF, Cranefield PF:** Electrophysiology of the Heart. New York, McGraw-Hill, 1960
2. **Rosen MR, Wit AL, Hoffman BF:** Electrophysiology and pharmacology of cardiac arrhythmias: cellular electrophysiology of the mammalian heart. Amer Heart J 88:380, 1974
3. **West TC:** Ultramicroelectrode recording from the cardiac pacemaker. J Pharmacol Exp Ther 115:283, 1955
4. **Wit AL, Rosen MR, Hoffman BF:** Electrophysiology and pharmacology of cardiac arrhythmias: relationship of normal and abnormal electrical activity of cardiac fibers to the genesis of arrhythmias. Amer Heart J 88:798, 1974
5. **Zipes DP, Fischer JC:** Effects of agents which inhibit the slow channel on sinus node automaticity and atrioventricular conduction in the dog. Circ Res 34:184, 1974
6. **Fozzard HA, DasGupta DS:** Electrophysiology and the electrocardiogram. Mod Conc Cardiovasc Dis 44:29, 1975
7. **Beeler GW Jr, Reuter H:** Membrane calcium current in ventricular myocardial fibers. J Physiol (Lond) 207:191, 1970
8. **Hoffman BF, Bigger JT Jr:** Antiarrhythmic drugs. In, Drill's Pharmacology in Medicine, fourth edition (DiPalma J, ed). New York, McGraw-Hill, 1971, p 824
9. **Weidmann S:** The effect of the cardiac membrane potential on the rapid availability of the sodium carrier system. J Physiol 127:213, 1955
10. **Massumi RA, Amsterdam EA, Mason DT:** The phenomenon of supernormality in the human heart. Circulation 46:264, 1972
11. **Singer DH, Ten Eick RC:** Pharmacology of cardiac arrhythmias. Prog Cardiovasc Dis 11:488, 1969
12. **Moe G, Mendex C:** Physiologic basis of premature beats and sustained tachycardia. New Eng J Med 288:250, 1973
13. **Rosen M, Hoffman B:** Mechanisms of action of antiarrhythmic drugs. Circ Res 32:1, 1973
14. **Myberg RJ, Stewart JW, Hoffman BF:** Electrophysiological properties of the canine peripheral AV conducting system. Circ Res 26:361, 1970
15. **Dreifus LS, deAzevedo IM, Watanabe Y:** Electrolyte and antiarrhythmic drug interaction. Amer Heart J 88:95, 1974
16. **Bigger T, Bassett AL, Hoffman B:** Electrophysiologic effects of diphenylhydantoin on canine Purkinje fibers. Circ Res 22:221, 1968
17. **Bigger JT Jr, Heissenbuttel RH:** Clinical use of antiarrhythmic drugs. Postgrad Med 47:119, 1970
18. **Bigger JT Jr, Mandel WJ:** Effect of lidocaine on the electrophysiological properties of ventricular muscle and Purkinje fibers. J Clin Invest 49:63, 1970
19. **Bigger JT Jr, Jaffee CC:** The effect of bretylium tosylate on the electrophysiologic properties of ventricular muscle and Purkinje fibers. Amer J Cardiol 27:82, 1971
20. **Mason DT, Braunwald E:** Mechanisms of action and therapeutic uses of cardiac drugs. In, Modern Trends in Pharmacology and Therapeutics (Fulton W, ed). London, Butterworths, 1967, p 112
21. **Mason DT, Spann JF Jr, Zelis R, et al:** The clinical pharmacology and therapeutic applications of the antiarrhythmic drugs. Clin Pharmacal Ther 11:460, 1970
22. **Rosen MR, Wit AL, Hoffman BF:** Electrophysiology and pharmacology of cardiac arrhythmias: cardiac effects of verapamil. Amer Heart J 89:665, 1975
23. **Conn HL Jr, Luchi RJ:** Some cellular and metabolic considerations relating to the action of quinidine as a prototype antiarrhythmic agent. Amer J Med 37:685, 1964
24. **Bigger JT Jr, Heissenbuttel RH:** The use of procainamide and lidocaine in the treatment of cardiac arrhythmias. Prog Cardiovasc Dis 11:515, 1969
25. **Wallace AG, Troyer WH, Lesage MA, et al:** Electrophysiologic effects of isoproterenol and beta-blocking agents in awake dogs. Circ Res 18:140, 1966
26. **David LD, Temte JF:** Effects of propranolol on the transmembrane potentials of ventricular muscle and Purkinje fibers of the dog. Circ Res 22:661, 1968
27. **Gibson D., Sowton E:** The use of beta-adrenergic receptor blocking drugs in dysrhythmias. Prog Cardiovasc Dis 12:16, 1969
28. **Fisch C, Knoebel SB, Feigenbaum H, et al:** Potassium and the monophasic action potential, electrocardi-

ogram, conduction and arrhythmias. Prog Cardiovasc Dis 8:387, 1966

29. **Watanabe Y, Dreifus LS:** Interactions of lanatoside C and potassium on atrioventricular conduction in rabbits. Circ Res 27:931, 1970

30. **Helfant RH, Lau SH, Cohen SI, et al:** Effects of diphenylhydantoin on atrioventricular conduction in man. Circulation 36:686, 1967

31. **Helfant RH, Scherlag BJ, Damato AN:** Protection from digitalis toxicity with the prophylactic use of diphenylhydantoin sodium. Circulation 36:119, 1967

32. **Rosati R, Alexander JA, Schaal SF, et al:** Influence of diphenylhydantoin on electrophysiological properties of the canine heart. Circ Res 21:757, 1967

33. **Damato AN:** Diphenylhydantoin: pharmacological and clinical use. Prog Cardiovasc Dis 12:1, 1969

34. **Mason DT, Zelis R, Lee G, et al:** Current concepts and treatment of digitalis toxicity. Amer J Cardiol 27:546, 1971

35. **Massumi RA, Amsterdam EA, Zelis R, et al:** The digitalis glycosides: contractile and electrophysiologic actions, clinical indications, precautions and toxicity. Semin Drug Ther 2:221, 1972

36. **Amsterdam EA, Gorlin R, Wolfson S:** Evaluation of long-term use of propranolol in angina pectoris. JAMA 210:103, 1969

37. **DeMaria AN, Fabregas RA, Gray D, et al:** Ventriculo-atrial conduction in pacing and digitalis-induced ventricular tachycardia: effects of vagal stimulation and vagotonic drugs. Clin Res 21:235, 1973

38. **Amsterdam EA, Hughes JL, Mansour E, et al:** Circulatory effects of practolol: selective cardiac beta adrenergic blockade in arrhythmias and angina pectoris. Clin Res 19:109, 1971

39. **Bacaner M:** Bretylium toxylate for suppression of induced ventricular fibrillation. Amer J Cardiol 17:528, 1966

40. **Mason DT, Spann JF Jr, Zelis R, et al:** Evolving concepts in the clinical pharmacology and therapeutic uses of the antiarrhythmic drugs. In, Cardiovascular Therapy: The Art and Science (Russek H, ed). Baltimore, Williams & Wilkins, 1971, p 112

41. **Amsterdam E, Mansour E, Hughes J, et al:** Present status of glucagon and bretylium tosylate. In, Changing Concepts in Cardiovascular Diseases (Russek H, ed). Baltimore, Williams & Wilkins, 1972, p 215

42. **Amsterdam EA, Massumi RA, Zelis R, et al:** Use of bretylium tosylate in the management of cardiac arrhythmias. Heart and Lung 1:269, 1972

43. **Zelis R, Mason DT, Spann JF Jr, et al:** Effects of ventricular stimulation and potassium administration on digitalis-induced arrhythmias. Amer J Cardiol 25:428, 1970

44. **Lazzara R, Abelleibra JL:** Intracellular recordings from infarcted canine endocardium. Fed Proc 31:387, 1972

45. **Solberg LE, Singer DH, Ten Eick RE:** Electrophysiological study of myocardial infarction in dogs. Fed Proc 31:387, 1972

46. **West TC, Amory DW:** Single fiber recording of the effect of quinidine at atrial pacemaker sites in the isolated right atrium of the rabbit. J Pharmacol Exp Ther 130:183 1960

47. **Pauley K, Weisfogel G, Damato A:** Sinus node reentry: the effect of quinidine. Amer J Cardiol 31:152, 1973

48. **Vera Z, Gray D, Massumi RA, et al:** Electrophysiologic aspects of quinidine poisoning. Circulation 48 suppl IV:227, 1973

49. **Vaughan-Williams EM:** The mode of action of quinidine on isolated rabbit atria interpreted from intracellular potential records. Brit J Pharmacol 13:276, 1958

50. **Szekeres L, Vaughan-Williams EM:** Antifibrillatory action. J Physiol 160: 470, 1962

51. **Atkinson JA:** Clinical use of blood levels of cardiac drugs. Mod Conc Cardiovasc Dis 42:1, 1973

52. **Miller R, Amsterdam E., Massumi R, et al:** Procainamide: reappraisal of an old antiarrhythmic drug. Heart and Lung 2:227, 1973

53. **Cooper JR, Berlin I, Rovenstine EA, et al:** The physiological disposition and cardiac effects of procainamide. J Pharmacol Exp Ther 102:5, 1951

54. **Ladd AT:** Procainamide induced lupus erythematosus. New Eng J Med 267:1357, 1962

55. **Taylor J, Kosowsky B, Lown B:** Complications of procainamide in a prospective antiarrhythmic study. Circulation 44 suppl II:43, 1971

56. **Hilmi KI, Regan TJ:** Relative effectiveness of antiarrhythmic drugs in treatment of digitalis-induced ventricular tachycardia. Amer Heart J 76:365, 1968

57. **Cohen LS, Rosenthal J, Horner D, et al:** Plasma levels of lidocaine after intramuscular administration. Amer J Cardiol 29:520, 1972

58. **Hollunger G:** On the metabolism of lidocaine. II. Biotransformation of lidocaine. Acta Pharmacol (Kobenhaven) 17:365, 1960

59. **Thomson P, Rowland M, Conn K, et al:** Critical differences in the pharmacokinetics of lidocaine between normal and congestive heart failure patients. Clin Res 17:140, 1969

60. **Koppanyi T:** The sedative, central analgesic and anticonvulsant action of local anesthetics. Amer J Med Sci 244:646, 1962

61. **Helfant RH, Seuffert GW, Patton RD, et al:** The clinical use of diphenyhydantoin (Dilantin) in the treatment and prevention of cardiac arrhythmias. Amer Heart J 77:315, 1969

62. **Helfant RH, Scherlag BJ, Damato AN:** Diphenylhydantoin prevention of arrhythmias in the digitalis-sensitized dog after direct-current cardioversion. Circulation 37:424, 1968

63. **Dill W, Kazenki L, Wolf L, et al:** Studies on 5-5' diphenylhydantoin in animals and man. J Pharmacol Exp Ther 118:270, 1956

64. **Kutt H, Louis S:** Anticonvulsant drugs. II. Clinical pharmacological and therapeutic aspects. Drugs 4:256, 1972

65. **Conn RD:** Diphenylhydantoin sodium on cardiac arrhythmias. New Eng J Med 272:277, 1965

66. **Unger AH, Sklaroff HJ:** Fatalities following intravenous use of sodium diphenylhydantoin for cardiac arrhythmias. JAMA 200:335, 1967

67. **Coltart DJ, Fibson DG, Shand DG:** Plasma propranolol levels associated with suppression of ventricular ectopic beats. Brit Med J 1:490, 1971

68. **Seides SF, Josephson ME, Batsford WP, et al:** The electrophysiology of propranolol in man. Amer Heart J 88:733, 1974

69. **Fitzgerald JD:** Perspectives in adrenergic beta-receptor blockage. Clin Pharmacol Ther 10:292, 1969

70. **Miller RR, Amsterdam EA, Mason DT:** The pharamacologic basis for clinical use of beta adrenergic blocking drugs. Ration Drug Ther 8:4, 1974

71. **Powell CE, Slater IH:** Blocking of inhibitory adrenergic receptors by a dichloro analog of isoproterenol. J Pharmacol Exp Ther 122:480, 1958

72. **Harrison DC, Braunwald E, Glick G, et al:** Effects of beta adrenergic blockage on the circulation with particular reference to observations in patients with hypertropic subaortic stenosis. Circulation 29:84, 1964

73. **Harrison DC:** Circulatory Effects and Beta-Adrenergic Blocking Agents. Amsterdam, Excerpta Medica, 1971

74. **Choquet Y. Capon R, Mason DT, et al:** Comparison of the beta adrenergic blocking properties and negative inotropic effects of oxyprenolol and propranolol in patients. Amer J Cardiol 29:257, 1972

75. **Frankl WE, Soloff LA:** Sotalol: a new, safe, beta-adrenergic receptor blocking agent. Amer J Cardiol 22:266, 1968

76. **Dunlop D, Shanks RG:** Selective blockage of adrenoceptive beta-receptors in the heart. Brit J Pharm 32:201, 1968

77. **Bagwell EE, Custy J, Steen RG, et al:** Beta receptor blocking and antiarrhythmic properties of tolamolol. J Pharmacol Exp Ther 191:496, 1974

78. **Gray D, Vera Z, Harter KW, et al:** Electrophysiologic actions of tolamolol on the canine heart. Circulation 50 suppl III:176, 1974

79. **Miller RR, Vismara LA, Amsterdam EA, et al:** Hemodynamic effects of tolamolol and comparison with propranolol in patients with coronary disease. Circulation 49 suppl III:78, 1974

80. **Amsterdam EA, Morrison SL, Lee G, et al:** Efficacy of intravenous tolamolol in the treatment of cardiac arrhythmias. In, Tolamolol (Lown B, Mason D, et al, ed). Amsterdam, Excerpta Medica, 1976, p 149

81. **Lucchesi BR:** The effects of pronethalol and its dextroisomer upon experimental cardiac arrhythmias. J Pharmacol Exp Ther 148:94, 1965

82. **Barrett AM. Cullum VA:** The biological properties of the optical isomers of propranolol and their effects on cardiac arrhythmias. Brit J Pharmacol 34:43, 1968

83. **Stanton HC, Kirchgessner T, Parmenter K:** Cardiovascular pharmacology of two new beta adrenergic receptor antagonists. J Pharmacol Exp Ther 149:174, 1965

84. **Parmley WW, Braunwald E:** Comparative myocardial depressant and antiarrhythmic properties of d-propranol, d-propranolol and quinidine. J Pharmacol Exp Ther 158:11, 1967

85. **Dohadwalla AN, Friedberg AS, Vaughan-Williams AM:** The relevance of beta-receptor blockade to ouabain-induced cardiac arrhythmias. Brit J Pharmacol 36:257, 1969

86. **Kleiger RE, Lown B:** Cardioversion and digitalis. II. Clinical studies. Circulation 33:878, 1966

87. **Tsolakas TC, Davies JPH, Oram S:** Propranolol in attempted maintenance of sinus rhythm after electrical defibrillation. Lancet 2:1064, 1964

88. **Stern S:** Conversion of chronic atrial fibrillation to sinus rhythm with combined propranolol and quinidine treatment. Amer Heart J 74:170, 1967

89. **Dreifus LS, Lim HF, Watanabe YL, et al:** Propranolol and quinidine in the management of ventricular tachycardia. JAMA 204:190, 1968

90. **Shand DG, Evans GH, Nies AS:** The almost complete hepatic extraction of propranolol during intravenous administration in the dog. Life Sci 10:1417, 1971

91. **Butcher RMK:** Cyclic 3,5-AMP and the lipolytic effects of hormones on adipose tissue. Pharmacol Rev 18:237, 1966

92. **Levey GS, Epstein SE:** Activation of adenyl cyclase by glucagon in cat and human heart. Circ Res 24:151, 1969

93. **Olson HG, Miller RR, Amsterdam EA, et al:** The propranolol withdrawl rebound phenomenon: acute and catastrophic exacerbation of symptoms and death following the abrupt cessation of large doses of propranolol in coronary artery disease. Amer J Cardiol 35:162, 1975

94. **Faulkner SL, Hopkins JT, Boerth RC, et al:** Time required for complete recovery from chronic propranolol. New Eng J Med 289:607, 1973

95. **Bacaner MR:** Treatment of ventricular fibrillation and other acute arrhythmias with bretylium tosylate. Amer J Cardiol 21:530, 1968

96. **Mansour E, Mason DT, Spann JF Jr, et al:** Clinical evaluation of antiarrhythmic and hemodynamic properties of bretylium. Circulation 42 suppl III:41, 1970

97. **Day HW, Bacaner MR:** Use of bretylium tosylate in the management of acute myocardial infarction. Amer J Cardiol 27:177, 1971

98. **Lown B:** Electrical reversion of cardiac arrhythmias. Brit Heart J 29:469, 1967

99. **Surawicz B:** Role of electrolytes in etiology and management of cardiac arrhythmias. Prog Cardiovasc Dis 8:364, 1966

100. **Ayres SM, Grace WJ:** Inappropriate ventilation and hypoxemia as causes of cardiac arrhythmias. Amer J Med 46:495, 1969

101. **Mason DT, Spann JF Jr, Zelis R:** New developments in the understanding of the actions of the digitalis glycosides. Prog Cardiovasc Dis 11:443, 1969

102. **Mason DT, Amsterdam EA, Massumi RA, et al:** Recent advances in antiarrhythmic drugs: clinical pharmacology and therapeutics. In, The Acute Cardiac Emergency (Eliot R, ed). Mount Kisco, New York, Futura, 1972, p 95

103. **Oakley C, Marsh BT, Mennie AT, et al:** International symposium on perhexiline. Postgrad Med J 49 suppl 3:1, 1973

104. **Ten Eick RE, Singer DH:** Effects of perhexiline on the electrophysiologic activity of mammalian heart. Postgrad Med J 49 suppl 3:32, 1973

105. **Drake FT, Singer DH, Haring O, et al:** Evaluation of antiarrhythmic efficacy of perhexiline maleate in ambulatory patients by Holter monitoring. Postgrad Med J 49 suppl 3:52, 1973

106. **Vera Z, Gray D, Harter KW, et al:** Electrophysiologic effects of perhexiline maleate (Pexid) in dog. Clin Res 22:309A, 1974

107. **Wit AL, Cranefield PF:** Verapamil inhibition of the slow response: a mechanism for its effectiveness against reentrant AV nodal tachycardia. Circulation 50 suppl III:146, 1974

108. **Zoli I, Baroncini S, Cornia G, et al:** 17-mono-chloroacetyl-ajmaline in the prophylaxis and treatment of cardiac arrhythmias. Minerva Cardioangiol 19:536, 1971

109. **Dalmastro M, Lang TW, Rubbins S, et al:** Antiarrhythmic effectiveness of 17-monochloroacetyl-ajmaline: hemodynamic and metabolic study. Amer J Cardiol 33:133, 1974

110. **Bojorges R, Pastelin G, Sanchez-Perez S, et al:** The effects of ajmaline in experimental and clinical arrhythmias and their relation to some electrophysiological parameters of the heart. J Pharmacol Exp Ther 193:182, 1975

111. **deAzevedo IM, Dreifus LS, Watanabe Y:** Electrophysiologic effects of new ester of ajmaline 17-monochloroacetyl ajmaline hydrochloride. Europ J Cardiol 2:321, 1975

112. **Vismara LA, Mason DT, Amsterdam EA:** Disopyramide phosphate: clinical efficacy of a new oral antiarrhythmic drug. Clin Pharmacol Ther 16:330, 1974

113. **Dreifus LS, Filip Z, Sexton DM, et al:** Electrophysiological and clinical effects of a new antiarrhythmic agent: disopyramide. Amer J Cardiol 31:129, 1973

114. **Befeler B, Castellanos A, Wells DE, et al:** Electrophysiologic effects of the antiarrhythmic agent disopyramide phosphate. Amer J Cardiol 35:282, 1975

115. **Vismara LA, DeMaria AN, Miller RR, et al:** Effects of intravenous disopyramide phosphate on cardiac function and peripheral circulation in ischemic heart disease. Clin Res 23:87A, 1975

116. **Mason DT, Amsterdam EA, Massumi RA, et al:** Combined actions of antiarrhythmic drugs: electrophysiologic and therapeutic consideration. In, Cardiac Arrhythmias (Dreifus L, Likoff W, ed). New York, Grune & Stratton, 1973, p 531

117. **Lister J, Cohen L, Bernstein W, et al:** Treatment of supraventricular tachycardia by rapid atrial stimulation. Circulation 38:1044, 1968

118. **Schnitzler R, Goldseyer B, Westura E, et al:** Demand coronary vein pacemakers for drug resistant supraventricular tachycardia. Circulation 44 suppl II:97, 1968

119. **Cobb FG, Blumenschein SD, Sealy WC, et al:** Successful surgical interruption of the bundle of Kent in a patient with Wolff-Parkinson-White syndrome. Circulation 38:1018, 1968

120. **DeMaria AN, Lies JE, King JF, et al:** Echographic assessment of atrial transport, mitral movement and ventricular performance following electroversion of supraventricular arrhythmias. Circulation 51:273, 1975

121. **Fisher RD, Mason DT, Morrow AG:** Restoration of sinus rhythm after mitral valve replacement: correlations with left atrial pressure and size. Circulation 37 suppl II:173, 1968

122. **Vismara LA, Hughes JK, Kraus J, et al:** Relation of ventricular arrhythmias in the late hospital phase of acute myocardial infarction to post-hospital sudden death. Amer J Cardiol 33:175, 1974

123. **Killip T, Kimball JT:** Treatment of myocardial infarction in a coronary care unit. Amer J Cardiol 20:457, 1967

124. **Kimball JT, Killip T:** Aggressive treatment of arrhythmias in acute myocardial infarction. Prog Cardiovasc Dis 10:483, 1968

125. **Miller RR, Hilliard G, Lies JE, et al:** Hemodynamic effects of procainamide in patients with acute myocardial infarction and comparison with lidocaine. Amer J Med 55:161, 1973

126. **DeSanctis RW, Kastor JA:** Rapid intracardiac pacing for treatment of recurrent ventricular tachyarrhythmias in the absence of heart block. Amer Heart J 76:168, 1968

127. **Koch-Weser J, Klein SW, Foo-Canto LL, et al:** Antiarrhythmic prophylaxis with procainamide in acute myocardial infarction. New Eng J Med 281:1253, 1969

128. **Epstein SE, Redwood DR, Smith ER:** Atropine and acute myocardial infarction. Circulation 45:1273, 1972

129. **Massumi RA, Mason DT, Amsterdam EA, et al:** Ventricular fibrillation and tachycardia after intravenous atropine for treatment of bradycardias. New Eng J Med 287:336, 1972

130. **Kouwenhoven WG, Jude JR, Knickerbocker CG:** Closed-chest cardiac massage. JAMA 173:1064, 1960

131. **Zoll PM, Linenthal AJ:** Termination of refractory tachycardia by external countershock. Circulation 25:596, 1962

132. **Lown B, Amarasinglham R, Neuman J:** New method for terminating cardiac arrhythmias. JAMA 182:548, 1962

133. **Tavel ME, Fisch C:** Repetitive ventricular arrhythmias resulting from artificial internal pacemaker. Circulation 30:493, 1964

134. **Vassauz C, Lown B:** Cardioversion of supraventricular tachycardias. Circulation 39:791, 1969

135. **Hurst JW, Paulk EA, Proctor HD, et al:** Management of patients with atrial fibrillation. Amer J Med 37:728, 1964

136. **Bjerkelund CJ, Oming OM:** The efficacy of anticoagulant therapy in preventing embolism related to D.C. electrical conversion of atrial fibrillation. Amer J Cardiol 23:208, 1969

137. **Hughes JL, Mansour E, Salel AF, et al:** Elective conversion of atrial fibrillation: relation of energy level, digitalis, and lidocaine to post shock rhythm. Amer J Cardiol 26:639, 1970

138. **Lown B, Kleiger R, Williams J:** Cardioversion and digitalis drugs: changed threshold to electric shock in digitalized animals. Circ Res 17:519, 1965

139. **Lown B, Wittenberg S:** Cardioversion and digitalis. III. Effect of change in serum potassium concentration. Amer J Cardiol 21:513, 1968

140. **Elkins RC, Vasko JS, Morrow AG:** Digitalis tolerance during atrial fibrillation and normal sinus rhythm. Amer J Cardiol 20:229, 1967

141. **Zipes DP, Wallace AG, Sealy WC, et al:** Artificial atrial and ventricular pacing in the treatment of arrhythmias. Ann Intern Med 70:885, 1969

142. **Pick A, Langendorf R, Katz LN:** Depression of cardiac pacemakers by premature impulses. Amer Heart J 41:49, 1951

143. **Zeft JH, Cobb FR, Waxman MB, et al:** Right atrial stimulation in the treatment of atrial flutter. Ann Intern

Med 70:447, 1969

144. **Braunwald E, Sobel BE, Braunwald NS:** Treatment of paroxysmal supraventricular tachycardia by electrical stimulation. New Eng J Med 281:885, 1969

145. **Braunwald E, Ross J Jr, Frommer PL, et al:** Clinical observations on paired electrical stimulation of the heart. Effects on ventricular performance and heart rate. Amer J Med 37:700, 1964

146. **Giannelli S Jr, Ayres SM, Gomprecht RF, et al:** Therapeutic surgical division of the human conduction system. JAMA 199:155, 1967

147. **Couch OA:** Cardiac aneurysm with ventricular tachycardia and subsequent excision of aneurysm. Circulation 20:251, 1959

148. **Mirowski M, Mower M, Denniston RH, et al:** Prevention of sudden coronary death through automatic detection and treatment of ventricular fibrillation using a single intravascular catheter system. Circulation 44 suppl II:124, 1971

149. **Nayler WG:** Calcium exchange in cardiac muscle: a basic mechanism of drug action. Amer Heart J 73:379, 1967

150. **Mixter CG, Moran JM, Austen WG:** Cardiac and peripheral vascular effects of diphenylhydantoin sodium. Amer J Cardiol 17:332, 1966

151. **Austen WG, Moran JM:** Cardiac and peripheral vascular effects of lidocaine and procainamide. Amer J Cardiol 16:701, 1965

152. **Mierzwiak DS, Shapiro W, McNalley MC, et al:** Cardiac effects of diphenylhydantoin (Dilantin) in man. Amer J Cardiol 21:20, 1968

153. **Nayler WG, McInnes I, Swann JB, et al:** Some effects of diphenyldydantoin and propranolol on the cardiovascular system. Amer Heart J 75:83, 1968

154. **Schumacher RR, Lieberson AD, Childress RH, et al:** Hemodynamic effects of lidocaine in patients with heart disease. Circulation 37:965, 1968

155. **Grossman JI, Cooper JA, Frieden J:** Cardiovascular effects of infusion of lidocaine on patients with heart disease. Amer J Cardiol 24:191, 1969

156. **Mason DT, Spann JF Jr, Zelis R, et al:** Effects of antiarrhythmic drugs on myocardial performance in man: assessment by the maximal velocity of contractile element shortening. Amer J Cardiol 25:114, 1970

157. **Nayler WG, McInnes I, Carson V, et al:** The effect of lignocaine on myocardial function, high energy phosphate stores, and oxygen consumption: a comparison with propranolol. Amer Heart J 78:338, 1969

158. **Harry JD, Kappagoda CT, Linden RJ, et al:** Action of propranolol on the dog heart. Cardiovasc Res 7:729, 1973

159. **Liang C, Hood WB Jr:** The myocardial depressant effect of beta-receptor blocking agents. Circ Res 35:272, 1974

160. **Kirchberger MA, Tada M, Repke D, et al:** Cyclic adenosine 3',5'-monophosphate-dependent protein kinase stimulation of calcium uptake by canine cardiac microsomes. J Mol Cell Cardiol 4:673, 1972

161. **Gaffney TE, Braunwald E, Cooper T:** Analysis of the acute circulatory effects of guanethidine and bretylium. Circ Res 10:83, 1962

162. **Markis JE, Koch-Weser J:** Characteristics and mechanism of inotropic and chronotropic actions of bretylium tosylate. J Pharmacol Exp Ther 178:94, 1971

INDEX

(continued)

(continued)

(*continued*)